The Complete Medical Guide
for the
Family Caregiver

The Complete Medical Guide

for the

Family Caregiver

The Authoritative, At-Home Companion for Giving the Best Care

Edited by

Jeffrey A. West, M.D.

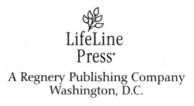

LifeLine
Press

A Regnery Publishing Company
Washington, D.C.

Library of Congress Cataloging-in-Publication Data on file.
Available on request.

ISBN 0-89526-119-7

Published in the United States by
LifeLine Press
A Regnery Publishing Company
One Massachusetts Avenue, N.W.
Washington, DC 20001

Visit us at www.lifelinepress.com

Distributed to the trade by
National Book Network
4720-A Boston Way
Lanham, MD 20706

Printed on acid-free paper
Manufactured in the United States of America

10 9 8 7 6 5 4 3 2 1

Books are available in quantity for promotional or premium use. Write to Director of Special Sales, Regnery Publishing, Inc., One Massachusetts Avenue, N.W., Washington, DC 20001, for information on discounts and terms or call (202) 216-0600.

The Complete Medical Guide for the Family Caregiver is designed to give you information on various medical conditions, medications, and procedures for your personal knowledge and to help you be a more informed caregiver and consumer of medical and health services. It is not intended to be complete or exhaustive, nor is it a substitute for professional medical counseling and care. All matters pertaining to your physical health and that of any person in your care should be supervised by a health care professional.

Contents

Contributing Editors and Writers

CONTRIBUTING EDITORS

Paul G. Auwaerter, M.D.

Assistant Professor, General Internal Medicine and Infectious Diseases
The Johns Hopkins University School of Medicine
Divisions of General Internal Medicine and Infectious Diseases
Baltimore, Maryland
Human Immunodeficiency Virus/AIDS

Dorothy I. Baker, Ph.D., M.N.

Research Scientist, Chronic Disease and Epidemiology
Yale University School of Medicine
New Haven, Connecticut
Falls and Mobility Problems

Susan P. Baker, M.P.H.

Professor of Health Policy and Management
The Johns Hopkins University School of Public Health
Baltimore, Maryland
Safety in the Home

Basia Belza, Ph.D., R.N.

Associate Professor of Biobehavioral Nursing and Health Systems
University of Washington, Seattle
Seattle, Washington
Self-Care for the Caregiver

Leslie J. Blackhall, M.D., M.T.S.

Medical Director, Center for Palliative Care
University of Virginia School of Medicine
Charlottesville, Virginia
End-of-Life Issues

Peter Calabresi, M.D.

Assistant Professor of Neurology
Maryland Center for Multiple Sclerosis, University of Maryland Medical Center
Baltimore, Maryland
Multiple Sclerosis

Betsy Campochiaro, R.N.

Coordinator, Macular Degeneration Center

Wilmer Eye Institute

The Johns Hopkins University School of Medicine

Baltimore, Maryland

Vision Disorders Older Adults

H. Ballentine Carter, M.D.

Professor of Urology and Oncology

Brady Urological Institute

The Johns Hopkins University School of Medicine

Baltimore, Maryland

Prostate Cancer

Lawrence J. Cheskin, M.D.

Director, Gastroenterology and Associate Professor
    of Medicine

Bayview Medical Center

The Johns Hopkins University School of Medicine

Baltimore, Maryland

Colorectal Cancer; Gastrointestinal Disorders;
    Nutrition, Feeding, and Eating Problems

Denise B. Corey, R.N., B.S.N., CRR.N.

Rehabilitation Evaluator/Drug Study Coordinator

J. Paul Sticht Center on Aging and Rehabilitation

Wake Forest University School of Medicine

Winston Salem, North Carolina

Stroke and Stroke Rehabilitation

Kathleen Costello, N.P.

Clinical Director

Maryland Center for Multiple Sclerosis

University of Maryland Medical Center

Baltimore, Maryland

Multiple Sclerosis

Emily Susan Crim, R.N.

Clinician II Registered Nurse

Digestive Health Research Center

University of Virginia Health Sciences Center

Charlottesville, Virginia

Fecal Incontinence

Arlene D'Alli, L.C.S.W.-C.

Clinical Social Worker

Parkinson's Disease Center

The Johns Hopkins University School of Medicine

Baltimore, Maryland

Parkinson's Disease

Marcia Day Childress, Ph.D.

Associate Professor of Medical Education

University of Virginia School of Medicine

Charlottesville, Virginia

End-of-Life Issues

William C. Dooley, M.D.

Director, Breast Institute

University of Oklahoma Health Sciences Center

Oklahoma City, Oklahoma

Breast Cancer

Charlotte Eliopoulos, Ph.D., M.P.H., R.N.C

President, American Holistic Nurses Association

Glen Arm, Maryland

Exercise and Physical Rehabilitation; Safety in the
    Home; Complementary and Alternative Medicine

Joseph A Eustace, M.B., B.A.O., B.Ch., M.R.C.P.I., M.H.S.

Assistant Professor of Medicine, Division of Nephrology

The Johns Hopkins University School of Medicine

Baltimore, Maryland

End-Stage Renal Disease

Betty Ferrell, Ph.D., R.N.

Research Scientist

City of Hope Medical Center

Duarte, California

Pain Management

Cynthia J. Finley, R.D., L.D., C.N.S.D.

Clinical Dietitian Specialist

The Johns Hopkins University Weight Management Center

Baltimore, Maryland

Nutrition, Feeding, and Eating Problems

Daniel E. Ford, M.D., M.P.H.

Associate Professor of Medicine, Epidemiology

Associate Professor of Medicine, Health Policy and Management

The Johns Hopkins University Schools of Medicine and Public Health

Baltimore, Maryland

Depression

Elizabeth M. Gibson, M.A.

Administrative Director, Center for Palliative Care

University of Virginia School of Medicine

Charlottesville, Virginia

End-of-Life Issues

Paul Godin, M.D.

Pulmonary and Critical Care Specialist

Palo Alto, California

Chronic Obstructive Pulmonary Disease

David C. Good, M.D.

Professor of Neurology and Medical Director of Rehabilitation

J. Paul Sticht Center on Aging and Rehabilitation

Wake Forest University School of Medicine

Winston Salem, North Carolina

Stroke and Stroke Rehabilitation

Margaret R. Gottschalk, M.S., P.T.

Research Therapist, Claude D. Pepper Older Americans Independence Center

Yale University School of Medicine

New Haven, Connecticut

Falls and Mobility Problems

Mikel Gray, Ph.D., R.N.

Associate Professor of Nursing, Assistant Professor of Urology

University of Virginia Health Sciences Center

Charlottesville, Virginia

Urinary Incontinence

Eric Hardt, M.D.

Clinical Director, Geriatrics and Associate Professor of Medicine

Boston University School of Medicine

Boston, Massachusetts

Substance Abuse Problems and the Elderly

Reena Kakka, Pharm.D.
Pharmacist
Stanford Hospital and Clinics
Stanford, California
Osteoarthritis

Holli Kang, Pharm.D.
Clinical Pharmacist
Stanford Hospital and Clinics
Stanford, California
Breast Cancer; Colorectal Cancer

William F. Kelly, P.A.-C.
Program Coordinator, Clinical Training
Division of Infectious Disease and AIDS Service
The Johns Hopkins University School of Medicine
Baltimore, Maryland
Human Immunodeficiency Virus/AIDS

Abby C. King, Ph.D.
Associate Professor of Health Research and Policy
    and Medicine
Stanford University School of Medicine
Palo Alto, California
Self-Care for the Caregiver

Michael J. Klag, M.D., M.P.H.
Director, General Internal Medicine and Assistant
    Professor of Medicine
The Johns Hopkins University School of Medicine
Baltimore, Maryland
*End-Stage Renal Disease; Hypertension (High
    Blood Pressure)*

Harlan Krumholz, M.D., M.P.H.
Associate Professor of Medicine
Yale University School of Medicine
New Haven, Connecticut
Coronary Artery Disease

Nancy E. Lane, M.D.
Associate Professor of Medicine, Rheumatology
University of California, San Francisco School of
    Medicine
San Francisco, California
Osteoarthritis

Melissa Levine, M.S.W.
Berkeley, California
Medication Management

Kimberly E. Loman, R.N., C.D.E.
Diabetes Nurse Educator
Department of Medicine, Division of Endocrinology
The Johns Hopkins University School of Medicine
Baltimore, Maryland
Diabetes Mellitus

Simeon Margolis, M.D., Ph.D.
Professor of Medicine and Biological Chemistry
The Johns Hopkins University School of Medicine
Baltimore, Maryland
Coronary Artery Disease; Diabetes Mellitus

Louise M. Nett, R.N., R.R.T.
Information Specialist
National Lung Health Education Program
Denver, Colorado
Chronic Obstructive Pulmonary Disease

John K. Niparko, M.D.

Director, Division of Otology, Neurotology and Skull Base Surgery
Professor of Otology
The Johns Hopkins University School of Medicine
Baltimore, Maryland
Hearing Disorders in Older Adults

Joel Pearlman, M.D., Ph.D.

Assistant Chief of Service, Wilmer Eye Institute
The Johns Hopkins University School of Medicine
Baltimore, Maryland
Vision Disorders in Older Adults

Thomas L. Petty, M.D.

Professor of Medicine
University of Colorado
Denver, Colorado
Chronic Obstructive Pulmonary Disease

Peter V. Rabins, M.D., M.P.H.

Professor of Psychiatry and Behavioral Sciences
The Johns Hopkins University School of Medicine
Baltimore, Maryland
Alzheimer's Disease

Victoria Rand, M.D.

Assistant Clinical Professor of Medicine
University of California, San Francisco
San Francisco, California
Complementary and Alternative Medicine

Stephen Reich, M.D.

Director, Parkinson's Disease Center and Associate Professor of Neurology
The Johns Hopkins University School of Medicine
Baltimore, Maryland
Parkinson's Disease

Barbara Riegel, D.N.Sc., R.N.

Professor of Nursing
San Diego State University
San Diego, California
Coronary Artery Disease

Lillie Shockney, R.N., B.S., M.A.S.

Director of Outreach and Education
The John Hopkins University Breast Center
Baltimore, Maryland
Breast Cancer

Peter Staats, M.D.

Director, Division of Pain Medicine and Associate Professor, Anesthesiology and Critical Care Medicine
The Johns Hopkins University School of Medicine
Baltimore, Maryland
Pain Management

William D. Steers, M.D.

Professor and Chairman, Department of Urology
University of Virginia Health Sciences Center
Charlottesville, Virginia
Urinary Incontinence

Kerry J. Stewart, Ed.D.

Director of Cardiac Rehabilitation and Associate
Professor of Medicine
The Johns Hopkins University School of Medicine,
Bayview Medical Center
Baltimore, Maryland
Exercise and Physical Rehabilitation

Mary E. Tinetti, M.D.

Professor of Internal Medicine (Geriatrics) and
Epidemiology
Yale University School of Medicine
New Haven, Connecticut
Falls and Mobility Problems

Lana Witt, Pharm.D.

Clinical Assistant Professor
University of California San Francisco School of
Pharmacy
San Francisco, California
*Chronic Obstructive Pulmonary Disease; Coronary
Artery Disease; Gastrointestinal Disorders;
Human Immunideficiency Virus/AIDS; Medication
Management*

Laurence Witt, Pharm.D.

Clinical Assistant Professor
University of California San Francisco School of
Pharmacy
San Francisco, California
*Diabetes Mellitus; Human Immunideficiency
Virus/AIDS*

Laura Hope Wolfe, M.D.

Staff Physician
County of San Mateo Mental Health Services
Palo Alto, California
Depression

Karen Wolf, R.N.

Manager, Special Care Unit
Keswick Multicare Center
Baltimore, Maryland
Alzheimer's Disease

Mark Worthington, M.D.

Associate Program Director and Associate Professor
of Medicine (Gastroenterology and Hepatology)
University of Virginia Health Sciences Center
Charlottesville, Virginia
Fecal Incontinence

Eileen Wright, R.N.

Manager, Ambulatory Services, Gastroenterology
and Endoscopy Services
The Johns Hopkins University School of Medicine,
Bayview Medical Center
Baltimore, Maryland
Gastrointestinal Disorders

Hunter Young, M.D., M.H.S.

Assistant Professor of Medicine
The Johns Hopkins University School of Medicine
Baltimore, Maryland
Hypertension (High Blood Pressure)

MEDICAL WRITERS

Mark Giuliucci

Huntersville, North Carolina

Chronic Obstructive Pulmonary Disease; Hearing Disorders in Older Adults; Nutrition, Feeding, and Eating Problems; Osteoarthritis; Pain Management; Vision Disorders in Older Adults

Randi Henderson

Pylesville, Maryland

Breast Cancer; Multiple Sclerosis; Parkinson's Disease; Stroke and Stroke Rehabilitation; Substance Abuse and the Elderly

Matthew Hoffman

Albuquerque, New Mexico

Falls and Mobility Problems; Gastrointestinal Disorders

Janet Farrar Worthington

Free Union, Virginia

Colorectal Cancer; Fecal Incontinence; Prostate Cancer; Urinary Incontinence

Lyn S. Yonack, M.S.W., M.A.

Great Barrington, Massachusetts

Alzheimer's Disease; Depression; Self-Care for the Caregiver

Acknowledgments

I would like to acknowledge the many individuals who helped to create this work. First, I had the privilege of working with international experts in caregiving and medicine; I hope you enjoy their wisdom in the following chapters.

Second, numerous individuals played critical roles in the origination and execution of the work. Ron Sauder, an accomplished health editor, led the recruitment of authors and oversaw editorial review of the chapters. Sigrid Metson, an innovative publishing executive, helped in all facets of editorial review, production, promotion, and placement of the work. Many individuals at CareThere, a pioneering online health care company focusing on caregivers, supported the project: Andy Thompson, George Savage, Chris Guinn, Scott Roeth, Lana Witt, and others too numerous to mention.

Finally, Paul Godin, M.D., contributed to the original vision of unique medical content crafted for caregivers and formulated for print and digital media.

—Jeffrey A. West, M.D.

Introduction

Family members are an underutilized but key element in the well-recognized health care triad of the health care professional (doctor, nurse, allied health professional), the system (hospital, office), and the patient and family members. Family members are fundamentally patient advocates, pushing for appropriate and timely access to medical care and aiding in implementation of the treatment plan. Health care professionals and organizations, however, rarely provide specific, practical information that can be easily used and applied by the family members who care for individuals with chronic disease and disability.

With the aging of the U.S. population, the importance of family caregivers cannot be underestimated. Currently, over 25 million family caregivers in the United States alone care for an elderly, disabled, or chronically ill family member. More than 23% of American families care for an adult care recipient. Caregiving is a demanding calling—the average caregiver is a 45-year-old woman who works outside the home, has children, *and provides 22 hours of care each week to a relative with chronic illness and disability*. With the aging of the baby boomer generation, the prevalence of family caregivers will only increase.

Family caregivers seek practical, useable information about the *disease* or *condition* that their loved one faces. Family caregivers and their care recipients need answers to fundamental questions: What exactly is the disease or condition? How is it diagnosed? What can I expect if my loved one has this disease or condition? How is it treated? How can it be prevented? What research is being done? What should I do now?

Some of the finest minds in medicine today have come together to answer those very questions and offer guidance through the maze of modern medicine. For the past three years I have worked with this brilliant and caring group of international experts in all aspects of diseases and conditions that affect the elderly and those who care for them to create this comprehensive, evidence-based, practical manual for family caregivers. Drawing from the disciplines of medicine, nursing, pharmacology, psychology, rehabilitation, and numerous other health disciplines, these experts in common conditions that impair health have created a foundation for understanding complicated medical issues.

The Complete Medical Guide for the Family Caregiver is for family caregivers who want to understand complex conditions and to apply that understanding to better care for their loved ones. To that end, the information in this volume focuses directly on the perspective of the caregiver, explaining the reality of each condition in relation to how it affects the caregiver.

And because family caregivers struggle with the emotional, physical, and intellectual demands of caring for those with chronic illness and disability, we also address the critical issue of how family caregivers can better take care of themselves.

With increasing fiscal pressure on health care systems despite the ever-increasing needs of an aging population, physicians, patients, and their families will need to forge a more cohesive team. *The Complete Medical Guide for the Family Caregiver* can help family caregivers become strong advocates for their loved ones and more effective members of the health care team by providing practical, comprehensive medical information in an easy-to-understand format. Accurate, up-to-date information leads to awareness and understanding, the first steps toward behavior change and effective health care.

—JEFFREY A. WEST, M.D.
September 2002

PART 1
Diseases
and
Conditions

Alzheimer's Disease

SIGNS & SYMPTOMS

- Progressive mental difficulties
- Forgetfulness, perhaps coupled with attempts to hide or compensate for difficulties
- Impaired ability to use good judgment or to understand reason
- Difficulty planning, organizing, and reasoning
- Recognition and perception difficulties
- Apraxia—the inability to perform purposeful motor activities even though there is nothing wrong with coordination or muscular system
- Sudden or unusual language difficulties
- Personality changes
- Aggression
- Anxiety and agitation
- Extreme frustration
- Paranoia and suspicion
- Depression
- Absent-minded wandering

Someone you love—an older member of your family—seems to be forgetting things repeatedly. He cannot seem to focus or to think straight. At times, he seems like a totally different person: irritable, irrational, moody, withdrawn, maybe a little depressed. At first you chalk it up to getting old. After all, who doesn't forget where they put the car keys, or parked the car, for that matter? And what's the big deal about mistaking the neighbor for someone else or one grandchild for another? We're all irritable from time to time. And goodness knows, we've all known times when we just couldn't concentrate no matter how hard we tried.

So, maybe what you notice in your father or your brother or your wife isn't so serious. But there's that nagging doubt in the back of your mind. What if it *is* serious?

Not too long ago, senility was viewed as a natural part of getting old. The older a person gets, the worse his memory gets. Right? *Wrong.* Today, we know that forgetfulness and confusion are not part and parcel of old age. Rather, impairment in cognitive or intellectual functioning—what's called dementia—is usually a sign of some other illness.

The truth bears repeating: Severe memory loss is not an inevitable consequence of growing older. Studies show that only about 5% of all those over age 65 and about 20% of those over 80 experience severe dementia. Most elderly people retain their intellectual capacities and live rich, active lives.

For millions of people in the United States, though, the news isn't so optimistic. For these adults, dementia is a fact of everyday life. And for each person who suffers from dementia, the effects ripple out and wash over numerous family members.

WHAT IS IT?

Dementia is a general term used to refer to the development of impairment in at least two areas of cognition with an intact level of consciousness. Dementia is characterized by memory loss, disorientation, and general intellectual impairment. In short, dementia is "brain failure." There are at least seventy-five conditions that cause dementia, several of which are treatable, that is, in which the confusion and memory difficulties are reversible. For example, depression, thyroid disease, and certain medications can diminish cognitive functioning, and these conditions can be corrected. On the other hand, most of the disorders that cause dementia are persistent and irreversible.

Alzheimer's disease is the most frequent cause of irreversible dementia. Defined by a specific set of symptoms, Alzheimer's disease is characterized by a progressive intellectual impairment that tends to move from forgetfulness to complete incapacity. Over time, it impairs a person's ability to reason, remember, and control his behavior.

At present, Alzheimer's disease can be identified conclusively only through autopsy, which reveals particular microscopic abnormalities of the brain. Yet, even in the absence of a pathologic diagnosis, an accurate diagnosis can be made on a clinical basis. This irreversible neurologic disorder affects an estimated four million Americans, most of whom are over 65. The majority of Alzheimer's patients live at home and are cared for by family. The National Institute on Aging estimates that Alzheimer's costs the United States $80 to $100 billion a year in medical care and lost productivity.

In its early stages, Alzheimer's disease is heralded by mild memory difficulties and sometimes by personality or mood changes. By its end phase, many people with Alzheimer's are completely incapable of caring for themselves.

It is imperative, therefore, to take note of any changes in an older adult's intellectual functioning, and not to dismiss these changes as a natural function of old age. Noticing such changes may be the first step toward identifying just what's causing them and, on occasion, to correcting them.

Even when the underlying condition cannot be reversed, as in the case of Alzheimer's, many of the symptoms can be addressed, and day-to-day living can be made better for the older person and for you, the caregiver. Therefore, just as you would call your doctor with any unexplained physical ailment, it is essential that you contact a doctor promptly whenever an older person experiences any mental difficulties.

WHAT CAUSES IT?

Autopsies show structural changes in the brains of people who die from Alzheimer's disease. Yet exactly what causes those changes is unknown. That's the short answer. Currently, researchers are looking into several possible theories, ranging from a genetic abnormality to a slow-growing virus, from environmental toxins to a neurochemical imbalance. That's the longer answer. But the real, more complicated and still evolving answer begins at the beginning of the last century when this particular form of dementia was identified by a German psychiatrist.

In 1907, Alois Alzheimer discovered the disease that would carry his name. He was examining under a microscope brain tissue that belonged to a mentally disabled patient who died at age 55. Before she died, she suffered from suspicion, difficulty speaking, and forgetfulness. As he looked at the tissue, Alzheimer noticed two abnormalities: first, clusters of proteins scattered in the gaps between nerve cells; second, tangled strands spewing out from lesions. Apparent only in autopsy, these two abnormalities are the markers of Alzheimer's.

It took fifty years after Alzheimer's discovery for clinicians to agree that what had been commonly called senile dementia was actually Alzheimer's disease. It may take even longer for scientists to agree about the dynamics of the dementia. In the last few years, the race to uncover the course and the cause of Alzheimer's has reached fever pitch. And indeed the stakes are high. The companies that discover the source of Alzheimer's will be in the position to develop appropriate treatments, specifically drugs to prevent, slow, or cure the disease. And as people live longer, the numbers of those who develop Alzheimer's will mushroom. According to the Alzheimer's Association, by the year 2050, the number will increase to almost fourteen million Americans. As a result, solving this medical mystery could translate into millions of more productive lives.

The Alzheimer's debate that permeates laboratories and academic offices around the world these days is quite complicated. To put it simply, most research revolves around the thick clumps of protein called plaques, which accumulate in brain tissue, and the gnarled tangles of former neurons called tau. The question is: Just what accounts for the death of the nerve cells in the brain?

In the 1980s, scientists were able to isolate the proteins that make up Alzheimer's plaques. These proteins are called beta-amyloid. While scientists agreed that beta-amyloid must have a natural function (amyloid is present in the cell membranes of all neurons, or nerve cells), they were not able to figure out just what that function is. However, they could determine that beta-amyloid is cut into two lengths when neurons in the brain degenerate. The slightly longer form of beta-amyloid is what accumulates into plaques. Shortly after the proteins were isolated, scientists were able to identify a gene on chromosome 21 that is responsible for making the beta-amyloid protein. And scientists noticed that beta-amyloid was a segment of a larger protein, which they named the amyloid-precursor protein, or APP.

This discovery was linked to a general observation. For a long time, scientists recognized that a rare form of Alzheimer's, called early-onset Alzheimer's, seemed to run in families. Once the APP gene was identified, scientists began to look for a mutant APP gene. In 1991 researchers in England found a mutant APP gene in a family with early-onset Alzheimer's disease.

Soon after that, two other mutant genes associated with early-onset Alzheimer's were identified by researchers at the University of Washington in Seattle—presenilin-1, on chromosome 14, and presenilin-2, on chromosome 1. Because these genes, like APP, are dominant, anyone who receives one mutant gene from either parent will eventually get the disease.

In the early 1990s, Dr. Allen Roses, at Duke University, reported a different type of genetic linkage. He and his colleagues found a relationship between the apo-E4 gene on chromosome 19 and Alzheimer's disease in which a variant of the apo-E lipoprotein appears to render a person more vulnerable to late-onset

Alzheimer's. Apo-E lipoprotein normally functions to transport cholesterol throughout the body, and is known to increase a person's risk for heart disease.

As the Duke researchers showed, one form of the apo-E gene called E4 is a major risk factor for Alzheimer's disease. But the E4 gene is a susceptibility gene, unlike APP and the presenilins, which are dominant genes. The degree of risk as well as the age of onset seems to reflect the number of copies of E4 that have been inherited. One study found that the presence of the E4 gene can advance the age of onset by as much as 17 years. However, scientists have also learned that having even two copies of E4 does not mean someone is necessarily doomed to develop Alzheimer's; there must be other risk factors, as well.

Today, conventional thinking ascribes between 30 and 60% of late-onset Alzheimer's cases to the apo-E4 gene. But what about the remainder? Researchers are looking for other genes that may be implicated in Alzheimer's disease.

Another area of research focuses on tau, the protein composing the neurologic tangles that appear along with beta-amyloid plaques in the brain tissue of an Alzheimer's patient.

Scientists have long recognized the role that tau plays within brain cells. Tau proteins make up neurofibrillary structures that act like a skeleton to support the axons, the long protrusions that transmit electric signals from one nerve cell to another. When tau becomes corrupted, the filaments become tangled, and the axons atrophy. In one particular form of dementia, scientists have found, patients do not develop the characteristic plaques of Alzheimer's, but instead exhibit the neurologic damage associated with mutant tau.

Other research is focusing on the enzymes that serve to clip off pieces of beta-amyloid in the first place. Two such enzymes, gamma-secretase and beta-secretase, have been identified, and much evidence points to a possible identification of gamma-secretase with presenilin-1, produced by one of the genes that codes for early-onset Alzheimer's. By stopping the action of these enzymes, researchers hope to slow or prevent the production of new beta-amyloid plaques. Yet presumably, these enzymes also serve normal functions that are necessary for good health. So it is hard to predict what side effects might be involved in taking drugs to block these enzymes for the long periods of time that would be required to prevent the development of Alzheimer's. Still other researchers are trying to understand

Alzheimer's as the product of a chronic inflammation response. On the one hand, nerve cells in the brain called microglia react to inflammation by producing excess amounts of a chemical called interleukin-1, which may be involved indirectly in the formation of beta-amyloid plaques. On the other hand, some researchers believe that the microglia could be involved in responding to and actually cleaning up the plaques, and that they could be activated by a vaccine. To say the least, the picture is complex. Research is under way to test both sides of the coin.

THE COURSE OF ALZHEIMER'S DISEASE

Alzheimer's disease usually develops gradually. It may have taken you some time to realize that something was wrong; this may lead some people to think that the disease appeared suddenly. Sometimes the person himself can draw attention to the problem with statements like, "I just can't find the right words," or "Thoughts fly out of my head." And then sometimes an Alzheimer's patient seems completely oblivious to the changes going on in his mind.

During the early stages of Alzheimer's, many people try to conceal their problems, or seem unaware of them. They may deny that anything is wrong, or use lists to compensate for their failing memory, or blame others for their mistakes. Sometimes the first signs of dementia look like signs of depression: listlessness, apathy, withdrawal, or irritability.

On average, people live between nine and 11 years after Alzheimer's disease first appears, with the condition gradually progressing. Memory deficits typically show up first and for the first three or so years tend to be the most pronounced problem. In the last several years, physical problems such as incontinence, swallowing difficulty, and speech troubles usually become more apparent.

THE STAGES OF ALZHEIMER'S DISEASE

In the early stage of Alzheimer's disease, the symptoms are usually mild and therefore easy to miss. Marked by repeated or increased instances of memory loss and confusion, these intellectual difficulties may begin to interfere with job performance or the ability to complete day-to-day tasks. The person may get lost easily, for example. He may forget names of everyday items or have difficulties with numbers or other kinds of abstract reasoning. You may notice that his personality seems to have changed. Perhaps he is easily distracted and lacks energy for the simplest of tasks. He is uninterested in his normal pursuits. These changes usually prompt a family member to schedule a medical examination, which leads to the diagnosis of dementia.

The middle stage usually lasts three or four years. Memory difficulties increase. Typically, the person's attention span seems to shorten dramatically. He may not be able to recognize friends and family. He may have trouble gathering his thoughts in an organized way and speaking logically. During this phase, he may wander off and get lost. He may find it more difficult to deal with such ordinary tasks as dressing or washing himself. He may turn on the stove to cook something and then forget it is on. A type of paranoia may creep into his thinking and into his behavior; he may become suspicious and hide things or accuse others of stealing from him. He may become agitated on a regular basis, often around sundown—called "sundowning," a common symptom in people with dementia. He may have delusions, and his sleep may become more disturbed and irregular.

The final stage also usually lasts several years. The person with Alzheimer's will have extreme difficulty communicating verbally or understanding words. In all likelihood, he may not recognize any of his family. In many cases, the person cannot recognize his own image in the mirror. He may have difficulty eating or swallowing, and even if he is eating adequately, he may lose weight. He will probably not be able to bathe, dress, or groom himself; nor will he be able to control his bowels or bladder. Many Alzheimer's patients become totally bedridden at this point. It is not uncommon for Alzheimer's patients to die from aspiration and pneumonia.

WHO IS AT RISK?

Age. The single most significant risk factor in developing Alzheimer's disease is old age. As mentioned earlier, about 5% of all those over 65 and about 20% of those over 80 experience severe dementia. An estimated 50 to 60% of all cases of dementia are caused by Alzheimer's disease. The National Institute on Aging estimates that there are approximately 360,000 new cases of Alzheimer's each year in the United States and says that number will rise as the population ages.

Race and gender. Whereas the incidence of Alzheimer's is about the same for all races, the disease afflicts more women than men, partly because they live longer.

Genetics. Alzheimer's disease tends to run in families, yet the genetic component is not well understood. Family history seems to play a role, especially in instances of early-onset Alzheimer's; about 40% of people with early-onset Alzheimer's have a parent or sibling who developed Alzheimer's. Yet even in families in which several members have had Alzheimer's, most do not develop the disease.

High blood cholesterol. Although inconclusive, studies suggest that when high blood cholesterol is not corrected, people may be at higher risk for developing sticky plaques in their brain cells; such plaques are thought to contribute to the Alzheimer's process.

Environment. Because many people with Alzheimer's disease appear to have no genetic risk, it is likely that environmental factors cause or predispose one to Alzheimer's. Head injury is the one proven environmental risk factor but there must be others. Although autopsies reveal traces of aluminum in the brains of some patients with Alzheimer's, scientists do not believe there is any link between the disease and our usual exposure to environmental sources of aluminum such as antacids, antiperspirants, cookware, or drinking water. Having little formal education may also be a risk factor.

HOW IS IT DIAGNOSED?

Learning that a loved one has Alzheimer's disease can be frightening to say the least. Yet, living with someone who has all the symptoms without knowing exactly why can be even more burdensome to all involved. For that reason alone, consulting a health care professional and getting the condition accurately diagnosed are very important.

A number of conditions other than Alzheimer's could lie at the root of the memory and thinking difficulties. For example, research indicates that older people typically need more time than a young person to process new information. So what you notice in an older adult may be perfectly expectable. Also, if a person has problems with vision, hearing, or coordination, he can seem forgetful, distracted, or confused. Stress, depression, and grief can and do cause intellectual difficulties. In fact, depression regularly impairs concentration, memory, and clear thinking.

However, when an older person has persistent memory problems, especially when these problems get worse as time passes, it is very likely that something more serious lies at the root. Confusion and forgetfulness can arise from infections, thyroid problems, low blood sugar, or medication side effects. Tumors and stroke can lead to cognitive difficulties. Many of these conditions can be effectively treated, and the intellectual problems thus reversed. That's why it's crucial to have the root of such problems identified early.

The diagnostic process usually involves taking a detailed history, performing a physical and neurologic examination, and ruling out other physical or emotional problems that could be interfering with a person's ability to think straight.

A diagnostic examination usually begins with a comprehensive medical history. The doctor will review present and past medical conditions as well as all medications currently being used. The review should include an assessment of family history, alcohol use, substance use and abuse, physical activities, and possible exposure to toxins.

The doctor will perform a mental status examination and observe the person's behavior for signs of confusion and disorientation. During a conversation, the doctor may ask basic questions such as "Where do you live?" "What year were you born?" or "Who is the current president?" to determine the extent of the person's impairment. If the person makes mistakes about widely known facts, Alzheimer's may be indicated. The doctor will also look for a relatively specific pattern of cognitive difficulties: problems with language, recognition and perception, and praxis, that is, the inability to use objects properly, such as knife and fork, pen or pencil, shirt buttons, or hair brush, even though there is no apparent physical impairment.

A physical examination is a key step in the diagnostic process. During the exam, other conditions can be ruled out and important clues uncovered. If a person has mild or moderate Alzheimer's disease, he will typically have a normal neurologic examination result; there will be no evidence of stroke, for example. In addition, people with Alzheimer's have a characteristic walk. Perhaps you have noticed that your loved one walks stooped over with legs spread, hands curled at his side, thumbs pointing inward. Reflexes can also indicate the presence of Alzheimer's. Place pressure on the bottom of the foot, for example, and a person with Alzheimer's often curls his toes. Scratch the palm of his hand and he may tense up around his neck.

SIGNS AND SYMPTOMS

- Progressive mental difficulties
- Forgetfulness, perhaps coupled with attempts to hide or compensate for difficulties
- Impaired ability to use good judgment or to understand reason
- Difficulty planning, organizing, and reasoning
- Recognition and perception difficulties; inability to identify objects despite normal vision
- Apraxia—the inability to perform purposeful motor activities even though there is nothing wrong with coordination or muscular system
- Incontinence
- Sudden or unusual language difficulties
- Personality changes
- Aggression
- Anxiety and agitation
- Extreme frustration
- Paranoia and suspicion
- Depression
- Absent-minded wandering

DISTINGUISHING BETWEEN ALZHEIMER'S AND OTHER CONDITIONS

Vascular dementia

Vascular dementia is probably the second most common form of irreversible dementia. Also known as multi-infarct dementia, it is caused by a series of strokes within the brain that may be so small that there are few apparent signs of changes, yet they destroy areas of the brain tissue and affect memory and other cognitive functions. Like Alzheimer's, it is irreversible. It may be that between 15 and 25% of all cases of dementia actually arise from vascular disease.

Parkinson's disease

This disease, caused by a deficiency of the neurotransmitter dopamine, affects the area of the brain that regulates body movement. People with Parkinson's disease have neurologic problems that cause tremor, body rigidity, and difficulty walking. Over time, between one-third and two-thirds experience a decline in cognitive functioning. There is no cure for Parkinson's, but medication can help to control the symptoms in the early and middle stages. (See the Parkinson's Disease chapter on p. 431.)

Lewy body disease or Lewy body dementia

This illness is caused when microscopic abnormalities, called Lewy bodies, build up in the cerebral cortex. Clinically, the course of Lewy body dementia is similar to Alzheimer's, but may also be characterized by Parkinson-like symptoms and hallucinations. The condition is irreversible and may count for as much as 5 to 10% of cases of dementia, although it was recognized only in the 1980s.

Other forms of irreversible dementia

Several other forms of irreversible dementia produce Alzheimer's-like symptoms and can make diagnosing the cause of the dementia all the more difficult.

Creutzfeldt-Jakob disease. Exceedingly rare, Creutzfeldt-Jakob disease affects only one in two million people a year, most over the age of 55. Although some of the symptoms—personality changes, anxiety, hallucinations, walking problems, and difficulties with speech and memory—can resemble Alzheimer's, its rapid progression (death usually occurs within eighteen months) is the most telling sign. Muscle twitching and stiffness distinguish Creutzfeldt-Jakob disease diagnostically from Alzheimer's. Also, autopsy shows spongy brain tissue as opposed to the lesions and plaques of Alzheimer's.

Creutzfeldt-Jakob disease is caused by an abnormal formation of a prion protein that causes microscopic holes to develop throughout the brain. It can be transmitted through grafting corneas and brain tissue from infected donors and from contaminated natural growth hormone. However, careful screening and the use of genetically engineered human grown hormone have lessened the risk. Recent cases have been linked to infected meat. This has been called "mad cow disease" and affects primarily young adults. Some cases may have a hereditary root.

There is no cure for the disease, although medications can control some of the behaviors and muscle problems. Most people succumb to pneumonia soon after contracting the infection.

Korsakoff's syndrome. Also called Wernicke-Korsakoff syndrome and Korsakoff's psychosis, this neurologic disorder is characterized by severe memory loss, but otherwise normal cognitive function. (Technically, therefore, it is not a dementia, because only memory is affected.) It is usually caused by a deficiency in the B vitamin thiamin, which plays a role in metabolizing glucose to generate energy to fuel brain activity. This disease is typically associated with chronic alcoholism, but may be caused by malnutrition, toxic or infectious brain illnesses, or severe head injury. Korsakoff's syndrome can be transient if treated early with thiamin, but some cases are chronic.

Korsakoff's syndrome tends to affect short-term memory. Like Alzheimer's, it can produce confusion, apathy, inattentiveness, and agitation.

Korsakoff's syndrome is extremely rare, but it is likely that the disease is underreported and underdiagnosed. Based on clinical research, between 22 and 29% of people with dementia were found to be heavy drinkers or alcoholics and 9 to 23% of elderly alcoholics in alcoholism treatment were found to also have dementia. Although Korsakoff's syndrome is treatable with thiamin replacement therapy if caught early enough, the death rate from it is relatively high at about 10 to 20%.

Frontotemporal disease or Pick's disease. Pick's disease is a progressive dementia that usually begins between the ages of 50 and 60. Characterized by early changes in personality and social behavior, Pick's disease (and other, closely related frontotemporal disorders) damages the frontal lobe of the brain, which affects the ability to plan, control behavioral and emotional responses, and monitor performance, and the temporal lobe, which is responsible for speech and language comprehension. It is believed to account for about 5% of the cases of irreversible dementia.

The cause of Pick's disease is unknown. Currently, there are no treatments to halt the progression of the disease. The drugs used in the treatment of Alzheimer's disease do not work for frontotemporal dementia. On the contrary, they make the aggression associated with the disease worse. Pick's disease may progress rapidly; most patients die two to ten years after it appears.

Reversible causes of dementia

Many other physical and emotional conditions cause confusion and forgetfulness in older adults. Depression, for example, is somewhat common in older people and can produce symptoms that mimic Alzheimer's disease, specifically the inability to remember, concentrate, and reason clearly. However, memory loss and other cognitive problems that arise from depression usually clear up once the depression lifts or in response to antidepressive medications.

Other conditions that can induce dementia-like symptoms include infections, drug interactions, dehydration, malnutrition, and specific types of vitamin deficiencies. When dementia is a result of any of these conditions, it can usually be addressed effectively.

LABORATORY TESTS AND FINDINGS

Analyses of blood and urine samples can rule out thyroid and other glandular problems. An electroencephalogram can provide a detailed picture of the brain's activity and indicate whether a brain tumor, seizure, or stroke is at root of the cognitive difficulties. A computerized tomography (CT) scan can identify abnormal structural changes in the brain, such as a tumor, a blow to the head, or small strokes that have produced the symptoms. In some instances, a CT scan can reveal severe shrinkage or atrophy of the brain.

In the end, though, Alzheimer's can be diagnosed with 100% certainty only through autopsy or biopsy of the brain tissue. When brain cells from people who had Alzheimer's are examined under a microscope, there are abundant neurologic fibers, the ridges on the outside of the brain appear deeper and wider than normal, and the brain's inner ventricles, or fluid-containing sacs, seem enlarged.

HOW IS IT TREATED?

Currently, the goal of treatment is to manage the symptoms of Alzheimer's disease. In other words, treatment aims at reversing, lessening, or slowing the mental and behavioral processes of dementia and easing the emotional upset that often accompanies the disease. At present, though, Alzheimer's cannot be prevented or cured. What new drugs have been developed are designed only to treat symptoms, not to cure the disease.

Because Alzheimer's symptoms are exacerbated by the presence of other medical conditions such as urinary tract infections, depression, delirium, heart or lung problems, and vision or hearing problems, those will be treated. In addition, many older adults may have severe reactions to medications, including over-the-counter drugs. Often adjusting the dosage or changing the drug or drug combination can reduce Alzheimer's symptoms.

Sometimes medications can be used to modify the behavioral symptoms of Alzheimer's, such as sleeplessness, wandering, anxiety, agitation, and depression. Antidepressants, such as sertraline (Zoloft), are often prescribed to address those. In addition, three drugs have proven moderately successful in modifying the effects of Alzheimer's on memory and other intellectual functioning. These drugs may maintain, stabilize, and slow the decline. Actual improvement is not common and often is short-term, measured in weeks. The first such drug approved by the FDA, tacrine (Cognex) is not generally used any more because of liver complications.

Donepezil hydrochloride (Aricept) was approved in 1996 for use with mild to moderate symptoms of the disease. It appears that Aricept increases the availability of acetylcholine in the brain. Taken once a day at bedtime, Aricept can cause nausea, diarrhea, and fatigue. These side effects are usually mild and of short duration.

Another acetylcholinesterase inhibitor is rivastigmine (Exelon). Prescribed for the treatment of mild to moderate Alzheimer's disease, Exelon has been shown to improve thinking, daily functioning, and behavior. However, rivastigmine can cause vomiting and nausea serious enough to cause patients to lose weight even when they are eating well.

In early 2001, the FDA issued its approval for yet another drug in the same class, galantamine (Reminyl), which bolsters the transmission of nerve impulses in the brain. Tests showed that galantamine enhanced Alzheimer's patients' ability to carry out the activities of daily living and improved their behavior. In one recent study, this medication slowed patients' decline in their functional status.

Donepezil is given at bedtime; rivastigmine should be given with food to lessen the common side effects of nausea, vomiting, and weight loss; and galantamine is given after meals. Dosages should be increased slowly until the optimal level for each patient is reached. Patients who fail at one agent may respond better with another. Drug trials are necessary to find the right drug at the right dosage for each person. It is important to continue a drug for a period long enough to assess the drug's effectiveness, preferably at least six months. It is worth noting that treatment of the Alzheimer's patient benefits their caregivers as well by reducing caregiver burden. A study in 2000 by the Institute for the Study of Aging showed less difficulty in doing caregiving tasks and lowered time demands and distress for the caregiver, leading to improved quality of life for both patients and caregivers.

At the same time, it should be noted that some commonly used drugs in older persons may depress cognitive functioning, and should be avoided in Alzheimer's patients. These drugs include diphenhydramine (Benadryl), often used as a sleeping aid, and oxybutynin (Ditropan), often prescribed for bladder spasms.

Other medications used to treat symptoms and decrease discomfort include:

Divalproex (Depakote) and carbamazepine (Tegretol). Antiseizure drugs that take the edge off agitation and anxiety and decrease irritability, restlessness, and emotional instability. Gabapentin (Neurontin) is also occasionally used for this purpose.

Risperidone (Risperdal), olanzapine (Zyprexa), and quetiapine (Seroquel). Antipsychotic medications used to calm agitation and paranoia and to treat aggressive behavior and hallucinations.

Lorazepam (Ativan) and trazodone (Desyrel). For insomnia.

Usually, behavioral techniques and environmental modifications are used in conjunction with drugs. It is mandatory that medications be started at low dosages and increased slowly. Side effects must be closely monitored.

Finally, many older adults have other illnesses, and when they have dementia as well, they are more vulnerable to other health problems. It is therefore essential that other conditions be diagnosed, treated, and kept under control in order to ease mental and behavioral problems associated with Alzheimer's disease.

WHAT RESEARCH IS BEING DONE?

For years, Alzheimer's research has yielded little more than frustration and false starts. Recently, however, research has moved into a very promising and exciting phase. The search to understand Alzheimer's disease—what causes it to develop, what exactly are the dynamics of the disease, and how it can be prevented and treated—is being conducted on many fronts.

Vaccine. Some of the most tantalizing research centers on developing a vaccine to prevent and possibly reverse the damaging effects of Alzheimer's. The basic principle of a vaccine would be to introduce a disease-causing substance into the body that would prompt the immune system to mount a defense against it. And in 1999, scientists at Elan Pharmaceuticals announced that they had vaccinated mice that were genetically engineered to develop plaques, with a fragment of beta-amyloid. Specifically, one group of mice received a vaccine made from a beta-amyloid called AN-1792 and other groups received no vaccine. While the untreated mice had a steady buildup of plaques over a period of thirteen months, the mice who received the immunization did not develop beta-amyloid plaques in their brains. Furthermore, when scientists treated the mice who had developed beta-amyloid plaques with AN-1792, the plaques cleared up after seven months. Results from a recent trial held in the United States indicate that the vaccine is safe for patients with mild to moderate forms of the disease. Further trials will be conducted in the United Kingdom.

Gene therapy. Scientists at the University of California, San Diego, have had some success in reversing brain cell degeneration in monkeys using a new kind of gene therapy. The scientists implanted cells that were altered to deliver human nerve growth factor into the brains of monkeys. Here, the chemical nourished the cells and, according to the study, effectively restored brain cells responsible for memory, attention, and other aspects of thinking. In April 2001, with FDA approval, a UCSD neurologist implanted genetically engineered skin tissue, designed to release nerve growth factor, in the brain of a 60-year-old woman. The pioneering procedure will help to determine whether the treatment is safe, prior to larger-scale research that will determine whether it is effective.

Nonsteroidal anti-inflammatory drugs. Researchers have long noticed that Alzheimer's disease is less common in people who have arthritis—who typically take large amounts of nonsteroidal anti-inflammatory drugs (NSAIDs). A 1996 National Institute on Aging study established a link between the use of NSAIDs and a lowered risk of developing Alzheimer's. Evidence suggests that people who regularly take NSAIDs, such as ibuprofen (Advil, Motrin), naproxen sodium (Aleve), and indomethacin (Indocin) have a lower risk of developing Alzheimer's than those who do not take painkillers. In fact, the study showed that use of NSAIDs lowered the risk of Alzheimer's by 30 to 60%. Scientists speculate that these agents curb the brain inflammation that occurs in the first stage of Alzheimer's, and thereby slow the development of the disease. However, it is unclear why neither aspirin, an anti-inflammatory drug, nor acetaminophen (Tylenol), had any such effect. Before NSAIDs can be recommended, however, more studies need to be completed.

NSAIDs can cause serious side effects, including stomach irritation, ulcers, and internal bleeding. New studies are designed to compare the effects of a relatively newer class of drug, COX-2 inhibitors, which have fewer side effects, against those of NSAIDs.

Estrogen. Scientists have known for many years that the hormone estrogen has positive effects on memory and cognitive function in women. Some studies of estrogen replacement therapy in women after menopause have found that it cuts their risk of developing Alzheimer's disease by up to half. However, other studies have found that estrogen was not helpful in slowing the progression of Alzheimer's in postmenopausal women who were already showing symptoms of the disease. Most recently, Boston University researchers compared more than 112,000 women who took estrogen with 108,000 women who did not and found the two groups developed an identical number of cases of Alzheimer's. Research in this area will continue.

Antioxidants. Scientists are looking at several ways of slowing Alzheimer's symptoms early in the disease. One such study involves the use of vitamin E and a compound called selegiline (Eldepryl). Selegiline is currently being used to treat people with Parkinson's disease. Both vitamin E and selegiline are antioxidants, chemicals that seem to limit cell damage by helping to mop up toxic molecules called "free radicals," which are produced by normal cell metabolism.

In 1997, a study published in the *New England Journal of Medicine* suggested that vitamin E slowed the progression of Alzheimer's disease once it had begun. However, it did not improve memory. The benefits were seen on large doses of vitamin E—2,000 international units per day. There is no evidence that vitamin E supplements can prevent healthy people from developing Alzheimer's. Some doctors recommend vitamin E rather than selegiline because they were equally effective and because vitamin E is safer and less expensive.

Neurotransmitters. A key neurotransmitter (or chemical messenger between nerve cells) called acetylcholine is gradually lost in the brains of Alzheimer's patients. It is very important for the formation of memories and for learning. All of the drugs approved to date for the treatment of Alzheimer's are designed to inhibit, or stop the action of, an enzyme that chemically breaks down acetylcholine. Researchers continue to look for ways of preventing the breakdown of this neurotransmitter and replacing the missing chemical once Alzheimer's disease has set in.

All this research is yielding great promise. According to the National Institute on Aging, fifty to sixty drugs and compounds are currently being tested in human trials. However, drug development is an exacting process, and it will be years before most of these new agents come to market—assuming they can pass the hurdles for safety and efficacy that their manufacturers are required to clear.

WHAT YOU CAN DO NOW

CARING FOR SOMEONE WITH ALZHEIMER'S DISEASE

It is a bit of an understatement to say that if you love someone with Alzheimer's disease, your life can be full of emotional ups and downs. A person who was once so well known and predictable now seems to fade in and out of his body. Traces of his familiar self rise to the surface, only to sink back into obscurity just moments later.

And if you are responsible for your loved one's care, the emotional and physical weight can be unwieldy at times. You spend hours involved in every aspect of his day-to-day life, yet as time passes, you recognize him less and less. Relationships become topsy-turvy. If it's your parent who has Alzheimer's, you may find yourself acting as a parent and he as a child. If it's your spouse, you may find yourself longing for the emotional and sexual partnership you once had or perhaps grieving the relationship you never had. Yet the demands of caregiving mean that instead of focusing on yourself and your feelings, you must attend to his needs, and with endless patience, as if you were tending to a child.

And yet the person is not a child. Nor is he always agreeable, grateful, cooperative. Instead, he may become easily upset or hostile, aggressive or hurtful. Many times, no amount of coaxing, reasoning, explaining, or goading will get him to yield or comply, even when his own safety is at stake.

Your loved one is frustrated, and much of the time, so are you. How do you take care of someone with Alzheimer's and take care of yourself at the same time? However hard it may be to take care of yourself while you're taking care of another, it can be done. First, you need information.

Medical information

For complete and comprehensible medical information, turn to your physician. A doctor can provide a medical evaluation and possibly an explicit diagnosis, which will serve as your baseline. Don't assume that your loved one has Alzheimer's or any other form of dementia without a medical evaluation. On the other hand, no matter how troubling it is to hear the words "Alzheimer's disease," just knowing what you're dealing with, and why your loved one is acting the way he is, will make coping and planning that much easier both now and in the long run. Your doctor can give you some idea of how far along the condition is, and based on the history and observation, make an educated guess as to how things will progress and what you can expect.

If you're dealing with Alzheimer's, it's important to acknowledge that the disease is a chronic, progressive, long-term condition. As the condition progresses over time, the ways in which you render care will naturally change. Indeed, the manifestations of the disease can shift from moment to moment, and an Alzheimer's patient's needs will change, sometimes from day to day. It is therefore essential that you stay somewhat flexible. If you develop a good relationship with the person's physician, she might notice and assess the changes, and help you respond appropriately.

In fact, a good relationship with your loved one's doctor will ensure that he gets good, regular general medical care. When someone has Alzheimer's, obtaining good medical care is important for a number of reasons. First, even though the underlying condition cannot be treated, many of the expressions can be, thus alleviating much of the discomfort and distress. Second, people with Alzheimer's tend to have intense reactions to medications. When side effects seem severe, talk to the doctor who can either adjust the dosage or change the medication. And third, Alzheimer's symptoms tend to get worse when there is even a small medical problem, such as a urinary tract infection or a cold. Therefore, you will want to consult the doctor for seemingly minor illnesses.

Legal and psychosocial information

For legal and psychosocial information, turn to an attorney who specializes in elder law and perhaps to a geriatric social worker or case manager. You should have a will and trust for your loved one and for yourself. You will need to understand such concepts as durable power of attorney and advanced directives. A lawyer who knows her way around elder law and a specially trained social worker or case manager can help you consider such issues as what to do if the person becomes incompetent or whether to allow the use of ventilators, feeding tubes, and other heroic measures should there be a need. Special financial issues may also need to be weighed. All this should be discussed early in the course of the condition with your loved one, with other family members, and with professionals who know the ropes. In all such issues, the needs of family members as well as the wishes of the older adult should be factored in.

Practical information

Once you have a grasp on the medical, legal, financial, and psychosocial ramifications of the disease, you will be better able to manage the day-to-day particulars. Dealing with the emotional and behavioral manifestations of Alzheimer's is never an easy matter. But there are ways of managing, in fact managing quite well.

First, just as each older individual has his own way of being in the world, each case of Alzheimer's takes on its own distinct shape. Focus your care on the singular shape of your loved one's illness. Be aware of the special difficulties he has. Is he paranoid or suspicious? Does he have hallucinations? Is he depressed, withdrawn, or overactive? Is he still driving? How is he eating? Tailor your care to him and his illness. At all times, maintain a problem-solving attitude. Break things down to their parts: "What is the problem at the moment, and how can we solve it?"

THE STAGES OF CAREGIVING

Alzheimer's disease is a progressive condition. Many researchers and clinicians divide the progression of the disease into stages. Others describe a continuum of symptoms. However the disease is characterized, the degree and type of care you provide will progress and change. As the condition progresses, as different symptoms appear or fade, you will have to tailor your caregiving accordingly.

The early phase

The first step involves consulting with a doctor to have the condition diagnosed.

Once a diagnosis has been made, begin to think long term. Talk to your loved one, other family members, and perhaps geriatric or medical professionals about the practical issues involved. Determine at what point financial responsibilities should be turned over, what treatment options are preferred, and what legal plans need to be made. Look into supplemental caregiving resources such as adult day care and home health aides, and begin to consider the possibility of nursing home placement at some time down the line.

• As your loved one begins to make mistakes or becomes forgetful, do not correct him. This can be frustrating for you and perhaps embarrassing to your loved one.

• Keep important items, such as keys, glasses, emergency phone numbers, calendar, and the clock, in an obvious place. Make sure the environment is organized and predictable.

• Help the person stay in touch with friends and keep physically active as much as possible.

• Keep a close eye on his driving ability to make sure he still drives safely. This may become one of the most difficult issues you have to face. Eventually, every Alzheimer's patient must stop driving. In the early stages of the disease, the American Medical Association advises that patients drive only in the daytime, never at rush hour, and with the aid of a "co-pilot," or passenger with intact memory. Later, it may become necessary to remove the person's car (out of sight, out of mind), obtain a "prescription" from his doctor that orders him to stop driving, ask him to surrender his license, and/or take away the keys.

• Monitor the person's use of all medications.

The middle phase

If you haven't already done so, start looking into residential care facilities, just in case.

• If your loved one has become confused about everyday items, use labels to guide and clarify. Label drawers, closets, rooms, appliances, and hot- and cold-water faucets. Put names on photographs.

• Safety-proof the house.
  ✔ Make sure hallways and bathrooms are well lit at night and furnished with support rails.
  ✔ Make sure the bathtub has grab rails and a skid-proof mat.

✔ Make sure you have working fire and smoke alarms.

✔ Control the temperature on your water heater to prevent scalding.

✔ Use plastic plug guards in unused electrical outlets.

✔ Electric stoves can be equipped with timers and automatic shut-off devices to limit the hours in which they can be turned on.

•Simplify your loved one's surroundings so that they are familiar, predictable, and calming.

✔ Encourage him to be as independent as he can be, to do whatever he's capable of doing, but be careful not to make unreasonable demands on him.

✔ Take away car keys and make other transportation arrangements. Also, take away credit cards and checkbooks to guard against uncontrolled phone donations and purchases.

✔ Install alarms and special door locks if he has a tendency to wander. Equip the person with an ID bracelet that will facilitate his return if he goes off and can't find his way home. Register him with the Alzheimer's Association Safe Return program.

✔ Use gentle reminders and coaxing to address issues of personal hygiene and grooming.

The late phase

If your loved one has moved into a nursing facility, maintain contact and involvement.

• Arrange to have someone come in and tend to the person's personal hygiene, such as hair, nails, and perhaps dental needs.

• Consider how aggressively you want medical problems treated; minimize unnecessary medical tests and painful procedures.

• Seek out help and support for yourself as the condition worsens or the end nears.

MANAGING THE BEHAVIOR AND PERSONALITY CHANGES

Now and then, people with Alzheimer's disease will act in ways that are extremely frustrating, if not altogether maddening. Or, even if their behavior is mostly tolerable, their personality may seem a bit odd. As you've probably figured out by now, arguing or even reasoning with someone who has Alzheimer's does little good. But distraction often works. Try shifting the focus of attention when things get intense, frustrating or even a bit dangerous.

At the same time, people with Alzheimer's are still adults. They should be treated with the respect one would show an older adult. They should be encouraged to do for themselves whenever they can. And perhaps most important, no matter how debilitated adults become, they still need to be treated with love and kindness.

One of the most obvious and perhaps troubling changes wrought by Alzheimer's disease involves the individual's personality. Some people become paranoid, usually because they're misplacing and forgetting things. So, for example, your father may forget that his wife has died, and instead insist that she's running around on him. Your wife may forget that you've put her jewelry in a safe deposit box, and insist that the home health care aide has stolen it.

Some people become angry and aggressive. Anger and aggression can be expressions of extreme frustration. Many Alzheimer's patients engage in repetitive behaviors: they check doors and windows time and again, ask the same question over and over, pick objects up only to set them back down, tug at their clothes. As spoken language becomes more problematic for them, repetitive behaviors can be the voice of their discomfort. Possibly the person needs to go to the bathroom. Possibly she's hot or cold. Possibly she's in pain. Sometimes increased confusion or lethargy is a sign of illness. If you know that these types of behaviors have meaning, you may find them less irritating.

Many times, difficult behaviors can be managed through understanding their meaning. When this fails, distraction can work wonders to redirect a person's attention, defuse his frustration, and soothe his anxiety. Help your loved one engage in activities that he enjoyed at an earlier time. Repetitious activities are usually the best. All activities must be safe and supervised. Such activities include gardening, for example, or making the beds. Some people enjoy washing the car or fiddling with a simple mechanical task. Some derive pleasure from washing dishes, dusting, or wiping down counters. Cradling a baby doll can be soothing as well. While it may be unsettling to see your elderly mother wandering about with a baby doll in her arms, or to watch your father engaged in what appears to be a meaningless task, such activities can be enormously comforting to them.

Another source of comfort for Alzheimer patients is music—playing a favorite song or singing. In fact, anything that's predictable and repetitious can be calming: hearing the same songs, eating the same foods, walking the same path, taking the same drive, wearing the same clothes. In other words, people with Alzheimer's disease do best when their environment is simple and predictable, never frenetic or overstimulating or confusing. Nor should the demands placed on them exceed their capability.

When talking to a person with Alzheimer's, make eye contact and use gestures to make him understand. Touch him if he can tolerate touch. You may be tempted to make decisions for the person without asking because you anticipate resistance. You might be in the habit of making announcements like, "Let's take a bath now," or "Let's go for a walk." But whenever possible, give your loved one the opportunity to make his own decisions. While too many choices can be overwhelming to someone with Alzheimer's disease, you can limit choices to two or, at the most, three options, thus giving the person a feeling of control and involvement. When helping your loved one dress, for example, offer a choice between two outfits instead of picking for him or letting him rummage through a whole closet full of clothes. Offer a choice between taking a bath or a shower. Inevitably, caring for someone with Alzheimer's disease means making many of his decisions. But it's important that he feels part of the process.

Alzheimer's patients have been known to use inappropriate language or touch in inappropriate ways. If this should happen with your loved one, calmly try to change the behavior or divert his attention. The fact is that a person with Alzheimer's is incapable of understanding why certain language or behaviors are inappropriate.

And just when you think you've figured out how to cope with Alzheimer's, things change. In many cases, personality shifts are temporary. As the dementia progresses, the person may lose contact with his earlier self and forget that he ever remembered. For some this brings on an air of calm. Some seem to withdraw altogether. Others seem completely vacant. You may be left with absent-minded wanderings and incontinence, and perhaps a new sense of loneliness.

Finally, practically speaking, as long as the person is living at home, make sure the environment is safe. Remove scatter rugs and make sure electrical wires and extension cords are out of the way. If the person sleeps in an upstairs bedroom, consider moving her to a downstairs room so she can avoid going up and down stairs.

TAKING CARE OF YOURSELF

Every phase of Alzheimer's disease touches all those involved in different and meaningful ways. In the early stages, the person with Alzheimer's can be painfully aware of differences in their ability to remember and think clearly. You, the caregiver, may see the pain this causes, and experience the expressions of frustration, agitation, and anxiety. After a while, though, many become mercifully unaware of their memory lapses. Your loved one may actually forget that he was ever able to remember. While this may bring a degree of peacefulness to him, it can be painful for family members.

You may remember what your mother was like before, for example, or how intelligent and capable your husband used to be. And you will miss the conversations, the give-and-take of your earlier relationship. Taking care of someone with Alzheimer's can be taxing, physically, emotionally, and financially. And many times, the Alzheimer's patient is never able to show appreciation for your efforts.

FINDING SUPPORT AND HELP

Loving and taking care of someone with Alzheimer's naturally entails a significant amount of emotional stress. While the emotional needs of caregivers vary greatly depending on the relationship with the patient and the amount of time and responsibility invested, research shows that the rate of emotional distress is three times greater in people who take care of loved ones with dementia than in the general population. Caregivers may experience a range of shifting emotions, including depression, anxiety, exhaustion, shame, demoralization, worry, irritability, anger, sadness, and grief.

Many find support groups helpful. Such groups afford people who are experiencing similar challenges the opportunity to share encouragement and empathy as well as specific suggestions and information. Even if your loved one is living in a nursing home, you may benefit from group meetings with other Alzheimer's families. The Alzheimer's Association can help you find such a group nearby. And perhaps individual counseling will be beneficial, especially if you are feeling overwhelmed.

In addition, from time to time you will need support and additional help with the practical matters of caregiving. Options to help ease the burden of care and to improve the quality of life for the patient include adult day care, home care aides, alternative housing arrangements such as supervised group home living, and nursing homes. Some people find home health care or an adult day care program helpful. When looking for a substitute or relief home care provider, find someone who has training and experience working specifically with people with dementia. If possible, ask the home health aide to spend time with the person with dementia before hiring, to make sure that both are comfortable with the arrangement.

Respite care may be available in your area, through a residential facility or home health care agency, or the Alzheimer's Association or Society so that you can arrange for substitute care for a longer period of time. In some instances, as time progresses, the Alzheimer's patient can live in a nursing facility part of the time and at home part of the time. In other instances, respite arrangements provide at-home care so that the family caregiver has a chance to get away from the responsibilities for a weekend or longer. If you allow yourself occasional breaks from your caregiving responsibilities, you will no doubt be more patient and effective overall. However, whenever you leave the person in the care of another, be sure that you leave clear, detailed instructions, perhaps written down, about what he needs and expects.

CONSIDERING NURSING HOME PLACEMENT

Whether you want it or not, at some point, institutionalization—placing your loved one in a nursing home—may become necessary. Up to 80% of all Alzheimer's patients eventually need nursing home care. It is a myth that families "dump" Alzheimer's patients in nursing homes. On the contrary, most families resist placement, many times to the detriment of the patient. Indeed, many patients actually get better once they are moved to a nursing home. Because they get the constant medical and psychosocial attention they need, in addition to a predictable environment, many feel better emotionally; they become less agitated, less anxious, or less depressed. Many behave better; they seem able to exercise greater control over their behavior. And many function better, perhaps benefiting from structured activities and finding comfort being among other Alzheimer's residents. As for the family, once they are freed up from the physical and emotional demands of day-to-day care, many find that they suddenly have more time and internal resources to relate with the patient in a loving and meaningful way. Most family members stay involved in the resident's care in the nursing home, but now they can relate to the patient as a loved one and not a mere responsibility.

It is time to consider a nursing home when your own stamina seems to be waning and your physical and emotional health seem to be at risk. If you live with someone with Alzheimer's, chances are that he doesn't sleep well, and nor do you. You may be constantly on guard, vigilant that he doesn't wander off late at night, or leave the stove on, or, even worse, the gas. If he is incontinent, which is often the case, accidents mean a slippery floor in unexpected places, increasing the likelihood that he, or perhaps you, will fall. If he paces, there is an increased chance that he will fall eventually. And your home could pose risk of injuries, between the steps, and the scatter rugs, spills, and pets running underfoot.

Of course, you may believe that you should be able to care for your mother or your wife, or your brother, but the truth is that Alzheimer's sometimes makes sticking with it impossible. Even with the help of adult day care and home health care, placement in a nursing home may be the best step for all involved.

CHOOSING A RESIDENTIAL CARE FACILITY

When choosing a nursing home, look at more than one facility. Be sure the facility offers a safe and pleasant environment for people with all levels of dementia. The staff should seem competent, caring, and up-to-date when it comes to overseeing people with dementia. Ask the administrator or head of nursing or social services to describe their specific approach for working with residents, regardless of their particular health needs.

- What types of programs do they offer?
- How involved in programs and activities is the typical resident?
- To what degree are treatment and caregiving individualized?
- Are there different levels of care to match different levels of functioning?
- How do they deal specifically with people who have Alzheimer's?

Be ready to describe your loved one's behavior and ask how the staff typically respond to such behavior. Look around you and notice how people are treated. Do the residents seem content, alert, well cared for? If possible, talk to doctors, nurses, aides, residents, and family members. Deliberate and thoughtful investigation early on will go a long way to ensure that a residential care facility will eventually become a comfortable and caring home for your loved one.

ADDITIONAL RESOURCES

ORGANIZATIONS AND ASSOCIATIONS

Administration on Aging
330 Independence Avenue, SW
Washington, D.C. 20201
202-619-7501
www.aoa.dhhs.gov

Aging Network Services
4400 East-West Highway Suite 907
Bethesda, MD
301-657-4329
www.agingnets.com

Alzheimer's Association
919 North Michigan Avenue Suite 1100
Chicago, IL 60611-1676
800-272-3900
312-335-8700
Fax 312-335-1110
www.alz.org

Alzheimer's Disease Education and Referral Center
PO Box 8250
Silver Spring, MD 20907-8250
301-495-3311
800-438-4380
www.alzheimers.org

American Association for Geriatric Psychiatry
7910 Woodmont Ave.
Suite 1050

Bethesda, Md. 20814
301-654-7850
www.aagpgpa.org

American Geriatrics Society
770 Lexington Ave.
New York, New York 10021
212-308-1414
800-247-4779
www.americangeriatrics.org

American Association of Homes and Services for the Aging
901 E St., N.W.
Washington, D.C. 20004-2937
202-508-9420

AARP
The American Association of Retired People
601 E St., N.W.
Washington, D.C. 20049
800-424-3410
www.aarp.org

American Society on Aging
833 Market St.
Suite 511
San Francisco, CA 94103
415-974-9600
800-537-9728
www.asaging.org

Medicare

800-MEDICARE (800-633-4227)

www.medicare.gov

National Institute on Aging

Building 31, Room 5C27

31 Center Drive, MSC 2292

Bethesda, MD 20892

301-496-1752

www.nih.gov/nia

National Institute on Aging (Age Pages)

P.O. Box 8057

Gaithersburg, MD 20898-8057

301-496-1752

National Citizens' Coalition for Nursing Home Reform

1224 M St., N.W., Suite 301

Washington, D.C. 20005

202-393-2018

National Association of Area Agencies on Aging

927 15th St., N.W., Sixth Floor

Washington, D.C. 20005

202-296-8130

fax 202-296-8134

www.n4a.org

Eldercare Locator

800-677-1116 weekdays

National Association for Home Care

519 C Street, N.E.

Washington, D.C. 20002

202-547-7424

National Association of Professional Geriatric Care Managers

1604 North Country Club Drive

Tucson, AZ 85716

602-881-8008

National Institute on Adult Daycare

National Council on Aging

409 Third Street, S.W., Second Floor

Washington, D.C. 20024

202-479-1200

BOOKS AND ARTICLES

American Medical Association. *Guide to Diagnosis, Management, and Treatment of Dementia.* Internet on-line. http://www.ama-assn.org/ama/pub/category/4789.html [May 20, 2002].

American Psychiatric Association. *Diagnostic & Statistical Manual of Mental Disorders (DSM-IV.)* Washington, D.C.: American Psychiatric Press, 2000.

Davies, Helen D., and Michael P. Jensen. *Alzheimer's: The Answers You Need.* Forest Knolls, Calif.: Elder Books, 1998.

Gray-Davidson, Frena. *Alzheimer's Disease Frequently Asked Questions: Making Sense of the Journey.* Lowell House, 1999.

Gray-Davidson, Frena. *The Alzheimer's Sourcebook for Caregivers: A Practical Guide for Getting Through the Day.* Lowell House, 1996.

Kaplan H., and B. Sadock. *Kaplan & Sadock's Synopsis of Psychiatry: Behavioral Sciences - Clinical Psychiatry.* Baltimore: Lippincott Williams & Wilkins, 1998.

Mace, Nancy L., and Peter V. Rabins. *The 36-Hour Day: A Guide to Caring for Persons With Alzheimer's Disease, Related Dementing Illnesses and Memory Loss in Later Life.* Baltimore: Johns Hopkins University Press, 1999.

Morris, Virginia, and Robert Butler. *How to Care for Aging Parents.* New York: Workman Publishing, 1996.

Nash, J. M. The New Science of Alzheimer's, *TIME* Magazine, August 1, 2000.

National Institute on Aging. *Progress Report on Alzheimer's Disease 2000: Taking the Next Steps.* Internet on-line. http://www.alzheimers.org/pubs/prog00.htm. [May 5, 2002].

Pierce, Charles. *Hard to Forget.* New York: Random House, 2000.

Powell, Lenore S., and Katie Coutice. *Alzheimer's Disease - A Guide for Families.* Cambridge, Mass.: Perseus Press, 1993.

Tanzi, Rudolph E. *Decoding Darkness: The Search for the Genetic Causes of Alzheimer's Disease.* Cambridge, Mass: Perseus Press, 2000.

Young, Ellen P. *Between Two Worlds: Special Moments of Alzheimer's and Dementia.* New York: Prometheus Books, 1999.

Breast Cancer

SIGNS & SYMPTOMS

- Swelling in the breast or underarm area
- Lump in the breast or underarm area
- Skin irritation or dimpling of the breast or nipple
- Nipple pain
- Nipple retraction (turning inward)
- Redness or scaliness of the nipple or skin of the breast
- Discharge from the nipple (other than breast milk in a lactating woman)
- Any change in the contour of the breast

A few statistics paint a vivid picture of breast cancer:

- Approximately 180,000 women in the United States are diagnosed each year with invasive breast cancer, about 110 cases per 100,000 women per year. Another 30,000 are diagnosed with noninvasive breast cancer. It is the most common cancer among women (not including skin cancer) and the second deadliest. In the United States, a woman is diagnosed with breast cancer every three minutes, and one dies of the disease every eleven minutes. (Men can also get breast cancer, but it is very rare; less than 1% of cases are in men, and most of the information in this discussion is directed at women.)

- Nearly 30% of new cancers diagnosed in women each year are cancers in the breast.

- In 1998, 43,500 women died of breast cancer in the United States. The American Cancer Society estimated that in the year 2001, 40,200 women would die of breast cancer.

By the time we reach middle age, many of us will know at least one woman who has had breast cancer. Increasingly, these women are likely to be breast cancer survivors. A woman diagnosed with breast cancer today has a greater than 80% chance of living at least five years after diagnosis, and the odds for long-term survival rise to 95% for cancer diagnosed early and contained within the breast in early stages. Many women who have had breast cancer live decades after their successful treatment for the disease. Merely a generation ago, the diagnosis of breast cancer was a potential death sentence. The cancer often spread to other parts of the woman's body before the primary tumor was even diagnosed. But now, extensive public education campaigns have resulted in early breast cancer detection through widespread screening and self-examination. New and evolving treatments offer a realistic hope for cure for many women.

But make no mistake, this is still a serious and sometimes deadly disease that marks the lives of women and their loved ones and caregivers in many different ways—physically, emotionally, psychologically, and sexually. And the course is not always clear. In some areas, there are disagreements and even controversies about the best approaches for treatment and prevention of breast cancer.

WHAT IS IT?

The breast is made up of as many as fifteen to twenty overlapping sections or lobes. Each lobe contains smaller sections called lobules, which branch into dozens of tiny bulbs capable of producing milk. The lobes and lobules are linked by a system of ducts that lead to the nipple. Breast development and growth are fueled by the hormone estrogen; it is the surge of estrogen in puberty that causes adolescent girls' breasts to grow. Most people don't think of the breast as an organ or gland, like the heart or pancreas, but it is—a gland, stimulated by hormones, with the very specialized function of feeding offspring. Throughout most of a woman's life, the milk-producing machinery within her breasts lies dormant. The hormones of pregnancy stimulate the breast to produce milk, and lactation can continue months or years after childbirth. Estrogen also figures prominently in the growth of many breast tumors.

Ductal carcinoma in situ. Breast cancer is an overgrowth of the cells in the breast, resulting in a tumor. Most often, cancer begins in the cells lining the milk ducts, and is known as ductal carcinoma in situ. The earliest stages of ductal carcinoma are confined to the lining of the duct; this is called noninvasive ductal carcinoma or ductal carcinoma in situ. When the malignancy breaks through the duct wall and into the fatty tissue of the breast, it has become invasive (or infiltrating) ductal carcinoma. Invasive ductal carcinomas account for 70 to 80% of breast cancers.

Lobular carcinoma. Cancer in the lobes is called lobular carcinoma. Lobular cancer is more likely to occur in both breasts at the same time. Lobular carcinoma in situ will increase a woman's risk of developing more invasive types of cancer. Invasive lobular carcinomas account for 10 to 15% of invasive breast cancers.

Inflammatory breast cancer. Very rare, inflammatory breast cancer accounts for about 1% of invasive breast cancer, and is very aggressive and quick-growing. The skin of the affected breast is often red, warm to the touch, thickened, with an orange-peel-like quality, and swollen. The inflammatory symptoms result from cancer cells blocking the lymph vessels in the skin of the breast.

Medullary carcinoma. In medullary carcinoma, which accounts for about 5% of all breast cancers, there is a clear-cut boundary between tumor and normal tissue.

Colloid (or mucinous) carcinoma and tubular carcinoma. These are two other uncommon and relatively slow-growing cancers of the breast.

Another kind of malignancy, called Paget's disease, is cancer of the nipple. Paget's disease is uncommon, accounting for about 1% of all breast cancers.

In recent years, a growing number of researchers have begun exploring the causes of breast cancer, but one fact predominates: For most cases of breast cancer, the cause is unknown.

Cancers are caused by either genetic or environmental factors or a combination of the two. It is most likely that someone has a genetic predisposition to the disease, which may then be triggered by environmental factors. Inherited cases of breast cancer are thought to make up only 5 to 10% of all cases. Two genes implicated in breast cancer—BRCA1 and BRCA2—have been identified on chromosome 17. Another group of genes, known as the p53 tumor suppressor genes, may also be involved in breast and other cancers. But the extent of involvement of these genes is unclear. The BRCA genes have many mutations, which makes testing for the gene expensive and complicated. The advisability of genetic testing is discussed below, in the section "What You Can Do Now."

Many scientists also believe that toxic chemicals in the environment have something to do with causing breast cancer. Some chemical compounds in the environment mimic the actions of estrogen, and studies are under way to determine the effects of long-term low-level exposure.

WHO IS AT RISK?

Any woman can get breast cancer. The biggest risk is just being a woman. Many women—70% of those diagnosed—get it with no other known risks at all. But it is important for a woman to know something about her personal risk of developing breast cancer. When caught early, breast cancer can nearly always be treated successfully. Women who know they are at risk can use the knowledge by performing breast self-examination, having their doctor perform a clinical breast examination at least annually, and taking advantage of screening and other diagnostic tests at an earlier age than women at lower risk. Other proactive preventive steps include taking the medication tamoxifen, a hormonal treatment that blocks the activity of estrogen, and preventive mastectomy.

NONCONTROLLABLE RISK FACTORS

Age. One of every eight women in this country will develop breast cancer in her lifetime. This is probably the statistic most commonly used to describe the prevalence of breast cancer, but it is somewhat misleading. It is true that over the course of a long lifetime, a woman has a 1 in 8 chance of getting breast cancer, but through the years, her chances vary, depending on her age. For example, according to the National Cancer Institute, a woman's risk of developing breast cancer during her lifetime are these:

- To age 30: 1 in 2212
- To age 40: 1 in 235
- To age 50: 1 in 54
- To age 60: 1 in 23
- To age 70: 1 in 14
- To age 80: 1 in 10
- Ever: 1 in 8

As you can see from these numbers, age is a significant risk factor. The older a woman gets, the more likely she is to get breast cancer.

Family history. Other uncontrollable risk factors are in our genes and family histories. Fifty to sixty percent of women with inherited BRCA1 or BRCA2 mutations will develop breast cancer by age 70. The risk is also increased in

BREAST CANCER STAGING

If left untreated, breast cancer will spread from the original tumor site to other sites in the breast, and out of the breast to the rest of the body. Most of the time, the cancer cells move through the axillary (underarm) lymph nodes, and microscopic dissection of lymph nodes will provide a fairly reliable indication of whether the cancer has spread or not. If the nodes are negative for cancer and the tumor was small, there is an excellent (more than 90%) chance that the cancer has been contained in the breast. If the nodes are positive for cancer, the malignancy has begun to spread and may have made its way to distant parts of the body.

Cancer spreads in the body through the bloodstream or the lymphatic system or both. The bloodstream circulates blood through the entire vascular system: arteries, capillaries, and veins. The lymphatic system circulates a clear infection-fighting fluid through the body via lymph vessels and nodes. The extent of spread is measured in stages, from 0 to IV. Tumor size also figures into the staging of breast cancer:

Stage 0. Carcinoma in situ. Abnormal cells are confined to the lining of the duct of the breast.

Stage I. The invasive tumor is contained within the breast and is less than 2 centimeters (about three quarters of an inch) at its largest dimension.

Stage II. The tumor remains smaller than 2 cm but has spread to the lymph nodes, or the tumor is greater than 2 cm and less than 5 cm in size and the lymph nodes are negative for cancer.

Stage III. The tumor is greater than 5 cm and the lymph nodes are negative, or a tumor of any size has spread to the skin or chest wall, or there is evidence of lymph node involvement, but no spread beyond the lymph nodes to other organ sites.

Stage IV. There is evidence that the tumor (regardless of size) has spread beyond the lymph nodes, to other parts of the body. The most common organs to which breast cancer spreads are lungs, bone, and liver.

women with family histories of the disease, whether they know their genetic status or not. This applies to relatives on both sides of the family, both paternal and maternal. A woman with one first-degree relative (mother, sister, daughter) with breast cancer is twice as likely to develop breast cancer herself as a woman with no family history. A woman with two first-degree relatives who have had the disease has five times increased risk. The more close relatives who have been affected, the greater the risk.

Previous cancers. A woman who has had breast cancer has a threefold to fourfold increased risk of developing a new cancer in her other breast. This risk equals about 15% risk over her remaining lifetime. This is a sobering thought for women who have fought the battle once, with good outcome, but know they must remain vigilant for the rest of their lives, or as long as they have a remaining breast or breasts. Even short of cancer, women who have had breast biopsies and been diagnosed with proliferative breast disease have one and a half to five times increased chances of getting breast cancer, with the higher odds for biopsies that found abnormal cell growth in the cells that were studied. Dense breast tissue, in which the tissue appears white on a mammogram and abnormalities are very hard to see, also implies an increased risk because it is harder to detect cancer early by mammography, the primary method used for screening.

Radiation therapy for another cancer in the chest area (for example, Hodgkin's disease, non-Hodgkin's lymphoma) or for treatment of a childhood disease such as adenoiditis also increases the risk for breast cancer later in life. The younger a woman is when she receives radiation treatment, the greater her chances of getting breast cancer.

Lifetime exposure to estrogen. We know that many breast cancers are related to lifetime exposure to estrogen, which increases when a girl begins to menstruate. Therefore, early onset of menstruation (before age 12) or late menopause (after age 50) gives a woman a slightly increased risk of developing breast cancer. Race may have some effect on the odds of getting breast cancer. White women have a slightly higher rate of the disease than black women, but rates are considerably lower for Hispanic women and lowest for American Indian women. American Indian women have a rate nearly four times lower than whites. Reasons for these differences are unknown. One ethnic group with a particularly high rate of breast cancer is Ashkenazi Jews, women with Jewish ancestors from central or Eastern Europe. In one study, 2% of Ashkenazi Jewish women had BRCA1 or BRCA2 mutations—a high percent for a gene mutation in an ethnic group.

Interestingly, one study has found that left-handed women have a higher risk for breast cancer than right-handed women. This analysis of more than four thousand women found a "modest" association between left-handedness and increased risk. Left-handedness has been linked to intrauterine hormone exposures, and researchers speculated that the same factor may be involved with breast cancer.

CONTROLLABLE RISK FACTORS

Knowing we have some control over some risk factors is empowering. For some controllable risk factors, most notably, hormone replacement therapy in post-menopausal women, there is confusion and uncertainty about the role they play, and further research is needed before these factors are fully understood. Researchers suspect that women who take hormone replacement therapy and develop hormone-sensitive breast cancer probably speeded up the arrival of the cancer by a decade.

Not giving birth. Women who have not had children, or had their first child after the age of 30, are at slightly increased risk for breast cancer. It appears that the more menstrual cycles a woman experiences in her youth, the higher her risk due to hormone exposure and its relationship to breast cancer growth.

Overweight. Being overweight after menopause seems to increase the risk of breast cancer. In one study of more than 25,000 Asian women, the heaviest 20% had twice the breast cancer rate of the thinnest 20%.

Smoking and drinking. Smoking and drinking both appear to increase the risk of breast cancer. The relationship with cigarette smoking is not clear, but some studies show higher rates of disease in women who smoke. And risk is also related to alcohol consumption. Women who have three or more drinks a day double their risk of getting breast cancer. Moderate drinking (less than two drinks a day) does not seem to increase the risk of breast cancer, but what is a safe intake is far from clear. And it doesn't matter if the alcohol comes from beer, wine, or hard liquor—they all have comparable effects. One study found that increased folate intake offset the alcohol factor. Folate is a vitamin B nutrient that we get from dark-green leafy vegetables, peas and beans, nuts and seeds, eggs and liver, and fortified cereals in our diets, and from supplementary vitamins.

Sedentary lifestyle. A sedentary lifestyle may be another risk factor for breast cancer. Researchers have found that exercising one hour three times a week can reduce the risk by as much as 20%.

Oral contraceptives. Some studies have looked at whether the use of oral contraceptives increases breast cancer risk. Results show that risk is increased slightly during the time a woman takes birth control pills, but it returns to normal when she stops taking them. However, taking oral contraceptives for more than five years may increase the risk.

Hormone replacement therapy. Many women use hormone replacement therapy (HRT) during and after menopause to alleviate menopausal symptoms and reduce their risks of osteoporosis, heart disease, Alzheimer's disease, and other conditions related to aging. Hormone replacement regimens supply estrogen and usually progesterone, another female hormone. (While estrogen provides the benefits of this therapy, its use alone has been linked to high rates of uterine cancer in women who have not had a hysterectomy. Adding progesterone decreases that risk.) Because breast cancer is related to estrogen exposure, researchers have studied breast cancer rates in women taking HRT and documented slightly increased breast cancer risks in women on HRT for ten years or longer.

HOW IS IT DIAGNOSED?

Breast cancer is a disease that usually arrives without notable symptoms. The most common sign is a lump in the breast or under the arm, but many lumps are not cancerous, and many cancers are detected by mammogram before anything can be felt, even by an experienced health care provider. In less than 10% of cases are any symptoms painful. The American Cancer Society advises women to become familiar with their breasts through breast self-examination beginning at age 20, and to have a clinical breast examination by their health care provider at designated intervals—every three years beginning at age 20 and every year by age 40. In addition, women should consult their health care providers if they notice any of the following:

- Swelling in the breast or underarm area
- Lump in the breast or underarm area
- Skin irritation or dimpling of the breast or nipple
- Nipple pain
- Nipple retraction (turning inward)
- Redness or scaliness of the nipple or skin of the breast

- Discharge from the nipple (other than breast milk in a lactating woman)
- Any change in the contour of the breast

Remember, though, that any of these symptoms can indicate benign breast disease or another breast disorder. They are a sign of the need for professional consultation, but they do not necessarily mean cancer.

BREAST SELF-EXAMINATION

The American Cancer Society recommends that women begin a methodical monthly breast self-examination (BSE) at age 20. This takes only a few minutes and, quite literally, saves lives. The best time to do the exam is three days to a week after the end of the menstrual period, when breasts are their least tender and swollen. Women who no longer get periods can examine themselves on the same day each month.

Some women, particularly those at high risk for breast cancer, find it difficult to be conscientious and consistent about BSE. Who wants to look for what she doesn't want to find? It is important to overcome this psychological barrier, however, because BSE, when properly done (see Sidebar), has been proven to lead to earlier detection of malignancies and a reduced risk of death from breast cancer. And the sooner cancer is detected, the less treatment is needed for cure.

MORE ABOUT HRT...

Some scientists believe supplying postmenopausal estrogen increases the risk of breast cancer by 20 to 40%, and recent studies of combined therapy (estrogen and progesterone) have found that the progesterone further increases the breast cancer risk. Recent studies have also found that HRT does not provide as much protection against heart disease as was once thought. In deciding whether to take HRT, a woman must weigh many factors—her risks for osteoporosis, heart disease, and other diseases, and the severity of her menopausal symptoms—in addition to her risk for breast cancer. In many cases, the woman at high risk for breast cancer or who already has had breast cancer will find that these increased risks outweigh the potential benefits of HRT. This is an individual decision that a woman must make in consultation with her health care providers. There is no hard and fast rule to follow. Lifestyle changes and other medications can prevent osteoporosis and heart disease and help to manage menopausal symptoms.

BREAST SELF-EXAMINATION (BSE)

Women should examine each of their breasts lying on their back in bed or standing in the shower. Some women find that soap and water make it easier to move their fingers on the surface of the breast to probe what's within.

• Raise the arm on the side of the breast you are examining and place it behind your head. This spreads the tissue, making it easier to feel any abnormalities.

• Using the pads of the three middle fingers of the opposite hand (i.e., left hand on right breast), with soft, medium, then deep pressure and small circular motions, check the breast and surrounding area for lumps. You are also looking for any puckering, swelling, discharge, or change in size or shape.

• Move your fingers in either a circular, wedge, or linear (up and down, back and forth) pattern, feeling the tissue of the breast. Use the same pattern every time you do a BSE. Include the area above the breast, from armpit to collarbone, and below. Most women have what feels like a ridge in the lower curve of each breast. Get to know the feeling of your breasts, so you can recognize any changes. The key word is "change": you are looking for any change in your breasts from last month to this month.

• Now do a visual exam. Look at your breasts in a mirror. First with your arms over your head and then with your hands on your hips, look for dimpling of the skin, changes in the nipple, redness, change in the size or contour of your breast, or the presence of discharge.

• If anything seems abnormal about your self-exam, make an appointment to consult your health care provider about it.

CLINICAL BREAST EXAMINATION

Clinical breast examination is an examination of a woman's breasts by a health care provider: gynecologist, nurse practitioner, primary care physician, physician's assistant, or any trained medical professional. The health care professional will inspect the breasts visually, then palpate (feel) them in much the same way as in a BSE. Usually the clinical breast exam is done at the time of an annual gynecological exam. If a woman has questions about BSE, this is a good time to ask for some guidance and instruction.

The American Cancer Society recommends that women aged 20 to 39 have a clinical breast exam every three years and women 40 and older have the exam annually.

MAMMOGRAPHY

A mammogram is a specialized x-ray of the breast. Mammography has become the most commonly used method of medical imagery that leads directly to lowering mortality from disease. Mammograms and other methods of imaging the breast now account for at least 10% of all radiological examinations.

Mammography is used for two different purposes:

Screening mammography. This looks for breast disease in women who have no symptoms. The National Cancer Institute and the American Cancer Society both recommend that a woman get regular mammograms after the age of 40. There has been some dispute about this recommendation, and about how often to get mammograms, but most health care providers and health care institutions recommend beginning mammograms annually at age 40.

Diagnostic mammography. This allows a closer look at a breast problem or abnormality, including any abnormality found on a screening mammogram.

For either purpose, the basic technique of mammography is the same. The x-ray machine (which is specialized for this purpose and not used to x-ray any other part of the body) includes two compression paddles that flatten and spread the breast, which is positioned on a small platform on the machine. The compression is necessary to get the best view of the tissue of the breast and is the only part of the procedure that might be painful. Many women with

WHAT MAMOGRAMS FIND

A mammogram can turn up a number of different findings of abnormalities in breast tissue:

• **A solid mass.** Mammograms can detect a tumor as small as about a quarter of an inch. A mass can be benign (i.e., noncancerous), as in the case of a cyst, which is fluid-filled; or it may be malignant (i.e., cancerous).

• **Calcifications,** or tiny calcium deposits. Most calcifications are benign, but a type called microcalcifications, or clusters of tiny specks of calcium, can be an early sign of cancer.

• **Distortion** in the structure of the breast. This may indicate the presence of some disease process, even if there is no discernible mass.

sensitive breasts find this a rather unpleasant experience, but it only lasts a few seconds. Breasts are usually most tender the week before and during a menstrual period, so a mammogram should not be scheduled for that time. Taking an over-the-counter pain reliever such as Advil an hour before a mammogram can help reduce this discomfort.

Mammography has evolved in the past thirty years so that only very low levels of radiation—about 0.1 to 0.2 rad dose per x-ray—are necessary to get the pictures. The risk of this dose causing cancer is considered insignificant. Yearly

MAMMOGRAMS: HOW OFTEN ... AND FOR WHOM?

In recent years, there has been some debate about when a woman should begin getting mammograms. Women with a family history or other increased risk factors that concern them should begin getting mammograms in their 30s, or even earlier if that is the family history. All women should have a "baseline" mammogram between the ages of 35 and 40. The radiologist will look for abnormalities on the film, but also will note any changes in the appearance of the breast tissue between the "baseline" mammogram and the current one. But the breast tissue is dense in younger women, making it difficult to get useful pictures. The greatest benefits of regular mammography are for women over 50, whose breast tissue is easier to view and who are more likely to get breast cancer. Data from large population studies indicate that when women between 50 and 69 receive regular mammograms, breast cancer deaths are reduced by about 30%. For women in their 40s, it is little more than half that effective, with 17% fewer deaths.

Still, breast cancer is the leading cause of death for women in their 40s in the United States. Nearly 20% of breast cancer cases are in women under 50, and 13% of deaths are women in their 40s. And the percentages and risk/benefit ratios don't seem very important if you or a loved one is a woman who in her 40s had her life extended by detecting a malignancy in early stages. Or, more tragically, died young because a malignancy was not detected. For years, there was debate about the benefits of screening women in their 40s. *The National Cancer Institute (a division of the National Institutes of Health) recently reaffirmed their recommendation that women aged 40 or older get screening mammograms every one to two years. The American Cancer Society recommends annual mammograms for women over 40.*

mammograms from age 40 to age 90 would expose a woman to a lifetime total of 10 rads, which is about the amount of radiation a person receives from riding in a car for 300 miles. This is compared with the several thousand rads that are administered when radiation is used as a treatment for cancer.

The only advance preparation necessary for a mammogram is not to apply underarm deodorant, powder, or lotions on the day of the procedure because they can affect the pictures. It's more convenient to wear a shirt or blouse, rather than a dress, because women undergoing mammograms are asked to undress from the waist up. The procedure is done by a radiology technologist, almost always a woman. Pictures will be taken with the paddles in both horizontal and vertical positions to get a variety of views. The technologist will look at the pictures immediately and may want to take additional shots if the images are not clear enough. But the technologist will not discuss whether the mammogram shows a possibility of cancer. That is done by either the woman's referring doctor or a radiologist associated with the mammography facility. Some facilities provide immediate consultation; at others, the woman undergoing the procedure will return home not knowing the results of her mammogram. Mammography facilities are regulated by the Food and Drug Administration. Do not get a mammogram at a facility that is not FDA-certified and accredited by the American College of Radiology. The FDA requires that women be notified of their results in writing within thirty days. If there is a suspicious spot on the mammogram or anything that requires follow-up, the patient should be notified within five days.

For many women, it's difficult to avoid feelings of anxiety associated with getting a mammogram. It might be helpful to keep this reassuring statistic in mind: Only one or two screening mammograms of every thousand (i.e., 0.1 to 0.2%) lead to a diagnosis of cancer. Even when a mammogram indicates the necessity for a biopsy (see below), 80% of biopsies do not subsequently find malignancies.

SCINTIMAMMOGRAPHY

Scintimammography is a refinement of mammography that uses nuclear medicine to better define a mass in the breast. A tiny amount of radioactive material (called technetium 99m Sestamibi), which collects in tumor tissue, is injected intravenously and then viewed with a special nuclear medicine camera. Radiologists are still working out the best uses for scintimammography, but it is likely this will be a valuable tool for evaluating women whose mammograms are difficult to interpret.

DIGITAL MAMMOGRAPHY

The latest advance in mammography is the digital mammogram, which produces digital images rather than the standard analog photographic image. The FDA approved the first digital mammography system in January 2000. Although a digital system does not seem to have any advantage in finding malignancies, it allows for easier storage and retrieval of images, remote evaluation by distant specialists, and a larger range to examine all areas of the breast despite varying densities. The conventional mammogram sometimes needs additional exposures at different settings to assess areas of different density in the breast.

A mammogram is used to rule out cancer, although, like most tests, it is not 100% accurate. By itself, though, it cannot definitely diagnose cancer. Other diagnostic tests are available for that purpose.

BREAST ULTRASOUND

An ultrasound of the breast is a painless test that uses high-frequency sound waves to determine the nature of a lump and to differentiate a cyst from a solid mass. It is often used to supplement diagnostic mammography at the same office visit. The radiologist or technician smears a cool conducting gel on the breast and moves a wand over the area. The wand transmits the sound waves to a computer that translates them to an image on a computer screen. Ultrasound does not pick up calcifications, which is one of the reasons it is not used for screening purposes.

DUCTOGRAM

To determine the cause of a nipple discharge, a dye is injected into a plastic tube that has been inserted into the duct opening in the nipple. When this is x-rayed, it will show the shape of the duct and whether there is a mass or blockage within it.

MAGNETIC RESONANCE IMAGING (MRI)

Magnetic fields and radio waves produce images for this procedure, which is widely used for other parts of the body. MRI highlights the soft tissues of the body, and is used with the intravenous injection of a special dye, which highlights abnormalities. The use of MRI for screening and diagnosis of breast cancer is still mostly experimental, but a number of studies have shown results equal to or better than mammograms. Best results come from an MRI machine specially designed to look at the breast, but these are usually not found except in large medical centers conducting research trials. Expense is a major barrier to more widespread use of this technique. MRI also does not detect calcifications. But it can ascertain valuable cancer markers such as blood flow to a tumor and the size and appearance of the mass. Some researchers think the MRI can play a important role in evaluating women at high risk for breast cancer. The role of the MRI in diagnosing breast cancer will be further defined in coming years as additional studies are completed.

BIOPSY

A biopsy removes tissue from inside the breast so that it can be examined under a microscope to determine the exact nature of the cells. There are several different types of biopsies, ranging from less to more invasive.

Fine-needle aspiration biopsy. Fine-needle aspiration biopsy uses a very thin, hollow needle (about the size of a needle used in a vaccination shot) to extract a small amount of fluid and/or tiny pieces of tissue from the breast for analysis. Only a local anesthetic is needed. Fine-needle aspiration biopsy can also be used to drain fluid from a noncancerous cyst. The disadvantage of this method is that it might not remove sufficient tissue to include a malignant sample, leading to a false-negative diagnosis. If the lab report is negative and the health care provider is still suspicious about a specific lump or area on the mammogram, a larger biopsy may be taken.

Core needle biopsy. Here a little larger needle (about the size of a needle used to draw a blood donation) is used to remove a larger cylinder of tissue. It is also done in a doctor's office, with local anesthetic. Usually about three to five core samples of tissue are removed during the procedure, each about 1/16 of an inch in diameter and half an inch long. A woman may feel a little sore for a couple of days after undergoing a core biopsy.

Surgical (excisional) biopsy. As the name implies, surgical biopsy is a larger incision than that needed for a needle biopsy. It is used to remove a larger mass or area containing calcifications, which is surgically removed with a margin of healthy-looking breast tissue around it. This procedure is usually done by a surgeon in an outpatient center with local anesthesia, and sometimes intravenous sedation is given. Only 3 to 5% of biopsies today need to be done as an open surgical biopsy; most others can be performed using minimally invasive techniques that eliminate the need for an incision.

WHAT SHOULD YOU EXPECT?

Many statistics have been generated about the likelihood of survival from breast cancer, according to the type of cancer, the stage when diagnosed, and several other factors. But statistics paint a broad picture that can't necessarily be applied at the personal level. Numbers can give an idea of the impact of a disease on a population, but at the individual level, each case follows its own course and few outcomes can be definitively predicted. We have all heard stories of people with advanced cancer who responded to treatment, or improved for unknown reasons, and went on to live many years beyond what had been predicted. And there is the other side, also, people who do not do as well as the statistics predict. So remember that statistics can give important context to thinking about this disease, but they do not foretell the future.

That said, it is encouraging to see that survival statistics for breast cancer continue to improve. Death rates continue to decline. Fewer than one-third of women diagnosed with breast cancer will die of the disease. With every technological advance and new insight into treatment, the prognosis brightens. Looking at all women who get breast cancer, the American Cancer Society presents the following survival statistics:

- 85% of women live five years after diagnosis
- 71% of women live ten years after diagnosis
- 57% of women live fifteen years after diagnosis
- 52% of women live twenty years after diagnosis

Cancer stage. The factors that most predict outcome and survival for women with breast cancer are the stage of the disease when diagnosed (see the sidebar on Stages on p. 35), size of the tumor, hormone receptor status of the tumor, and other prognostic factors, such as the her2/neu receptor (see below). The lower the stage, the better the prognosis, but there are exceptions. An early stage does not guarantee a cancer-free outcome. Twenty-five to 30 percent of women with lymph nodes negative for cancer (stage 0 or I) will have a recurrence of the disease at some point in their lives. Survival rates improve for women who undergo chemotherapy or take hormonal therapy.

According to stage, the five-year survival rates for breast cancer are:

- Stage 0 to I: 96%. (In the 1940s, nearly 30% of women diagnosed with localized breast cancer were dead in five years.)
- Stage II to III: 77%. For stage II patients with cancer extending to the axillary (armpit) lymph nodes, the most important predictive variable is the number of nodes involved—the more that are involved, the lower the survival rates.
- Stage IV: 21%. Nearly four of five women diagnosed with metastasized breast cancer will die of the disease within five years.

Age. Age at onset is another factor that influences the course of breast cancer. Younger women have lower survival rates, although the differences are not dramatic. Women diagnosed when they are 45 or younger have an 81% chance of surviving five years, whereas women older than 65 have an 86% chance. For women between 45 and 65, the rate is 85%. Younger women are more likely to have more aggressive cancers, and they are also more likely to have cancers that are unresponsive to hormone therapy. Some researchers believe that these characteristics of breast cancer in younger women point to a need for more aggressive treatment for these patients (for example, chemotherapy as well as surgery) even when diagnosed at an early stage.

Other genetic, cellular, and biological factors determined in laboratory tests also may be related to outcome, but it will take further studies to be able to more reliably predict outcomes. As we learn more about the biological and genetic activities of tumors, we can apply that knowledge to treatment decisions.

HOW IS IT TREATED?

The treatment options for breast cancer fall into several categories:

- Surgery (with or without reconstruction)

- Radiation
- Chemotherapy
- Hormone treatment
- Immunotherapy

A woman's treatment decisions will be guided by her health care provider and her own personal preferences. All of the factors discussed in the previous section will figure into the therapy she selects. The goals of treatment are to get rid of the cancer and prevent it from returning. But treatments also have risks, and knowledge about these is another factor in treatment decisions. Many women decide upon a combination of two or more types of treatment to increase their odds of cancer-free survival. Surgery and radiation are considered local treatments, confined to the site of the cancer; chemotherapy, hormonal treatment, and immunotherapy are called systemic treatments, and are given orally or through injection into the bloodstream to attack cancer cells that may have gotten out of the breast.

SURGERY

There are two types of surgery to remove cancers of the breast: mastectomy, or removal of the entire breast; and lumpectomy, which removes only the tumor and surrounding tissue. Axillary node dissection (see below) usually accompanies either procedure. In the case of lumpectomy, a second incision under the arm is necessary to remove the lymph nodes. In choosing a surgeon and facility where the surgery will be performed, look for experience. Studies show that the more procedures done by a surgeon and the higher the volume of these procedures at a medical center, the better the outcomes and survival rates.

Lumpectomy

About 70% of women diagnosed with breast cancer are candidates for lumpectomy or breast-conserving surgery and need not lose their breast. About half of all breast cancer patients who have surgery now choose breast-conserving therapy. Most tumors smaller than 2 centimeters are candidates for lumpectomy; this accounts for 80% of breast cancer diagnoses. Lumpectomy or partial or segmental mastectomy is also known as breast-conserving surgery. Often, these procedures can be performed with only local anesthetic and do not require overnight hospitalization.

Although there may be a change in the shape of a woman's breast after lumpectomy, this type of surgery spares a woman the emotional trauma of losing a breast, preserves sensation in the skin and nipple, and usually gives a very good cosmetic result. Years of studies have found that in patients with stages I and II invasive breast cancer, treatment with lumpectomy and follow-up radiation or mastectomy results in equal rates of metastases outside the breast and equal survival rates. However, lumpectomy patients do have an increased risk of cancer recurrence in the treated breast—the recurrence is 1% per year, which means that in ten years, 10% of women who have breast-conserving surgery will develop another tumor in the same breast. Early detection of these recurrences keeps them from affecting long-term survival, but women who have lumpectomies may eventually need mastectomy. These lifetime recurrence rates are one reason a younger women might choose mastectomy over lumpectomy.

In recent years, a growing number of patients have been deemed candidates for lumpectomy with the use of chemotherapy before surgery to shrink their tumor to a size that will allow removing the tumor and preserving the breast. This is called neoadjuvant chemotherapy. However, there are a number of situations in which lumpectomy is not recommended:

- More than one tumor in the breast.
- Tumor is so large or breast is so small that the results would not be cosmetically acceptable.
- Tumor extends beyond the margins of the original surgery.
- The woman has had radiation to the affected breast or chest area.
- The woman is unwilling or unable (usually because of distance from the facility) to have subsequent radiation therapy. Radiation is usually given five days a week for six to eight weeks after surgery.
- The woman has a connective tissue disease that makes her particularly sensitive to side effects of radiation.

In addition, some women may opt for mastectomy because they feel a greater comfort level and think they have a better chance of beating their cancer by having the entire breast removed.

BREAST CANCER AND PREGNANCY

While breast cancer is primarily a cancer of older women, the incidence is increasing in women of childbearing age. Two major questions must be answered when considering breast cancer and pregnancy:

• What is the effect of treatment on a woman diagnosed during pregnancy?

• What is the advisability of becoming pregnant for a woman who has been treated for breast cancer?

Diagnosis during pregnancy

About 2% of breast cancers are diagnosed in women who are pregnant. There is no evidence that terminating a pregnancy will lead to a better outcome from cancer. However, some women may want to end their pregnancies so they have more treatment options. Special care during pregnancy is necessary to ensure maximum benefits and least risk for both mother and fetus.

Because the breasts of pregnant women are tender and engorged, a lump is not as apparent, and the tendency is for pregnant women to get diagnosed at a later stage than nonpregnant women. There is very little data on breast cancer diagnosis and treatment during pregnancy, so each woman and fetus must be closely monitored. For diagnosis, ultrasound and biopsy with local anesthetic are usually safe and effective for pregnant women. Physicians are cautious about using mammograms during pregnancy; if done, the fetus is shielded. Nuclear scans should be avoided, so there is no fetal exposure to radiation.

Little is known about the effect of breast surgery on pregnancy. A little more is known about chemotherapy, but there have been few long-term follow-up studies of children born to mothers treated for breast cancer. Different drugs appear to have different effects and risks to the fetus. Chemotherapy is most likely to

Mastectomy

Mastectomy—surgical removal of the breast—is the oldest procedure to treat breast cancer and has evolved through the years to involve less disfigurement and discomfort than it once did for women. Many medical centers now do mastectomies on an outpatient basis and don't require overnight hospitalization for the procedure. In these cases (called ambulatory surgery), a combination of local and "twilight" anesthesia (meaning the patient is sedated but not under heavy seda-

cause birth defects in a fetus, or even fetal death, when given in the first trimester of pregnancy. Second- and third-trimester exposure to chemotherapy drugs may affect the baby's growth and development, especially in the brain. Methotrexate, a chemotherapy drug classified as an antimetabolite, should be avoided during pregnancy since it inhibits cell reproduction, causing birth defects. Radiation may also cause damage to the fetus.

Women receiving chemotherapy should not breastfeed because these drugs can be excreted into breast milk. Side effects such as depressed immune function from chemotherapy drugs have been seen in breastfeeding infants.

Becoming pregnant after breast cancer treatment

Younger women with a history of breast cancer may fear becoming pregnant, afraid that the elevated hormones of pregnancy will increase the risk of cancer recurrence. While there have only been a few studies on this, there appears to be no increased risk of getting cancer again if you get pregnant. Most oncologists advise women to wait two years after cancer diagnosis and treatment before becoming pregnant; in most young women, if there is breast cancer recurrence, it will be in the first two years.

Another concern for younger women is their ability to become pregnant, since treatment for breast cancer can affect the ability to conceive. Younger women who have had short-term courses of chemotherapy probably will not have difficulty conceiving. However, if a woman has been treated with high-dose chemotherapy and a bone marrow transplant, she probably will not be able to become pregnant, because those treatments cause ovulation to cease, or sterility. If a woman is nearing menopause, chemotherapy, particularly if it is long-term, will probably stop ovulation.

tion) is often used, and the patient is able to walk around less than an hour after the completion of surgery.

A mastectomy without reconstruction generally takes one to two hours in the operating room. The mastectomy operation may also include reconstruction of the breast; this is a longer procedure, depending on the type of reconstruction, and a hospitalization of several days is usually necessary. (See Breast Reconstruction sidebar on p. 56.)

There are four different versions of the mastectomy:

Total simple mastectomy. Removes entire breast, but no lymph nodes or muscle.

Modified radical mastectomy or Patey mastectomy. Removes the entire breast and some axillary lymph nodes. This is the procedure used most often and is sometimes called "total mastectomy with axillary sampling."

Halstead radical mastectomy. Removes the entire breast, axillary lymph nodes, and chest wall muscles under the breast. Once standard procedure, this is rarely used today, as the modified radical mastectomy has proved to be equally effective and much less disfiguring

Skin-sparing mastectomy. The newest variation of mastectomy. This procedure, in which breast tissue is extracted through a circular incision around the nipple, allows much of a woman's own skin to encase the material of reconstruction, which is done at the same time as mastectomy when this technique is used. Lymph nodes are removed through a second incision. Skin-sparing mastectomy is considered appropriate if there is an adequate cancer-free margin between the tumor removed and the tissue that remains. Several studies have shown that there is no higher recurrence rate when a skin-sparing procedure is used, but it may not be available at all medical centers.

Axillary lymph node dissection

Except in cases of ductal carcinoma in situ, when the tumor is confined to a small area, some underarm lymph nodes are almost always removed as part of either mastectomy or breast-conserving therapy. This can be done through the mastectomy incision for conventional mastectomies; a separate incision is needed in breast-conserving therapy or skin-saving mastectomy. A wedge of fat containing the nodes is removed and examined in the laboratory for evidence of whether the cancer has spread or not. Usually ten to fifteen nodes are removed. The information yielded by the lymph nodes will guide the staging of the cancer and decisions about postsurgery treatment.

Lymphedema

Surgery on the lymphatic system carries the small risk of lymphedema, a disruption of the lymph drainage process which can leave—in the case of axillary nodes—a woman's hand or arm fluid-filled and swollen, an uncomfortable or painful condition that can be irreversible. Nationally, the incidence rate is about 7 to 10% after breast surgery, but the true rate might be higher because not all hospitals track the long-term occurrence of lymphedema.

Most women resume a normal lifestyle after axillary dissection with just heightened awareness of additional changes to the affected arm. But lymphedema cannot be predicted and can occur days, months, or even years after surgery. It may be associated with an injury such as a cut or insect bite that would stimulate the lymph system to send its infection-fighting fluid to the site.Some precautions may prevent lymphedema and the American Cancer Society advises:

- Avoid having blood drawn or injections on the arm on the side of the surgery.
- Avoid getting blood pressure taken on that side.
- Pay close attention to the arm and be alert to any feelings of tightness or swelling. If detected early, serious lymphedema can often be prevented with a specialized type of massage.
- Wear gloves while gardening or doing other activities that could break the skin.

It has been theorized that limiting the removal of lymph nodes will lessen the risk of lymphedema. The first lymph node into which a tumor drains is called the sentinel node. The sentinel node can be identified by injecting a radioactive tracer into the tumor. This procedure is not available everywhere; it can be found at some major medical centers, and as part of treatment studies.

A negative sentinel node has been found to be an accurate predictor that all nodes will be negative; in the case of a positive sentinel node, more nodes are usually removed to determine the extent of spread. However, it has not been conclusively established that the less invasive dissection required for sentinel lymph node biopsy actually results in fewer cases of lymphedema. More research is necessary before that answer will be known.

RADIATION

Radiation, also called radiotherapy, is commonly used to treat cancers in the breast, particularly after lumpectomy. Treatment with strong, targeted particle

OTHER RISKS AND SIDE EFFECTS OF SURGERY

There are risks from anesthesia for any surgery, including allergic reaction and, in rare cases, death. Other risks of breast surgery include infection of the incision, accumulation of blood in the incision (hematoma), and accumulation of clear fluid—serum—in the incision (seroma). The risks of hematoma and seroma are very low and usually easy to reverse. Many women also experience numbness in the underarm and upper arm area; this may be permanent.

beams has long been known to kill cancerous tumors and is part of the therapy for nearly half of all cancer patients. Radiation can be used to shrink a tumor before surgery, to remove cancer cells after surgery, and to shrink tumors to relieve pain at sites of metastases. Use of radiation translates to a twofold to fourfold reduction of breast cancer recurring locally. And today's technologically advanced techniques allow more tightly focused rays that hit the tumor but spare surrounding healthy tissue. Sometimes markers are placed at the time of biopsy to provide a precise target for the radiation.

In some cases, particularly when lymph nodes are positive, a woman's doctor will recommend radiation following a mastectomy. Radiation is always recommended after breast-conserving surgery, to begin as soon as the incision is healed, usually by twelve weeks after surgery. If a woman is also going to get chemotherapy, she should talk to her health care providers, including the radiation oncologist, about the most beneficial sequence of the treatments. Usually the formula is chemotherapy before radiation, with the underlying philosophy: "Save your life before you save your breast."

Types of radiation. There are two types of radiation used today. External beam, the most common to treat breast cancer, is focused from a machine outside the body. External beam radiation is painless; it is usually administered five days a week, for a period of about six to eight weeks. The other type is called brachytherapy, or internal radiation. For this procedure, radioactive materials are surgically placed directly into the breast, on the tumor or next to its site. Brachytherapy for breast cancer is currently considered experimental but has the promise to shorten the period of treatment and lessen side effects.

Side effects. Fatigue is the most common side effect from radiation. It is usually most noticeable during the last two weeks of therapy, because radiation has a cumulative effect. Women undergoing radiation therapy may also notice sunburn-type changes on their skin where the ray entered, and some swelling and heaviness in the breast. Sometimes the breast becomes smaller and firmer after radiation. Radiation is also associated with an increased rate of lymphedema in women who have had axillary node dissection.

CHEMOTHERAPY

Chemotherapy is body-wide treatment with drugs to fight cancer. It is designed to kill any cancer cells that remain in the breast or have escaped into the body, whether they can be detected or not. It is either given through intravenous injection or taken orally. For cancers that have spread by the time of diagnosis, chemotherapy may be the primary treatment. For breast cancers found earlier, chemotherapy is a supplemental or "adjuvant" treatment after surgery. Studies have found that adjuvant chemotherapy improves survival in most cases.

Chemotherapy is also being used before surgery, often to shrink a tumor enough so that it can be safely removed by lumpectomy rather than mastectomy. This is called neoadjuvant chemotherapy. Neoadjuvant chemotherapy also gives the oncologist to chance to see how the tumor reacts to anticancer drugs. One disadvantage with neoadjuvant chemotherapy, however, is that the pathologist is not able to accurately stage the disease. Since the aim of chemotherapy is to shrink the diameter of the tumor, the true stage of the disease originally may never be known.

Chemotherapy is usually given in cycles, and each treatment is followed by a rest period to recover from side effects. For example, the patient may get a several-hour chemotherapy infusion, and then another three weeks later. The drugs used for chemotherapy are toxic to cancer cells, but they are also toxic to normal cells, and this results in lowered white blood cell counts and decreased resistance to infection in people getting chemotherapy. The body's blood counts need a chance to recover before the patient receives another dose. Adjuvant chemotherapy usually lasts from three to six months, depending on what drugs are used. Chemotherapy used as the primary treatment for advanced breast cancer may continue for much longer.

Usually a combination of drugs is used. The choice depends on stage of the cancer and other individual factors. Patients should discuss with their health care provider which regimen is best for them, and why, and what the side effects are for each drug to be used. Some regimens are more popular in certain areas of the

continued on p. 58

BREAST RECONSTRUCTION

About half of women who have a mastectomy also have breast reconstruction—the building of an artificial breast using either a synthetic implant or a woman's own body tissue. Women who do not choose reconstruction usually wear an external breast form, or prosthesis, which fits into a special bra or attaches directly to the chest using an adhesive. Women who will use a prosthesis should seek out an experienced professional for fitting. The nurses or social worker at the breast center where you had your surgery can provide you with a recommended list of mastectomy supply shops with certified fitters.

Most women who have mastectomies are eligible for reconstruction. The number of women choosing reconstruction is increasing. Surgical reconstruction can be done at the time of mastectomy, or some time later, after healing from mastectomy is complete. When to have reconstruction depends on the type and stage of the tumor, the need for radiation or chemotherapy, and a woman's personal preference. Some women may feel they need more time to make the decision about reconstruction and postpone it until after mastectomy, when they know more about their cancer and prognosis. About 39% of reconstructions are done with the mastectomy.

The advantages of having simultaneous mastectomy and reconstruction are the need for only one surgery and the elimination of the feeling of the loss that can come with any amputation. However, because the reconstructed breast lacks sensation and may be different in appearance, a woman may still experience some degree of mourning of the loss of her natural breast. A breast is a strong part of any woman's identity and femininity, and learning to live without one, especially along with the burden of a cancer diagnosis, can extract a heavy emotional toll. Compounding the emotional issues is the fact that this is happening to a part of the body that is generally not discussed, except with embarrassment or sexual innuendo. In generations past, the high mortality for women with breast cancer was—in part—a reflection of the secrecy that surrounded this body part.

If reconstruction is performed at the same time as mastectomy, a general anesthetic will be used and a plastic surgeon will take over from the breast surgeon while the patient is still under anesthesia. An implant reconstruction takes about an hour. Reconstruction with the patient's own tissue—called a flap—is a much more complicated procedure and can take up to eight hours.

After the reconstruction is healed, if a woman wishes, she can complete the procedure with a nipple reconstruction. The nipple is sculpted, usually with skin grafts from the thigh, and later tattooed to match the opposite breast. The final result can be very realistic looking, but it will not, of course, have the sensation of a natural nipple.

Reconstruction with breast implants

Two types of synthetic material are used for implants: silicone gel or saline. There has been a great deal of publicity in recent years about the dangers of silicone, although scientific investigation has not definitively associated it with any disease. But some health care professionals think that there have been too many reports of problems for there not to be an association, even though the link has not yet been found. Some medical centers offer silicone implants, others do not.

The implant is usually placed under a layer of the pectoral muscle. If it is small, the skin's natural stretchability can handle it. For larger implants, though, a temporary expander is used, a silicone balloon with a valve that will gradually expand the skin and muscle. This is done with periodic injections of saline into the balloon to stretch the skin and muscle over the next three to six months, when the permanent implant can replace the expander. The injections are done in the surgeon's office and are not painful.

Flap reconstruction

Increasingly, patients choosing reconstruction are selecting a flap, which usually looks more natural and does not place foreign material in the body. In the traditional abdominal or TRAM (transverse rectus abdominus myocutaneous) flap, skin, fat, and a piece abdominal muscle are tunneled through the abdomen to form a breast, with an intact blood supply to the area where the tissue graft was obtained. In the free TRAM, the skin, fat, and muscle are detached completely and grafted to the chest area, and blood vessels are attached through microvascular surgery, in which the surgeon uses a microscope to reconnect tiny arteries and veins. Studies show comparable complication rates for the two procedures.

In another procedure, the LAT flap, the large, flat latissimus dorsi muscle from the back is used. Except for smaller breasts, an implant is often necessary with a LAT flap, since there is only a small amount of fat from the back to be transplanted. The newest type of flap is a gluteal flap, which uses tissue from the buttocks to make a breast.

In choosing a procedure, one of the most important things to consider is the experience of

continued on p. 58

BREAST RECONSTRUCTION (CONTINUED)

the plastic surgeon. If the surgeon is not comfortable performing the procedure the patient prefers, the patient has the option of reconsidering that particular surgery or seeking a surgeon who is experienced in this procedure.

Risks and complications

Both implants and flaps have risks and potential complications. First, any surgery has possible complications. Because the flap operations are long procedures, taking as long as eight hours to perform, these surgical risks may be magnified. The most common specific complication of implants is capsular contracture, which occurs when the scar tissue (or capsule) around the implant begins to contract, squeezing the implant. This may require removal or scoring of the scar tissue, to release the tightness, or the removal or replacement of the implant. Much more rarely, implants develop infections and may need to be removed until the infection heals. On

rare occasions, implants may also push out through the incision.

One of the possible problems with a TRAM flap is that sometimes the blood supply to the grafted tissue is not adequate and the tissue dies, generally within the first thirty-six hours while the patient is still in the hospital, and must be removed. Also, the abdominal tissue is removed through a hip-to-hip incision, and for many patients this provides the added benefit of a "tummy tuck." But because a piece of muscle is removed, many women experience abdominal weakness, and sometimes abdominal bulging or hernia. Women who are poorer candidates for flap surgeries are smokers, women who have a history of cardiac disease, who have diabetes that is difficult to control, or who have had several previous abdominal surgeries that may influence the blood vessels.

country than others. The different combinations are given for different lengths of time, and that may influence the patient's decision about which drugs to use.

The drug names are tongue-twisters and the regimens are usually referred to by initials. Following are the most commonly used drugs against breast cancer, and the combinations in which they are used.

- Cyclophosphamide (cytoxan), methotrexate, 5-fluorouracil (5-FU), called CMF

- Cyclophosphamide (cytoxan), doxorubicin (Adriamycin), 5-fluorouracil (5-FU), called CAF
- 5-fluorouracil, Adriamycin or epirubicin, cyclophosphamide, called FAC or FEC
- Adriamycin, cyclophosphamide, called AC
- AC followed by paclitaxel (Taxol) or docetaxel (Taxotere), called AC/T

Different drugs and regimens have various actions, but in reviewing the results of many studies of its effect, it is clear that adjuvant chemotherapy extends lives and prevents recurrence in women with breast cancer.

Side effects. When chemotherapy was first used to fight cancer, decades ago, the side effects of the drugs were so severe that patients were often hospitalized for the treatments. People are still sometimes hospitalized for chemotherapy, but the majority now get their treatments at outpatient clinics or doctor's offices and then resume their normal lives, often going to work the day of or day after a treatment.

Chemotherapy drugs attack the fast-growing cells in the body—which includes any cancer cells it can find. But it also includes hair follicles, blood cells, and the mucousy lining of the stomach or mouth. This is the reason for the wallop of unpleasant or even disabling side effects associated with chemotherapy. But now there is a whole new generation of drugs to fight the side effects. Each chemotherapy drug has its own side effects. They include low blood counts, nausea and vomiting, mouth sores, numbness in fingers and toes, and menstrual changes such as premature menopause. Some drugs also cause heart problems in the long-term, so doctors will keep track of the cumulative doses of doxorubicin, a toxic drug to the heart, that a patient receives. Chemotherapy can even cause another cancer to develop. The low red blood cell counts cause fatigue, and the low white cell counts increase chances of infection. In many regimens, an antibiotic is given preventively during the time of the chemotherapy cycle when white blood cells are at their lowest level, to prevent infection. A number of different drugs are used to prevent and treat nausea and vomiting, some administered intravenously or by mouth along with the chemotherapy.

The drugs to alleviate chemotherapy side effects are largely effective and chemotherapy is not the sentence of misery it once was. But these are potent drugs and sometimes have side effects of their own. Patients are advised to talk to their health care providers (doctors, pharmacists, and nurses) about the potential side effects of any drugs they may be taking, alert themselves to the possibilities, and report any problems they might have.

One side effect that cannot be countered is alopecia, or hair loss. Almost everyone taking Adriamycin loses her hair, and other drugs also attack the quick-growing hair follicles. This can be emotionally troubling to many women, especially if they are also coping with the loss of a breast. Attractive, realistic-looking wigs are now relatively inexpensive. Oncologists can prescribe a "scalp prosthesis," and in some states, insurance companies are required to cover up to $350 for a wig purchased under these circumstances. And the hair loss is only temporary. A few months after the end of chemotherapy, new hair begins growing back, and for many women it represents the new lease on life that surviving cancer gives you.

High-dose chemotherapy and bone marrow or stem cell transplantation

With the theory that higher doses of chemotherapy will have a greater effect against cancer cells, clinical researchers have been studying whether doses two to twenty times higher than standard chemotherapy can knock out widely spread advanced cancers.

High-dose chemotherapy also wipes out the recipient's bone marrow, killing the stem cells, which produce blood, and making patient extremely susceptible to potentially lethal infections. Therefore a process was created to remove bone marrow or stem cells from patients before the high doses; treat the patients in isolation, without exposure to infectious diseases; and then reintroduce the patient's own bone marrow or stem cells—called an autologous transplant—to stimulate the body's ability to again produce blood cells.

This is an extreme treatment used for extreme cases: women who have advanced breast cancer spread to distant sites in the body, cancer that has not responded to more conventional chemotherapy doses, or a large number of positive lymph nodes, which could indicate that the cancer may have spread microscopically. However, the consensus at this point is that the treatment is no better than standard chemotherapy in most patients and should be approached cautiously. This is not the "magic bullet" some hopeful researchers once thought it was. Study results show, at best, modest increases in survival from the high-dose treatment. Some studies show no survival benefits at all from what is a very intense and difficult treatment. Studies continue on the success of high-dose chemotherapy with autologous bone marrow transplant or stem cell replacement, but it will be years before the role of this treatment for breast cancer is clearly defined. The risk of complications is higher with this type of treatment and therefore patients must remain hospitalized an average of four weeks during treatment.

HORMONAL TREATMENT

We now know that estrogen, a hormone produced by the ovaries, plays a role in the growth of many breast cancers. With this knowledge, therapies have been developed to attack the disease on this level. Data collected over the years shows that hormonal treatments play a very useful role, not only in treating breast cancer, but also in preventing it. (See Prevention, below.) As you might expect, the hormone therapies are effective against cancers with receptors that are hormone-positive, but not against hormone-negative cancers.

Historically, the first hormonal treatment against breast cancer was removal of the source of the hormone, the ovaries. Today this can be done surgically or by radiation, and has been shown to be a beneficial treatment for pre-menopausal women, with the most benefits seen for the youngest women. Much more common, though, is treatment with tamoxifen (Nolvadex), an antiestrogen drug that binds to cells' estrogen receptors, thus keeping estrogen from getting into the cells.

Tamoxifen, a selective estrogen receptor modulator or SERM, is taken in pill form, usually for five years. It has been used for more than 25 years and studies have shown that it fights breast cancer in a number of ways. It reduces recurrence rates of invasive breast cancer, causes tumors to shrink in advanced stages, and prevents breast cancer in high-risk women. It is often prescribed for women who had cancer in one breast, and has been shown to prevent cancer in the other. In one large study, women taking tamoxifen who had previously had breast cancer had a 50% reduction in risk of cancer in the other breast.

Hormonal treatment is gentler than chemotherapy's assault on the body, but there are a number of potential negative side effects from tamoxifen. Many women find it intensifies the symptoms of menopause, particularly hot flashes. It is also associated with weight gain, mood swings, blood clots, and cataracts. Most seriously, it is linked to twofold to sevenfold increases in rate of cancer of the

MORE ON HORMONE THERAPIES...

As scientists learn more about the intricate biochemistry of hormone receptors, they are working to design other hormonal agents that might be more effective with fewer side effects. Among the drugs that are being tested:

• Toremifene (Fareston) is an antiestrogen drug similar to tamoxifen, but it has less associations in endometrial cancer and may be useful for women who do not respond to tamoxifen.

• Anastrozole (Arimidex) uses a different mechanism, blocking an enzyme needed for estrogen production. One of several aromatase inhibitors that are being tested, anastrozole may have a role treating metastasized breast cancer, or in a regimen with other front-line drugs, or for prevention. Common side effects include nausea and hot flashes.

• Megestrol (Megace) acetate is a synthetic hormone modeled after progesterone. It is used to treat cancers that do not respond to tamoxifen, or for cancers that recur after treatment with tamoxifen. Common side effects include weight gain, slight hair loss, nausea, dry skin, and cessation of menstrual periods.

endometrium, the lining of the uterus. Women taking tamoxifen should be alert to any unusual vaginal bleeding, which is an early sign of endometrial cancer.

IMMUNOTHERAPY

Immunotherapy uses the body's own immune system to fight cancer. An example of this is the formulation of a drug called a monoclonal antibody, which attacks a specific target. Human epithelial growth factor receptor 2, called HER2/neu, is a growth-promoting protein, which is overly abundant in about one-third of breast cancers. Cancers with an excess of HER2/neu are apt to be very aggressive. A drug called trastuzumab (Herceptin) was formulated that blocks the HER2/neu receptor and also interacts with the immune system to kill cancer cells.

Herceptin was approved for use by the FDA in September 1998, a "fast-track" drug given priority attention because it did well in testing and offered hope for women who were dying of advanced stage breast cancer. It is given in weekly intravenous infusions, which take about a half-hour. Investigators are now looking at how Herceptin works with other drugs, and early data show that it is even more effective when used in combination with chemotherapy drugs such as paclitaxel (Taxol) and docetaxel (Taxotere). The side effects are much milder than chemotherapy. However, there have been some signs that it is toxic to the heart, so oncologists are cautious in prescribing Herceptin along with Adriamycin, which is also toxic to the heart in large doses.

WHAT RESEARCH IS BEING DONE?

Breast cancer is the focus of some of the most intensive and extensive research in medical science. The National Cancer Institute currently lists 165 clinical trials related to breast cancer, and those are only the research projects that enroll patients for their studies. Many hundreds more efforts are ongoing in laboratories. Breast cancer research is also funded by private sources such as the American Cancer Society and the Susan G. Komen Foundation. The U.S. Army funds another research endeavor that is even bigger than that of NCI. Beginning in 1993 with a small program that looked at military women's health, Congress responded to grassroots demand and lobbying by the National Breast Cancer Coalition, and has now appropriated more than $500 million to the Army to disperse to scientists for breast cancer research.

Investigators are examining every conceivable aspect of breast cancer, from prevention in individuals and in large populations, to state-of-the-art diagnostic techniques, to treatment of late-stage disease. Breast cancer research is a fertile field, and lab work that has moved expeditiously to the clinic in the past decade clearly can be credited for adding years to many women's lives. Researchers are gaining new insights into the genetic and biochemical mechanisms of breast cancer, and applying their results to early detection, treatment, and prevention. But the search for a cure remains elusive, and despite a barrage of possible treatments, women with metastasized breast cancer today don't have much better survival odds than their mothers or grandmothers did.

A major focus in treatment research is on combination therapies—surgery and chemotherapy, chemotherapy and hormonal, chemotherapy and radiation, radiation and hormonal, hormonal and immunotherapy, chemotherapy and immunotherapy, and many different combinations of different drugs and procedures. As we learn more, the benefits of certain treatments will become clear, as will understandings of which treatments work best for which patients. However, the unfortunate truth is that advances are being made on the slower growing cancers (usually hormone receptor-positive), but the more aggressive and deadly hormone receptor-negative cancers remain resistant to the various treatment options available. Following are some of the current highlights of breast cancer research:

New chemotherapy drugs. Many new chemotherapy drugs are under investigation. These include variations of current drugs and new classes of drugs. Drugs that prevent tumor growth by blocking blood flow are one of the exciting areas of research. Also under study are "antisense" drugs, which in the lab turn off the genes needed for cancer cell growth. Emerging drugs with promise have longer actions and milder side effects.

Current chemotherapy drugs. Meanwhile, drugs currently being used are under study to determine optimal doses, regimens, and combinations.

Delivery methods. New delivery methods are under investigation for various types of treatment. These include oral chemotherapy, implanted chemotherapy agents, and implanted radiation.

Side effects. Researchers are also looking at drugs to prevent and treat the side effects and health-threatening aspects of chemotherapy.

HRT. Hormone replacement therapy is an area of active research in several arenas, including breast cancer. Scientists are examining the role of HRT in contributing to the growth of breast cancer, whether it can be successfully given to breast cancer survivors and women at risk for breast cancer, and other issues related to hormone influence on breast cancer development.

Raloxifene. Raloxifene (Evista) is a hormonal drug similar to tamoxifen that was tested in large numbers of study participants to see if it prevented osteoporosis. In finding that raloxifene did, indeed, prevent bone fractures, it was also noted that the group taking the drug had a significantly lower rate of breast cancer. Raloxifene also does not appear to cause the uterine stimulation that leads to endometrial cancer. Since breast cancer reduction was not a primary goal of the study, researchers agree that trials designed to test for this specifically are needed. In 1999, STAR (Study of Tamoxifen and Raloxifene) was launched, a 22,000-woman study to compare the effectiveness of raloxifene and tamoxifen in preventing breast cancer. Raloxifene has also been found to be "modestly" effective in treating advanced breast cancer.

Surgery. Surgical techniques to remove breast cancers are continually being refined, and then studied to see which offer the best survival benefits.

High-dose chemotherapy. While high-dose chemotherapy and bone marrow transplant has not been as successful as many had hoped, many ongoing studies continue to look at a role they might play. Generally transplants in which the donor and host are the same person are safer because they avoid the host immune system attacking the transplant. But a new approach in bone marrow transplant is considering whether this attack mechanism can be used so that a transplant from another donor, usually a close relative, can trigger the immune system in a way that attacks the cancer cells.

Vaccines. One vaccine, Theratope, has already proved to be safe and to have some usefulness. It targets a protein, MUC-1, which is found on many breast cancer cells, and stimulates the immune system to develop an immune response against the malignancy. Theratope is being tested on women who have had metastatic disease.

Molecular research. In the laboratory, scientists are studying cancer at the molecular level to find the genes that influence a cell to turn cancerous, and the genes that change when this happens.

Imaging. Enhanced imaging has the goals of detecting breast cancer earlier, giving a better idea of the size and spread of the tumor, evaluating the lymph nodes, finding microscopic disease, and using an image to target chemotherapy or radiation. Nuclear medicine provides many new techniques to be applied to imaging, including magnetic resonance imaging and positron emission tomography scanning.

Ductal lavage. This minimally invasive way of looking at the breast has the potential to detect cancer earlier than any current method in use. In this technique, sometimes referred to as a Pap smear of the breast, a catheter is threaded through a duct in the nipple and a salt solution is injected. The fluid that is then washed out of the duct contains thousands of cells that can be examined for cancer or precancerous conditions. Many medical centers across the country are now investigating this promising new technique.

Complementary therapies. Alternative or complementary therapies are coming under increasing scrutiny by researchers to see what role they can play in treating breast cancer and other diseases. Among the alternative methods being investigated are foot reflexology for relaxation and antianxiety, acupressure for nausea, spiritual healing, herbal remedies, dietary methods, massage, traditional Chinese medicine, and mind-body approach in support groups.

HOW CAN IT BE PREVENTED?

In 1998, the National Cancer Institute ended a study fourteen months ahead of its projected completion date because the results were much better than expected. The study was an investigation of tamoxifen as a preventive against breast cancer in healthy but high-risk women. The Breast Cancer Prevention Trial included 13,388 women and found a 45% reduced rate of breast cancer in the women who took tamoxifen. What had been suspected and seemed logical was now proven—tamoxifen prevents breast cancer.

This was exciting news in the breast cancer world, but only the tip of the prevention iceberg. Much more information is needed before we know exactly how tamoxifen can best be used and which women can best benefit from it, and there is much controversy over giving this potent drug to healthy women. Other prevention efforts stir up other controversies and questions. We have a long way to go before we know how to prevent breast cancer, but considerable work continues and we're hopeful that women today will see the results of this work spare their daughters and granddaughters.

TAMOXIFEN AND SIMILAR HORMONAL TREATMENTS

Tamoxifen and other selective estrogen receptor modulator (SERM) drugs like it will probably play a large role in the prevention of breast cancer. But even that is not totally clear: Other studies with the drug have not produced as definitive a result as the Breast Cancer Prevention Trial. And tamoxifen carries with it a number of serious risks that can be as potentially dangerous as breast cancer. One of the interests of research into developing other SERM drugs is to minimize these risks in new drugs.

The most serious risks associated with tamoxifen are endometrial cancer and blood clots. Formulas have been devised to balance a woman's risk for breast cancer against the risks of the drugs. Because the adverse effects of the drug increase with age, it appears to be most beneficial for women under 50 who have higher than average risk of developing breast cancer.

Raloxifene, another SERM, is used to prevent osteoporosis, and some studies show it also seems to protect against breast cancer without the stimulating effects on the uterus that cause endometrial cancer. With funding from the National Cancer Institute, a large Study of Tamoxifen and Raloxifene (STAR) is in progress to compare the effects of these two drugs on preventing breast cancer, but it will be several years yet before the results are known.

PHYTOESTROGENS AND OTHER DIETARY APPROACHES

Several dietary components might have an effect on breast cancer, but information is conflicting and insufficient to warrant recommendations. A low-fat diet is a diet known to promote general health and prevent a number of diseases, and studies have found lower rates of breast cancer (and other cancers) in groups with low-fat diets. But the evidence is not clear that reducing dietary fat actually prevents breast cancer, or that high fat intake causes it. One recent lab study found different actions of different fats. Polyunsaturated fatty acids stimulated development of breast cancer cells, while omega-3 fatty acids (such as those found in fish) seem to prevent it. Another lab study found that increasing dietary calcium and vitamin D reversed changes in breast tissues that were linked to high fat.

Phytoestrogens are estrogen-like compounds that occur naturally in certain plants, specifically legumes. Soy is one of the best natural sources of phytoestrogens. Populations (for example, Asian women) with high rates of soy in their diet have low rates of breast cancer. Some studies in laboratory animals have found that dietary phytoestrogens impede the growth of breast cancer, but others have found no effect. Many women also find that phytoestrogens reduce symptoms of menopause such as hot flashes. But some women at high risk for breast cancer are as wary of phytoestrogens as they are of estrogen replacement. A great deal more research is needed before definitive answers are known to questions about environmental estrogens, both natural and man-made.

PREVENTIVE MASTECTOMY

The most effective measure to prevent breast cancer is the simplest to understand—but it is also the most extreme. An increasing number of women, knowing they are at high risk for breast cancer, sometimes knowing for certain they have a genetic "marker" for breast cancer (BRCA1 or BRCA2 mutation), choose to have their noncancerous breasts removed. Often in these cases, cancer has developed in one breast, and the woman elects to have both removed—a bilateral mastectomy. A woman can have reconstruction after a preventive mastectomy, with the same options as after any mastectomy. (See Breast Reconstruction sidebar on p. 56.)

Preventive mastectomy removes the entire breast and nipple. However, about 2% of breast tissue invariably remains in the body, so this procedure does not completely eliminate the risk of breast cancer. Preventive removal of the ovaries—called oophorectomy or ovariectomy—is another surgical option for premenopausal women. Removal of the ovaries can serve two purposes: to prevent the production of estrogen in the body that might fuel breast cancer growth, and to prevent ovarian cancer, which is sometimes genetically related to breast cancer.

One of the few studies of preventive mastectomy determined that the risk of breast cancer was reduced by at least 90% in women who had the surgery. However, it is not common enough to have been systematically studied, and it is not known if preventive mastectomy actually saves lives. This is a fairly drastic option filled with potential emotional and psychological ramifications. In a study of about six hundred women who had undergone preventive mastectomy, about 70% reported they were satisfied with their decision, and 75% said it lessened their concerns about getting cancer. But 20% said they were unhappy with their decision and 25% said they felt less feminine after the operation.

A decision about preventive mastectomy must be made on a very individual basis, taking into consideration a woman's unique risks and characteristics. Preventive mastectomy will probably be used less in the future as prevention with hormonal treatment becomes better understood and more widely used.

OTHER PREVENTION METHODS

Indole-3-carbinol and sulforaphane are chemicals found in large amounts in cruciferous vegetables such as broccoli and cabbage that have decreased breast cancer in laboratory animals. These are fairly non-toxic substances and preliminary studies are under way to see if they have any preventive effect on women at high risk for breast cancer.

Melatonin, a hormone secreted by the body's pineal gland and available as an over-the-counter dietary supplement, is best known for its role in regulating the body's sleep cycle. But lowered melatonin production has been linked to breast cancer, while supplementary melatonin given to lab animals was found to protect against breast cancer. Scientists are beginning to test the preventive effects of melatonin in the lab and in the clinic.

EARLY DETECTION

Finding cancer early doesn't prevent it, but it can prevent spread of the cancer and the generally gloomy prognosis that is still predicted for most cases of metastasized breast cancer. This is called secondary prevention, and it may prevent death from this disease. So it's important for women over 40 to do regular breast self-examination and get regular mammograms.

WHAT YOU CAN DO NOW

Many women who have been diagnosed with breast cancer notice that their experience encourages their female friends and relatives to get a mammogram, when it is something they have been putting off. This is a very positive response to a not-so-positive situation. All women older than 40 should have annual screening mammograms to look for breast cancer. Eating healthy and exercising is good advice to prevent any disease, and breast cancer is no exception.

If a woman is diagnosed with breast cancer, she must give careful consideration to where she will receive treatment, and from whom. While breast cancer certainly represents a health crisis, it is not an emergency and should not be treated as one. A few days or even weeks before treatment will not change the course of the disease. A woman must feel free to get a second opinion if she feels her doctor is rushing her into treatment, and she is not sure of her options. In any case, she should be treated by a breast cancer specialist. The best results and long-term outcomes come from the health care providers and facilities that have the most experience treating this disease.

Once breast cancer is diagnosed, patients may find it helpful to speak to survivors about their experiences. Today, there are many breast cancer survivors who can personally demonstrate successful passage through treatment and resumption of their normal lives. For information about what the treatment will be like, look for a survivor who has recently been treated, because treatments are quickly changing and evolving. But it can also be very heartening to speak with a long-term survivor, to realize that breast cancer does not have to limit the years of a woman's life. Volunteer organizations or a multidisciplinary cancer center (one with health care providers in each treatment division of breast cancer, including medical oncology, surgical oncology, radiation oncology, pathology, genetics, radiology, nursing, and social work) can help put patients in touch with breast cancer survivors. Support groups can also be very beneficial. Some studies show that breast cancer survivors who participate in support groups live longer than those who do not.

Many women who have strong family histories of breast cancer may want to get a genetic test to find out if they have a gene that causes breast cancer. From a patient's point of view, all that is involved for this test is giving blood to be analyzed. In general, knowledge is power, but women should not rush into this test without considering how and whether they are prepared to act on the results. And be aware that if the gene is not found, that doesn't mean the woman is not at risk for breast cancer. Genetic alterations account for only a small percentage of breast cancer cases.

If the breast cancer gene is found, a number of preventive options are available, ranging from increased frequency of mammograms to taking tamoxifen to prophylactic mastectomy. It is important for a woman to discuss these options with an experienced and qualified health care provider, and get a second or even third opinion if she is having trouble making a decision. Another issue related to genetic testing is whether the woman wants her insurance company to know if genes positive for breast cancer are found. Many women who have the test pay for it themselves, so they don't have to let their insurance companies know the results.

OTHER POSTTREATMENT ISSUES

Having breast cancer changes a woman's life. For most women, diagnosis, treatment, and then trying to resume a normal life influence priorities, goals in life, and even relationships. A woman who has had breast cancer will have a different view of her body. Depending on her stage (how advanced the cancer was), she may have different attitudes about her future and what she wants to accomplish in her life.

A posttreatment issue that everyone faces is fear of recurrence. This can be converted to positive action. Women who have had breast cancer are not likely to miss their regularly scheduled mammograms, for example, and may be more diligent about breast self-examination. They are attuned to their bodies. But this fear can also be paralyzing, and make a woman lose trust in her own body. Many women who develop breast cancer—or any type of cancer—feel their bodies have betrayed them. And the unfortunate fact is, once a woman has had breast cancer, she is at higher risk than average for developing another breast cancer, and other types of cancer as well.

But it's also important for these women to resist the feeling that every physical symptom they have is related to cancer recurrence—most of the time, it isn't. As time passes, these fears will fade, although it is unlikely they will ever fully disappear. Again, a support group or talking with survivors may help women deal with these emotional and psychological problems. Women are encouraged to talk to their doctor about any symptoms they have, but they should try to wait out routine aches and pains for a few days, because most of the time they will go away on their own. Any persistent problem should be brought to the attention of their health care provider. Women with breast cancer have probably been treated by a team of doctors—i.e., gynecologist, surgeon, oncologist— and should arrange among them a sequential schedule of visits with the following frequency:

- First three years after diagnosis: Every three to six months.
- Fourth and fifth year after diagnosis: Every six to twelve months.
- Fifth year and after: Annually.

Women who have had breast cancer may also face long-term problems related to chemotherapy or radiation. If they were premenopausal when diagnosed, chemotherapy or hormonal treatment will often cause menopause, and this sudden menopause usually brings with it more intense hot flashes and other symptoms than the more gradual natural menopause. Along with this may come decreased sexual desire, which may be related to negative feelings about their body and sexuality. If intimate relations suffer, it is important that women have open communication with their partner, and seek counseling and medical advice if they can't handle the problems on their own.

ADDITIONAL RESOURCES

ORGANIZATIONS AND WEB SITES

The American Cancer Society's
Breast Cancer Network
800-ACS-2345
www.cancer.org

Avon's Breast Cancer Awareness Crusade
800-FOR-AVON
www.avoncrusade.com
BCN, Breastcancer.net
www.breastcancer.net

Cancer Care, Inc.
275 Seventh Ave.
New York, NY 10001
212-302-2400
800-813-HOPE
www.cancercare.org
email: info@cancercare.org

The Cancer Information Service
of the National Cancer Institute
31 Center Drive
Bethesda, MD 20892-2580
800-4-CANCER
www.cancer.gov

Centerwatch Clinical Trials Listing Service
www.centerwatch.com

The Susan G. Komen Foundation
National Office
5005 LBJ Freeway, Suite 370
Dallas, TX 75244
800 I'M-AWARE
972-855-1600
www.komen.org

Living Beyond Breast Cancer
610-645-4567
www.lbbc.org

Mothers Supporting Daughters with Breast Cancer
(MSDBC)
21710 Bayshore Road
Chestertown, MD 21620
410-778-1982
email: msdbc@dmv.com
www.mothersdaughters.org

The National Alliance of Breast Cancer
Organizations (NABCO)
Nine East 37th St., 10th floor
New York, NY 10016
212-889-0606 or 888-806-2226
www.nabco.org
email: nabcoinfo@aol.com

Patient Advocacy Foundation (PAF)
Suite B
753 Thimble Shoals Blvd.
Newport News, VA 23606
800-532-5274
email: help@patientadvocate.org
www.patientadvocate.org

Women's Information Network Against
Breast Cancer (WIN ABC)
19325 East Navilla Place
Covina, CA 91723
626-332-2255
www.winabc.org

Y-ME

212 West Van Buren St.

Chicago, IL 60607-3908

312-986-8338

800-221-2141 (24-hour national hotline)

email: info@y-me.org

www.y-me.org

BOOKS

Berger, Karen J., and John Bostwick III. *A Woman's Decision: Breast Care, Treatment & Reconstruction.* New York: St. Martin's Press, Quality Medical Home Health Library, 1998.

Link, John. *The Breast Cancer Survival Manual: A Step-By-Step Guide for the Woman With Newly Diagnosed Breast Cancer.* Owl Press, 1998.

Love, Susan M., et al. *Dr. Susan Love's Breast Book.* New York: Pegasus Press, 1995.

Rich, Katherine Russell. *The Red Devil: To Hell with Cancer—And Back.* New York: Crown Publishers, 1999.

Shockney, Lillie. *Breast Cancer Survivors' Club: A Nurse's Experience,* Loveland, Colo.: Real Health Books, 2001.

Chronic Obstructive Pulmonary Disease

O f the top ten causes of death in the United States, only one remains on the rise: chronic obstructive pulmonary disease, or COPD. This year, COPD will kill an estimated one hundred and fifteen thousand Americans, up more than 5% since 1997 alone. More than one in every twenty-five deaths in this country is now caused by COPD.

The reason for this rapid growth is clear. Simply put, the nation is paying the price for a half-century of increased cigarette smoking. COPD is a smokers' disease, almost always brought on by lung damage caused by years of smoking. In advanced stages, the disease leaves the lungs unable to deliver oxygen to the body, resulting in a gradual decline in quality of life and, after twenty to forty years, death.

COPD is not curable, nor are its effects truly reversible. Yet caregivers and people with the disease can choose from a growing array of treatments, lifestyle changes, and medication that can both increase the lifespan of the patient and make that life more productive and enjoyable. In addition, researchers are working on several new treatment methods that could advance the fight against COPD. With proper guidance and motivation, some people with COPD can continue functioning at a relatively high level for many years.

WHAT IS IT?

After the brain, lungs are the most complex organs in the human body. They are responsible for delivering life's most important catalyst—oxygen—from the outside world to all cells within. Without a constant supply of oxygen, the body would be unable to digest food, repair tissue, keep a heartbeat, maintain brain function, or even move muscles for more than a matter of seconds.

To capture oxygen, lungs employ a huge net of specialized tissues. Air enters the chest through the windpipe, also known as the trachea. The trachea then splits into two tubes called bronchi, one leading to each lung. These bronchi again split in half, then continue to divide twenty more times until the bronchi end in what are called terminal bronchioles. Attached to these bronchioles are tiny passageways called alveolar ducts, which look like very small, spiral staircases. These ducts lead to the alveoli, tiny, folded sacs where oxygen molecules are transferred from the air to the bloodstream. Together the alveoli and alveolar ducts unwind and unfold as the lungs inflate.

The 300 million or so alveoli in a set of lungs compose incredibly thin membranes, across which the oxygen passes to waiting capillaries. These membranes are one-fiftieth the thickness of a piece of tissue paper. If all the membranes and other lung tissue were laid out flat, they would cover an area of about 100 square yards—bigger than a tennis court.

COPD attacks the lungs in several different places, depending on the particular course of the disease. There are three main types of COPD, which overlap to varying degrees in all patients.

EMPHYSEMA

Emphysema does its damage in the alveoli. Usually caused by cigarette smoking, emphysema breaks down these air sacs and makes them lose their elasticity. This means the lungs are unable to expel old, spent air and take in new, oxygen-rich air. At the same time, the alveolar walls are destroyed, making the air-to-blood transfer of oxygen more difficult. When the elastic scaffolding of the lungs that holds the air sacs open breaks down, air gets trapped in the air sacs and can no longer be fully expelled from the lungs. These conditions combine to hyperinflate the lungs, resulting in the telltale barrel-chested appearance of people with the disease.

In addition to oxygen deprivation, people with emphysema also suffer from an excess of carbon dioxide in their bodies in advanced stages of disease. This gas is the byproduct of the body's metabolism, and is usually exhaled through the lungs.

When the lungs are damaged, a dangerous buildup of carbon dioxide that can be life-threatening, known as respiratory acidosis, can result.

Researchers believe that an enzyme called neutrophil elastase is released in great amounts by certain cells of the immune system to combat the irritation caused by cigarette smoke. This enzyme breaks down damaged lung tissue so that the lungs can repair themselves. Too much elastase, however, ultimately leads to massive destruction of lung tissue.

Less commonly, emphysema also can be caused by a genetic disorder called alpha-1-antitrypsin (AAT) deficiency. People with this condition are unable to produce a substance called alpha-1-antitrypsin—the "off" switch that inhibits the

QUITTING SMOKING FOR GOOD

With a support network and nicotine replacement or other drug therapy in place, smoking cessation can begin. Here are some key pointers that can make quitting last forever:

Pick a quit date. Telling family, friends, and co-workers about your intention to quit can help create a supportive and positive environment for the smoker.

Commit to quit. Cold turkey is the best way to go. Tapering off rarely works in the long run.

Tough out the first week. Cravings are their strongest during the first seven days or so of smoking cessation. This is a good time to tap that new network of family, friends, and other non-smokers.

Avoid tempting situations. Sitting among smokers, drinking alcohol, keeping cigarettes in the house, and other related situations all can cause relapses. Learn to identify past habits and avoid these triggers during the first weeks or months of smoking cessation.

Don't sweat the weight gain. Most people who quit smoking gain weight. In the majority of cases, it's less than 10 pounds, although about 10% of people who quit will gain upwards of 30 pounds. Almost always, the extra weight poses a negligible health risk—especially when compared with the dangers of smoking. Nicotine replacement therapy may delay the weight gain for the first few months, although people usually gain weight after stopping the gum or patches.

Be persistent. It can take as many as seven attempts to finally quit smoking. People learn a little more each time, and those who keep their eyes on the goal usually succeed.

work of elastase. It's also believed that smoking may block the effectiveness of AAT, giving elastase more chance to destroy lung tissue.

CHRONIC OBSTRUCTIVE BRONCHITIS

Chronic obstructive bronchitis is defined as a chronic cough with expectoration and reduced airflow for at least three months per year in two consecutive years. It usually begins as an inflammation of the small airways in the lungs, and often progresses to the larger bronchi. The swelling is usually accompanied by mucus, which further restricts the air spaces in the lungs. Spasms in the muscle walls of the bronchi can make breathing even more difficult. While chronic obstructive bronchitis can be caused by repeated lung infections, the leading cause is irritation from cigarette smoke. It differs from the more common simple chronic bronchitis in that the airways are partially blocked by the swelling and mucus.

ASTHMATIC BRONCHITIS

Asthmatic bronchitis differs from chronic obstructive bronchitis in only one major respect. In chronic obstructive bronchitis, the patient responds little, if at all, to medications designed to open airways in the lungs. People with asthmatic bronchitis, however, get partial relief from their condition by using medications like inhaled beta-agonists, corticosteroids, anticholinergics, and methylxanthines. People who respond completely to these drugs are not considered to have COPD. Over time, people with asthmatic bronchitis may stop seeing benefits from asthma medications, leading to permanent restriction of their airways. Asthmatic bronchitis is also marked by breathing difficulties brought on by walking or other activity (exertional dyspnea).

Most patients with COPD have a combination of these conditions.

WHO IS AT RISK?

About sixteen million people in the United States have been diagnosed with COPD, and another fifteen to sixteen million have the disease but show no symptoms and have yet to be diagnosed. By comparison, the number of Americans diagnosed with all forms of cancer in 1995 was about 7.4 million.

Smokers. COPD has been called a smokers' disease, and, in fact, the great majority of people with COPD are cigarette users. Researchers believe the actual figure may run as high as 80 to 90%. Smokers are ten times more likely to die from COPD than are nonsmokers.

Not all smokers will develop COPD, however. It's believed that only 10 to 20% of people who smoke get the disease. The reasons for this remain mysterious. There does appear to be a threshold beyond which smoking becomes more likely to cause COPD. This is expressed by a term called pack-years, which is related to the number of packs of cigarettes smoked in a person's lifetime. People who smoke ten or more pack-years—the equivalent of one pack per day for ten years, two packs per day for five years, etc.—are at a far greater risk of developing COPD than lighter smokers.

For decades, gender was believed to be a strong predictor for COPD. Men developed the disease and died from it at a far higher rate than women. But that gap has closed rapidly as more women become regular cigarette smokers. Between 1992 and 1997, mortality from COPD rose 10.9% in men—but jumped 27.9% in women.

In fact, scientists believe that women may be even more vulnerable than men to the effects of cigarette smoke. Women have smaller lungs and smaller airways than men. They also have less elastic recoil in their lungs. These factors combine to make it harder for women to escape the toxins from cigarette smoke. In addition, women are more likely than men to remain smokers into old age—a factor that may speed up the progression of COPD.

AAT deficiency. As discussed earlier, people with AAT deficiency are unable to produce enough of a protein that counteracts the destructive effects of elastase in the lungs. AAT deficiency plays a role in only 2 to 3% of all cases of COPD, but it remains the only clearly established hereditary risk factor for the disease. AAT deficiency is limited almost exclusively to people of Caucasian descent.

Even people with this disorder are not likely to develop COPD unless they smoke; those who develop COPD without smoking usually do so only late in life. Smokers with AAT deficiency, on the other hand, are likely to develop COPD at a younger age than other smokers.

Family history. COPD is known to cluster in families, whether AAT deficiency is present or not. A recent study of forty-four people with early-onset COPD found that close blood relatives had a higher risk of also developing the disease. This indicates that there may be other genetic components to COPD, although none has been clearly established.

Other family-related factors—especially the likelihood of children of smokers to become smokers themselves—are important risk factors. A family's socioeconomic status may play a role as well. People from poorer backgrounds are somewhat more likely to develop COPD, even after controlling for higher smoking levels. Again, the effect is weak when compared to smoking.

Childhood lung infections. There's some evidence that smokers who had respiratory infections as children may be predisposed to develop COPD later in life. While the infections themselves were not enough to cause COPD, researchers believe they may make lungs more vulnerable to tobacco smoke later.

Allergies and asthma. People who are susceptible to allergies and asthma are believed by some researchers to be at a higher risk of developing breathing obstructions and COPD. This possible link, known since the 1960s as the Dutch hypothesis, is not generally considered a major risk factor for COPD unless the person in question is also a smoker.

Occupational dusts. Exposure to coal dust is a known risk factor for COPD, although this problem has lessened with the advent of cleaner mining techniques. Dust from grain processing is also believed to cause COPD in some people whether or not they smoke. Unlike coal dust, grain dust can cause an allergic reaction in susceptible workers. This leads to hyper-reactivity in the lungs, which, over time, can restrict the amount of airflow in and out of the body. Other airborne particles, such as mites and fungi, may also lead to COPD, but this hasn't been proven.

Air pollution. Canadian studies have shown that smokers who live in cities with high air pollution levels are more likely to develop COPD than those who live in areas with cleaner air. But this effect is small, and the role of air pollution is considered minor compared to smoking itself.

Poor diet and alcohol consumption. Neither of these has been clearly proven as risk factors, although some evidence does exist. Some researchers believe that diets low in antioxidants—vitamins C and E, plus beta-carotene—may leave smokers at greater risk of lung destruction through oxidation. The link with alcohol is sketchy, since it's hard to determine whether alcohol or passive smoke in bars contributes more to the development of COPD.

HOW IS IT DIAGNOSED?

COPD takes years, even decades, to run its course. In the early stages, people with the disease usually don't notice any symptoms. Even when they visit the doctor for other reasons, the condition almost always goes undetected. Routine examinations with stethoscopes rarely reveal any abnormalities, and even chest x-rays appear normal.

As the lungs continue to deteriorate, people begin to notice mild symptoms. Usually, these include a chronic cough and a shortness of breath on exertion. Typically, the onset of these symptoms occurs when a person reaches his late 40s or early 50s. Even at this stage, most people still ignore the symptoms, attributing the shortness of breath to just "getting older." Many people still consider themselves healthy and are unaware that they have curtailed their exercise levels substantially in response to their worsening condition.

It's only when the symptoms begin to interfere with simple tasks, like walking, that people with COPD see a doctor for diagnosis. This typically occurs when a person reaches his late 50s or early 60s (in some cases, including those involving AAT deficiency, serious symptoms arrive much earlier). Doctors will then perform a series of tests and procedures to determine whether COPD is present, or whether the symptoms are caused by something else.

HISTORY

The physician usually will start the diagnosis by taking a detailed health history. This will include numerous questions about smoking: how long the person has smoked, how many packs per day, whether or not she has quit and, if so, when. These questions help give the doctor an idea of how many pack-years the person has been a smoker, to see if the diagnosis of COPD is possible.

The doctor is also likely to ask the patient about other possible risk factors for COPD. His questions might include some or all of the following:

Have you ever worked in a dusty occupation?
Have you been continuously exposed to second-hand smoke?
Do you live in an area with high levels of air pollution?
Do you have a chronic cough and, if so, how long have you had it?

Do you produce sputum when you cough?

Do you ever wheeze?

Have you ever had bronchitis, pneumonia, or other chest infections?

How long have you had a shortness of breath, and when do you notice it most?

Of course, the doctor also will ask about family history, since COPD tends to cluster in families. (*Do any family members have COPD? Do you know of any family member who has AAT deficiency?*)

In many cases, a doctor will ask the patient to fill out a questionnaire that asks about day-to-day activities and how the person feels about the general state of his health. This will help him determine how much COPD may already have affected lifestyle and emotional well-being. It usually will include questions about whether the patient has trouble with everyday tasks like grocery shopping, walking, and cleaning the house, plus questions about whether he has been feeling worn out, unhappy, depressed, or nervous.

PHYSICAL EXAMINATION

After taking a complete health history, the doctor will begin looking for the physical signs of COPD. She will use a stethoscope to check for unusual noises in the lungs and heart. While the patient breathes out, the doctor will listen for wheezing or crackling in the lungs. The doctor also will listen for abnormal heart sounds, which often accompany COPD in advanced cases. The doctor probably will tap lightly on the chest (a technique called percussion) to listen for a hollow sound that would indicate that the lungs are hyperinflated. Many of these symptoms will be absent in people with early, or even mild, stages of COPD.

In advanced cases of COPD, other physical signs become obvious. Hyperinflation occurs when the lungs are constantly expanded because they are unable to expel air. It becomes harder to hear the heartbeat and breathing sounds while using a stethoscope. The diaphragm is held in a low position, since the lungs are full and taking up an abnormal amount of space. The doctor also may notice pursed-lip breathing—a technique people sometimes use to increase the amount of air they can remove from the lungs. This involves tightening or puckering the lips into a whistling position while exhaling. Doing so helps force out air more efficiently.

SPIROMETRY

If a doctor has reason to suspect COPD, she will likely begin a series of tests to confirm the diagnosis. The most important of these is a painless office procedure called spirometry. This involves blowing into a machine called a spirometer, which measures the amount of air a patient can exhale from his lungs.

Everyone's lungs begin to lose power and capacity with age. A typical 5-foot-10 man, for instance, may be able to blow out 4.5 to 4.8 liters of air in one second at age 20, but only 3.5 to 3.8 liters at age 50. Similarly, a 5-foot-5 woman may blow out more than 3.5 liters at age 20, but only 2.5 to 2.8 liters thirty years later. The rate of decline averages 0.3 liters per decade in healthy people.

Smoking—and, in rare cases, other problems like dust exposure and AAT deficiency—can speed this normal decline rapidly. In fact, the loss of lung capacity can be two to four times faster in smokers, depending on the number of cigarettes smoked and an individual's susceptibility to the effects of smoke. Quitting smoking can increase lung capacity in the short run; the rate of decline then returns to normal levels associated with aging after several years.

The spirometer is used to see how far a person's lungs have declined compared to healthy subjects. The doctor will ask a patient to place a tube in her mouth and blow as hard as possible for about six to ten seconds. The spirometer will calculate how much air the patient expels in the first second—a number known as Forced Expiratory Volume in one second (FEV1). The machine also will record the total amount of air exhaled, a figure known as Forced Vital Capacity (FVC). The test is usually repeated three times or so to make sure the numbers are accurate.

Once the numbers are determined, the doctor will divide the FEV1 figure by the FVC figure to create a ratio known as FEV1/FVC. This tells the doctor what percentage of the air is exhaled in the first second. In healthy people, the ratio is 0.70 to 0.75; that means that nearly three-fourths of all the air is exhaled during the first second.

Anytime the ratio falls below 0.70, COPD is suspected. This lower ratio indicates that the lungs are losing elastic recoil and can't exhale properly. In other words, it's taking too long for the lungs to blow out all the exhaled air containing carbon dioxide and other byproducts of normal metabolism. This is usually caused by airflow obstruction that results from emphysema or chronic bronchitis. The doctor usually retests the patient's lungs after giving him an inhaled bronchodilator, a medicine designed to open up the bronchi. If the ratio improves after taking the medicine, it usually means that asthma is playing a role in the condition.

In addition to the FEV1/FVC ratio, the FEV1 number itself can reveal important information about the progression of COPD. Anytime the FEV1 number falls below 80% of normal for people of the same sex, height, and age as the patient, COPD is suspected. For instance, a 50-year-old man who stands 5-foot-10 normally has an FEV1 of about 3.6 liters. If the FEV1 drops to 2.9 liters or less, COPD is probably the cause. An average 50-year-old woman who stands 5-foot-5 has an FEV1 of about 2.7 liters; any FEV1 reading below 2.2 liters indicates COPD.

People with COPD begin to notice symptoms like shortness of breath (dyspnea) when the FEV1 reaches about 1.5 liters.

COPD can be divided into three stages using FEV1 numbers. When the FEV1 figure is 50 to 80% of normal, a person is considered to have stage 1 (mild) COPD. At this point, the disease causes minimal symptoms, and usually can be handled by a primary care doctor. When FEV1 is 35 to 49% of normal, stage 2 (moderate) COPD is diagnosed. At this level, people notice significant symptoms, such as shortness of breath during minor exertion. A person in this range may or may not need supplemental oxygen to improve their condition.

When FEV1 falls below 35% of normal, stage 3 (severe) COPD is diagnosed. This is the most severe stage, where people almost always need oxygen and may have trouble breathing even when at rest. Pulmonary specialists usually care for these patients when they reach stage 3.

FEV1 measurements also can give patients an idea of their relative lung age. This is a powerful concept that tells people how much faster their lungs are deteriorating than the rest of their body. For example: A 40-year-old woman who stands 5-foot-5 normally has an FEV1 of about 3.0 liters. But if a woman's FEV1 measurement is 2.5 liters, she essentially has the lung capacity of someone who is nearly 60 years old. Doctors have found that using lung age with patients can motivate them to stop smoking, so that their lung capacity can start declining at a slower rate.

LABORATORY TESTS

In addition to spirometry, the doctor may order a series of additional tests to determine what complications, if any, have already arisen from COPD. A chest x-ray will not show signs of COPD except in advanced emphysema. In that case, the x-ray will reveal overinflation of the lungs, and possible strain on the heart and arteries caused by the extra burden COPD puts on the circulatory system. More importantly, the chest x-ray can help doctors determine if other problems exist along with COPD—most notably lung cancer.

An electrocardiogram (ECG) test or an echocardiogram may help to determine if COPD has caused any damage to the heart. This usually only occurs in advanced stages of emphysema. The most common heart problem associated with COPD is called cor pulmonale. Because emphysema breaks down the capillaries in the alveoli, the heart must pump extra hard to collect oxygen from the lungs. This leads to high blood pressure in the pulmonary circulation and an enlargement of the right ventricle in the heart, which is the chamber that pumps blood from the heart to the lungs.

It may also be necessary to take a few blood tests. If a person has signs of COPD at an early age—usually 50 or younger—the doctor may want to test for the concentration of AAT in the bloodstream. Too little of this protein can lead to breakdown of lung tissue by the enzyme elastase. Another blood test will screen for a condition called erythrocytosis. This is an excess buildup of red blood cells; the bone marrow creates these cells, which carry oxygen through the bloodstream, in an attempt to make up for the lack of oxygen delivered by the blood. The doctor also may draw blood from an artery in the wrist to check for the amount of oxygen, carbon dioxide, and pH (acidity) of the blood. This is usually only done to determine whether a person needs to use supplemental oxygen to breathe more effectively. Supplemental oxygen can be delivered in various ways. (See Oxygen Therapy on p. 93.)

WHAT SHOULD YOU EXPECT?

COPD is a progressive disease that can take forty or more years to run its course. In general, the damage done by cigarette smoke and other factors is permanent. After years of harm from smoke, the lungs simply are not able to heal and regenerate; once lung function deteriorates past a certain point, death from COPD is almost inevitable. When FEV1 falls to 1 liter or less (as measured by spirometer), about 50% of patients die within five years. When the volume drops to 0.75 liter, mortality is 30% at one year and 95% at ten years. Death usually occurs through a complication of COPD: pneumonia, heart arrhythmia, or pulmonary embolism, a blockage in a blood vessel within the lung.

These bleak numbers underscore the need for early detection and treatment of COPD. While the damage may be irreversible, it's often possible to slow the rate of decline in the lungs. The caregiver's and patient's roles in effective COPD treatment are enormous. The single most important factor in treatment—smoking cessation—is wholly reliant on the patient's motivation and desire to overcome the disease.

A growing number of other treatments and therapies, including regular vaccinations, bronchodilators, dietary changes, exercise, portable oxygen, and lung-reduction surgery, can also slow the progression of COPD. The use of each treatment depends on the age of the patient and the stage of the disease.

HOW IS IT TREATED?

SMOKING CESSATION

Without question, quitting smoking is the most important step anyone can take to slow the progression of COPD. People who continue to smoke after being diagnosed with the disease will continue to lose lung capacity at a dangerous rate. Stopping will improve lung function in the short run—and then return the rate of decline to that of a nonsmoker in most cases.

A massive study on smoking cessation bears out this good news. The Lung Health Study tracked 5887 middle-aged COPD patients in America and Canada to see what effect smoking cessation had on lung function. The average patient in the study had smoked nearly thirty pack-years of cigarettes and had mild COPD (an average FEV1/FVC ratio of 63.5%). People who quit smoking enjoyed a slight increase in FEV1 measurements during the first two years of the study. Their lungs then began losing capacity at a rate similar to that of nonsmokers—about 0.3 liter per decade. Those who were unable to quit smoking declined faster than nonsmokers, indicating that COPD was growing worse.

Quitting smoking will not return a person's lungs to normal capacity, but it can add years to one's life. And it's never too late to quit. Studies have even shown that smoking cessation in COPD patients 65 or older may extend life significantly.

Of course, quitting smoking is a major challenge. Heavy smokers are addicted to nicotine, a chemical stimulant contained in cigarette smoke. Seven of ten smokers report that they want to quit and have made at least one "serious" but unsuccessful attempt to do so. Even people who have already been diagnosed with COPD find it hard to give up the habit, even though they are aware of the consequences. Fewer than one in ten people who try to quit succeed in the long run.

Fortunately, there are ways to improve the odds significantly. A combination of counseling, social support, and nicotine replacement therapy or other drugs can double the chances of quitting for good.

Getting started

People who have been diagnosed with COPD have special motivation to quit smoking. But getting started can be a confusing proposition. That's why it's important to gather as much information as possible before getting the process under way.

The family doctor is a good place to turn first. Primary care physicians are in a unique position to help patients quit smoking. Their knowledge and influence can help convince smokers to at least make an effort to stop. And even a token effort can make the difference. About 10.2% of patients will quit smoking just because a doctor advises them to do so; that figure is a modest increase from the 7.9% of those who get no such advice.

It's also a good idea to start gathering information from other sources. The American Lung Association, National Cancer Institute, and other groups publish self-help pamphlets, books, and videotapes that offer sound advice for quitting (See Additional Resources.) While these self-help guides can be a good starting point, however, they're not enough by themselves to ensure success. In fact, studies show that people who use nothing but self-help materials are only slightly more likely to quit for good than the average smoker.

Counseling and support

Family physicians can point patients toward smoking cessation programs. The federal Agency for Healthcare Research and Quality has developed guidelines for successful programs. These include at least four to seven sessions, with each session lasting at least twenty to thirty minutes; a duration of at least two weeks, preferably as long as eight weeks; and counseling that helps patients deal with common problems encountered by smokers who are trying to quit—such as dealing with friends and spouses who smoke, nicotine cravings, and weight gain.

Counseling sessions have been shown to help people quit. Whether in a group or individual setting, counseling can improve the success rate to about 15%—twice that of people who do not undergo the sessions.

In addition to formal counseling sessions, people also can benefit from informal support groups. The appendix lists several resources that will help people locate groups near their homes. It's also important for people to tap whatever support they can find among family and friends.

Drug therapy for smoking cessation

Nicotine replacement therapy. The use of nicotine substitutes can greatly improve the odds of quitting. Replacement nicotine can help reduce cigarette cravings during the first eight to ten weeks of cessation.

Nicotine replacement is now available in several forms, in both prescription and nonprescription forms.

Gum containing nicotine has been available over the counter (without prescription) since 1996. The gum is sold under the brand name Nicorette, and is available in 2 mg and 4 mg dosages. The nicotine is released slowly and absorbed through the lining of the mouth during chewing.

Nicotine gum has been shown to increase the odds of quitting in more than fifty studies. People who use the gum are 40 to 60% more likely to stop for at least twelve months than those who use no nicotine replacement method. Among heavy smokers (twenty or more cigarettes per day) the 4 mg dosage is usually more effective.

When using the gum, it's important to remember a few guidelines. First, chew the gum slowly. Each piece will release nicotine for at least thirty minutes. Since the nicotine is absorbed by the mouth lining, it's best to leave the gum sitting between the gums and cheek when not actively chewing. Don't eat anything for fifteen to twenty minutes prior to chewing, as this inhibits the body's ability to absorb the nicotine. And since the nicotine is released slowly, it's a good idea to start chewing the gum upon awakening, so that nicotine is available in the body when cravings arise. Never smoke while using nicotine gum. This may increase the risk of a heart attack.

While nicotine gum can be effective, it does have a few drawbacks. The taste is not pleasant to all chewers. Some people find it hard to chew with the proper technique. And others find it difficult to quit using the gum after the first few months. One study found that, when given free access to the gum, patients are likely to continue using it for at least a year.

Nicotine patches also have been available without a prescription since 1996. They are sold under the brand names Nicoderm, Habitrol, ProStep and Nicotrol. With this method, users apply an adhesive patch, similar to a large BAND-AID®, to the body. The patch releases nicotine at a constant rate throughout the day. Studies have found that using the patch can double the rate of success during the first year. Many people find it easier to use the patch than gum, since all they have to do is apply the patch once each day.

Typically, the patch is used for a period of about eight weeks. The over-the-counter brands use a step-down method, starting at 15 to 22 mg per day and working down to 5 to 11 mg per day. Users apply the patch first thing each morning; it can be placed on any relatively hairless surface, so that it can be used discreetly. The patch can be removed at bedtime if you notice sleep disorders.

About one-half of people who use the patch develop a minor local skin rash. It may be a good idea to rotate areas where the patch is applied. Topical hydrocortisone cream usually clears up the irritation, although about 5% of people must stop using the patch because of worsening rashes. It's very important not to smoke while using the patch, because the amount of nicotine from the combined sources greatly outweighs the dosage people get from cigarettes alone.

Nicotine replacement therapy also is available in two prescription forms, an inhaler and a nasal spray, which require more frequent dosing than patches. Although they have not been studied as thoroughly as the gum or patch, it's believed that they can significantly improve a smoker's chances of quitting when used properly. The recommended doses of these inhalers should never be exceeded. Nasal and throat irritation is common.

People using any of these forms of nicotine replacement must keep them out of the reach of children and pets. Even used patches and spray containers may have enough nicotine in them to poison a child or pet if ingested.

Antidepressants. The U.S. Food and Drug Administration has approved the use of the antidepressant bupropion for smoking cessation. This drug is available by prescription only, and is sold under the name Zyban. It also carries the name Wellbutrin when used as an antidepressant.

Doctors aren't sure why Zyban works. When used to treat depression, the drug allows the mood-uplifting brain chemical serotonin to function longer before being absorbed. Some believe that nicotine may act as an antidepressant, and feel that Zyban may work on the same brain receptors that nicotine usually occupies.

Whatever the mechanism, Zyban appears to work. A study of more than six hundred smokers found that 23.1% of people using a 300 mg daily dose of the drug for the first seven weeks of smoking cessation were still nonsmokers after one year. This was nearly double the 12.4% of people who were given a placebo during the trial. Not everyone can use Zyban, however, including people with uncontrolled hypertension, seizure disorders, and eating disorders (anorexia and bulimia). Zyban may be used in combination with nicotine replacement therapy but users must check for possible increases in blood pressure.

VACCINATIONS

Two common diseases—influenza and pneumonia—can have devastating consequences for people with COPD. Both attack the lungs, which may not be able to handle the stress because of the damage caused by the underlying airway obstructions.

For this reason, the Centers for Disease Control and Prevention recommend that all people with COPD receive vaccinations. The flu shot is an annual vaccine that is geared to stop strains of influenza that are likely to predominate in a given year. It can prevent 30 to 80% of all flu cases among high-risk groups such as COPD patients. The only people who should be wary about flu shots are those who have severe allergies to egg proteins, which are part of the vaccine. In highly sensitive people, this can cause a life-threatening shock response called anaphylaxis.

Thinking has changed on how often to receive pneumonia vaccines. While a one-time shot was the standard regimen, most experts now recommend booster shots every five to six years. This is especially true for people who have underlying immune weakness (such as those who have had their spleens removed). Just how effective the vaccines are in preventing pneumonia remains questionable.

Some studies show no benefit among high-risk groups, while others show an effectiveness of 65 to 84%. In most cases, however, the potential benefit is powerful enough to warrant the vaccine.

BRONCHODILATORS

Most people with COPD have some degree of airflow reversibility; that means that they respond to drugs that temporarily open their lungs to accept more air. Bronchodilating drugs are used for this purpose. These are the same drugs commonly used by asthma patients to get relief from attacks.

BRONCHODILATORS

Here's a list of common bronchodilators:

• **Beta-agonists:** albuterol (brand names Ventolin, Proventil), salmeterol (Serevent), terbutaline (Brethine), metaproterenol (Alupent, Metaprel), pirbuterol (Maxair).

• **Anticholinergics:** ipratropium bromide (Atrovent).

• **Combination:** ipratropium plus albuterol (Combivent).

It's important to note that bronchodilators do not affect the underlying disease process or progression, but can extend life.

The medication is delivered in two ways, either through an inhaler or in pill form. The two main types of inhaled bronchodilators are beta-agonists and anticholinergics. The beta-agonists tend to act most quickly, but are not as effective as the anticholinergics. A new product combines both types of bronchodilators, and is an option for many people.

Bronchodilators are usually inhaled through a device known as a metered-dose inhaler. These provide an exact dose each time they're used, but can be tricky to operate. Doctors, nurses, or other health care workers should provide instructions and training prior to use.

The pill form of bronchodilators can be used alone or in combination with the inhaled varieties. The most common drug in this class is theophylline, and is marketed under the brand names Slo-Bid, Slo-Phyllin, Theo-Dur, Uniphyl, and others. These drugs have a mild bronchodilating effect, and also help relieve fatigue in muscles used for breathing.

Bronchodilators can have unpleasant side effects, including nervousness, headache, insomnia, and rapid heartbeat. It's important to notify a doctor if any of these symptoms arise during early usage of the drugs.

ANTIBIOTICS

When bacterial infections settle in the lungs, antibiotics may help fight the infection. Antibiotics, however, are not cure-all drugs. In general, they work against bacterial infections like pneumonia but not against viral infections like influenza (although some viral infections will include a secondary, bacterial infection as well). Usually, bacterial infection is present when sputum changes color from white or gray to yellow or green. When accompanied by difficult breathing and chest tightness, the condition is known as acute purulent bronchitis.

On doctor's advice, people with chest infections can take an antibiotic like amoxicillin, erythromycin, trimethoprim-sulfamethoxazole or doxycycline. Secondary antibiotics may be used in persistent or unusual cases. Antibiotic therapy is taken for a week or so.

Antibiotic use is more controversial when dealing with chronic bronchitis. Some research shows that rotating through a series of antibiotics every two weeks can help control constant sputum production. Antibiotics are usually given only when the cough, sputum production, and shortness of breath from chronic bronchitis begin to interfere with a person's ability to function.

CORTICOSTEROIDS

Corticosteroids are anti-inflammatory drugs that doctors usually only prescribe during severe COPD flare-ups. The most common drug is prednisone. This is a powerful drug that is usually given for a period of ten to fourteen days.

Studies are under way to see if long-term use of corticosteroids can improve airflow or at least reduce the decline in FEV1. Doctors may provide low-dose, long-term regimens for patients who show improvement from corticosteroids.

Prednisone causes a number of dangerous side effects, which are the main reason for the limited use of the drug. Sustained use can lead to osteoporosis, glaucoma, and cataract formation. Inhaled corticosteroids are generally free of these side effects, but may not be as useful in controlling COPD exacerbations. Studies are under way to determine their effectiveness.

OTHER DRUGS

Depending on a patient's symptoms, doctors can prescribe a number of other drugs as well. These include mucolytics, which help clear excess mucus from the lungs. These drugs are sometimes combined with guaifenesin, an expectorant that helps patients cough up mucus from the lungs. Diuretics, a form of blood pressure medication, can help reduce swelling in the extremities that may accompany the use of corticosteroids like prednisone. And some patients will receive digoxin, a drug used to treat heart failure or irregular heartbeat. This drug does not improve problems with cor pulmonale (enlarged right heart muscle and high blood pressure in the lungs), the most common heart trouble associated with COPD.

OXYGEN THERAPY

In advanced cases of COPD, supplemental oxygen can help patients live longer and more productive lives. For people with chronic hypoxemia (insufficient oxygen in the blood) and cor pulmonale, long-term oxygen therapy may extend life for five years or more. Oxygen is the only therapy that has been positively proven to slow the progression of advanced COPD.

The theory behind oxygen therapy is simple. Since the air we breathe is only about 21% oxygen, adding extra oxygen to the mix increases the amount available in the lungs. This allows people with damaged lungs to absorb more oxygen into the bloodstream, allowing body processes to proceed more smoothly. Studies even show that oxygen therapy can raise a person's IQ level several points over a year-long period.

People with mild or moderate cases of COPD do not generally need supplemental oxygen, although it may be used during exacerbations. The threshold for using oxygen is a blood-oxygen saturation level of less than 88%. This measurement is usually taken with a device called a pulse oximeter. The oximeter clips on a patient's finger or ear lobe and uses infrared light to measure the amount of oxygen in the bloodstream. Doctors also measure the pressure oxygen exerts in the bloodstream. Levels below 55 mm Hg usually indicate the need for oxygen therapy. Most people on oxygen therapy use a lightweight, plastic delivery tube called a nasal cannula. This tube leads from the oxygen source, wraps behind the ears, and has two small prongs that fit inside the nose. While it's the standard method of oxygen delivery, it does have drawbacks. The oxygen can cause dryness in the nose and the tube can become uncomfortable to wear after a period of time. In addition, many people dislike the appearance of the cannula.

In some cases, people can choose a different method: transtracheal oxygen. A small incision is made in the windpipe, allowing a permanent tube to be placed in the throat. This can be easily concealed with a shirt or scarf, although it must be carefully cleaned to avoid infection. The transtracheal system may deliver oxygen more efficiently than the cannula, since its direct connection to the windpipe may aid with breathing. In addition, there's some evidence that people with a transtracheal system are more likely to use oxygen continuously than those who use a nasal cannula.

Supplemental oxygen comes from three main sources. Tanks of compressed oxygen (oxygen bottles) can work for people who don't use oxygen all the time. But their size and weight, plus the need to replace them frequently, make the tanks inconvenient for active people. Liquid oxygen stores the gas in liquid form at a very low temperature. The oxygen returns to gaseous form as it warms. This system is lightweight and highly portable, and can be refilled from a larger, stationary unit. An oxygen concentrator draws oxygen from the surrounding air. It's useful for people who use oxygen while sleeping or while staying in one place for long periods of time. The main drawback is that it's a large and heavy unit; although concentrators can be used in cars, people cannot take them on trips where no power source is available.

Research shows that the more hours a person uses oxygen during each day, the more effective the treatment becomes. Recent improvements in oxygen systems make it possible for patients to remain on oxygen almost constantly, as opposed to when they are sleeping or sitting in the house.

MECHANICAL VENTILATION

When a patient suffers a bout of acute respiratory failure, it may be necessary to use a mechanical ventilator to deliver oxygen to the body. Mechanical ventilation is used when the patient is no longer able to do the work of breathing and needs help. This usually involves sedating the patient, placing a plastic tube in the windpipe, and using a machine called a ventilator to move air in and out of the lungs. In less severe cases, a less invasive form of respiratory support can be used, where a patient can wear a tight-fitting mask instead. Mechanical ventilation is usually used in cases where respiratory failure would otherwise lead to cessation of effective breathing, followed by death.

It's important to note that 90% of COPD patients survive episodes of acute respiratory failure—and the majority of people who go on a ventilator will be weaned off the machine after the crisis passes. In fact, one recent study has found that patients who use ventilation are not at a higher risk of dying in either the short term or long term than those who do not use it during acute flare-ups of COPD. It is important that patients remember this before telling the doctor that they don't want to be placed on "life support," of which a mechanical ventilator is one form.

LUNG TRANSPLANT SURGERY

In very rare cases, people with COPD may receive a transplanted lung from a deceased donor. Only a thousand to twelve hundred such transplants are done each year in the United States, mostly because of a lack of donors, prohibitive cost, and problems finding suitable recipients for the organs.

Most people who receive transplants are under 60 years of age and have few underlying health problems besides COPD. Because most surgeries replace only one lung (because of both the shortage of lungs and the increased risks of replacing both lungs), the patient must be free of lung infections that could spread to the new lung. Patients undergo exercise therapy before and after surgery, to strengthen the body's ability to accept the new lung.

Transplant surgery has a high success rate—as much as 90% after one year. But transplants are not seen as a large-scale solution to COPD, since few lungs are available and a small percentage of COPD patients are suitable recipients.

AAT REPLACEMENT THERAPY

A small percentage of people develop COPD because they lack alpha-1-antitrypsin, a protein that helps protect the lungs from the destructive effects of the enzyme elastase. Injections of AAT could help these people ward off COPD.

The procedure is still considered experimental; clinical trials are now under way to judge how effective AAT replacement therapy will be. The AAT is delivered intravenously on a weekly, twice-weekly, or monthly basis. Replacement therapy can cost twenty thousand to forty thousand dollars per year, although insurance sometimes covers the expense. More convenient inhaled sprays are now being tested to see if they can effectively replace the intravenous method.

Unfortunately, replacement therapy probably will help only those who are unable to produce AAT. Smoking has been shown to shut down AAT function in people without AAT deficiency, but there's no evidence that adding more of the protein will reverse this effect.

WHAT RESEARCH IS BEING DONE?

Even though it affects tens of millions of people in the United States alone, COPD remains a medical mystery. Researchers still don't understand why COPD attacks some smokers and not others, or why certain drugs are effective and others aren't. Although progress is being made to this end, many doctors are frustrated by the slow pace. Some experts believe that COPD receives less research attention than it should, mainly because the disease is viewed as largely untreatable and partly because it's caused by cigarette smoking, a known risk factor that people choose to continue despite the effects.

Research into COPD focuses on several key areas.

Genetics. AAT deficiency is a clear risk factor for COPD. But it's likely that some smokers carry additional genetic markers that make them more prone to develop the disease. For instance, it's believed that an unusual change in one gene causes overproduction of tumor necrosis factor, a protein that helps kill cancer growth but also leads to inflammation in the lungs. Another genetic marker, for production of the enzyme microsomal epoxide hydrolase, may be associated with a four-fold to five-fold increase in COPD and emphysema. Fortunately, advances in genetic research and engineering make more progress likely. This may help doctors identify high-risk smokers and help treat them before COPD sets in.

Smoking cessation. Nicotine replacement therapy has helped hundreds of thousands of people quit smoking. But nicotine itself may have harmful side effects in the body—especially in the heart. So research is focusing on ways to turn off the body's desire for nicotine altogether. This might be done by blocking the brain receptors that link with nicotine. Zyban is one step in this direction, although no one is sure exactly how it works. Other drugs being studied are different types of antidepressants, including nortriptyline.

Drugs. Bronchodilators do not cure or even stop the progression of COPD. But they can make breathing easier for people by opening the air passages in the lungs temporarily. While many bronchodilators are available now, research is under way to find drugs that work more effectively. One promising drug is tiotropium bromide, which may work for as long as seventy-two hours per dose. Clinical trials are now looking at how well people with COPD tolerate the drug.

Research also is looking at new drugs that may ease the chronic inflammation in COPD, or even shut down the action of neutrophil elastase and other chemicals in the body that work to break down tissue and damage lungs.

Tissue repair. It's not possible to fix alveoli in the lungs once they're destroyed by emphysema, nor may it ever be. But scientists have discovered at least one substance, retinoic acid, that has slowed the progress of lung deterioration in laboratory animals. Another chemical, called hepatocyte growth factor, is known to spur the creation of alveoli in human fetuses. It may be possible one day to teach adult bodies to respond to hepatocyte growth factor and start building new alveoli.

Lifestyle changes. Researchers are continually trying to fine-tune treatments for COPD. Exercise therapy and diet are both being studied for their effects on COPD. One recent analysis found that eating high amounts of certain types of fish may limit the damage caused by moderate cigarette smoking. The study followed Japanese-American men who ate diets high in fish that contained omega-3 fatty acids—cold-water fish like salmon, tuna, mackerel, cod, and herring. High levels of fish intake reduced the loss of FEV1 among smokers by as much as one-half. Heavy smoking (more than thirty cigarettes per day) tended to negate the effects of the fish intake, however.

Diets high in the antioxidant vitamins C and E also may blunt the effects of COPD, although no specific recommendations on intake have been created. And researchers are seeking to control malnutrition in COPD patients, a common problem in advanced cases. It's possible that anabolic steroids or other hormones may offer help someday. This would be an important finding, since nutritional supplements do not appear to ward off malnutrition once the disease has progressed.

Lung volume reduction surgery. Emphysema tends to cluster in the upper reaches of the lungs. When the alveoli there fail to deflate when exhaling, the rest of the lungs have less room to inhale fresh, oxygen-rich air. Experiments are now being done to see if removing these damaged sections will help the healthier portions of the lungs operate more efficiently. Lung volume reduction surgery is considered investigational, and is being studied by seventeen centers across the country as part of the National Emphysema Treatment Trial (NETT).

HOW IS IT PREVENTED?

Preventing COPD is as simple—and as monumentally difficult—as convincing people to stop smoking. Since 80 to 90% of all cases involve smokers, eliminating smoking would drastically reduce the number of people who develop the disease. This could save the nation a huge portion of the twenty-four billion dollars spent annually on health care for people with COPD.

Toward this end, a coalition of government agencies and physician organizations has created the National Lung Health Education Program (NLHEP). NLHEP reaches out to both doctors and patients to educate them about the dangers of smoking and the need for testing. The group's motto, "Test your lungs, know your numbers," encourages patients to become aware of their FEV1 and FEV1/FVC ratios. It also educates primary care physicians about the great benefits of regular screening and spirometry exams for their patients who smoke.

Spirometric tests give doctors a strong tool to help convince patients to stop smoking: the lung-age concept. Comparing a person's FEV1 reading to that of an average nonsmoker can show the patient how much smoking has "aged" his lungs. A 50-year-old male smoker with FEV1 readings equal to that of a non-smoking person of 75 years old gets a powerful message: that smoking has given him the lungs of an old man. About 11% of people who are given repeated spirometry tests stop smoking, a significantly higher number than those who do not. Lung age is used for comparative purposes only; there's no accurate way to link lung age with life expectancy, since countless other factors also come into play.

WHAT YOU CAN DO NOW

Patients who have been diagnosed with COPD need to remember this: They can live with the disease. It may take mental adjustments, lifestyle changes, and a few hard decisions, but the work will be worth it. Many people live for years with COPD, remaining active, productive, and happy all the while.

Here are some of the major issues patients will face in the years to come, and some possible solutions.

Fatigue and pacing. Many people with COPD tire easily, in part because they don't get regular exercise. Studies have shown that even mild exercise can increase oxygen intake and reduce fatigue. The best form of exercise is usually simple walking. Patients should start off slowly; if they can't walk for more than a minute or so before tiring, that's fine. Doing that several times a day will build up strength. It's best to increase the walking time gradually. It's okay for patients to find themselves short of breath, but they should not walk so much or so fast that they develop sore muscles or other problems. It might be useful and fun to keep a diary that tracks how often and how long the walks are each day, and keep notes about things like the weather and how the patient felt while exercising.

Exercise has benefits beyond gaining energy. It may help patients sleep better, lose weight (if necessary), ease anxiety and depression, and even handle the stress of quitting smoking.

Any number of other activities—from gardening to bowling to bicycling—are perfectly acceptable for people with COPD. Patients should always talk to their doctor before beginning an exercise routine.

Because people with COPD tend to tire easily, it pays to think ahead when facing a task. Make a list of things that need to be done, and try to be as efficient as possible. If a patient needs to do little things around the house, like get the mail, pick up the laundry, and turn on the television, try to do them in a circle—so that they can make a loop around the house and return to their seat or other resting place without having to continually go back and forth. Patients should always take a break when they feel tired—pushing will only cause more fatigue. It's best to plan so that they don't exert themselves right after meals. Patients might try to take their medication shortly before beginning tasks. The medicine may provide just the boost they need to finish the job.

Poor sleep. In some cases, people with COPD have more trouble feeding oxygen to their bodies while sleeping. This can lead to a shortage of oxygen in the bloodstream. Doctors aren't entirely sure why this happens, although people seem to breathe less when they're in rapid eye movement, or dream state, sleep. Again,

BREATHING EXERCISES FOR SHORTNESS OF BREATH

Dyspnea, or shortness of breath, is one of the hallmarks of COPD. Two breathing methods can help you cope.

Pursed-lip breathing. This allows you to exhale more fully, so there's more room in your lungs for fresh air. Start by relaxing your neck and shoulders. Then breathe in through your nose for about two seconds. Once you've finished inhaling, pucker your lips as if you were going to whistle. Then exhale slowly through your mouth for at least four seconds. With a little practice, you'll find it much easier to grab a full breath. Pursed-lip breathing is especially useful when you exercise or find yourself short of breath when climbing the stairs. You may get training from a specialist, such as a pulmonary nurse or a respiratory or physical therapist.

Abdominal breathing. This helps take the strain off your upper chest muscles, which work overtime in people with COPD. This method teaches you to use your diaphragm, the powerful muscle under your lungs that helps to take in and push out air. People with emphysema often lose the full use of their diaphragm because their lungs are overinflated, which pushes the diaphragm lower and keeps it from functioning.

Start by lying on your back in a comfortable position. Put one hand on your belly and one hand on your chest. Inhale slowly through your nose, and imagine that the air is being pulled into your lungs and into your abdomen. As you breathe in, you should feel the abdomen rise while the upper chest remains in the same position. When it's time to exhale, purse your lips, tighten your abdominal muscles and breathe out slowly. Push in and up with the hand that's on your belly. Again, you should feel the abdomen move while the upper chest remains in the same place.

Practice breathing this way until it becomes natural. Then try it while standing, then sitting, and finally while moving. It's the best way to breathe at all times.

regular exercise seems to help people sleep better. Talk to the doctor if sleep problems persist. Supplemental oxygen may help the patient get better rest.

Coping with supplemental oxygen. Oxygen therapy is a proven way to live longer in advanced cases of COPD. But it takes a little getting used to. Oxygen is not dangerous if used properly. Keep the oxygen supply tank at least five feet from electrical appliances, heaters, furnaces, stoves, and radiators. Avoid using vapor rubs, petroleum jellies, and aerosol sprays while the oxygen is turned on. These are very flammable. While oxygen itself doesn't burn, it can make other things burn more freely. So always keep oxygen supplies away from open flames. Never smoke while using oxygen.

Oxygen use takes a little planning when travelling. If flying, notify the airline ahead of time. Patients won't be able to bring their oxygen tank on board, but the airline can provide oxygen—usually for a fee. If riding in a car, open a window a bit and never allow anyone in the car to smoke. Public transportation (buses and trains) usually allows passengers to use their own oxygen on board; be sure to call and check before starting out on the trip. Finally, if the patient is going on a cruise, check with the cruise line at least four to six weeks ahead of time. A note from the doctor and a few other things might be required before they can take their oxygen on board.

Eating right. Most people with COPD lose weight as the disease progresses. The best way to deal with food is to eat a full and balanced diet. Don't limit intake of carbohydrates; they provide immediate energy and are vital to any diet. While it's true that digesting carbohydrates in large amounts may lead to a buildup of carbon dioxide in the blood, it's almost impossible to eat enough to cause any trouble.

• Drink lots of fluids. Drinking as much as a gallon of water per day can help make mucus thinner and easier to cough up.

• Take vitamin supplements. Supplements, particularly those that contain the antioxidant vitamins A, C, and E, are usually a good idea. A multivitamin once per day is probably enough, although some people may benefit from a higher dosage of vitamin C—as high as 500 to 1000 mg per day. This may help ward off chest colds and might even reduce bronchial spasms, although this is not proven. It's very important to talk to the doctor before taking vitamin supplements, because they may not react well with medications or other underlying health conditions.

If there is trouble with shortness of breath while eating, try switching to lighter meals. It's perfectly fine to eat smaller amounts more frequently—in fact, it may help the patient maintain a healthy weight more easily.

Sexual dysfunction. COPD can interfere with a person's sex life, but the reason is usually psychological and not physical. It's highly unlikely that sex will cause any problems. Still, it pays to take a few precautions. Try to use a bronchodilator shortly before sexual activity. If the patient is using supplemental oxygen, it's usually a good idea to keep it hooked up. And experiment a little with different sexual positions and techniques—some may prove less demanding than others. It's best to avoid trying to have sex when the patient has a chest infection, is especially tired, or has just finished a large meal.

Depression and anxiety. COPD can be difficult to handle emotionally, too. Depression is a frequent symptom of the disease. If a person with COPD feels blue, is having trouble eating or sleeping, or just feels overwhelmed, talking with a loved one or their doctor can be helpful. Professional or informal counseling can ease fears and help patients deal with anxiety. Many cities have COPD support groups, where people with COPD meet and talk with others about how they deal with the disease. It's comforting when they know they're not the only one having trouble.

End-of-life decisions. Although people routinely live for years with COPD, it's wise to make plans in case of serious complications. Most people with the disease have not talked with their family or doctor about whether they wish to be placed on a ventilator or other life support (see Mechanical Ventilation on p. 94), whether they want doctors to use heroic methods to revive them, or whether they wish to have food or water withheld when recovery becomes unlikely. While it's hard to think about these issues, it's even harder for family members to face them without being able to consult the person with the disease. The best way to handle things is to speak openly with the doctor about quality-of-life issues and the patient's prognosis. Patients can also work with an attorney or other professional to create advanced directives, durable powers of attorney, or living wills. These will clearly state the patient's desires, so that everyone knows ahead of time how end-of-life situations will play out. Keep in mind that patients can always change their mind about these issues as time passes.

COPD AND LUNG CANCER

COPD has been strongly linked to another serious smoking-related disease: lung cancer. Studies suggest that people who smoke and have an airflow obstruction are at the highest risk to develop lung cancer of any group. A landmark 1987 study compared data on lung cancer collected by the National Heart, Lung and Blood Institute and the Johns Hopkins Lung Cancer Project. All told, the study looked at 4395 men who had varying degrees of lung obstruction as measured by

FEV1. The average man in the study was about 62 years old, had smoked cigarettes for a total of about 60 pack-years, and had an FEV1 between 36 and 46% of that predicted for men his age.

The researchers compared the percentage of men with COPD who developed lung cancer with those who did not have COPD but developed lung cancer anyway. The result: People with any degree of airflow obstruction were six to seven times more likely to get lung cancer. About 4.2% of heavy smokers (61 or more pack-years) with COPD developed cancer—roughly ten times more than lighter smokers (40 or fewer pack-years) without COPD. This link between lung cancer and COPD has been confirmed in other studies as well.

Scientists do not fully understand the reason the two diseases often occur together. Both COPD and lung cancer tend to affect the upper half of the lungs, and most researchers believe the diseases both result from oxidative damage and/or cell destruction caused by the enzyme elastase. Lung cancer could be more prevalent in people with COPD because they are unable to clear cigarette smoke and the carcinogens it contains from their lungs as well as other smokers can.

Lung cancer screenings are not routinely performed in the United States. This policy resulted from studies in the 1970s that found that x-rays and other tests did not significantly improve survival rates for people with lung cancer. But doctors have revisited these studies in recent years, and some believe that screening smokers over the age of 45 every year could save fourteen thousand lives per year, a 10% drop in mortality from lung cancer. A study from Japan, where lung cancer screenings are encouraged, seems to confirm this belief. It found that the screenings detected lung cancers at earlier stages, when they could be more effectively treated. While only one of three Japanese lung cancer patients survived for five years or more before the screenings became routine, about six of ten now make it.

While doctors may be hesitant to screen for lung cancers, it may be wise to push for the tests. Some experts recommend the following: People over the age of 40 who have smoked at least 30 pack-years should have an annual screening. This is particularly important in people with an FEV1 that's less than 70% of predicted, or an FEV1/FVC ratio that's less than 70%. The screening should include a procedure called sputum cytology, where a sample of fluid from the lungs is tested for cancer cells or precancerous cells.

ADDITIONAL RESOURCES

WEB SITES

American Lung Association

www.lungusa.org

National Cancer Institute

www.nci.nih.gov

National Heart, Lung, and Blood Institute

www.nhlbi.nih.gov

National Lung Health Education Program

www.nlhep.org

BOOKS AND PAMPHLETS

Around the Clock with COPD. New York: American Lung Association.

COPD: Living with a Chronic Lung Condition. San Bruno, Calif: The Staywell Co.

Medical Health Annual. *Chronic Obstructive Pulmonary Disease: Insights and Advances.* Chicago: Encyclopedia Brittanica Inc., 1997.

Petty T. L., and L. M. Nett. *Enjoying Life with Chronic Obstructive Pulmonary Disease.* Cedar Grove, N. J.: Laennec Publishing, 1995.

Colorectal Cancer

In its early stages, colon cancer often has no symptoms, which is why screening for this disease is so important. But some common symptoms may point to abnormal bowel function.

- change in bowel habits: constipation; difficulty having a complete bowel movement; a change the appearance of stool; or diarrhea.
- red blood in the stool or black, tarry stool
- intermittent bleeding from the rectum
- frequent gas pains, or a constant "crampy" feeling
- urge to have a bowel movement even when it's not needed

If your family has been affected by colorectal cancer, or the fear of it, you're not alone: Colorectal cancer is the second leading cause of cancer deaths in the United States. This year, 130,000 Americans will find out that they have colorectal cancer; this year, too, an estimated 56,300 Americans will die from the disease, according to the American Cancer Society. Sobering statistics, indeed—and yet, *there is much good news*: Of all cancers, colon cancer is one of the most treatable and easiest to cure, if caught early. And thanks to the increasing awareness of this disease and emphasis on early screening, doctors are finding and treating colorectal cancer earlier than ever before, removing intestinal polyps (growths in the colon and rectum that can lead to cancer) before they have a chance to do any harm.

In the United States, almost certainly because of what we eat—the typical Western diet has too much fat and red meat, and not enough fruits and vegetables—colorectal cancer looms large on the list of diseases to worry about. In Asia, where the average diet is basically the opposite—not much meat, hardly any fat, and a lot more grains and vegetables—colorectal cancer is a much rarer phenomenon.

WHAT IS IT?

Colorectal cancer is an umbrella term used to describe cancer found in the colon (the large intestine) and in the rectum. (If there is cancer in the rectum, the doctor will probably still refer to it as colorectal cancer.) Many doctors use the words "bowel" and "intestine" interchangeably. By any name, colorectal cancer refers to a malignant tumor, the uncontrolled growth of abnormal cells lining the colon or rectum into surrounding healthy tissue and, potentially, into other sites in the body.

And what, exactly, is the colon? It's an impressive entity that takes up most of the abdomen, a large, coiled, muscular tube that, if stretched out, would be about six feet long. Briefly, the colon is the second-to-last stop of food's journey through the body; before it gets here, any food that is swallowed first must go through the esophagus to the stomach, and then to the small intestine. The colon is the body's final food-processing center, where salts and water are removed and absorbed. (Most other nutrients are absorbed before they reach the colon, in the stomach and small intestine.) Food enters the colon as mostly liquid, and leaves it as a mostly solid form (stool) traveling through the sigmoid (the S-shaped tail end of the colon) and on to the rectum. The rectum is a storehouse, the holding area from which, during defecation, food passes from the body (by way of the sphincter, or muscular door, in the anus).

Normally, stool should be solid or well formed, but not hard or rough, and the effort of passing it should not involve cramps or pain. Some people make several bowel movements a day; others have only three or four each week—and both of these extremes fall within the range of what's considered "normal." Thus, bowel habits in and of themselves are not nearly so important as any change in those habits that lasts for more than a few days and can't be explained by any other reason. (Sometimes this could signal colorectal cancer. If you notice such a change in yourself or a family member, talk to your doctor. For more specific warning signs, see "How Is It Diagnosed?")

Colorectal cancer begins, like all cancer, with tiny mutations in the genes—in this case, in the tissue lining the colon and rectum. In most people, these mutations take years to develop, and are most likely the result of decades of damage—most likely caused by diet. Although scientists aren't sure what foods definitely contribute to cancer and which definitely prevent it, at least one likely culprit is red meat.

Remember, scientists have honed in on diet as a major culprit in colorectal cancer because the disease is so much more common in Western countries than in Asia and Africa. However, among the things that still aren't understood is whether this cancer is caused by harmful foods that Westerners eat too much of—such as high-fat foods, red meats, and low-fiber processed foods—or stems from a lack of beneficial foods, such as vitamin- and fiber-rich fruits, vegetables, and grains, which we don't eat enough of.

One of the genes involved is called the APC gene, for adenomatous polyposis coli. This gene is a regulator, a checkpoint that controls cell growth. When it mutates and can't do its job anymore, at least two other genes are damaged as a result, and this is the start of a cascade of events that leads to rampant cell growth—in other words, cancer. In some families prone to colorectal cancer, this APC gene is damaged before birth. (More on this below, in "Who Is at Risk?")

POLYPS

The normal bowel is smooth on the inside, and pink. Polyps, mushroom-shaped growths that sprout inside the tissue lining the colon and rectum, are not normal, although not all of them are bad. The "good" ones are called hyperplastic polyps; they're usually small and lumpy—resembling a grape, or just the cap of the mushroom (without a stalk)—and they are benign; that is, they don't develop into cancer. The growths to worry about, called adenomatous polyps, are the ones with stalks. These don't have all the mutations they need—yet—to become cancerous, but they're well on their way, and should be removed immediately. The larger adenomatous polyps, those greater than half an inch in diameter, tend to bleed, and for purposes of early detection, this is good, because it's a helpful warning sign. In some people, cancer starts on the right side of the body, in some, the left. Right-sided lesions (your doctor may use this term and the word "cancer" interchangeably) tend to appear as cauliflower-shaped masses, and often bleed more than lesions on the left side of the body (and thus, are more likely to be detected by a fecal occult blood test—see "How Is It Diagnosed?"). Left-sided cancers, in contrast, often appear as "apple-core lesions," so named because of their appearance on a barium enema test, in which the colon is nearly obstructed by a wrap-around tumor that grows from both sides of the colon wall.

Smaller adenomatous polyps may not bleed, but they can be just as dangerous—and worse, may give no signal to announce their presence. Not all adenomatous polyps become malignant, or cancerous; in fact, many of them do not. However, there is currently no way to distinguish the adenomatous polyps that will remain benign from those that will become harmful.

Polyps grow slowly. It may take a minimum of five years for an adenomatous polyp to turn into a full-fledged, invasive tumor. This is plenty of time for detection with regular screening, and plenty of time to stop cancer before it starts. Removing these polyps is the best way to prevent colon cancer now. Other strategies for long-term prevention are discussed below.

WHO IS AT RISK?

Colorectal cancer doesn't discriminate; it cuts across both genders, affecting men and women equally. The average American has a 6% lifetime risk of developing the disease. What does this mean? For most people—about 90% of those who develop colorectal cancer—the risk goes from being very small before age 50 to becoming increasingly significant with each birthday thereafter. For most people, in fact, the biggest risk factor for cancer in the colon and rectum is age. Basically, the older you get, the more susceptible you are, although there are some dietary and lifestyle changes you can make now that may lower your odds of developing it (see "How Can It Be Prevented?").

GENETICS

Only about 10% of those who develop colorectal cancer are under age 50. Most of these people have a strong family history of the disease, one of the hereditary forms discussed below. However, it should be pointed out that not having a family history of colorectal cancer doesn't mean someone in your family hasn't had it. It may be that the polyps were not diagnosed, or that your older relatives died of other causes. Which, again, is why early screening is so important (see "What You Can Do Now").

Even if you don't have a strong family history, but someone in your immediate family has developed colorectal cancer, your own risk rises: Colorectal cancer in one first-degree relative (a parent, sibling, or child) increases your odds of developing the disease by three times. Colorectal cancer in two first-degree relatives means your risk is nine times greater. People who already have inflammatory bowel disease (especially ulcerative colitis) have a higher risk of developing colorectal cancer, too. Finally, if cancer just seems to run in your family, you may also be at increased risk. There is some evidence that a family history of certain cancers—particularly breast, ovarian, prostate, and uterine—means you may be more susceptible to colorectal cancer.

If you fall into one of these "higher-risk" categories, you should begin screening sooner, at age 40 (see "What You Can Do Now").

At highest risk are those with inherited forms of colorectal cancer. Cancer—any form of cancer—is a chain reaction, a "domino effect" that happens when one genetic mutation leads to another, and then another. Among the very earliest events is the downfall of the APC gene. This gene provides a genetic version of "quality control," and its job is to regulate cell growth. In most people who develop colon cancer, it takes years for this gene to go bad. If, as scientists suspect, every cheeseburger we eat strikes a small blow at the body's defenses against cancer, it takes decades for red meat and other harmful foods to chip away this gene's resistance. But some people are born with the deck stacked against them: They're born with a bum gene—a defective copy of APC—and for them, colorectal cancer is almost a certainty. The two main forms of hereditary colorectal cancer, familial adenomatous polyposis and hereditary nonpolyposis colorectal cancer, are described below.

Familial adenomatous polyposis

The diagnosis of familial adenomatous polyposis (FAP) is made when a gastroenterologist finds at least one hundred adenomatous polyps. In FAP, which can be inherited from either parent, the polyp-making process is on fast-forward, and the risk of developing colorectal cancer in those who inherit the bad gene is 100%. The best treatment for FAP is to remove the entire colon prophylactically—which means removing the colon before cancer necessitates doing the same thing. Many people live normal lives without a colon; they also have normal bowel movements (because the small intestine is connected directly to the rectum, and there is no need for a colostomy, or bag).

In FAP, polyps—hundreds or even thousands, too many to count and definitely too many to manage without surgery to remove the colon—carpet the colon and rectum. These polyps can manifest themselves as early as age 16, and colon cancer in people with FAP who are not screened and treated early is diagnosed, on average, at age 39. Polyps may appear elsewhere, too—in the stomach and duodenum (part of the small intestine). These polyps may also become cancerous. If one member of your family has FAP, it is not a certainty that you will develop it, too. However, the stakes here are so high that you should begin screening for colorectal cancer early, and vigilantly. The definition of FAP has been enlarged in recent years to include manifestations outside the colon and rectum. (Note: If someone in your family has been diagnosed with Gardner's or Turcot's syndrome, these are other inherited conditions that increase the risk of certain cancers, including the adenomatous polyps that can lead to colorectal cancer, and also require careful screening and follow-up care.) Because some of the same genes that protect against colorectal cancer also help prevent disease elsewhere in the body, people with FAP are often prone to other problems that may include benign growths in the bones and skull; subcutaneous (below the skin) cysts in the face, scalp, arms, and legs; and tumors in the pancreas, thyroid, and nasopharynx. A rare form of liver cancer called hepatoblastoma—which can be cured if caught early—also may develop in very young children.

If FAP runs in your family, your children should begin screening at age 10 with yearly flexible sigmoidoscopy (see "How Is It Diagnosed?"). If nothing abnormal is found, at age 25, this can be downgraded to every other year and at age 35, to every three years. If your children make it to age 50 with no sign of trouble, their risk of developing colorectal cancer drops significantly, to the level of the average American's. If you have FAP—even if you have already been treated for colorectal cancer—you should have a thorough physical and follow-up monitoring at least once a year.

Some families with FAP are being helped by an anti-inflammatory drug called sulindac (Clinoril), which has been found to shrink some polyps and get rid of others altogether. Sulindac—a drug in the same family of drugs as ibuprofen (Advil, Motrin)—shows promise as a means of reducing or preventing some of the other growths associated with FAP. (Note: Most people who take sulindac have few side effects; however, about 2% experience significant rectal bleeding, and some of these must discontinue the medication.) Celebrex (celecoxib) has been approved by the Food and Drug Administration for FAP families, as well. Another drug like it is rofecoxib (Vioxx), which is a viable alternative for patients who have sulfonamide allergies and cannot take celecoxib. However, although both of these drugs can shrink polyps, it is not yet clear whether either can prevent colorectal cancer.

Genetic testing. Genetic testing is available for FAP, and can spot mutations in an estimated 70 to 80% of families. Here's how it works: The process itself involves a simple blood test, starting with someone in your family known to have FAP. If the testing laboratory can detect a genetic mutation—an "index," or yardstick that it can use as it searches the DNA (genetic material) of other members of your family—then the rest of your family can be tested with nearly 100% accuracy. If the lab can't spot anything abnormal in the blood of this "index case," then the testing won't be helpful for your family. *Not finding a mutation doesn't mean that your family isn't at risk of FAP. It simply means that the testing technology is not yet sophisticated enough to pinpoint every mutation, because some are terribly subtle.* If no mutation is found, all family members should still be screened.

Hereditary nonpolyposis colorectal cancer

Like FAP, hereditary nonpolyposis colorectal cancer (HNPCC) can be inherited from either parent. Unlike FAP, however, HNPCC is characterized by only one or a very few cancerous sites in the colon or rectum. In this disease, the problem is with damage in one of six "mismatch repair" genes. These genes are like "spell-checkers," designed to fix tiny problems that crop up when cells replicate.

HNPCC is responsible for at least 5% of all cases of colorectal cancer, and the defective gene also makes people with HNPCC more susceptible to cancer elsewhere, including the stomach, liver, small intestine, kidney, ureters, ovaries, and endometrium. Because HNPCC causes colorectal cancer to develop at an earlier age, and because the interval between the development of a polyp and the point at which it becomes cancerous is shorter, if it runs in your family, you should begin screening at age 25 with a full colonoscopy every two years. A colonoscopy offers a better chance of earlier detection than a flexible sigmoidoscopy, because it offers a thorough examination of the colon, not just the lower end of it (see "How Is It Diagnosed?").

Genetic testing. Genetic testing is available for HNPCC, but it's less successful in finding the mutation—it finds nothing abnormal in about 50% of affected families. As with FAP, a person known to have HNPCC is tested first, usually the youngest person in the family who has had cancer. If the mutation is found—and the lab then knows what specifically to look for—then the rest of the family can be tested with 100% accuracy. Again, *not* finding the mutation doesn't mean that families are off the hook; all family members should still be screened every two years with colonoscopy.

HOW IS IT DIAGNOSED?

Too often, in its earliest and most curable stages colon cancer is "silent." It has no symptoms. There are no lumps to feel, no telltale warning signs so distinct that they can only point to one diagnosis. Instead, all of its symptoms can be attributed to other conditions, which is why screening for this disease is so important (see "What You Can Do Now"). Some people experience a change in bowel habits: constipation; difficulty having a complete bowel movement; a change in the way the stool looks—pencil-thin stool, for instance—or, conversely, diarrhea. If there is any change in normal bowel habits that lasts more than a few days and can't be explained by anything else, such as a bout of stomach flu, food poisoning, or reaction to medication, talk to your doctor.

Some people notice red blood in the stool or black tarry stool (darkened by the presence of blood), or bleeding from the rectum. There can be intermittent bleeding with colorectal cancer; therefore, even if the bleeding seems to clear up on its own, it is important to see a doctor and figure out what has caused the bowel to bleed. In some people, however, the bleeding is in such tiny amounts that it can't be seen without a special test (called an FOBT test; see below). Some people may experience frequent gas pains, or a constant "crampy" feeling, or the urge to have a bowel movement even when they don't need to.

SYMPTOMS OF COLORECTAL CANCER

- Any unexplained change in bowel habits that lasts more than a few days
- Constipation
- Difficulty having a complete bowel movement
- A change in the appearance of stool; particularly, pencil-thin and/or darkened stool
- Blood in the stool or rectal bleeding—even if the bleeding is intermittent
- Diarrhea
- Frequent gas pains or cramps
- The frequent urge to have a bowel movement, even when it isn't needed
- Unexplained weight loss
- Or, there may be no symptoms at all

In more advanced cancer, there may be abdominal pain, bowel obstruction or perforation (a tumor eating a hole through the bowel), a palpable mass, and unexplained weight loss. About 15% of people with colon cancer are diagnosed because they have one or more of these problems—most often, bowel obstruction.

TESTS TO DETECT COLORECTAL CANCER

Fecal occult blood test (FOBT)

The most painless way to spot colorectal cancer early is with a simple test, available in a kit (such as the Hemoccult Test) which can be purchased over-the-counter and used at home, that looks for hidden, or "occult," blood in the stool. One out of four people who have a positive test turn out to have either a precancerous or cancerous lesion. The good news is that, for those who do have cancer, it's almost always in the earliest stages and therefore easiest to cure. Thus, although the FOBT isn't the most sensitive test on its own (it's almost always accompanied by sigmoidoscopy), it does find cancers, and the ones it spots are usually the most curable.

Although some polyps bleed enough to be seen with the eye, others bleed in microscopic amounts. The fecal occult blood test, a low-tech card with windows on each side, can spot the tiniest traces of blood. If you are at average risk of developing colorectal cancer, you should begin having this yearly at age 50. People at higher risk should begin sooner, at age 40, and members of families prone to hereditary colon cancer should begin it at age 25.

It is best to avoid red meat and peroxidase-containing vegetables and fruits (broccoli, radishes, cauliflower, cantaloupe, turnips) for about three days before taking this test, and stop taking iron pills and vitamin C supplements: All of these can interfere with the results. Also, be aware that the tests finds blood in the stool—any blood. Its approach is "better safe than sorry." Thus, it is not able to distinguish between swallowed blood (if you have a nosebleed, for example, or bleeding gums) and colon cancer.

What you need to do. This test is designed to find blood in your stool. *If the stool falls into the water of the toilet, the blood may be washed away; also, any cleaner or chemical in the water can affect the test, creating a false positive.* To prevent this, place one or two pieces of plastic kitchen wrap around the toilet seat, and have the patient defecate on it. This will need to be repeated two times more over the next day or two, so you can give the doctor three sequential samples. Open the flap on the "patient side" of the card. Dip the wooden applicator (it looks like a Popsicle stick) in the center of the stool. (This may vary, depending on the doctor's instructions; some doctors want one sample from the outside of the stool, and another from the inside.) *If you see any blood, take the sample from there.* Then close the flap, and dispose of the stool and plastic wrap. (Although you can flush the stool as soon as you finish the test, *do not flush the plastic wrap*; it can clog your toilet.) The last step is to get this to the doctor, as directed. Finally, if you—like many patients—recoil at the idea of sending the doctor a stool sample, it may help to know that the doctor opens the other side of the card, applies chemicals to amplify any blood that may be present, and never even looks at the patient side (and thus, doesn't see the smear).

Flexible sigmoidoscopy

This is the "condensed version" of a colonoscopy. It's fairly quick (usually lasting about 20 minutes), does not require sedation or anesthesia, can be performed right in the doctor's office, and is the main screening test for colorectal cancer. The American Cancer Society recommends that people who are at average risk—that is, who do not have a family history of early colorectal cancer nor a personal history of specific diseases like inflammatory bowel disease which put them at higher than average risk—should undergo a "baseline" sigmoidoscopy at age 50, and repeat the procedure every five years afterward.

Sigmoidoscopy is performed with the patient lying on his left side. The sigmoidoscope—a flexible, lighted tube, as wide as a forefinger and about as long as an arm—is lubricated and inserted through the rectum. As its name suggests, the instrument examines the rectum and the sigmoid—the S-shaped part of the colon—and reaches a few inches beyond. The sophisticated scope (like a long, thin periscope) features a miniature video camera, which can photograph any abnormal findings. If the patient has any suspicious-looking tissue or polyps, the doctor will take a sample, called a biopsy, and send it to a pathologist for further study. (Note: Just because a biopsy is done doesn't automatically mean that the patient has cancer; many biopsies are found to be negative.) One drawback to the sigmoidoscope is its relatively short length. If even one polyp is found, the patient will need to have a full colonoscopy, so the doctor can do a more thorough exploration of the colon.

What you need to do. In order for the doctor to have the best chance of seeing any polyps, the colon must be clean. Depending on the doctor's specific instructions, the patient may be asked to flush the colon with two cleansing enemas, or to take a laxative, and not to eat or drink anything after midnight.

Risks. The risk of complications with sigmoidoscopy is extremely low—about one in twenty thousand. There is a minimal risk of infection with this (or any) procedure; there is also a very slight risk of bleeding, and of developing a tiny hole or rip (called a perforation) in the tissue lining the colon. This may heal by itself, or may require surgery. To minimize the risk of bleeding, the patient will also be asked not to take aspirin, or nonsteroidal anti-inflammatory drugs, like ibuprofen (Advil, Motrin), coumadin, or any blood-thinning drug (including vitamin E) for at least two or three days ahead of time. Avoid over-the-counter herbal remedies, if you haven't already discussed them with your doctor and received your doctor's approval to take them. (Talk to the doctor before skipping a dose or two of any medicine—even aspirin—to be sure this is safe.)

The most common reaction to sigmoidoscopy is discomfort from the air that's pumped into the colon (this makes more room for the scope and enlarges the field of vision, giving the doctor a better chance of spotting any abnormal growths). The patient may feel abdominal distension or cramps during the procedure, but the good news here is that this lasts only a short time and resolves immediately afterward, as soon as he begins to pass the excess air. Some people report feeling abdominal tenderness for a few hours after the procedure. Another common feeling during the procedure is the need to have a bowel movement. This is an illusion, because there's nothing in there but the sigmoidoscope, and it, too resolves as soon as the scope is removed.

Colonoscopy

This is the "gold standard" of colorectal cancer screening. The colonoscope looks much like the sigmoidoscope—except this flexible, lighted tube, equipped with its own tiny video camera, is more than twice as long, reaching nearly five feet, and is able to examine the entire colon. (Because there is a slightly higher risk of complications with colonoscopy, this procedure should only be performed by a board-certified or board-eligible gastroenterologist.) In colonoscopy, this scope is lubricated and inserted through the rectum; the procedure lasts about forty-five minutes and is done while the patient is lying on his left side. During this procedure, as with sigmoidoscopy, the doctor can insert a cutting tool through the tube and remove a tiny sample of tissue, called a biopsy. This tissue will be sent to a pathologist and examined for the presence of cancer. But the colonoscope is not just a tool for diagnosis; it's also an excellent, minimally invasive means of fixing problems. Not only can it biopsy a polyp, it can snare it (using a wire loop, threaded through the scope) and electrocauterize any remaining cells. Among other tasks, it can cauterize areas of bleeding, dilate a stricture (a narrowing caused by scar tissue), and inject medication (with very long needles) directly into the colon.

Colonoscopy is done with "conscious sedation"—the patient will be anesthetized, but awake the whole time, and probably won't remember later what happens during the procedure itself, even if the doctor explains every step and the patient maintains a steady conversation the whole time. A few minutes before the colonoscopy begins, the patient will be given an intravenous sedative such as diazepam (Valium) or midazolam (Versed), plus a narcotic (to anesthetize the colon) such as meperidine (Demerol) or fentanyl (Sublimaze) to make him feel drowsy. (Because this can hamper judgment and slow reflexes, plan on having someone drive the patient home afterward, or taking a taxi. Some hospitals, in fact, will cancel the procedure or perform it without sedation—which is definitely uncomfortable, and may be painful, especially for people with irritable bowel syndrome—if the patient does not have a ride home. In some rural areas, patients with no other means of getting home make plans to spend the night at a nearby hotel.)

As with sigmoidoscopy, air is pumped into the bowel. This makes more room for the colonoscope and enlarges the field of vision, giving the doctor a better chance of spotting any abnormal growths. Thus, the patient may feel abdominal distension or cramps during the procedure (it is this, more than the presence of the scope itself, that can be painful without anesthesia), but fortunately this lasts only a short time and resolves immediately afterward, as soon as the patient begins to pass the excess air. The patient will probably be asked to change position from time to time, as the scope makes its way through the bowel. The doctor may take x-rays during the procedure, as well.

The colonoscope itself should not hurt at all, although its presence in the intestine may give the patient the false sensation that he needs to have a bowel movement. This feeling will go away as soon as the instrument is removed.

What you need to do. It is essential that the bowel be as close to squeaky-clean as possible. For one reason, this will give the doctor the best chance of finding any abnormalities. For another, if electrocautery is needed to remove a polyp or stop it from bleeding, cleaner is just plain safer. Hygienically speaking, there is a world of difference between the colon-cleansers required for colonoscopy and those required for sigmoidoscopy. With enemas and laxatives, some vestiges of stool or lingering pockets of gas may linger—which is why few doctors attempt any form of electrocautery during sigmoidoscopy, because of the risk that these may ignite, explode, and injure tissue.

From the patient's standpoint, the biggest part of colonoscopy is the unpalatable job of preparing the colon for it—by drinking a four-quart jug of a bowel-cleansing solution, such as Go-Lytely or Colyte, which flushes everything out of the digestive tract from the top on down. And there's even preparation for this task (which is usually done the night before): At least two hours before the patient plans to start drinking the solution, don't eat any solid food. At least one hour before starting, if the patient regularly takes any evening medication, take it now—because if it's in the body for less than an hour, it won't be absorbed, and will be rinsed out along with everything else.

Although the manufacturers of these colon-cleansers have tried to make them as appealing as possible—new flavors include pineapple—the truth is that nobody would call these drinks a treat; in fact, they may make the patient feel nauseated. Many people have found it helpful to drink the solution when it is ice-cold. Submerge the jug in ice for a couple of hours before starting. The patient shouldn't try to drink it all at once. Drink just a few sips at a time, keeping the jug on ice or in the refrigerator in between sips.

A colon-cleanser called Fleet's Phospho-Soda involves a lot less drinking—it's only three ounces plus two glasses of water, instead of a gallon. However, it is not for everybody; people with certain medical conditions including heart disease and kidney problems, for example, should not take it. Ask your doctor if this is a good option for you or your loved one.

Risks. The risk of complications is very low—about one in one thousand, but it increases slightly if other procedures (such as removal of a polyp) are performed. About 1% of people experience some gastrointestinal bleeding (which manifests itself either as rectal bleeding, or blood in the stool) afterward. This may happen immediately, or you may notice blood several days later. Do not worry if there are trace amounts of blood in the stool; this is very common. However, if there is significant or persistent bleeding, call the doctor immediately: an emergency colonoscopy may be needed to find and cauterize the damaged tissue. Note: As with sigmoidoscopy, to keep the risk of bleeding to a minimum, for two or three days ahead of time the patient should not take aspirin, coumadin, or any blood-thinning drug (including vitamin E) or any other over-the-counter herbal remedies that haven't been discussed with the doctor. (Talk to the doctor before skipping a dose or two of any medicine—even aspirin—to be sure this is safe.) Finally, as with any procedure, there is a small risk of infection.

Barium enema

Barium is an opaque dye that is visible on an x-ray. In a barium enema, which shows the entire colon and rectum, defects in the lining of the bowel show up as silhouettes. To illustrate the difference between a barium enema and one of the above procedures involving a scope, imagine yourself making shadow pictures on the wall. The barium test shows only the shadows, which a doctor then must interpret; sigmoidoscopy and colonoscopy shed light on what's really making those shadows. A barium enema can show polyps, but it may miss small ones. Because this test depends on interpretation, a remnant of stool can sometimes be mistaken for a polyp. Another problem is that because the S-shaped sigmoid overlaps itself, it is often difficult to see exactly what's in there. For these reasons, most doctors do not feel a barium enema provides enough information; it should be accompanied at least by sigmoidoscopy. (Although if a cancerous polyp is then found in sigmoidoscopy, the patient will need a third procedure, colonoscopy, in order to remove it.)

What you need to do. Getting ready for a barium enema is much like the preparation for sigmoidoscopy. The patient will probably be asked to take a laxative the night before, and one or two enemas the morning of the procedure. During the procedure, barium is pumped into the colon through a soft tube inserted in the rectum. The patient will probably be asked to change position from time to time during the procedure; also, the doctor may press on the abdomen in an effort to move the barium further into the colon. As with the other tests, air is pumped into the bowel. This allows for clearer, more detailed x-rays, giving the doctor a better chance of spotting any abnormal growths. Thus, there may be feelings of abdominal distension or cramps, but fortunately this lasts only a short time and resolves immediately afterward, as soon as the patient begins to pass the excess air. The barium enema is a very safe procedure, with a one in one thousand risk of complications. There is a slight risk of a tear or tiny hole in the lining of the bowel or rectum (which may heal on its own or require cauterization to repair), and a slight risk of infection.

HOW IS IT TREATED?

The treatment of colorectal cancer depends entirely on its stage—the point at which it is caught, and the extent of the cancer. Many pathologists use a system called Dukes' classification for staging colorectal cancer, which assigns letter grades to tumors. It takes about four years for a tumor to progress from Stage A to Stage D. Fortunately, more than 85% of polyps diagnosed in people who are "asymptomatic" (who have no symptoms) are in the earliest, most curable stages, Dukes' A and B. (An alternative staging system, called TNM, is also widely used and is more common internationally, although many hospitals in the United States may use the two staging systems interchangeably. The "T" refers to the status of the tumor, the "N" to the extent of cancer cells' spread into surrounding lymph nodes, and the "M" to the degree of distant metastasis, or spread elsewhere in the body. Tumors are classified in stages of severity corresponding roughly to the Dukes stages.)

STAGE A

This is the easiest to treat and cure. Stage A cancer is a polyp only, confined to the cells lining the bowel. Treatment is performed at the time of diagnosis—removing the polyp (this is called a polypectomy) and cauterizing the site—so by the time the diagnosis is made, the cancer has already been removed. Follow-up monitoring may vary (depending on several factors including how many polyps were found, and whether they were cancerous or precancerous, for example). At minimum, the patient will need to undergo colonoscopy again in a year, and then every one to three years, depending on the physician and insurance company. Or, the doctor might be more conservative, and want to see the patient within a few months for a repeat colonoscopy—and in fact may inject India ink (a harmless dye) to mark the exact spot where the polyp used to be, to check for any residual cancer. In most cases, however, there isn't any cancer left; in fact, there's less than a 5% chance that further treatment would be needed.

STAGE B1

In stage B1, cancer is still confined to the bowel, but it has extended into the layers of tissue lining the colon. A polypectomy is not enough here, because it doesn't go deep enough. Treatment for B1 cancer is to remove the diseased portion of the bowel, but this is sometimes more complicated than it sounds, because of the plumbing—the blood supply—of the bowel. Imagine you wanted to plant a garden on a vacant lot in a neighborhood. The houses on either side are hooked up to the city's water supply, but there are no pipes running through your lot, and there's no way for you to connect to the water. Anything you planted on that lot would wither and die. Surgeons working with the bowel face a similar problem. The most meticulous surgery in the world won't work if the tissue will promptly die because blood can't get to it. Thus, there may be a small area of cancer, but the surgeon may have to take out a bigger piece, in order to hook up two good sections of bowel that have a working blood supply. (One benefit of the surgeon taking out more bowel is that more lymph nodes will be removed along with it. The more lymph nodes that are examined by pathologists and found not to have cancer, the greater the confidence that the cancer hasn't spread.)

Surgery to remove part of the bowel and reconnect the remaining parts is called an anastomosis. Studies have shown that side effects and complications from surgery (such as bowel perforation, an emergency condition in which stool leaks into and contaminates the peritoneum, the abdominal cavity, and could be fatal if not corrected immediately) go up significantly with every anastomosis. Thus, it is better for the surgeon to take out a large portion—even the entire left colon, or entire right colon—than to take out snippets here and there and turn the bowel into a patchwork quilt. Most patients who have large stretches of bowel removed do not require a permanent or temporary colostomy (a bag, worn outside the body, to collect stool—see below). Amazingly, the body can handle losing a large portion of the colon without any noticeable changes in bowel function.

After bowel surgery, it is very important to keep things moving, and avoid constipation. Keep bowel movements gentle with a stool softener such as Colace (docusate sodium) or fiber supplement such as Metamucil or Citrucel, if need be. Drink lots of water, exercise (which can promote healthier bowel movements), and eat plenty of fruits and vegetables. Note: Talk to your doctor first before you take a laxative or enema; both of these disrupt the normal functions of the bowel, and can irritate the intestinal lining. Worse, overuse of laxatives (or home remedies such as castor oil) can eventually make constipation worse, and make the patient dependent on outside help to move the bowels. For those with stomas (temporary or permanent openings from the end of the part of the colon not removed by surgery to the outside through the skin) consultation with an expert in stoma care (an enterostomal therapist—usually a nurse) is often very helpful. The care of the stoma and any changes in diet required because of the stoma can be discussed.

STAGE B2

In stage B2, cancer has penetrated not only the lining of the colon, but also the entire wall of the colon, and has spread into the abdomen. Treatment is primarily surgery, with adjuvant chemotherapy (discussed below). Sometimes, the cancer erodes a hole in the bowel wall, creating a perforation. This is a surgical emergency, because if stool leaks into the peritoneum (the abdominal cavity), it could cause massive infection, sepsis, and may even be fatal if not treated immediately. If there is a perforation, the surgeon will remove the damaged section of bowel, and insert a temporary or permanent colostomy (an external bag for stool; see below) to give the bowel a chance to heal.

If the cancer is in the rectum. Unlike the colon, the rectum has less of a "buffer zone" of muscle and tissue around it. Thus, it's easier for cancer to spread to nearby structures in the pelvis (including the bladder and, in men, the prostate). In order to determine the extent of the cancer, a transrectal ultrasound is needed—a painless imaging technique that can detect differences between cancerous and normal tissue by the way it sounds. As its name suggests, transrectal ultrasound uses a probe, inserted in the rectum.

The operation to remove cancer in the rectum varies, depending on where the cancer lies in the rectum. If it's in the upper and middle rectum, it may be possible for the surgeon to perform what's called a "sphincter-sparing" resection (also called a "low anterior" resection), in which the anal sphincter is preserved, allowing for normal defecation. If the cancer is in the lower part of the rectum, however, it may be necessary to remove the sphincter and surrounding tissue, resulting in a permanent colostomy (see below). If the rectal cancer is in stage A or B1, with minimal invasion of surrounding tissue, it may be possible for the surgeon to use a technique called "transanal excision." Operating through the anus, the surgeon pulls down the rectal wall, removes the bowel tissue around the tumor, and sews the remaining rectum back together.

STAGE C

In this stage, cancer has invaded the nearby lymph nodes. The treatment is to remove the cancerous portion of the colon, plus adjuvant chemotherapy (described below). Before surgery, the doctor will want to test the patient's levels of an enzyme called carcinoembryonic antigen (CEA), which is a tumor marker for colon cancer. If the level is very high, the doctor may suspect liver metastases (or spread to the liver), and may order a CT scan of the liver. (A CT, or computerized tomography, scan is a special set of x-rays that take very fine cross-sectional pictures) You may also need "liver function tests," which measure specific liver enzymes called alanine aminotransferase (ALT; also known as SGPT) and aspartate aminotransferase (AST; also known as SGOT) in the blood. (When the liver is injured or disrupted, these enzymes can leak into the bloodstream.) If the surgeon suspects that cancer has spread, the patient may undergo ultrasound testing during surgery.

STAGE D

Cancer is no longer confined to the colon or local lymph nodes in stage D; it has metastasized, or spread, to distant sites. Cancer in the lower rectum can spread to the liver or lungs; cancer that is higher in the colon typically spreads to the liver first, and then the lungs. Treatment depends on several factors, including the extent to which cancer has spread, and the patient's general health. About 20% of people who have "liver involvement"—cancer that has spread to the liver—have minimal cancer there. If there is just a single site of cancer, or cancer involving only one lobe of the liver that is small enough to be considered "resectable" (which means it's confined enough to be removed with surgery), then the cancer may still be cured with surgery and adjuvant chemotherapy (see below). With improved surgical techniques, the definition of "resectable" has become broader in recent years. Traditionally, the five-year survival for stage D cancer was 10%. However, this is improving, with more aggressive treatment, new and better chemotherapeutic drugs, and new uses of old drugs (see "Adjuvant Therapy" and "What Research Is Being Done?," below).

If you are in pain. There is often a vicious cycle with cancer, and it starts with pain: Your loved one is hurting. He doesn't eat. He loses weight. If there is depression, it gets worse. He may become bedridden. His body becomes weaker, and he's less able to fight off the cancer. So he hurts worse, and still doesn't eat—and so on.

The first step is to go after the pain. There is no reason for anyone with cancer to suffer from pain. If your loved one is hurting despite painkillers, then clearly, either your doctor isn't prescribing enough medication, or—perhaps in some noble attempt to be stoic, and not complain about how bad it is—the patient isn't taking enough. You're not alone. There are a lot of cancer patients out there who could be more comfortable than they are. If your loved one is suffering, talk to your doctor. If the patient is being seen by a group practice—where perhaps his pain is "falling through the cracks" because no one physician is looking after it—ask that one doctor be put in charge of his pain management. Or consider changing doctors. Try to find one who treats many cancer patients, and understands the particular, agonizing pain so many of them endure in the course of their illness.

Don't worry that if the patient takes more pain medication now, he'll become tolerant to it, and the "heavy-duty" medication won't be there later if the pain gets worse. With the strongest painkillers, such as morphine, the doctor can always increase the dosage to a level that provides better relief. You may want to contact the National Hospice Organization, which is dedicated to helping patients "carry on an alert, pain-free life and to manage other symptoms." If patients are prescribed narcotics such as Percocet, Vicodin, or Lortab, which contain acetaminophen (Tylenol), they should not take more than 4 grams of acetaminophen per day (amounting to approximately 2 extra-strength tablets 4 times per day). This is to prevent liver toxicity. To avoid side affects of acetaminophen—or if the pain is not being relieved—patients can ask their doctor for a prescription for the narcotic alone.

ADJUVANT THERAPY FOR STAGE B2, C, AND D CANCERS

Traditionally, colorectal cancer at any point past stage A has been what doctors call a "surgical disease." In other words, the best chance to cure the cancer is to cut it out of the body. But for as many as 40% of people with the higher stages of colorectal cancer—Dukes' B2 (particularly patients with vascular or lymph node involvement, and/or bowel perforation), C, and D—before they ever set foot in the doctor's office, before the diagnosis of cancer, before any treatment at all, the cancer has already escaped the local tumor site and made its way to one or more distant sites. It has done this silently, in bits so tiny—called micrometastases—that they're invisible even under the microscope.

How can this be? Cancer changes over time. It gets smarter, and it gets restless. It looks for new neighborhoods, and it travels by public transportation—the bloodstream. These micrometastases are undetectable by current means, although scientists are working on new ways to predict which cells will roam, and seeking better ways of attacking this invisible enemy.

Because right now there's no way to tell who has micrometastases and who doesn't, the best way to lower the odds that cancer may spread is simply to assume that it will, or that it already has. Which brings us to adjuvant chemotherapy before or after surgery and, for rectal cancer, preoperative radiation therapy. This is one of the most exciting areas of colorectal cancer research, and the two approaches described here are the proverbial tip of the iceberg. Over the next decade, advances may include targeted drug delivery—injecting cancer-killing drugs directly into the area of metastases (in the liver, for example)—new and better drugs, gene therapy, and immunotherapy. (For more on this, see "What Research Is Being Done?," below.)

Chemotherapy. Several drugs and drug combinations are currently being tested. One of the oldest and most successful is 5-fluorouracil (5FU). Colorectal cancer cells are most susceptible to this drug when they are dividing. Animal studies have suggested that the act of surgery to remove a tumor stimulates any cells that might be left behind, shifting them into a phase of active dividing—and making them particularly vulnerable to a chemical strike. But scientists have found that 5FU is even more effective when given in combination with another drug, most notably, folinic acid. The combination of these two drugs in recent trials has more than doubled the tumor response rates.

This chemotherapy is not pleasant, and is not without its own risks and side effects, which include nausea, vomiting, diarrhea, suppression of the immune system, hair loss, and mucositis or sloughing of the lining of the gastrointestinal tract—depending on the duration of the infusion. Thus, doctors don't take this step lightly. But the greater risks—of micrometastases setting up shop in the lungs, liver, or elsewhere, ticking away like tiny time bombs—and demonstrated benefits (a lower rate of cancer coming back, or recurring, and an improved rate of survival) make this a step worth taking in people who are healthy enough to withstand it. Recently, in three large phase III clinical trials (designed to test the effectiveness of new drugs versus older or established treatments), colorectal cancer patients were randomly assigned to one of two groups—either surgery alone, or surgery followed by 5FU and folinic acid. All of them have found improved three-year, disease-free survival rates in the groups receiving the adjuvant therapy—as much as a 30% decrease in the odds of dying of colorectal cancer.

Scientists are still working out the dosage of these drugs (which are administered intravenously), and the length of time they should be given; one recent North American study, for example, found that getting the chemotherapy for six months is just as good as getting it for twelve months, but it's a lot less expensive, and a lot better in terms of quality of life.

For rectal cancer, radiation therapy. For surgeons attempting to cure rectal cancer, the terrain of the region itself poses quite a few challenges. The good news is that about half of rectal cancer that recurs after surgery is in the local area. The tricky part is that the cancer is in other important organs in the pelvis. The scalpel can't attack all these cancer cells—but the radiation beam can. A Swedish Rectal Cancer Trial, of rectal radiation therapy administered before surgery, found a 61% decrease in local recurrence of cancer, and an improvement in overall survival. (Giving the radiation before, rather than after, surgery seems to be more successful, and to have fewer side effects.) Scientists are currently exploring whether the addition of 5FU makes tumor cells more vulnerable and increases the cancer-killing power of radiation.

COLOSTOMY

A colostomy is a surgically created opening in the abdominal wall that makes an alternative outlet for stool; it drains to a small plastic bag that's attached to the skin. For some people, a colostomy is temporary; it gives an injured or recovering colon a chance to heal. For others, it's permanent, and although it takes some getting used to, it doesn't have to slow people down or change their lives in any significant way. About fifteen thousand Americans are "ostomates," with one of several forms of ostomy. Many of them are young—people with bowel disease, or FAP, an inherited genetic disorder that causes colon cancer (see above)—and they have found that you can ski, dance, ride a horse, get pregnant and have a baby, even play professional-level sports with an ostomy.

Before we discuss the procedure, we should add that it is completely normal, and very common, for people to have doubts about their ability to function with a colostomy, and to be worried about their quality of life—body image, sexuality, even the mundane task of emptying the bag at work. Most hospitals have an enterostomal therapist and home health nurses who can help you or your loved one deal with these issues; there may be a local ostomy support group, as well.

In a colostomy, part of the colon is brought outside the abdominal wall through the hole made by the surgeon, and sewn in place; this outer ring is called the stoma. The procedure is performed using general anesthesia, and it requires several days of hospitalization. After surgery, the area around the stoma will be swollen, but the stoma itself should be pink or dark red. (The color shows the health of the tissue; the doctor will monitor it for several days—by shining a light inside it, or looking with an endoscope, a thin tube much like a sigmoidoscope—to make sure the tissue is healing, and to make sure that there is not a stricture, or narrowing caused by scar tissue.) Complications can include development of a stricture, or scar tissue, which may need treatment (it can be dilated during colonoscopy).

It may take several days for the bowel to begin functioning normally—for the muscle contractions involved in moving food down the intestinal tract to start working again. It will help if the patient resumes eating normal food as quickly as the doctor allows; this stimulates the colon. Once the normal digestive process resumes, the product that appears in the bag should look like normal stool. And, since the only thing that's different is where the stool comes out, if a person usually has trouble with constipation, he or she probably still will. (Using bulking agents like Metamucil or stool softeners like docusate sodium, eating a high-fiber diet, and drinking lots of water may help.)

WHAT RESEARCH IS BEING DONE?

Although much research in colorectal cancer is aimed at understanding the genetic processes that cause it, scientists are also working to find new ways to kill cancer that has escaped the colon and rectum.

Regional adjuvant therapy. A tiny bit of cancer has escaped into the liver. It's small—less than 3 mm wide—and small lesions like this are believed to be fed by the portal vein. Scientists are testing a targeted approach to chemotherapy—injecting 5FU (a drug used in adjuvant therapy, discussed above) directly into the liver through this portal vein (this is called portal vein infusion therapy) for five to seven days after the main cancer is removed from the colon or rectum. So far, this remains experimental therapy.

Another approach is to take out the metastasis, or spot of cancer, in the liver (as well as the main tumor), and then administer chemotherapy—this time through the hepatic artery. (Research suggests that over time, as a liver metastasis becomes more established, its blood supply comes from the hepatic artery instead of the portal vein.) In two small patient trials, this approach has had promising results: In one, one hundred fifty-six patients who had a liver metastasis removed were divided into two groups. One group received fluorodeoxyuridine (floxuridine or FUDR) and dexamethasone (Decadron) directly in the hepatic artery, plus systemic chemotherapy (5FU and folinic acid [leucovorin], given intravenously, so it affected the entire system). The other group received only the systemic chemotherapy. Both groups were treated for six months. The people who received the regional chemotherapy (directly in the liver) as well as the systemic medication did better, had a higher two-year survival rate, and were more likely to have a cancer-free liver.

In a similar study, people were divided into two groups—this time, those who received surgery to remove the liver metastasis, and those who received surgery plus regional and systemic chemotherapy. In this study, the people who received both forms of chemotherapy in addition to surgery had a significantly lower rate of recurrence.

New drugs on the horizon. Several new chemotherapy drugs are being tested—some in combination with 5FU, and some instead of it. Two of these will soon be tested in combination with 5FU and folinic acid: Oxaliplatin (not yet approved in the United States, but available abroad in the United Kingdom and France) works by interfering with the nucleus of cancer cells. Its main side effect is reversible numbness and tingling in the hands and feet. (The tingling stops when the course of treatment is over, or when the drug is discontinued.) Irinotecan (Camptosar), in early tests with 5FU and folinic acid, has been shown to improve survival in advanced disease better than 5FU and folinic acid alone. Oral fluoropyrimidines, now being tested against 5FU and folinic acid in two large studies, may be just as good as the drugs administered intravenously.

Immunotherapy. The idea here is to beef up the body's own immune system and strengthen its ability to fight off cancer. One form of immunotherapy being tested is called IgG2A; it's an anti-colorectal cancer antibody. It targets colorectal cancer cells, and encourages the body's disease-fighting cells nearby to kill them. (Basically, it's akin to someone standing in a crowd and saying, "That's the bad guy—get him!") It is being tested in patients with stage B and C colorectal cancer in several ways—as an alternative to surgery, and as adjuvant therapy—by itself, as well as combined with 5FU and folinic acid.

Gene therapy. Several strategies are being studied here. One of them uses a genetically altered virus. The virus invades the body, but only switches on in cancer cells, which it then destroys. Another benefit here is what scientists call a "bystander effect," in which not only the cancer cells, but the cells in the immediate vicinity are killed (similar to when a weed-killer kills the intended weed and a few blades of grass nearby as well)—yet the rest of the body is not harmed. This approach will soon be studied, in combination with other medications, in colorectal cancer patients with liver metastases.

HOW CAN IT BE PREVENTED?

For now, the best way to prevent colorectal cancer is to begin regular screening (see "What You Can Do Now," below) at age 50, or earlier if you are at higher risk of the disease, to find out if you have polyps—and have them removed immediately.

TAKE AN ASPIRIN A DAY

Another good means of prevention is probably sitting in your medicine cabinet already—aspirin. Just as aspirin may help prevent heart disease, it can also help protect the body against cancer. If you take an aspirin a day, starting now and for the rest of your life, you could cut your risk of developing colorectal cancer, and dying from it, in half. Note, however, that the use of aspirin and other nonsteroidal anti-inflammatory drugs (NSAIDs) is not recommended for everyone, despite the fact that aspirin and some other NSAIDs are available without a prescription. Aspirin and other NSAIDs can cause side effects that range from mild to serious, and can also worsen certain pre-existing medical conditions. Always consult your doctor before taking any NSAIDs.

Aspirin can be helpful in two ways: First, it inhibits certain enzymes involved in inflammation, which also play a key role in polyps and colon cancer, so it may stop polyps from forming. But another benefit of aspirin is that it inhibits platelets, which help the blood clot. It's a "blood-thinner," and encourages bleeding. Thus, it may make any polyps you do have more likely to bleed—and more likely to be detected—or may simply help by their effect on hormonal agents called prostaglandins. If this is the case, other drugs that inhibit prostaglandins, such as the COX-2 inhibitors discussed previously, may also be as effective as the more irritating aspirin—although this is still an active area of research and controversy. NSAIDs such as ibuprofen are also under study and may be less irritating to the stomachs of some patients.

GET YOUR FOLIC ACID

Folates, found in leafy green vegetables and orange juice (and in many multivitamins and folic acid supplements and fortified cereal) seem to protect the body against colorectal cancer. Evidence from the Physicians' Health Study and the Nurses' Health Study (large studies involving thousands of people, followed over many years) suggests that high levels of folate can reduce your risk by as much as 40%. Higher intakes of calcium have also been associated with a lower risk of colorectal cancer.

DON'T EAT MUCH RED MEAT

Although scientists still don't know exactly how red meat makes the body more susceptible to colorectal cancer, they're increasingly certain that it does. The

MAKE A FEW LIFESTYLE CHANGES

Cut alcohol consumption. Having a drink or less a day can reduce the risk; beer and ale have been linked to colorectal cancer.

Quit smoking. Smoking seems to raise the risk, as well. If you stop, you can reduce your chances of developing colorectal cancer by 20%.

Get regular, vigorous exercise. Over a long period of time, exercise can cut your risk of colon cancer by as much as 40%. Obesity also seems linked to an increased risk of colorectal cancer, although it is not clear whether this is an effect of a high-fat, low-fiber diet, or obesity as an independent risk factor.

Take a multivitamin. This one has no immediate effects, but over time, it can lower your risk. In the Nurses' Health Study, scientists found no noticeable drop in risk from taking a multivitamin for five years, but a 20% reduction after ten years, and a fourfold reduction after fifteen. Some researchers have also reported a reduction in risk of colorectal cancer for individuals taking dietary supplements of selenium.

Eat fiber anyway. For years, scientists believed fiber protected the body against colorectal cancer. This has turned out to be one of the classic disappointments in medical research: Five huge studies have not found the slightest suggestion of a link between fiber and colon cancer prevention. In the Health Professionals' Study, which has followed the health of fifty-four thousand physicians since 1986, scientists have found no difference in the rate of colon cancer between those who consumed the most fiber (an average 33 grams a day) and those who ate the least (about 14 grams a day). Still, fiber is good for the colon in other ways—namely, it promotes regularity and healthier bowel function. It lowers cholesterol, and if you're eating fiber, you're probably not eating as much of other foods that aren't so good for you.

Eat more fish. Fish is rich in polyunsaturated fatty acids, which some researchers believe are protective against malignancies.

Nurses' Health Study suggests there may be a threefold higher risk in people who eat red meat several times a week than in people who eat it less than twice a week.

WHAT YOU CAN DO NOW

In addition to the prevention measures described above, the best thing you can do is to be screened for colorectal cancer. How often, and what do you need? This depends on your risk (see "Who Is at Risk?").

If you are at average risk. Beginning at age 50, have a fecal occult blood test (FOBT) yearly, and a baseline flexible sigmoidoscopy, which should be repeated every three years. Or, if your insurance covers it, have a full colonoscopy every ten years

If you are at higher risk. Beginning at age 40, have an FOBT yearly and full colonoscopy every ten years

If you are at highest risk. If FAP runs in your family, your children should begin screening at age 10 with yearly flexible sigmoidoscopy. If nothing abnormal is found, at age 25, this can be downgraded to every other year, and at age 35, to every three years. If your children make it to age 50 with no sign of trouble, their risk of developing colorectal cancer drops significantly, to the level of the average American's. If you have FAP—even if you have already been treated for colorectal cancer—have a thorough physical and follow-up monitoring at least once a year

If HNPCC runs in your family. Begin screening at age 25 with a full colonoscopy every two years.

ADDITIONAL RESOURCES

WEB SITES

American Cancer Society, Colon and Rectum Cancer Resource Center
www.cancer.org

American Gastroenterological Association
www.gastro.org/public/digestinfo.html

National Cancer Institute
www.cancernet.nci.nih.gov

National Colorectal Cancer Research Alliance
www.nccra.org

Coronary Artery Disease

SIGNS & SYMPTOMS

Symptoms of a heart attack typically begin suddenly. The pain lasts longer than thirty minutes and is not relieved by rest or nitroglycerin. **When these symptoms arise, call 911 immediately**.

- Chest pain that is crushing, squeezing, vise-like, or heavy, like an elephant sitting on the chest
- Sweating
- Nausea
- Vomiting
- Weakness
- Dizziness
- Shortness of breath
- Extreme anxiety accompanied by a feeling of impending doom

Symptoms of early coronary artery disease are discussed within the chapter.

Coronary artery disease (CAD) is the single most common cause of death among both men and women in the United States. Many people mistakenly believe that breast cancer is the primary cause of death in women, but it is not—CAD is. About six million Americans have angina, and about 4.5 million have one of the major complications of CAD, heart failure or an abnormal heart rhythm. Every year in this country, about one million people have a heart attack and nearly half a million people die of CAD. Despite these frightening figures, the encouraging news is that the death rate from CAD has declined over the past forty years as the result of better measures to prevent heart attacks and improved treatment once a heart attack occurs.

WHAT IS IT?

Coronary artery disease is caused by a narrowing of one or more of the coronary arteries that supply blood to the heart. When an artery is narrowed enough (usually by 75% or more), the blood supply to the heart may be inadequate to meet its oxygen requirements. This condition is known as myocardial ischemia. Ischemia occurs most often when a narrowing does not allow blood flow to increase enough to meet the heart's need for a greater supply of oxygen during physical activity or emotional stress. Ischemia may be accompanied by chest discomfort known as angina. Conditions that limit the amount of oxygen carried in the blood, such as anemia, or speed the heart rate excessively, like an overactive thyroid gland (hyperthyroidism), can worsen angina. Ischemia may also be silent (especially in diabetes), and the discomfort of angina can be felt in the jaw, arms, abdomen, and back. Complete blockage of an artery in the heart, usually when a blood clot forms at a site where the artery is already narrowed, causes irreversible damage to the heart. This condition is called a heart attack or myocardial infarction.

CAD is caused by hardening of the arteries (atherosclerosis). The first signs of atherosclerosis are fatty streaks, slightly raised, yellowish areas on the surface of large arteries. Fatty streaks result when cholesterol from the blood accumulates in cells within the walls of arteries. The next, more advanced stage of the atherosclerotic process is the formation of plaques, which contain large amounts of fibrous tissue, as well as the cholesterol-laden cells. In the final stage, the plaque is covered by fibrous tissue and often contains deposits of calcium, which can be seen with imaging techniques. An artery becomes completely blocked when a break in the covering of the plaque exposes its interior to the blood and results in the formation of a blood clot.

WHO IS AT RISK?

Although everyone is at risk for CAD, certain inherited and lifestyle features, called risk factors, determine the likelihood that a person will develop CAD. These risk factors can be divided into modifiable factors, which you can change, and nonmodifiable factors, which you can't.

NONMODIFIABLE RISK FACTORS

If a first-degree relative (parent, sibling, or child) had CAD before the age of 55 if a man and before age 65 if a woman, this a risk factor. The risk of a clinical manifestation of CAD (for example, a heart attack) increases with age; about four out of five heart attacks occur after age 65. Compared with men, women are relatively protected from CAD before menopause, unless they smoke and take oral contraceptives. These two factors in combination increase the risk of premature CAD in women. The outcome of CAD is worse in younger women as compared with younger men.

MODIFIABLE RISK FACTORS

Smoking. Cancer is generally regarded as the greatest danger faced by smokers. But smoking, especially cigarettes, may also be the greatest risk factor for CAD. The risk increases with the number of cigarettes a day and the duration of smoking. Unlike the situation with lung cancer, the risk of CAD diminishes progressively after smoking cessation and reaches the level of a nonsmoker after about five years.

Cholesterol and triglyceride levels. Cholesterol and triglycerides, the two main blood fats or lipids, are combined with proteins to form complexes known as lipoproteins. Fasting blood always contains three lipoproteins, named very low density lipoprotein (VLDL), low-density

RISK FACTORS FOR CORONARY ARTERY DISEASE

Nonmodifiable:
- Family history of premature CAD
- Increasing age
- Male gender

Modifiable:
- Smoking
- Abnormal blood lipids
- Elevated LDL cholesterol
  - Low HDL cholesterol
  - Elevated triglycerides
- Elevated blood glucose
  - Impaired fasting glucose
  - Diabetes
- High blood pressure
- Obesity
- Sedentary lifestyle
- Elevated lipoprotein(a)
- Elevated homocysteine
- Elevated C-reactive protein

lipoprotein (LDL), and high-density lipoprotein (HDL). VLDL carries most of the blood triglycerides; LDL transports most of the cholesterol. LDL is associated with higher risk. Its oxidation, by highly reactive free radicals formed during the course of normal metabolism, promotes atherosclerosis because the oxidized LDL, along with its cholesterol, is then taken up by cells within the arterial walls. By contrast, HDL protects against atherosclerosis and CAD by removing cholesterol from the arterial wall and carrying it back to the liver for disposal. Thus, high levels of LDL and low levels of HDL are risk factors for CAD. Elevated blood triglycerides are also a risk factor. They are not only associated with low levels of HDL, but also with a type of LDL, called small dense LDL, that is an especially dangerous form of LDL.

Diabetes and impaired fasting glucose. Blood glucose levels below 109 milligrams per deciliter (mg/dL) are normal. Fasting glucose levels between 110 and 125 mg/dL are defined as impaired fasting glucose; diabetes mellitus is diagnosed when two or more fasting glucose levels are 126 mg/dL or higher. The risk of CAD is increased twofold in men and fourfold in women with diabetes. Premenopausal women with diabetes lose their relative protection against CAD. A number of studies have shown that people with impaired fasting glucose are also at increased risk for CAD.

High blood pressure. High blood pressure (hypertension), defined by blood pressures above 140 mm Hg systolic or 90 mm Hg diastolic, is a major risk factor for CAD, stroke, and kidney failure. Isolated systolic hypertension (high systolic pressure with normal diastolic pressure) is a common problem in the elderly and a significant risk factor for CAD. And studies have shown that mortality is reduced when systolic blood pressure is lowered in people with isolated systolic blood pressure. The National Institutes of Health have recently recommended the use of systolic blood pressure as the standard measure for the detection and treatment of hypertension, especially for middle-age and older adults.

Obesity. Obesity is now recognized as a major risk factor for CAD. In fact, it is a risk factor by itself and also contributes to CAD by complicating other risk factors, such as high blood pressure and diabetes. In addition, people who are obese are usually sedentary, another independent risk factor for CAD. A large study found no significant increase in CAD in overweight individuals, but the risk of CAD increased with greater amounts of obesity. Compared to control subjects of "normal" weight, CAD was twice as prevalent in the heaviest men and three times more prevalent in the most obese women.

Obesity is especially dangerous when excess fat accumulates within the abdomen. Abdominal obesity can be detected with a tape measure around the lower abdomen at the level of the top of the hip bones. A circumference of 40 inches or more in a man or 35 inches or more in a women has been defined as abdominal obesity. Abdominal obesity is associated with resistance to the action of insulin and a set of abnormalities, known as Syndrome X, and as the metabolic or hyperinsulinemic syndrome, which includes elevated insulin and triglyceride levels, low HDL cholesterol, high blod pressure, diabetes, and accelerated hardening of the arteries (atherosclerosis).

Sedentary lifestyle. Lack of exercise is recognized as an independent risk factor for CAD and one that is associated with other risk factors. Sedentary people are almost twice as likely to develop CAD as those who exercise. People who exercise are less overweight, and have better glucose control and lower blood pressure than those who do not.

OTHER RISK FACTORS

Several more recently recognized risk factors for CAD include lipoprotein(a), homocysteine, and C-reactive protein. High levels of lipoprotein(a) are thought to increase the risk of CAD by preventing the removal of clots that may form on atherosclerotic plaques. Strong evidence links elevated levels of homocysteine with an increased risk of coronary, cerebral, and peripheral vascular disease. Homocysteine levels tend to be higher in people who are deficient in two particular vitamins: folate and possibly vitamin B6.

An early study showed that higher levels of C-reactive protein, a "marker" of inflammation, are correlated with an increased risk of CAD events that occurred as much as six years later. We now know that inflammation plays an important role in the development of atherosclerosis. So, the findings in this study suggest that higher levels of C-reactive protein are the result of inflammation within arterial walls. This evidence of inflammation can serve as a predictor of later CAD events. Recent studies have verified that C-reactive protein, and other markers of inflammation, are elevated many years before the occurrence of a CAD event (heart attack, stroke). In an interesting new development, some studies have found an association between certain infectious agents, like viruses and bacteria, and atherosclerosis. This discovery has raised the possibility that atherosclerosis and its complications may be in part due to an infection. Studies are under way to determine whether antibiotics might protect against the development of atherosclerosis and its complications.

At the moment lipoprotein(a), homocysteine, and C-reactive protein measurements are best used to make decisions on whether to initiate aggressive preventive measures.

HOW IS IT PREVENTED?

Preventive measures can be broken down into those directed toward people without evidence of coronary artery disease (primary prevention) and those with known CAD (secondary prevention). Since the impact of risk factors is multiplied when more than one is present, preventive measures must address all risk factors. Primary prevention is discussed first to emphasize the advantage of preventing CAD over treating it. Secondary prevention is covered in a later section.

CIGARETTE SMOKING

The best way to prevent CAD is to stop smoking. Smoking cessation is difficult and many people stop smoking temporarily several times before they manage to quit permanently. Doctors and other health care providers (for example, nurses and pharmacists) have been asked to urge smokers to stop at the time of each patient encounter. (For information and guidance on how to quit smoking, see the section on smoking cessation in the Chronic Obstructive Pulmonary Disease chapter on p. 75.)

CHOLESTEROL AND TRIGLYCERIDE LEVELS

The National Cholesterol Education Program (NCEP) has recommended that dietary and drug measures to lower total and LDL cholesterol should be based on the combination of the number of risk factors and the level of LDL cholesterol. A cholesterol-lowering diet is recommended when LDL cholesterol exceeds 160 mg/dL, even in low-risk patients (one or no risk factors) or 130 mg/dL in those with two or more risk factors. For people who have known CAD, a cholesterol-lowering diet is started if the LDL exceeds 100 mg/dL.

The major components of a cholesterol-lowering diet are total fat less than 30% of total calories, saturated fats (e.g., butter, the fat in red meat) less than 10%

DO YOU NEED CHOLESTEROL MEDICATION?

NCEP Guidelines for Drug Treatment Based on LDL cholesterol

Risk status	Initiation level	Minimal goal
Low risk (men under 45, premenopausal women)*	> 220 mg/dL	< 190 mg/dL
Low risk (men over 45, postmenopausal women)	> 160 mg/dL	< 160 mg/dL
Two or more risks	> 130 mg/dL	< 130 mg/dL
Very high risk	> 100 mg/dL	< 100 mg/dL

* Optional

of total calories; and dietary cholesterol (found in eggs, for example) to less than 300 mg per day. About 10 to 15% of calories should come from monounsaturated fats. A serious try at following a low-fat, low-cholesterol diet should be made before beginning drug therapy unless the cholesterol levels are higher than 240 mg/dL. Such a diet is recommended even when drug therapy is prescribed. Recommendations for when to start drug treatment if targets are not reached by diet are shown in the sidebar above.

A group of drugs called statins are the most effective drugs to lower total and LDL cholesterol. Blood triglyceride levels above 200 mg/dL are considered elevated. Weight reduction, in addition to the dietary measures to lower cholesterol, is the best way to reduce triglyceride levels. Fibrates lower triglycerides more than any other drug. Lifestyle measures to raise HDL cholesterol include exercise, weight control, and smoking cessation. The most effective drug to raise HDL cholesterol is niacin, which also lowers LDL cholesterol and triglycerides. Statins and fibrates also raise HDL cholesterol by about 10%.

DIABETES

Although it is critical to control blood glucose levels in patients with diabetes to reduce the risks of kidney, eye, and nerve damage, blood glucose control has little to do with preventing CAD in people with diabetes. By contrast, several studies have clearly shown that controlling blood pressure and lowering LDL cholesterol reduces CAD events in patients with diabetes.

HIGH BLOOD PRESSURE

In general, the goal is to lower systolic pressures to less than 140 mm Hg and diastolic pressures to less than 90 mm Hg. Because of their greatly increased risk of CAD, target blood pressure readings in people with diabetes or renal disease are even lower: less than 130 mm Hg systolic and less than 85 mm Hg diastolic. For patients with high blood pressure, some lifestyle measures may help lower blood pressure without the need for medication:

- Get regular exercise
- Strive to lose weight, particularly in cases of upper body obesity
- Limit alcohol intake to no more than two drinks a day
- Restrict salt intake to less than 6 grams a day
- Quit smoking
- Increase potassium intake by eating fresh fruits and vegetables

When lifestyle changes are not sufficient to lower blood pressure, several different categories of drugs can be used to lower blood pressure. Diuretics, beta-blockers, ACE inhibitors, angiotensin II receptor blockers, calcium channel blockers, alpha-blockers, central and peripheral adrenergic antagonists, central alpha-agonists, and direct vasodilators are all popular and common choices, depending, of course, on how severe the condition is and the physical condition of the patient. ACE inhibitors are considered the drugs of choice in people with diabetes because they protect against kidney disease in addition to lowering blood pressure. There is some concern that diuretics and beta-blockers may lead to the development of type 2 diabetes. A March 2000 report in the *New England Journal of Medicine* described a six-year follow-up of 12,550 subjects, ages 45 to 64. Among the 3,804 participants taking a medication for hypertension, there was no increase in the development of type 2 diabetes in those taking a diuretic, ACE inhibitor, or calcium channel blocker. By contrast, the risk of developing diabetes was 28% greater in those taking a beta-blocker. The people with hypertension became diabetic twice as often as the people with normal blood pressure. In addition, a recent report described an increased incidence of heart failure and other cardiovascular problems in patients taking the alpha-blocker doxazosin for the treatment of hypertension.

Each type of antihypertensive medication works in a different manner, so drug combinations are often needed and effective in achieving desirable blood pressures.

And combinations of low doses of several drugs may control blood pressure with fewer side effects than with a large dose of a single medication.

Lipoprotein(a)

Except for niacin, cholesterol-lowering diets and drugs do not lower lipoprotein(a) levels. Estrogen replacement lowers lipoprotein(a) slightly in postmenopausal women. No studies have yet been done to determine whether lowering lipoprotein(a) helps to prevent CAD.

Homocysteine

Many studies have found that supplements of folate (and pyridoxine in some studies) lower homocysteine levels modestly. Most studies have shown that 0.4 mg of folate gives as great an effect as larger doses. It is recommended that 0.2 to 1 mg of vitamin B12 also be taken by people using folate supplements. This is done to avoid the danger of developing unrecognized pernicious anemia, a disorder of vitamin B12 absorption that causes anemia and irreversible nerve damage, because folate supplements can prevent the early warning signs of anemia. Most multi-vitamin pills contain appropriate amounts of folate and pyridoxine, but not vitamin B12. Folate has been added to breakfast cereals to prevent neural tube defects in the fetuses of pregnant women, as well as to lower blood homocysteine, but the amounts of folate in these products are too small to lower homocysteine levels adequately.

Homocysteine appears to be a marker for CAD but no studies have been completed yet to show whether lowering homocysteine levels helps to prevent cardiovascular disease. On the one hand, folate and B12 are safe, and taking a supplement is reasonable for those who are worried or know their homocysteine levels are high. On the other hand, they should not be used as a "silver bullet" in place of the more proven methods of reducing coronary heart disease, such as lowering one's LDL cholesterol, quitting smoking, and controlling blood pressure.

Hormone replacement

Estrogen has beneficial effects on total, LDL, and HDL cholesterol. It is one of the most potent agents for raising HDL cholesterol and also modestly reducing LDL cholesterol. Because it raises triglyceride levels, however, estrogen must be used with some caution by women with high triglyceride levels. Many studies have found that postmenopausal women who took estrogen alone had a highly significant reduction in their risk of CAD events, particularly if they had a history of CAD. But estrogen replacement increases the risk of uterine and breast cancer, so it should be used with caution. The risk of uterine cancer can be eliminated by taking estrogen along with progestational agent (which tends to lower HDL cholesterol).

Even though no studies had proven that estrogen prevented CAD, many doctors began to prescribe hormone replacement, either with estrogen alone or with the combination of estrogen and a progesterone in those menopausal women with a uterus. After all, they thought, estrogen diminishes or stops menopausal symptoms, helps to prevent osteoporosis, and might reduce the risk of CAD. Although some evidence indicates that long-term estrogen use increases the incidence of breast cancer, CAD is the main cause of death after menopause. In 1998, however, the National Heart, Lung and Blood Institute published the results of their important Heart and Estrogen/Progestin Replacement Study (the HERS trial). The results posed a major setback for the use of hormone replacement to prevent the recurrence of CAD events. This randomized clinical trial of postmenopausal women with known CAD placed half of the women on placebo and the other half on a combination of an estrogen (Premarin) and a progesterone (Provera) for an average period of 4.1 years. Hormone replacement reduced LDL cholesterol by an average of 11% and increased HDL cholesterol by 10%. Nevertheless, there was no overall difference in the rate of CAD events in the two groups.

It is too early to make definitive statements about hormone replacement therapy because more research is needed. However, the finding of the HERS trial that women on hormone replacement had more events in the first year, but fewer events in the last two years of the study, suggests that women should continue on their hormone replacement if they have been taking it for a few years or more. Recent guidelines from the American Heart Association recommend that estrogen plus a progestin should not be started in postmenopausal women after a heart attack, but women can continue with the hormone replacement if they were taking it at the time of a heart attack. Many physicians are still prescribing hormone replacement in postmenopausal women who have no history of CAD. Women deserve thorough information and advice on the benefits and risks of hormone replacement;

TIPS FOR PATIENTS AND CAREGIVERS

Take-home summary for patients

• Stop smoking. Quitting is a process that requires repeated attempts. Don't be disappointed if you fail after your first few attempts. Keep trying until you succeed.

• Become more active. Even minor increases in activity (parking the car farther away from the door when shopping, taking short walks) provide health benefits.

• Start with minor changes in your diet. Dietary changes are difficult but minor changes (more fruits and vegetables, smaller portions, water instead of soda) can have a big effect.

• If you are overweight, becoming more active and changing your diet are even more important. Do not put off losing weight because it is more difficult the older we get. Make slow and steady changes to achieve a goal of slow and permanent weight loss.

• Be religious about taking the medicines that your physician or nurse practitioner prescribes. These medicines cannot help you if you do not take them. Develop a system of cues that will help you remember your pills.

Take-home summary for caregivers

• Stop smoking. If you smoke, it will be even more difficult for your loved one to quit.

• Become more active. Exercise is more enjoyable when it is a shared activity. Take walks together.

• Makes changes in the family diet. If you are the person responsible for planning meals, shopping, and cooking, you have a great opportunity to help everyone in the family to improve their diet. Buy fewer chips and high-fat products. Make fruits available for snacks. Serve smaller portions.

• If you are overweight, changes to your diet and activity will be easier when they are shared with your loved one.

• Loved ones often want to help when the other has been diagnosed with a health problem. It is okay to help him or her remember pills or to eat fruit instead of dessert, but avoid taking responsibility for the other's behavior. Talk about your concerns. And most of all, avoid being critical if your loved one wants a hamburger!

the preferences of the patient are the most important factor in reaching a decision.

Another study casts doubt on the use of hormone replacement. The effect of hormone replacement was studied in three hundred and nine postmenopausal women with CAD (one or more coronary arteries narrowed by at least 30%). The diameter of the narrowing was measured before and after an average of 3.2 years of treatment with estrogen alone, estrogen plus a progestin, or a placebo. Despite major improvements in LDL and HDL cholesterol levels, there was no significant improvement in the progression of coronary atherosclerosis in the hormone-treated women.

The results of these two studies indicate that physicians need to be more thoughtful when considering hormone replacement to prevent CAD. The beneficial effects of estrogen on CAD for women without heart disease remain uncertain.

Antioxidants

Laboratory, animal, and population studies all suggest that antioxidants such as vitamins E and C, beta carotene, and selenium may prevent the development of CAD. The strongest epidemiologic evidence is for the possible benefits of vitamin E. But clinical trials have been disappointing. Three large controlled trials in the United States showed that beta-carotene supplements did not decrease the risk of developing CAD in people without CAD at the start of the study. Two large, five-year, controlled trials have found that vitamin E supplements did not reduce the incidence of coronary events in people with known CAD. It is still possible that long-term supplements of vitamin E may prevent the initial development of CAD, but this remains unproven.

HOW IS IT DIAGNOSED?

SIGNS AND SYMPTOMS

Angina

Angina refers to two types of chest discomfort due to CAD: stable and unstable angina. Because most people with angina have a characteristic set of symptoms, the most important initial step in making a diagnosis of angina is a careful evaluation of a patient's symptoms.

Stable angina. Stable angina is the most common form of angina. People with stable angina are at increased risk for a heart attack but may go on for many years with only chest discomfort associated with a predictable amount of physical exertion.

Patients use a variety of terms to describe their symptoms of angina: pressure, tightness, constriction, strangling, burning, suffocating, heaviness, aching, and even indigestion. The discomfort usually begins beneath the middle of the breastbone, sometimes in the upper abdomen, and often extends into the shoulders, lower jaw, and arms, most often the inner aspect of the left arm. Women and elders are now recognized as experiencing unusual types of angina. Common factors that initiate angina are exercise, strong emotions, and eating. Discomfort is often worse in the morning and when exercising in cold weather. Relatively minor arm movements like shaving, raking leaves, or mopping can trigger angina.

Anginal symptoms tend to come on gradually, reach a peak in a few minutes, and rarely last less than a minute or longer than twenty minutes. Relief is most often noted within five minutes with rest or the use of nitroglycerin placed under the tongue. Some people have a variant of angina that occurs at rest, often in the middle of the night, that is thought to be the result of spasm of either a healthy coronary artery or more often one already partly narrowed by an atherosclerotic plaque. Shortness of breath without pain can be another manifestation of myocardial ischemia. If a person should experience angina, the type of discomfort experienced and its location should be noted and watched for in the future.

Unstable angina. More serious than stable angina, unstable angina is intermediate in severity between stable angina and a myocardial infarction (heart attack). Like a myocardial infarction, unstable angina requires hospitalization and emergency treatment. Unstable angina commonly results from the rapid narrowing of a coronary artery due to the formation of a clot on top of an atherosclerotic plaque. The most recent information available, from 1996, indicated that unstable angina was responsible for more than a million hospitalizations each year in the United States. Between 6 and 8% of such patients have a nonfatal heart attack or die during the year following the diagnosis. Unstable angina has several distinctive features: pain may occur at rest and persist for more than twenty minutes, the angina may be a new occurrence that severely limits ordinary activity, or unstable angina may present as a change in pattern of stable angina that is more severe or frequent, or occurs with distinctly less exertion than in the past.

Heart attack or myocardial infarction

Symptoms of a heart attack typically begin suddenly with chest discomfort similar to angina, but more severe. The pain may be described as crushing, squeezing, vise-like, or heavy, like an elephant sitting on the chest. As with angina, pain is usually centered beneath the breastbone or upper abdomen and can extend to shoulders, arms, jaw, and back. The pain lasts longer than thirty minutes and is not relieved by rest or nitroglycerin.

Other frequent symptoms are sweating, nausea, vomiting, weakness, dizziness, shortness of breath, and extreme anxiety accompanied by a feeling of impending doom

It is important to note that not all persons experiencing a heart attack have the distinctive pattern of symptoms noted above. Many have "discomfort" that does not follow this classic pattern. Others experience symptoms that are uncomfortable but not so severe that they cannot "take it." Many of these people delay going to the hospital. But delay is a major problem because the sooner the symptomatic person gets to an Emergency Department, the sooner treatments like thrombolytics or angioplasty (both discussed below) can be administered.

Thrombolytic drugs are only effective when they are administered within the first few hours after symptoms occur. It is estimated that as many as 30% of people with a heart attack die suddenly, before they can benefit from any medical attention. By contrast, about an equal number of people, particularly older people and those with diabetes, have a painless heart attack that is only recognized later, during a routine electrocardiogram.

People are advised to chew a regular aspirin pill at the first sign of a heart attack. (An exception would be those who have severe allergies to aspirin.)

LABORATORY TESTS AND FINDINGS

Electrocardiogram

An electrocardiogram (ECG) detects the electrical impulses from the heart by means of small electrodes placed on the skin of the extremities and chest. An ECG is the first test used in an effort to make the diagnosis of either angina or a heart attack. Many people with stable angina have a normal ECG because the blood supply to their heart is adequate while they are at rest—they need to have an ECG during some form of stress that increases the heart's requirement for blood. Continuous (Holter) monitoring of the ECG can detect episodes of painless myocardial ischemia that occur during the course of a normal day. An ECG can also detect areas of damaged heart muscle caused by a previous myocardial infarction that may have gone unrecognized. Diagnostic changes in the ECG are present more often, but not always, during an acute myocardial infarction. The ECG is also useful for detecting abnormal heart rhythms that may complicate a heart attack.

Stress tests

Stress tests are done to diagnose CAD in several different situations:

- When CAD is strongly suspected as the cause of chest pain or shortness of breath even though the resting ECG is normal;
- In people at high risk despite the absence of symptoms of CAD;
- To determine cardiovascular fitness before a sedentary older person begins a strenuous exercise program.

Stress tests are not recommended in most young people who have no symptoms, because test results are falsely positive in about 20% of men under age 40 and in women under 50. False-positive tests often lead to unnecessary further tests, including invasive coronary angiography.

The risk of a stress test is small; possibly one in ten thousand patients may have a heart attack or die. A cardiologist and emergency drugs and equipment are always available during the test to provide immediate help should a serious complication arise. The risk is somewhat greater when exercise stress tests are done in many patients before hospital discharge following admission for unstable angina or a heart attack.

Standard exercise stress test. In this test an ECG is recorded while the person either walks on a treadmill or pedals a stationary bicycle in order to increase the work of the heart and its requirement for oxygen. During the test a slow increase in the angle of the treadmill and its speed, or greater resistance to pedaling, further raise the work of the heart and its need for oxygen. Myocardial ischemia, detected on the ECG tracing, is evidence of CAD and is considered an abnormal test. The test is especially meaningful if an individual experiences his typical symptoms at the time when the ECG is abnormal. The test is stopped if an ischemic pattern appears on the ECG; the patient complains of chest pain, shortness of breath, or fatigue; or the blood pressure falls or rises too much. Otherwise the test is continued with an effort to reach the maximal heart rate recommended for the individual's age. The test results may not be considered adequate if this heart rate is not achieved. A lower heart rate target (submaximal exercise test) is often chosen in patients about to go home after hospitalization for unstable angina or a heart attack.

Failure to detect CAD when it is present, that is, a false-negative test, occurs in about 15 to 20% of tests. A false-negative test is less likely when the ECG readings are accompanied by ultrasound measurements to detect abnormal motion of the left ventricular wall.

Nuclear stress test. This test involves monitoring and ECG during exercise and injecting a small amount of radioactive thallium into a blood vessel after the exercise is completed. Over a period of several hours the uptake of thallium by the myocardium is determined with a radioactive detector placed on the chest. Thallium is distributed uniformly throughout a normal heart, whereas an area of poor uptake indicates either ischemia due to CAD or heart damage from a prior heart attack. The two can be distinguished by a second injection of thallium following the clearance of radioactivity from the first dose. Persistence of the defect in thallium uptake long after the exercise indicates prior tissue damage rather than ischemia. The thallium stress test is not only more accurate than the standard exercise test in detecting CAD, but also adds information regarding the location of the ischemia and its extent. The small amount of injected radioactive material is not dangerous.

Because thallium tests are more expensive than the standard exercise test, they are usually done when strong suspicion of CAD persists despite a normal exercise test.

Dobutamine test

This test uses ultrasound to measure movements of the wall of the left ventricle (the most powerful contracting chamber of the heart) after the heart rate is temporarily increased by an injection of the drug dobutamine. Abnormalities of wall motion prior to the injection of the drug indicate a scar from prior heart damage. Evidence for CAD and ischemia is based on abnormal wall motion that appears only with the rapid heart rate induced by the dobutamine. The test is especially safe since there is only a short period of increased heart rate.

Ultrafast computed tomography

Ultrafast computed tomography (CT) scans detect the presence of calcium within the heart. Because atherosclerotic plaques can accumulate calcium, this test is an indirect measure of the extent of plaque formation within the coronary arteries. The amount of calcium, reported as the calcium score, undoubtedly increases as more plaques develop within the coronary arteries. However, small plaques, which are more likely to rupture and cause a heart attack, may contain little calcium, whereas larger plaques may be loaded with calcium and yet pose only a small risk of leading to a heart attack. Widespread publicity regarding ultrafast CT has led to a large number of people obtaining such tests. A low calcium score is certainly reassuring, and the risk is greater with a high calcium score. It is too soon, however, to know how well either a low or a high calcium score will predict the risk of a subsequent heart attack. Until this question is answered with ongoing studies, it makes sense to include the calcium score as yet another one of the factors used to consider how aggressive the individual and doctor should be in addressing the various risk factors.

Coronary angiography

Coronary angiography is carried out either after a heart attack or when an ECG or stress test suggests CAD. The procedure is usually done in a hospital catheterization laboratory, but may not require hospitalization. It involves the insertion of a catheter through a small incision in an artery in the groin. The catheter is threaded into one of the coronary arteries and contrast material is injected. X-rays show the location of the contrast dye and thus outline the arterial channels for blood flow. Coronary angiography takes about two hours, but pressure must be placed on the groin for six to eight hours after the procedure while the patient is in bed to avoid bleeding from the artery in the groin. Patients are typically awake for the procedure so that they can follow directions from the doctor. The procedure may be uncomfortable but patients rarely call it painful.

An angiogram is presently the best available technique to show narrowings of coronary arteries by atherosclerotic plaques. Its main use is to decide the need for coronary artery bypass or percutaneous transluminal coronary angioplasty. Indeed, patients are informed that angioplasty will be done, if indicated, at the time of catheterization. Angiography underestimates the amount of atherosclerosis because it only detects plaques that produce significant narrowing of the channels for blood flow. In addition, it is difficult to predict the risk of a heart attack since the smaller plaques are even more likely than the larger ones to rupture and lead to a blood clot that completely blocks an artery. Angiography is an invasive procedure that is associated with greater risk than stress tests either due to injury to an artery by the catheter or side effects from the contrast material.

Nuclear magnetic resonance

Advances in nuclear magnetic resonance (NMR) technology have enabled doctors to obtain images of the coronary arteries without the risks or inconvenience of coronary angiography. Thus far, the images are only satisfactory in about 60% of patients and the pictures are not as sharp as those obtained with angiography. It seems possible that further advances in the future will allow NMR to replace angiography in many patients.

Blood tests for heart attack

ECG abnormalities are the underpinning of the diagnosis of myocardial infarction, but in many cases the ECG is not diagnostic. In fact, even now, fewer than 30% of patients admitted to a coronary care unit are found to have a myocardial infarction although they were suspected of having a heart attack when admitted. The diagnosis can be made in the absence of characteristic ECG changes, and the extent of myocardial damage can be estimated by measuring blood levels of proteins that escape through the leaky membranes of injured heart muscle cells.

A widely used enzyme test for myocardial infarction is creatine kinase (CK). Large amounts of this enzyme are also found in skeletal muscle and the brain, but special methods allow measurement of the blood levels of the enzyme released from damaged heart tissue. Elevated blood levels can be detected after four hours, reach a maximum at about twelve hours, and then decline by the end of twenty-four hours. A newer test measures blood levels of troponin, a protein present in both skeletal and cardiac muscle. Troponin from the heart differs from the protein found in muscles so that specific tests can detect its release from the heart. Like

CK, troponin levels can be detected within about four hours after a heart attack. They reach their peak level in about twelve hours and then persist for several days. The level of these proteins correlates with the extent of heart muscle damage. A number of emergency departments are now equipped with bedside tests for troponin to make a rapid diagnosis of a heart attack. In many hospitals both CK and troponin levels are measured repeatedly during the period immediately following a suspected heart attack.

HOW IS IT TREATED?

STABLE ANGINA

Nitrogylcerin

Placement of a nitroglycerin tablet under the tongue (sublingual nitroglycerin) has been the tried and true treatment for anginal pain for over a century. Nitroglycerin and the other longer-acting nitrates work by widening veins in the extremities, thus decreasing the work of the heart by reducing the amount of blood returning to it, and by widening the coronary arteries. Another important role for sublingual nitroglycerin is the prevention of angina when taken shortly before exertion (but not sex because it may inhibit erection) or anticipated emotional stress. Nitroglycerin usually brings dramatic relief of pain within one to two minutes, and complete pain relief in five minutes, lasting for about thirty minutes. Should pain continue, the doctor should be called or the patient should go to an emergency room to rule out unstable angina or a heart attack. Patients with regular angina should keep nitroglycerin with them at all times. Keep another bottle at the bedside, and possibly one in the kitchen, but remember that the tablets are easily inactivated by heat or simply time. Their potency is best maintained by storage in a tightly stoppered, dark glass vial in a dry cool place. Even then it is necessary to get frequent small refills, at least every six months, to ensure the drug will work. The most common side effect is a headache. If the pills do not stop the discomfort, and they fail to produce any headache or at least a slight tingling under the tongue, they may no longer be active.

Nitrates

Longer-acting nitrate products include isosorbide dinitrate (Isordil and others) and isosorbide mononitrate (Imdur and others) pills as well as patches and ointments containing nitroglycerin. Although these pills do not relieve acute angina as quickly as sublingual nitroglycerin, they can protect against angina for as long as six hours and can be taken four to five times a day. Long relief of angina may also be obtained from the slow release of nitroglycerin from patches applied to the skin or by spreading a thin layer of a nitroglycerin ointment over the chest or arm. Long-acting nitrates can be supplemented with sublingual nitroglycerin when necessary. Since the effects of the long-acting nitrates tend to wear off when used continuously, an eight-hour period free from the drugs is recommended every day. Patients should remove patches or wipe off ointment, usually at bedtime, and take the last dose of Isordil in the afternoon.

Beta-blockers and calcium channel blockers

Beta-blockers are effective in relieving angina by slowing heart rate and reducing blood pressure, especially during exercise. Thus, they improve exercise tolerance by reducing the heart's requirement for oxygen. Possible side effects include fatigue, insomnia, erectile dysfunction (impotence), and an excessively slow heart rate. Beta-blockers should never be stopped abruptly because of the risk of causing unstable angina or a heart attack.

Calcium channel blockers can also reduce the workload of the heart and improve angina; calcium channel blockers can be used in combination with beta blockers. Some of the short-acting calcium channel blockers should be avoided because they may increase the risk of cardiovascular events. One of the more common side effects of calcium channel blockers is swelling of the feet due to fluid retention. Calcium channel blockers can slow or increase the heart rate, and constipation can be a problem with some.

Revascularization procedures

Revascularization procedures—coronary artery bypass surgery or percutaneous transluminal angioplasty—may be needed when medications do not control symptoms of angina.

Coronary artery bypass surgery (CABG). This surgery uses veins removed from a leg (venous graft) or the left internal mammary artery (LIMA graft) in the chest to carry blood around a narrowed segment of one or more coronary arteries. The procedure is done under general anesthesia while the heart is connected to a heart-lung machine that circulates blood to the rest of the body during the several hours when the heart is stopped to allow the surgeon to carry out the bypass. Venous grafts are started with the removal of a portion of a leg vein. One end of the graft is sewn into the aorta near the heart; the other end is attached to the obstructed coronary artery at a site past the blockage. Another conduit used is an internal mammary artery. The internal mammary artery is attached to a coronary artery at a point beyond the occlusion. Long-term results are better with a LIMA graft, which is less likely than a venous graft to become blocked by atherosclerosis.

More than 90% of patients experience dramatic or complete relief of symptoms after a CABG. Even though the grafts may become partly or totally blocked, the improvement in angina generally persists for at least ten years in arteries bypassed with a venous graft and possibly twice as long for a LIMA graft. CABG has been shown to improve survival when a blockage affects the left main coronary artery or when three or more arteries are occluded. Survival benefits are unclear when only two vessels are bypassed, and bypass of one coronary artery does not improve long-term survival.

Complications of bypass surgery include infections at the surgical sites, a heart attack in 3 to 5% of patients, and stroke, memory loss, or other neurological symptoms in about 6% of patients. About 1% of patients die as the result of an elective bypass; the mortality is higher for emergency procedures. In general, women have fewer acute complications of CABG than men but poorer long-term benefit.

Patients remain on a heart monitor in a cardiac intensive care unit for one to two days after the operation and can leave the hospital in four to seven days if there are no complications. Activity is gradually increased during the first two weeks after coming home. People with sedentary occupations can usually return to work after six to eight weeks, but up to three months of recuperation may be needed before going back to a job requiring heavy physical labor.

Some patients may be given the impression that a CABG has cured their CAD, so it is no longer necessary to follow preventive measures. Nothing could be further from the truth. Rather, it is important to recognize that after the operation atherosclerosis continues to develop in both the native coronary arteries and the bypass grafts. Studies have shown that lifestyle measures and medications can slow the progression of atherosclerotic plaques and delay the need for further revascularization procedures.

Percutaneous transluminal coronary angioplasty (PTCA). This procedure takes about an hour and is carried out in a cardiac catheterization laboratory, often at the same time as a diagnostic coronary angiography. It typically requires no more than an overnight stay. The patient is given a sedative and a local anesthetic to the groin, where a small incision is made in order to introduce a catheter with a balloon at its tip. Using x-ray images on a screen, the catheter is advanced into a coronary artery until the balloon is in the center of the obstructed area. The balloon is then inflated several times for as long as several minutes to widen the artery by squeezing the plaque against the arterial wall. Often a stent is placed to keep the artery open.

Nearly 90% of patients note immediate relief of anginal symptoms after angioplasty. One of the major problems of the procedure, however, had been clot formation and reobstruction of the artery at the angioplasty site in about 30% of patients in the three months after the procedure. Often the artery could be reopened with a second angioplasty. But today, the frequency of reobstruction has been significantly reduced by propping the artery open with a permanent mechanical device (stent) inserted at the time of angioplasty through a catheter at the site widened by the balloon. Administration of an antibody or synthetic compound (both called platelet IIb/IIIa receptor blockers) that binds to a receptor on the surface of platelets may prevent them from clumping and initiating the formation of a blood clot. Patients may continue on an oral antiplatelet agent afterward.

In one clinical study, people with diabetes been shown to have a poorer outcome from angioplasty than those who were not diabetic. Because outcomes were the same in the two groups after bypass surgery, a CABG is probably preferable to angioplasty in diabetics.

Lifestyle modification is extremely important after angioplasty. Just like with a CABG, patients often get the impression that the CAD is "cured" but again, this is not true. Smoking cessation, exercise, lipid lowering through diet and medications, blood pressure control, and weight loss are essential if the angioplasty is to last over several years.

Angioplasty is a relatively safe procedure, especially in the hands of cardiologists who have extensive experience with the procedure. The mortality is less than 1% and a myocardial infarction complicates closure of the artery in 2 to 5% of cases. Closure of an artery or a tear in its wall may require emergency bypass surgery in 1 to 2% of cases. Because of this possible need for an emergency bypass procedure, a surgical team must be available and angioplasty is only performed in hospitals equipped to do bypass surgery.

Transmyocardial laser revascularization and gene implantation. Here, a laser beam is used to form channels from the chamber of the left ventricle into the left ventricular muscle in patients whose angina had not responded to medical treatment and who have CAD that cannot be corrected with either CABG or angioplasty. In one study of ninety-one patients who were treated with this technique, angina had improved significantly in 72% compared with 13% of the one hundred and one patients assigned to medical therapy. An approach under active investigation is the injection of various genes to promote the growth of new blood vessels into a coronary artery or into the heart muscle close to a site of coronary artery blockage.

UNSTABLE ANGINA: HEART ATTACK

Unstable angina is an emergency situation that requires hospitalization and continuous monitoring of the ECG. In addition to bed rest, sedation, and nasal oxygen, treatment includes the use of beta-blockers, calcium channel blockers, and measures to prevent blood clots, usually with injections of the drug heparin for three to five days and with aspirin. Recent studies have shown that administration of the platelet IIb/IIIa receptor blockers reduces the complication rate in people with unstable angina. Nitroglycerin is given intravenously as well as under the tongue for acute symptoms. If the patient's condition is stabilized, an exercise stress test is often obtained before the patient is discharged from the hospital. If symptoms and ECG abnormalities persist, coronary angiography is carried out to evaluate the patient for angioplasty or bypass surgery.

Hospitalization

For those who reach a hospital with a heart attack, the death rate in the hospital has fallen from 30% to between 10 and 15% over the past thirty years. This dramatic improvement is the result of many factors, such as improved treatments and more effective drugs, but the most important factor is the establishment of coronary care units staffed by well-trained doctors and nurses who can respond immediately to any adverse change in a patient's status with proper medications and modern equipment.

A favorable outcome from a heart attack depends mostly on preventing or controlling the two major causes of death: heart rhythm disturbances (arrhythmias) and a decline in the ability of the heart to pump blood (pump failure). About half of the life-threatening arrhythmias (ventricular fibrillation is most common) occur during the first hour after a heart attack and are the reason that as many as 30% of all heart attack victims die before they can receive medical attention. Prevention of these sudden deaths depends largely on the rapid response of rescue squads or ambulance crews who have the training and equipment to monitor and support patients with cardiopulmonary resuscitation methods (CPR) until they arrive at a hospital.

Arrhythmias continue to be common over the next twenty-four hours, but they can usually be controlled with medications. Pump failure, now the most common cause of death both during hospitalization and afterward, is related to the extent of death of heart muscle cells. Preservation of heart muscle depends on rapidly re-establishing blood flow to the heart muscle supplied by the obstructed artery in order to save as much tissue as possible from irreversible injury.

These considerations clearly indicate how important it is for victims of a heart attack to seek immediate medical help. When a heart attack is suspected, an ambulance must be called for immediately and the patient (barring a known severe allergy to aspirin) should chew a regular aspirin, not a coated tablet like Ecotrin, to prevent further blood clot formation. The biggest holdups in starting treatment do not occur at the hospital but rather from delays on the part of patients in deciding whether to go to a hospital.

Monitoring

Upon their arrival at an emergency room, patients are quickly evaluated, often in a special chest pain unit dedicated to this task, to decide whether a heart attack has occurred. Immediate treatment includes relief of pain with sublingual nitroglycerin (or morphine if nitroglycerin does not work), oxygen, and sedation. An intravenous line is established and kept in place to allow rapid administration of medications in case of a complication. Patients are admitted to a coronary care unit, where their heart rhythm is constantly monitored. Preparations are started at once to eliminate the obstruction and restore coronary blood flow either with thrombolytic therapy or angioplasty. The need for rapid treatment is evident from the studies showing that mortality is cut almost in half when blood flow is restored within the first hour after the onset of symptoms. Treatment within the first one to three hours gives considerable reduction in mortality. It also reduces the amount of myocardial damage and preserves more of the pumping ability of the heart. Some benefit is still seen when restoration of blood flow is achieved within three to six hours after the onset of symptoms. These findings re-emphasize the importance of getting to the hospital quickly.

Therapy for blood clots

Thrombolytic therapy uses intravenous injections of streptokinase, tissue plasminogen activator, or newer agents to break up the blood clot that is blocking a coronary artery. Patients are also given aspirin and heparin continuously for two to five days to prevent further blood clot formation. Results of preliminary studies suggest that platelet IIb/IIIa receptor blockers will be used in the future along with thrombolytic therapy. The greatest danger of thrombolytic treatment is unwanted bleeding, especially into the brain, with a resultant stroke. Thrombolytic therapy cannot be used in patients who have had a recent stroke or surgical procedure, severe hypertension, or a history of a peptic ulcer. A recent observational study found that angioplasty did not benefit patients who are 75 years of age or older. A coronary angiogram is done if the patient does not respond to initial therapy or there is evidence of reobstruction of the involved coronary artery.

There is much debate about whether thrombolytic therapy or immediate angioplasty is the preferred treatment. Angioplasty appears to be as good as or better than thrombolytic therapy, but it cannot be carried out at many hospitals. In addition, angioplasty can be used in patients whose risk of bleeding makes thrombolytic therapy too risky.

Medication

Beta-blockers are started in the hospital and continued after discharge because they have been shown to reduce the risk of recurrent heart attacks and cardiovascular deaths in people who survive a myocardial infarction. Many patients are also started on an ACE inhibitor if there is any suggestion of heart failure or if the function of the heart is depressed.

Some clinicians have suggested that an ACE inhibitor should be taken by every person who has known CAD and by those with diabetes and other risk factors.

It is probably a good idea for patients to be given a statin drug to lower cholesterol, if it is elevated, at the time of hospital discharge. If this is not done, the patient's primary care physician may think the drug is not necessary, because the cardiologist did not prescribe it. Guidelines for a cholesterol-lowering diet should be discussed during hospitalization so that such a diet can be used immediately after discharge.

Recovery and rehabilitation

For many years patients were kept on complete bed rest for many days after a heart attack. We now recognize that bedrest is harmful because it deconditions patients and places them at risk for complications. The current approach is to keep patients mostly in bed during the first hospital day, but after that they are encouraged to get out of bed, first sitting in a bedside chair and then walking around the hospital ward. Most patients are discharged from the hospital after four or five days if the heart attack is uncomplicated.

Activity is increased gradually after patients leave the hospital, because it takes six to eight weeks for the heart damage to heal completely. Many patients are urged to enter a cardiac rehabilitation program for at least twelve weeks so that their heart function can be monitored as physical activity is increased. Cardiac rehabilitation programs also provide education about diet, home exercise, and stress reduction. An "exercise prescription," which provides advice on when and how much to resume activity, is guided by "risk stratification"—an effort to determine the status of a patient's CAD and heart function prior to hospital discharge.

The coronary arteries are often evaluated with a submaximal exercise stress test, but there is some debate as to which patients should undergo this procedure or wait for about six weeks after discharge to undergo a standard exercise test that is more likely to pick up signs of abnormal function. Some cardiologists believe a stress test should be carried out in all patients at discharge to guide the rate of resumption of activity; others think it unnecessary in those who have had a completely uncomplicated hospital stay. Left ventricular function is determined by estimating the ejection fraction (the fraction of the blood in the left ventricle that is pumped out with each contraction of the heart) with ultrasound (an echocardiogram) or using radioactive tracers.

After a heart attack, many patients and their partners are afraid to have sex. Before discharge from the hospital, patients would do well to have a frank discussion with their doctor concerning when sexual relations can be resumed.

WHAT YOU CAN DO NOW

For caregivers and care recipients alike, lifestyle changes can go a long way toward preventing heart disease and curbing the chances for additional damage to the heart.

Lots of risk factors can be reduced or even eliminated by following the recommendations below.

- Stop smoking
- Increase your activity level, even if it's just a little
- Eat a prudent, heart-healthy (low fat, low sodium) diet
- If your cholesterol and/or blood pressure levels exceed accepted limits, follow appropriate lifestyle measures. If they remain too high, speak to your doctor about medications
- Control your weight with diet and regular exercise
- Call an ambulance promptly for symptoms of a heart attack

For people with a prior heart attack, follow these recommendations:

- Stop smoking
- Take a regular aspirin (absent a known allergy)

- If LDL cholesterol is greater than 100, ask your doctor if you should be on a medication
- If a beta-blocker has not been prescribed, ask your doctor why not
- Suggest that family members and other caretakers enroll in a CPR course

PREVENTING RECURRENT HEART ATTACKS

Prevention is particularly important in people who have had a heart attack or other manifestation of CAD because they are far more likely than others to have a cardiovascular event. Secondary preventive measures include all those described for primary prevention. One difference is that in people with known CAD, stroke, peripheral vascular disease, or diabetes the target level for LDL cholesterol is less than 100 mg/dL.

Additional measures for people with CAD disease are beta-blockers, ACE inhibitors, and aspirin. Surveys have shown that a shocking number of patients have not had needed lipid-lowering medications, beta-blockers, or ACE inhibitors prescribed by their doctors. So patients need to ask about them.

The optimal dose of aspirin is not clear; recommendations vary from 82 mg/day (baby aspirin) to an adult aspirin daily or every other day. Less clear is the role of aspirin in people who do not have recognized CAD. Regular aspirin is probably a good idea for those with diabetes and some recommend regular aspirin in everyone over the age of 50.

ADDITIONAL RESOURCES

WEB SITES

American Heart Association

www.americanheart.org

National Heart, Lung, and Blood Institute

Cardiovascular Information for Patients and the General Public

www.nhlbi.nih.gov/health/public/heart/index.htm

Depression

Many people believe that growing older is inevitably a sad and sorrowful experience, and that given the losses associated with aging, depression is unavoidable. But this is not true. While change and loss are a part of living and growing older, depression is not inevitable. In fact, many people experience an increasing and deepening sense of satisfaction in their lives as they get older. An overview of studies published in the journal *Psychological Medicine* found that, on the whole, older people report less anxiety and depression than younger adults do. Having said that, it must be acknowledged that depression—whether it's a single episode or a chronic condition—is not uncommon in the population at large. Depression affects people of all ages. According to the National Institute of Mental Health, younger people are diagnosed with depression more frequently than elderly people. Nevertheless, depression in the elderly is not an insignificant problem.

What exactly do we mean when we say that someone is depressed or has a depression? Depression is not merely feeling sad. Everyone feels sad, discouraged, despairing, or downright hopeless every now and then.

SIGNS & SYMPTOMS

- Sadness, despair, listlessness, and fatigue
- When related to grief, feelings of sorrow, shock, disbelief, anger, protest, and despair lasting long beyond the actual loss
- Feelings of worthlessness, guilt, and irritability, perhaps accompanied by tearfulness
- Chronic pain or physical complaints with no apparent medical cause
- Sudden withdrawal from relationships
- Sleep problems, including difficulty going to sleep, staying asleep, waking too early, or sleeping too much
- Abrupt change in appetite and/or weight
- Dramatic changes in working and social patterns
- Alcohol or drug abuse
- Diminished concentration and/or memory
- Difficulties in coping with problems and demands of daily life
- Loss of interest or pleasure in most activities
- Depressed sex drive
- Reduced motivation
- Preoccupation with thoughts of suicide or death

Sometimes you know why you are feeling blue. At other times, you may have no idea why. Indeed, as we get older, we may experience more losses—the death of someone close to us, the loss of a job, the loss of a role when our children leave home. All those experiences will naturally evoke feelings of sadness. Still, that is not necessarily depression.

Depression is not mere sadness. It is not a fleeting emotion. Nor is it a weakness. Rather, depression is an illness. Brought about by a complex interplay of biological, social, and psychological factors, depression is characterized by certain feelings, thoughts, and behaviors that depart from the person's normal way of feeling and functioning.

Ultimately, the experience of depression, what it feels like from the inside, is quite individual. Indeed, there is no one way to describe the subjective experience of depression. Some have likened it to an impenetrable dark curtain descending, bringing with it a sense of profound and constant hopelessness and despair. In his memoir, *Darkness Visible: A Memoir of Madness*, the author William Styron writes of his descent into depression as an experience he can only describe as "connected to drowning or suffocation." Finally, he writes, "To most of those who have experienced it, the horror of depression is so overwhelming as to be quite beyond expression."

Feelings of hopelessness and despair distort every experience, perception, thought, action, and reaction. Feelings of sadness, emptiness, and worthlessness can be overwhelming, rendering life meaningless, at least for the moment. Moreover, while most people associate depression with low energy and low mood, depression can also stir up seemingly unreasonable irritation and agitation that can erupt in frustration and anger. Overall, such feelings have little relation to the reality of a person's life, or seem utterly out of proportion.

WHAT IS IT?

According to the *Diagnostic and Statistical Manual of Mental Disorders* (DSM-IV), depression is defined as a mental disorder in which a person's mood is persistently colored by sadness, despair, and hopelessness to the degree that it interferes with day-to-day activities, health, and general satisfaction with life. In order for a person to be diagnosed with depression, the depressed mood must last for most of the day for at least two weeks. In addition to a depressed mood, depression is characterized by irritability, poor appetite or overeating, sleep problems, lack of sexual interest, general lack of pleasure in life, low energy or fatigue, poor self-esteem, excessive guilt, self-criticism, difficulties concentrating and making decisions, feelings of hopelessness, and recurrent thoughts of death or suicide.

While depression, especially the first episode, may be set off by some life circumstance or event, usually the reaction seems greatly exaggerated. In general, depression has less to do with actual events than with an individual's inherent vulnerability to the condition.

Depression is a spectrum condition, meaning that it can be mild, moderate, or severe. Depression can drown out all other feelings and experiences in a person's life or it can exist as a constant mild undertow. It can be full blown, with a full array of symptoms, causing significant impairment and incapacity for a long period of time. Or it can be episodic, with fewer symptoms that last a few days or weeks, then disappear, only to recur.

However, even a minor depression can cause considerable impairment in older people. Studies show that between 13 and 27% of older adults who live out in the community on their own have some symptoms of depression. If these symptoms last longer than two weeks or seriously interfere with the person's usual activities, a health care professional should be consulted, since even seemingly minor symptoms can put a person at increased risk for a major depression, for physical disability, and for serious illness.

Major or clinical depression. Some people experience a major or clinical depression as a single episode. Usually, a major depression lasts for some time, with slight ups and downs throughout. In fact, a major depression can last longer than two years, in which case it's called "chronic." However, more often than not, clinical depressions occur periodically or cyclically.

Dysthymic disorder. Some people experience a milder, low-grade, intermittent or chronic depressive state called dysthymic disorder. Research suggests that this type of mood disorder can render a person more vulnerable to bouts of major depression. Thus, if you have dysthymic disorder, you may be more prone to serious depression when faced with certain life circumstances—the end of a relationship, retirement, moving away from home, illness, or the death of a loved one.

DEPRESSION IN THE ELDERLY

In some ways, depression in older adults can have a slightly different flavor. Clearly, the most prominent feature of depression is a depressed mood. However, when asked, older people are less likely to admit to feeling sad. For one, they may not notice that they are feeling particularly bad. Secondly, many have been brought up with a more stoic attitude—stiff upper lip, grin and bear it. As a result, older adults may be less likely to dwell on their feelings or may view any such feelings as weakness.

In fact they may say that nothing is wrong, but may experience other, less clear-cut symptoms of depression, such as:

- Sleep problems
- Somatic complaints or pain (in other words, physical symptoms that are not easily explained)
- Low self-esteem
- Poor concentration
- Poor appetite
- Lack of energy
- Sometimes, feelings of hopelessness

People around them, if they pay attention, may notice telling changes. They may appear agitated or anxious instead of sad. Or they seem apathetic. Statements such as, "Life is over," or "Things won't get better anyway," are signs of apathetic depression, a form particularly common in older adults. Similarly, depression in older people may manifest itself in feelings of self-blame and guilt—in complaints, for example, that they are "a burden, nothing but trouble."

While such signs are easily dismissed as part of getting older, they could well be indications of depression. Indeed, you may be tempted to nod your head in agreement, and discount these statements as typical of or even appropriate to old age. Yet chances are they reflect depression instead of a philosophical attitude.

Depression in the elderly is becoming an increasingly important and complicated issue for a number of reasons. According to the 1990 U.S. Census, adults 65 and older compose the fastest growing segment of our population. Therefore, the number of older adults affected by

Seasonal affective disorder. Some people experience a form of reactive depression called seasonal affective disorder, or SAD. More prevalent in northern parts of the country where climate extremes are greater, SAD occurs usually during the winter months. It is typically characterized by a depressed mood, fatigue, overeating, and oversleeping.

the depression will naturally continue to increase. And many of the medical conditions that affect the elderly may trigger, contribute to, or worsen depression. The existence of depression can worsen a co-existing medical condition.

The fact that older adults are often on multiple medications also complicates the matter. Older people are biologically more vulnerable to the side effects of medications, and many of the medications used by elderly can cause confusion, feelings of dissociation, depressed mood, lack of energy, sleep problems—all symptoms of depression.

For older people, other factors seem to come into play. These include:

- The loss of a loved one or series of losses
- Living alone or a sense of social isolation
- Worsening physical illness or chronic illness that is not managed effectively
- Moving from home—including relocating to a nursing home
- Retirement, especially when retirement means greater social isolation and inactivity

- Loss of such social roles as parent, worker, wife, or husband
- Abrupt loss of physical autonomy or impaired self-sufficiency
- Decreased cognitive function—imperfect memory, difficulties concentrating. In fact, 50% of all people with dementia or Parkinson's disease also have depressive symptoms.

Finally, because older adults are less likely to report depression, they are less likely to receive the treatment they need. In the elderly, even for those with few depressive symptoms, the impairment—the way in which depression interferes with day-to-day life—can be quite significant. And studies show that depression can and does worsen physical problems. It literally can make a person sick. Insofar as depression is under-recognized and under-treated in the elderly, it becomes a much more serious condition than it needs to be. This is truly unfortunate, because with effective treatment, there is no reason to suffer through depression.

Apathetic depression. People who have a history of either major depression or dysthymic disorder are more likely to experience depression in their later years. For older people, depression often takes on its own shape. Depression may announce itself in agitation, anxiety, or phobias instead of feelings of sadness. Or it may appear as an apathetic depression, in which older people casually but constantly claim that their life is over, or that things will never get better anyway. Also called melancholic depression, this type of depression commonly expresses itself in hypochondriasis (physical complaints without any obvious physical root), low self-esteem, a sense of worthlessness, self-accusations, paranoia, and suicidal ideation.

Bipolar disorder or manic-depressive illness. Some people who experience depression also experience intermittent episodes of euphoria or mania. This type of mood disorder is called bipolar disorder or manic-depressive illness. However, it is unusual for a person to have an episode of mania for the first time after the age of 65. Even for those who had manic episodes in the past, by the time they reach 65, manic swings tend to be uncommon or they may be a sign of an underlying medical condition.

Psychotic depression. Once in a great while, depression can be accompanied by psychotic features, specifically delusions and hallucinations. In most cases, these hallucinations and delusions center around guilt, sinfulness, worthlessness, failure, persecution, jealousy, and preoccupation with one's physical health or ailments. This type of depression is called psychotic depression.

Truth be told, no one knows exactly what causes depression. All indications, though, point to a complicated combination of biological, genetic, psychological, and environmental factors. There is little question that a family history of depression increases a person's vulnerability. In fact, people with first-degree relatives—a mother, father, sister, or brother—who have depression are two to three times more likely to develop a major depression at some point in their lives. A family history of alcoholism or suicide—remembering the stories of Uncle Jed, the family drunk, or great-grandmother Ruth who killed herself at 40—may uncover a predisposition toward depression.

Studies show that people who develop depression often have a biochemical imbalance. Neurotransmitters—substances such as norepinephrine or serotonin that transmit nerve impulses from one neuron to another across the synapses—are not efficiently regulated. Other studies point to a neuroendocrine dysfunction (or how the brain and adrenal system release hormones).

And of course, stress—the death of a loved one, a move, retirement, chronic illness, children leaving home, physical disability, a decline in cognitive abilities—all play a part in the development of depression in older adults. Indeed, the loss of a spouse is cited as the factor most likely to bring on depression.

WHO IS AT RISK?

Each year, depression strikes millions of people in the United States, regardless of education, income, ethnicity, or marital status. Studies indicate that as many as 26% of all women over the age of 18 and 12% of all men over the age of 18 experience at least one significant episode of depression in their lifetime.

For those with close relatives with depression—a mother, father, sister, or brother, the chances of suffering from depression are one and a half to three times greater. In addition, people who have other psychiatric or medical problems are at higher risk.

Depression is most likely to hit around the age of 40—that is the average age of onset. Almost 50% of all cases of clinical depression are diagnosed between the ages of 20 and 50. At younger ages, women are at greater risk for depression. According to the National Institute of Mental Health, women are almost twice as likely as men to suffer from depression. As they get older, though, the incidence of depression in men rises. The prognosis for those who develop depression after age 65 is variable. Most will recover but some can have frequent, recurrent episodes.

On the surface, depression seems less prevalent in the elderly. According to some figures, only 1% of people over the age of 65—1.4% of older women and 0.4% of older men—experience major episodes of depression. However, these numbers may be misleading. All too often, depression goes undiagnosed in the elderly because they are less likely to report feelings of sadness or despair. Instead they may complain of physical pain or problems, fatigue, faulty memory, inability to concentrate, lack of appetite—all less specific symptoms of depression. Thus they are frequently misdiagnosed.

Within the elderly population, the prevalence of depression is often tied to other factors. For example, between 7 and 36% of the elderly who are being treated for medical conditions on an outpatient basis report some symptoms of depression. Around 40% of those hospitalized for medical conditions have symptoms of depression. Although they would not necessarily be diagnosed with depression because they lack the classic symptoms, about 15% of older adults—both in the community and in nursing homes—have significant signs of depression. In addition, alcohol use and abuse can also mask depression in older adults.

Just about anyone can go through a period of depression. But there are a number of factors that appear to make a person more vulnerable. For reasons that are not altogether clear, women are twice as likely to experience depression than men. Divorce or separation makes individuals more vulnerable to depression. Although depression affects people from all socioeconomic groups, it seems that people whose limited income limits their access to resources are at higher risk. A person who lacks a strong social support network is more susceptible to depression. Certain medical conditions, such as chronic obstructive pulmonary disease, a history of stroke, a history of heart attack, or cancer seem to make individuals more susceptible to depression.

Finally, the psychologist Erik Erikson wrote about late adulthood as a time to reach a special type of integrity and life acceptance. It is important, he asserts, that older people find time to take stock of their lives. This type of life review means looking back and realizing that life was what it had to be—joys, sorrows, triumphs, disappointments, mistakes, and all. By recognizing that the course of life could have taken no other direction and that the past cannot be undone, people can derive a deep sense of satisfaction and meaning. Indeed, people who are able to look back and accept the choices made, life lived as necessary and inevitable, seem in some ways inoculated against depression. On the other hand, people who cannot discern meaning in their own lives appear to be at higher risk for despair.

Depression may begin at any age. Symptoms can develop over days or weeks; they may simmer like a low-grade fever that is hardly noticeable way before a full-blown condition makes itself known. Other conditions—an acute or persistent anxiety, panic or phobic reaction at the thought of leaving the house, for example—can signal the advent of depression. On the other hand, depression can come on abruptly, perhaps in response to some environmental stressor—a death in the family, for example, or retirement—and then fail to wane. If left untreated, depression typically lasts six months or longer.

Between 50 and 85% of all people who suffer a single episode of depression will eventually have another episode. Between 20 and 35% who have persistent depressive symptoms will continue to have residual symptoms even with treatment.

HOW IS IT DIAGNOSED?

Because an older person is less likely to report a depressed or blue mood, it may fall on you, as the caregiver, to pick up on other indications. It is a common misconception that depression is an unrelenting condition. However, depression does not operate like a light switch. Rather, it often comes in waves, so you may notice that your loved one's mood rises and falls. Nevertheless, if it consistently falls or plummets, pay heed.

Also, if it's obvious that suddenly your elderly loved one has lost interest in relationships or activities that once were the source of great pleasure, pay attention. These activities may include going to church or synagogue, spending time with grandchildren, sending out birthday cards, playing cards with friends, or gardening. Ask your loved one whether there are still things that get him excited or that he still enjoys; if the answer is "No," you have reason to be concerned.

In addition, physical complaints, especially when there is no clear physical cause, can be a sign of depression. Such complaints include pain, confusion, headaches, and sleeplessness. And while it is very often difficult to distinguish between depression and physical illness, depression could very well be at the root of many physical complaints.

Also, complaints about dementia-like troubles—problems with memory or concentrating—may be rooted in depression. When a decline in cognitive functioning is tied to depression, the condition is called pseudodementia.

At the same time, you should be on the lookout for stirrings of depression within you. In general, people who care for other people over extended periods of time are more likely to become depressed. Add to this the fact that if you have a parent who is depressed, or any close relative for that matter, you stand twice as great a risk of suffering from depression yourself. In order to counteract these pulls, be sure that you find ways of taking care of yourself:

- Ask others to help you care for your loved one.
- Stay engaged in activities that you find pleasurable.
- Carve out time for yourself.

You need diversions and other ways of taking care of yourself as you take care of another. If you are caring for a depressed loved one, though, finding the time to relax and care for yourself may not be so easy.

You may find yourself forever vigilant, wanting to take your loved one's emotional temperature constantly. Or you may find yourself on constant suicide watch.

(continued on p. 172)

SUICIDE IN THE ELDERLY

The incidence of suicide in older adults is actually quite high—approximately 40 elderly people in 100,000 successfully take their own lives each year. Loneliness, loss, and physical illness are the reasons most often cited. In addition, the presence of another psychiatric condition, such as anxiety or alcohol abuse, puts a person at higher risk for suicide.

On the lookout for signs of suicide

If you live with or love someone who suffers from depression, chances are that you constantly worry the depression will worsen. And perhaps you find yourself on the watch for suicidal behavior or gestures.

In fact, each year thousands of people, prompted by feelings of desperation and hopelessness, commit suicide. Some estimates put the number in this country as high as 30,000. And the number of people who attempt suicides may be eight to ten times higher.

Suicide is the eighth leading cause of death in this country. In the elderly, it is one of the leading causes. Women are four times more likely to make suicidal attempts, but men are more likely to be successful at it—perhaps because they tend to choose more efficient methods, such as jumping from high places, hanging, or shooting themselves, whereas women will typically use poison or drug overdose.

Older men are at greatest risk for suicide. Most male suicides happen after the age of 45. Women tend to be most vulnerable to suicidal behavior after the age of 55. Approximately 80% of all older people who commit suicide have evidence of depression.

Who is at risk for suicide?

When someone we love is profoundly depressed and wrapped in feelings of desperation, emptiness, or hopelessness, we may worry that he or she may attempt suicide. However, people who are profoundly depressed often lack the energy to kill themselves. Ironically, it is when a person is beginning to feel better, perhaps he is in treatment and starting to respond, that he is actually at higher risk for suicide. In other words, feeling better means regaining enough direction and energy to act.

Loneliness is cited as the most common reason that older people take their own lives. Other circumstances that seem to put older people at greater risk for suicide include:

• Living alone with few social connections

- Retirement, especially during the first few months, or unemployment
- A recent and significant loss
- Serious mental illness, such as clinical depression or schizophrenia
- Severe physical illness, chronic illness, or a critical accident that causes unremitting pain, diminished mobility, or disfigurement
- A personal and/or family history of suicidal behavior, depression, and/or substance abuse
- A personality or coping style that is somewhat rigid and narrow in its problem-solving ability

What to look for

If your loved one is not particularly ill, yet begins to exhibit certain new behaviors, you need to be particularly alert to the possibility of suicide. Pay attention if, for example, a person:

- Abruptly withdraws from normal activities and involvements
- Suddenly and profoundly changes
- Has no vision or plans for the future
- Starts giving away cherished possessions and becomes preoccupied with a will
- Talks with great specificity of killing himself

If you suspect that someone close to you is at risk for suicide, bring the subject up. Many people avoid the subject under the mistaken notion that by talking frankly about such thoughts and intentions, they will encourage the action. However, this is seldom true. Another popular misconception is that if someone threatens to kill himself, he will not act. However, suicidal threats are both a warning and a cry for help. They should always be taken seriously.

Suicide prevention centers and telephone hot lines throughout the country can help a person beyond the immediate crisis. Nevertheless, if there are signs that someone close to you is contemplating suicide, it is important to seek out treatment, even if it seems that the crisis has passed. One study of ninety-seven patients over age 50 who completed suicide in the Rochester, New York area found that half had seen a primary care provider in the past month. In only nineteen cases were psychiatric symptoms recognized and appropriate treatment provided. Only two of the patients were felt to be on appropriate treatment at the time of their suicide. Most suicides in older adults are not due to failure of treatment for depression, but to those with depression not getting adequate treatment.

SIGNS AND SYMPTOMS

Feeling blue, despondent, lethargic, negative, or hopeless—all feelings we normally associate with depression—is an inevitable part of life. Practically any kind of disappointment, change, or loss can trigger feelings of sorrow and despair. And while it is not always easy to judge where normal sorrow ends and clinical depression begins, as anyone who has been really depressed can tell you, depression is more than just sadness that won't go away.

Depression brings on feelings that are more intense and linger longer than what would be expected in response to the triggering event. In addition, some people respond to most every kind of stress with depressive symptoms, in which case, there is cause for concern.

Depression in older adults can have a very different flavor. Whereas the most prominent feature of depression is a depressed mood, in older people, the more prominent symptoms might be complaints of persistent pain, fatigue, sleep difficulties, or lack of energy. They may feel constantly agitated or anxious or, on the other end of the spectrum, apathetic. They may have cognitive difficulties—poor concentration, faulty memory—that are easy to dismiss as signs of old age. Or these symptoms may be mistakenly connected to a number of medical conditions or medications that are commonly associated with aging.

Depression in the elderly can be missed for another reason. As a whole, older adults seek help almost exclusively from their primary care physicians. Maybe as few as 15% of those over age 65 who are clinically depressed see a psychiatrist or psychologist who is specifically trained to treat mental illness or emotional problems. A general practitioner may be more likely to miss the signs of depression, looking instead for physical roots for the complaints. For that reason, family members or adult caregivers can be of tremendous help in reporting abrupt changes or specific patterns that may point beyond the physical to the emotional. Or, depression may be picked up by a home health aid, a social worker at a day care program, or an elder care worker.

The key to making an accurate diagnosis, especially in the elderly, is a thorough medical and psychiatric history. With such a history at hand, a clinician can connect more precisely the symptoms to emotional or physical sources. But, because the elderly typically have difficulty identifying feelings associated with depression, caregivers play an especially important role in the diagnostic process. Therefore, before your visit to the doctor, take the time to think about and be prepared to give such a history.

Significant information includes:

- Current signs and symptoms; when they began; how long they've persisted
- Description of mood
- Any and all recent stressors
- Any previous occurrences of the current complaint: has this problem surfaced before, when, and how it was handled?
- History of psychiatric problems, including anxiety, psychosis, alcoholism or drug abuse, eating disorders
- Past hospitalizations for medical, surgical, or psychiatric problems
- Use of psychotropic medications, including drugs for anxiety, depression, or psychosis
- History of electroconvulsive therapy, complete with dates
- Any suicide attempts
- Substance abuse, including cigarettes and alcohol
- Family psychiatric history
- Current medical condition
- Current medications. (It is extremely helpful to bring all bottles of current medications for the consultation—including over-the-counter medications and vitamins. Many medications can cause, contribute to, or worsen symptoms of depression. Some of the drugs commonly prescribed to treat high blood pressure or heart disease such as clonidine, metoprolol, and propranolol can actually make symptoms of depression worse.)
- Allergies to any medications
- Medical history—along with dates and treatment
- Names of all medical care providers

MEDICAL HISTORY

To rule out any medical condition that can produce or worsen depression, it is important to have a thorough physical examination. In fact, this cannot be emphasized too much: *It is essential that any medical condition, including medications, be ruled out as a factor in depression.*

Diagnosing clinical depression in older adults is made even more complicated by the fact that classic signs of depression—specifically memory impairment, poor concentration, irritability, slowed speech and movement—often mimic symptoms of dementia, that is, Alzheimer's disease, Huntington's disease, and Parkinson's disease. Then the condition is called pseudodementia. Indeed, when a person has his first episode of depression in the later years, he is more likely to experience significant cognitive impairments.

DISTINGUISHING BETWEEN DEPRESSION AND DEMENTIA

When you're dealing with the elderly, it is not always easy to tell if the confusion, agitation, or disorientation is caused by depression or some type of dementia. When someone says, "I feel like I'm in a fog" or "My mind just doesn't work the way it used to," you may wonder whether these statements are expectable given a person's age or a sign that something else is wrong. Even when a younger person is depressed, his thinking may not be as lucid or his mind as sharp. When depression begins to get better and all other symptoms abate, muddled thinking may be the last thing to clear up.

Although it is never easy to determine with great certainty whether a person is suffering from dementia or depression, you may be able to conjecture somewhat accurately. People who are depressed may complain about difficulties in thinking, focusing, and remembering; in contrast, people with dementia may not recognize their cognitive difficulties. In depression, there is often a preoccupation with physical complaints, which is not often the case in dementia. Moreover, a person who is depressed will, in all likelihood, respond to simple questions differently than a person with dementia. Notice the answer when you ask questions such as, "What is your phone number?" or "What is your granddaughter's name?" People with dementia are more likely to answer incorrectly while people with depression may avoid answering, saying "Don't bother me, I'm not interested," or "Let's do this later." Finally, in depression, most symptoms can be reversed by antidepressant medications, whereas the symptoms of dementia are, more often than not, irreversible. Nevertheless, studies show that the two conditions are linked in some ways. When a person is treated for depression, for example, the dementia may get a bit better along with the depression. On the other hand, if an older person has cognitive problems rooted in depression that improve in response to treatment, he may be at increased risk for developing Alzheimer's disease or some other form of dementia over time.

LABORATORY TESTS AND FINDINGS

A complete history and physical examination are crucial to rule out any possible medical problems that could be masquerading as or contributing to the depression, such as a urinary tract infection, hypothyroidism, overmedication,

SIGNS OF DEPRESSION—WHAT A CAREGIVER MIGHT OBSERVE

A caregiver or doctor may be aware of or notice signs of depression, even though an elderly person may deny feelings of sadness or despair.

- Lethargy and loss of interest in normal pleasures of life: family, friends, work, sports, hobbies, food, sex
- A family or personal history of depression or suicide attempts, alcohol or drug use
- Somatic preoccupations: persistent complaints about pain or illness with no apparent physical cause
- Sudden loss of energy
- Sleep problems such as early morning awakenings or multiple awakenings
- Diminished cognitive ability: thinking, problem-solving, decision making, focusing, concentrating, remembering
- A pattern of self-defeating, self-critical, negative, pessimistic thinking

- Suicidal ruminations or behavior
- Increased irritability, demandingness, dependency, and complaining

When to get help

Seek treatment when you observe any of the following.

- Mild symptoms of depression that seem constant and flare in reaction to most problems
- Depressive symptoms or acute grief that continues to worsen, does not lessen over time, or shows up in physical symptoms
- Dramatic weight loss or weight fluctuation that is not caused by a medical condition or by attempts to lose weight
- Persistent physical ailments and complaints
- Frequent outbursts of anger and frustration that seem exaggerated or uncharacteristic

tumors, or hearing problems. Once underlying medical conditions have been ruled out or treated, other tests may be administered to assess the extent and type of depression.

The Folstein Mini-Mental State Exam (MMSE), for example, can provide a pretty good picture of a person's orientation, attention, mood, and cognitive functioning. This relatively short test is often used to track progress or deterioration in cognitive function during and following treatment.

HOW IS IT TREATED?

Once depression is diagnosed, treatment aims at relieving and preventing a recurrence of symptoms. Today there is a wide range of treatment options. Studies suggest that older adults respond as well to treatment as do younger adults. Consequently, there is little reason for anyone to suffer through a depression for long when treatment can mean a better quality of life and greater ability to function.

Many times, treatment involves more than one approach, usually antidepressant medication combined with psychotherapy, at least in the beginning. On rare occasions, when a person is at risk of harming himself or someone else or when he is unable to care for himself, hospitalization may be necessary.

PSYCHOTHERAPY

Psychotherapy can be immensely helpful in treating depression. In cases of mild depression, therapy can work on its own. However, it is often used in conjunction with medication. While antidepressant medications can take the edge off the symptoms of depression, individual psychotherapy can identify and mitigate many of the stressors that prompted the depression as well as those inherent in growing older that can contribute to the vulnerability. In addition, the ways in which depression colors day-to-day life, what can precipitate depression, and what may lie beneath the symptoms are often the fodder of therapy sessions.

Even in cases of more severe depression, psychotherapy can provide the backbone for treatment. However, for psychotherapy to work, a person must commit to weekly sessions for at least six to ten weeks. And if the depression is severe, the course of therapy will likely take longer.

MEDICATIONS

Psychotropic medications, those medications prescribed for emotional problems and mental illness, aim to alleviate the symptoms of depression, to lift the veil of sorrow and return the person to a more reasonable level of functioning. Very often, they work effectively in conjunction with psychotherapy.

A number of antidepressant medications are now on the market that have proven quite effective. Usually, the doctor will choose a particular drug based on what the patient is likely to respond to, the history of response in the patient or a close relative, the likelihood of side effects, the presence of any coexisting medical illnesses, potential drug interactions, patient preference, and occasionally cost factors.

Selective serotonin reuptake inhibitors

For many clinicians, selective serotonin reuptake inhibitors (SSRIs)—fluoxetine (Prozac), sertraline (Zoloft), paroxetine (Paxil), citalopram (Celexa), and fluvoxamine (Luvox)—are the first choice for treating depression. They have been shown to be quite effective in treating mild-to-moderate depression without particularly troubling side effects. Specifically, these drugs improve a number of symptoms, including memory, energy level, and the general feeling of melancholy. The most common side effects are gastrointestinal discomfort, insomnia, anxiety or agitation, tremor, headache, and sexual dysfunction. Dry mouth, sweating, rash, decreased appetite, weight loss, and dizziness can sometimes occur as well. In general, SSRIs are taken in the morning to reduce the chance of insomnia and with food to cut nausea.

Tricyclic antidepressants

Although tricyclic antidepressants (TCAs)—imipramine (Tofranil), nortriptyline (Aventyl, Pamelor), amitriptyline (Elavil), clomipramine (Anafranil), doxepin (Sinequan), protriptyline (Vivactil), amoxapine (Asendin), and desipramine hydrochloride (Norpramin)—are highly effective, they can cause a number of troubling side effects. With the availability of newer, more easily tolerated medications, TCAs are seldom used these days as first-line treatment of mild-to-moderate depression. And when they are prescribed, nortriptyline and desipramine are usually preferred because they seem to cause less severe side effects. Side effects include dry mouth, constipation, blurred vision, urinary retention, and cognitive impairment.

Sleepiness and lack of energy can also result. Significant weight gain can occur with long-term use, and sexual dysfunction ranging from decreased desire to the inability to achieve orgasm occurs frequently. Finally, in rare cases, TCAs can increase the risk of heart failure, abnormal heart rhythms, and seizures. A TCA overdose may be lethal. Patients who have a history of suicide attempts are typically not given more than a one-week supply.

Monoamine oxidase inhibitors

The monoamine oxidase inhibitors (MAOIs)—phenelzine (Nardil), tranylcypromine (Parnate), and isocarboxazid (Marplan)—are used effectively with many patients whose depressions are consistently severe and have not responded to other treatments. However, people who take MAOIs must avoid foods that contain tyramine, an amino acid. The interaction can cause a hypertensive crisis, that is, headache, chest pain, palpitations, heart failure, or even stroke. Because tyramine occurs naturally in foods and is formed when proteins in foods break down over time, following a tyramine-restricted diet can be quite tricky. In addition, if a person is also taking decongestants, stimulants and weight-loss aids, SSRIs, or analgesics such as tramadol (Ultram) and meperidine (Demerol), there is a considerable risk for highly toxic drug interactions. As a result, MAOIs are no longer considered a first-line treatment for depression. The most common side effects include dizziness and lightheadedness upon standing, insomnia, stimulation, weight gain, swelling, muscle cramps, and sexual dysfunction.

Other medications

Other medications that are prescribed in ways similar to SSRIs to treat depression include:

Nefazodone (Serzone), trazodone (Desyrel), mirtazapine (Remeron) and venlafaxine (Effexor), bupropion (Wellbutrin). Possible side effects include sleep disruption, lightheadedness, agitation, dry mouth, fast heart rate, decreased appetite, headaches, rashes, and tremor gain. Wellbutrin can cause seizures and is therefore seldom prescribed for people who have a history of seizures or are at risk for seizures

Benzodiazepines. Although not antidepressants, benzodiazepines—Valium, Xanax, or Ativan—are prescribed for as many as 20% of older adults who meet the diagnostic criteria for major depression. While these antianxiety medications

TYPES OF PSYCHOTHERAPY

A variety of psychotherapies are available for treating depression.

Supportive psychotherapy. Here, the therapist can monitor medication and offer suggestions about managing and coping with depression. This type of therapy seems particularly effective when it furnishes practical information, and helps identify early warning signs of a possible relapse as well as stresses that might trigger an episode

Insight-oriented psychotherapy. Therapy that explores such factors as early experiences of loss, trauma, and the like that may provide the underpinnings for depression

Cognitive/behavioral therapy. Widely used to treat depression, this counseling technique considers and works to correct any negative and distorted thinking that typically underlies depression. While most people believe that the way they feel changes the way they think, this type of therapy operated on the assumption that the way people think can change the way they feel.

Life review therapy. In recent years, many therapists who work with older adults have used what is called reminiscent or life review therapy.

While at one time older people were dissuaded from dwelling in the past, today it is quite common for individual therapy, groups and programs to encourage life review. Such an approach encourages, allows people to reminisce, to share memories and stories, and generally to take stock of their lives in the presence of others. Studies show that this type of life review can enhance a person's self-awareness and self-acceptance, and in many cases prevent or ameliorate depression.

Family or couples' therapy. Living with depressive illness can cause problems for family members as well. Therefore, family or couples' therapy can be a helpful adjunct. A family therapist can offer practical information on living with the illness as well as discuss ways in which family patterns contribute to or worsen symptoms.

Group therapy. Many people with depression find group therapy helpful. In groups, people are able to cultivate mutual support, develop new friendships, and offer help to others. Groups seem to be especially helpful as a venue in which specific problem-solving skills and techniques are discussed.

can help alleviate anxiety and sleep problems, they are not effective at treating the underlying depression. They may have some short-term benefits, lasting between one and two weeks, but they have not been shown to improve long-term outcomes. In fact, benzodiazepines can worsen symptoms of depression. On the other hand, antidepressant medications can also treat anxiety but it usually takes longer to feel the benefits. Anyone over the age of 65 who is taking benzodiazepines should ask his doctor if an antidepressant might be a better choice.

Primary care physicians are the doctors who most frequently prescribe antidepressant medications for older adults. If you do not feel that your primary care physician can adequately answer your questions about these medications or the depressive symptoms are not improving over a period of one to two months, it is best to consult a psychiatrist or psychopharmacologist who is specially trained to evaluate and monitor the need for psychotropic medication.

When it comes to prescribing such medications, most doctors "start low and go slow" in order to minimize side effects and encourage compliance. The dose may be gradually increased until a beneficial response is seen. It is always best to use the lowest possible dose to achieve the greatest benefit. This is especially true with older adults since certain changes that come with age tend to diminish the body's ability to metabolize and excrete medications, resulting in a greater vulnerability to side effects.

All antidepressants take several weeks to be effective. For younger people, the effects of the medications may be felt in only six to eight weeks. For many older people, it may take as long as twelve weeks for antidepressants to produce their benefits. Whether young or old, it sometimes happens that a patient does not respond to the first medication prescribed. Medications may have to be augmented with another medication or switched altogether. Because every person and every depression differ, finding the most effective drug can sometimes mean a somewhat extended process of trial and error. While the process may be frustrating, eventually the right treatment will be found.

Regardless of the specific medication, antidepressants are nonaddictive. That means that patients who take antidepressants will not necessarily need larger doses of the medication to maintain the effectiveness. Nor will a person who is not depressed get "high" from taking antidepressants. Antidepressant medication does not change a person, but rather takes the edge off the symptoms. It will not make people feel happy, but it can *allow* them to experience happiness once again. Even once symptoms begin to subside, medications must be continued for at least six months to prevent relapse. For people with recurrent depression, most doctors recommend that the medications be continued for at least twelve months after recovery. Then, in most cases, the antidepressant is slowly tapered off as long as symptoms do not re-emerge. People who have experienced a number of episodes of depression are at high risk of recurrence; therefore, long-term antidepressant treatment may be considered.

ELECTROCONVULSIVE "SHOCK" THERAPY

While images of shock treatments can send chills down the spine, the fact is that electroconvulsive therapy (ECT) can be remarkably safe and effective. ECT is used primarily for symptoms of depression or mania when:

- symptoms are severe or persistent;
- the patient has not responded to medication;
- the patient cannot tolerate the side effects caused by the medications; or
- there is serious suicidal behavior or such psychotic symptoms as paranoid or persecutory delusions associated with the depression.

Electroconvulsive therapy passes electrical current through the brain to produce brief seizures. The seizures usually last between twenty-five and one hundred and fifty seconds and work to restore balance within the chemical makeup of the brain, thus relieving depressive and manic symptoms.

Patients must give informed consent before ECT is administered. This means that they understand the illness, the treatment, the reasons for recommending ECT, alternative treatments, and what will likely happen if ECT is refused.

Then, a comprehensive evaluation is conducted, including psychiatric, medical, and neurological assessments. Usually, the evaluation includes an electrocardiogram and complete blood analysis.

A short-acting general anesthetic is used during the procedure to prevent discomfort. A drug to dry secretions and a skeletal muscle relaxant to prevent injuries are administered. Electric currents are transmitted to the brain through two electrodes, which are placed either on the temples, on each side of the head, or both on the right side of the head. Treatment is typically given two to three times a week until symptoms begin to abate.

PHOTOTHERAPY

When depression is triggered by seasonal change, phototherapy or light therapy can relieve symptoms. A person sits under bright, full-spectrum light for specific periods of time each day.

HERBAL REMEDIES

Approximately 20% of people who suffer from depression take some type of alternative remedy to treat its symptoms. Far and away, St. John's wort is the most well-known and widely used alternative treatment. Touted as a natural agent, St. John's wort contains hypericin extract, which inhibits the reuptake of the neurotransmitters serotonin, norepinephrine, and dopamine. The plant also seems to slightly inhibit monoamine oxidase (MAO). Although St. John's wort seems to be somewhat effective in treating mild-to-moderate depression, few studies address its use in severe depression. Moreover, the Food and Drug Administration has warned that St. John's wort can interfere with the effectiveness of some drugs used to treat depression, as well as with some drugs used to treat AIDS, heart disease, seizures, certain cancers, or to prevent organ transplant rejection or pregnancy (oral contraceptives).

It is important, when considering taking an antidepressant, to tell the doctor if any herbal preparations are also being taken. In particular, it is not advisable to take St. John's wort along with an antidepressant medication.

DRUG THERAPY FOR MANIC-DEPRESSIVE ILLNESS

In most cases, treatment for manic-depression or bipolar disorder is the drug lithium, sometimes combined with psychotherapy. The goal of treatment is to stabilize a person's moods. A natural salt, lithium works to smooth out the highs and lows of the disorder, and in so doing to reduce the frequency and severity of manic episodes.

Use of the medication requires vigilant monitoring. This means measuring blood levels of lithium. It is also necessary to drink enough water to remain hydrated in order to guard against high blood concentrations of lithium. In addition, taking a synthetic hormone may be needed to counteract thyroid problems sometimes associated with lithium use.

Other possible side effects associated with lithium use include hand tremors, more frequent urination and increased thirst, acne, and weight gain. In most cases, side effects are mild.

If lithium is not effective, carbamazepine (Tegretol) or valproic acid (Depakote), both anticonvulsants, can be used to stabilize a person's mood.

It is crucial that these medications be used regularly. Otherwise, symptoms usually recur within a year and a half of stopping the drug.

WHAT SHOULD YOU EXPECT?

On the whole, depression can be effectively managed, especially when diagnosed early and treated aggressively. Seasonal affective disorder responds well to light therapy. In many cases, one course of treatment is sufficient to manage or remedy major depressive illness. In other cases, where depression is a chronic, life-long condition, continued or periodic treatment may be necessary.

Nevertheless, a number of factors pave the way for a poorer prognosis. Those factors include a long duration of illness and several prior episodes of depression, psychotic symptoms, poor social support, alcohol and other drug abuse, and anxiety.

On the other hand, people who have strong social supports tend to do better. In addition, if there are coexisting medical problems, treating depression can improve the course of the underlying medical problem. Conversely, treating the underlying medical problem can improve the course of the depression.

In general, depression tends to be chronic, and people who suffer from one depression may well experience periodic episodes, especially when stressed. It is therefore important to remain attentive to those stresses that are likely to trigger a depression. By being sensitive to typical catalysts and early signs that depression is brewing, you can contact the doctor before your loved one finds himself in a full-blown episode. People who can manage depression through therapy, medication, and lifestyle are much less likely to have it cast its shadow over everyone's life.

The course and prognosis for bipolar illness are a little more complicated. Manic-depressive disorder is a chronic illness that needs to be managed and monitored for life. Treatment is often more elaborate than for depression and it can feel unwieldy at times. However, it is crucial that the medications be taken regularly. Abruptly stopping can result in an acute manic episode that can prompt impulsive, reckless behavior or suicidal thoughts. When that happens, hospitalization, antipsychotic medication, and/or electroconvulsive therapy may be necessary. After the acute episode has subsided, medication may need to be monitored closely for a while to prevent another relapse.

WHAT RESEARCH IS BEING DONE?

While studies specifically on depression as it affects the elderly are few and far between, as a greater proportion of the U.S. population ages, more research is and will be conducted for this group. Some of the relevant and more interesting studies that have been done and are being done are described below.

• In 1998, the MacArthur Foundation published a study on Aging in America. In that study, they talked about the important role caregivers and home health care attendants have to play in spotting and monitoring depression in the elderly.

• Another study suggests that there are three crucial factors in preventing suicide in the elderly: immediate and aggressive treatment, monitoring, and follow-up.

• A recent study from the National Institute of Mental Health found that the combination of antidepressant medication and psychotherapy was more effective in preventing a recurrence of major depression in older adults than were either medication or psychotherapy by themselves. However, the improvement with both forms of treatment was not large.

• Researchers are studying whether programs based in primary care to identify and actively track patients with depression through phone calls or extra visits can improve treatment of depression and reduce suicides.

• Research shows that people who have a plan for dealing with depressive episodes—knowing how to recognize the symptoms early and who to ask for help—do much better, as do their loved ones.

• Medical research is now looking into who responds to which antidepressant medications so patients would not have to try as many different medications before finding the most effective medication.

• Studies are being conducted to determine more precisely when apathetic symptoms reflect depression and when they reflect tiny strokes. Research is also currently being done on the other possible mechanisms that may lead to depression in the elderly, such as inflammation and immune system dysfunction.

• Finally, studies are being conducted on the effectiveness of different types of psychotherapies in the elderly, and whether hormone replacement therapy can help improve mood in older women.

WHAT YOU CAN DO NOW

If your loved one tends to respond to environmental stressors with depressive symptoms, there are a number of things you—or he—can do. First, remember that depression does get better, and if depression is brought on by a specific event or situation—children moving away, selling the family home, an illness, or retirement—it will most likely diminish when the stress fades or the person adjusts to the new situation. Also, if certain types of events are likely to trigger such feelings—the approaching holidays, a visit to the doctor, for example—try to anticipate and prepare. When feelings arise unexpectedly, they can carry an additional power; learning to anticipate can drain some of the force from the depression.

Regular exercise and relaxation techniques can relieve or reduce symptoms of depression. And if you exercise along with your loved one, you may avoid exhaustion and perhaps even depression in yourself.

When a person is in the grips of a depression, supportive family and friends can make a world of difference. In cases of mild, transient depression, the emotional support of loved ones can be all that's needed. When a person experiences a seasonal depression, spending time outdoors every day, even during the winter, is essential. The amount of natural light in the house should be increased and, whenever possible, trips to warmer and sunnier climates should be planned. However, a more severe or persistent depression is an illness and, like other illnesses such as diabetes or hypertension, it requires medical attention.

SPECIAL NOTE TO CAREGIVERS: HOW TO TALK AND BEHAVE AROUND A PERSON WHO IS DEPRESSED

Honest discussions. Although you may not be doing it consciously, chances are that if you are caring for an older adult who seems depressed—a parent, spouse, relative, or neighbor—you are constantly taking his emotional temperature. On some level, you may be looking for upswings in his mood and simultaneously searching anxiously for signs of sorrow and despair, even thoughts of death and suicide.

But have you brought these concerns out into the open? Possibly not. There is a mistaken belief in our society that if we talk about depression and suicide, we could be promoting the very feelings and actions we fear. As a result, many who take care of older adults try to maintain a positive, optimistic, encouraging facade. But by not giving voice to your concerns, you can unwittingly leave yourself awash in feelings of anxiety and helplessness, and leave your loved one cut off and perhaps feeling more alone.

That's not to say you need to be full of gloom and doom. Indeed, you can hold out a vision of hope, yet not be falsely optimistic. As a person nears the end of his life—depressed or not—he will naturally entertain frequent thoughts of death and loss, regret and remorse. It's best not to try to cover over or make excuses when he admits to feeling blue, despondent, hopeless, or all alone. Rather than encouraging or positive, responses such as "Oh don't worry, you're doing just fine," may feel dismissive or inattentive.

Allow room for honest discussions (not just one) about death and suicide. In most instances, a candid talk that acknowledges and in some ways normalizes the person's feelings and difficulties can be reassuring. Moreover, by acknowledging the problem, you can begin to find solutions. For example, many such discussions have led to diagnosis and treatment—which means that the person is able to feel better soon.

Social contact. You may find it troubling to hear your loved one talk about his thoughts of death and loss. Indeed, for a number of reasons, many older adults find that their social support system has become limited to their caregiver—a child or spouse. It is natural for an older person to desire a certain amount of social withdrawal.

As older adults become more housebound as a consequence of increased disability or dementia, they will have diminished contact with peers. But contact with peers is important at this time since they are likely experiencing similar thoughts, questions, and concerns. It is necessary, then, that you, the caregiver, not take it all upon yourself, but instead encourage contact between your loved one and others.

Consider involving him in a day program at the local nursing home or community center. Help him identify other people he would enjoy talking to. Facilitate contact. Help with phone calls, schedule visits, even help set up e-mail correspondences.

Encouraging interaction. But that raises a question that inevitably figures into any discussion of caregiving: How much should you encourage independence in an older person and how much should you do for him yourself? How much do you heed the protestations that he doesn't want to anything, and how much do you gently coerce? The truth is that pleasurable activities are not just diversions; studies show that they can actually change the chemicals in the brain. (This, by the way, is the foundation of cognitive therapy.) By changing the way we think we can actually change our moods. So, whenever you can, encourage, coerce, gently force, cut a deal to get your loved one out of the house. Encourage him to go to the birthday party. Drive him to the card game. A movie, a drive, a family dinner out can make a world of difference. Getting out of the house means that he will have contact with other people, feel stimulated, and perhaps experience pleasure. Having fun can certainly mitigate feelings of depression, loneliness, and hopelessness.

Take precautions. Finally, if the person you are tending is depressed or appears to entertain suicidal thoughts, take precautions. Get guns out of the house. Most older men who kill themselves use guns. Keep an eye on medications. Most women who kill themselves do so by drug overdose.

Develop a plan. Discuss who your loved one can call when he is feeling especially despondent or isolated—a doctor, a friend, a relative, a suicide hotline. Finally, control your loved one's access to alcohol. When someone drinks too much, fatal accidents can happen—and suicide can seem like a more attractive option when intoxicated.

ADDITIONAL RESOURCES

WEB SITES

American Psychiatric Association Publications

www.psych.org/libr_publ

Internet Mental Health

www.mentalhealth.com

National Guidelines Clearinghouse

www.guideline.gov/index.asp

National Institute of Mental Health (NIMH)— Research Activities

www.nimh.nih.gov/research/index.htm

National Mental Health Association

www.nmha.org

ORGANIZATIONS

National Alliance for the Mentally Ill

Colonial Place Three

2107 Wilson Blvd., Suite 300

Arlington, VA 22201-3042

800-950-NAMI (-6264) (Help Line)

Front Desk 703-524-7600

Fax 703-524-9094

TDD 703-516-7227

www.nami.org

National Depressive and Manic-Depressive Association

730 N. Franklin Street, Suite 501

Chicago, IL 60610-3526 USA

800-826-3632

312-642-0049

Fax 312-642-7243

www.ndmda.org

National Institute on Aging

Building 31, Room 5C27

31 Center Drive, MSC 2292

Bethesda, MD 20892

301-496-1752

www.nih.gov/nia

BOOKS AND PAMPHLETS

American Psychiatric Association. *Diagnostic and Statistical Manual of Mental Disorders*, Fourth Edition, Text Revision. Washington, D. C.: American Psychiatric Press, 2000.

Bloomfield, Harold, and Peter McWilliams. *How to Heal Depression*. Los Angeles: Prelude Press, 1995.

Clinical Guidelines for Major Depressive Disorder. Washington, D.C.: Veterans Health Administration/Department of Veterans Affairs, 1997.

Detection of Depression in the Cognitively Intact Older Adult. Iowa City: University of Iowa Gerontological Nursing Interventions Research Center, 1998.

Kaplan, H., and B. Sadock. *Kaplan & Sadock's Synopsis of Psychiatry: Behavioral Sciences, Clinical Psychiatry*. Baltimore: Lippincott Williams & Wilkins, 1998.

Mathiasen, Patrick, and Suzanne LeVert. *Late Life Depression*. New York: Dell Publishing Company, 1998.

Prevention of Suicide. London, Ontario: Canadian Task Force on Preventive Health Care, 1994.

Sadavoy, J., L. Lazarus, L. Jarvik, and G. Grossberg. *Comprehensive Review of Geriatric Psychiatry II*. Washington, D. C.:American Psychiatric Press, 1996.

Styron, William. *Darkness Visible: A Memoir of Madness*. New York: Vintage Books, 1992.

Substance Abuse among Older Adults. Rockville, Md.: U. S. Department of Health and Human Services, Substance Abuse and Mental Health Services Administration, 1998.

Diabetes Mellitus

Diabetes mellitus is a disorder of metabolism that results from a deficiency of insulin, a hormone secreted by the particular cells in the pancreas, called "beta" cells.

There are two common types of diabetes:

- Type 1, formerly called juvenile diabetes or insulin-dependent diabetes mellitus
- Type 2, formerly referred to as adult-onset diabetes or non–insulin-dependent diabetes mellitus

Type 1 diabetes accounts for only about 5% of all patients with diabetes; the rest have the far more common type 2. Diabetes can also occur for the first time during pregnancy (gestational diabetes) and disappear after delivery. Women with gestational diabetes are at increased risk for the later development of type 2 diabetes.

The incidence of diabetes has grown dramatically over the past thirty years, in large part due to our national epidemic of obesity. It is now estimated that sixteen million Americans have diabetes and that nearly half of them are unaware they have the disorder.

WHAT IS IT?

Insulin is required for the removal of sugar (glucose) from the blood by muscles after a meal and to prevent the oversecretion of glucose from the liver during

189

periods of fasting. An inadequate amount or inefficient action of insulin leads to elevated blood levels of glucose, the hallmark of diabetes.

Type 1 diabetes is due to destruction of the beta cells of the pancreas by an autoimmune reaction (an attack on these cells by the body's immune system that normally works to fend off infections).

Type 2 diabetes results from a combination of resistance to the action of insulin and an inability of the pancreas to produce enough insulin to overcome the resistance.

The most common cause of insulin resistance is obesity, especially an excessive accumulation of fat in the abdomen (abdominal obesity). Abdominal obesity can be recognized with a tape measure. A man with an abdominal circumference of 40 inches or more, or a woman with an abdominal circumference of 35 inches or more, is obese. The consequences of insulin resistance stemming from abdominal obesity are often referred to as the metabolic syndrome or syndrome X, which is characterized by high blood pressure, elevated levels of blood triglycerides, low levels of high-density lipoprotein (HDL) cholesterol, an increased incidence of cardiovascular disease, and a high risk for the development of type 2 diabetes. Initially, the insulin resistance can be overcome by putting out more and more insulin, but in many people the pancreas is unable to keep up with the demand and diabetes follows.

Less often, type 2 diabetes can result from destruction of the beta cells by other disorders such as cancer of the pancreas, chronic pancreatitis, or an accumulation of iron in the pancreas due to a disorder called hemochromatosis.

Insulin resistance can also be caused by:

- Genetic factors
- Aging
- Some medications (beta-blockers, steroid hormones like prednisone)
- Overproduction of certain hormones (cortisol and epinephrine by tumors of the adrenal gland, growth hormone by tumors of the pituitary gland, and glucagon from tumors of the alpha cells of the pancreas)

Insulin is absolutely required for the treatment of type 1 diabetes. Most patients with type 2 diabetes can initially be treated with lifestyle measures or oral medications, but about 30% eventually require insulin. Control of blood glucose is important both to overcome the symptoms of high blood glucose (hyperglycemia) and to prevent some of the late complications of diabetes.

WHO IS AT RISK?

Type 1 diabetes was originally named juvenile diabetes because it tends to occur in young children and teenagers, but it is now recognized that it can affect people of all ages. Even though certain genetic factors increase the risk of developing type 1 diabetes, the disorder usually does not occur in other members of the family. Because type 1 diabetes often follows a viral illness, it is thought that the viral infection sets off the immune process within the body that destroys the beta cells in a person who is genetically susceptible. Type 2 diabetes was referred to as adult onset diabetes because it is far more frequent after age 40.

With the recent epidemic of obesity, type 2 diabetes is occurring more often in younger people and is now being recognized in a growing number of teenagers. Unlike type 1 diabetes, patients with type 2 diabetes often have other members of their family who are afflicted with the disorder. Type 2 diabetes occurs when a person with a genetic tendency to diabetes becomes resistant to the actions of insulin and is unable to secrete enough insulin to overcome this resistance.

HOW IS IT DIAGNOSED?

SYMPTOMS

The initial symptoms of diabetes are due to hyperglycemia (high blood glucose). High blood glucose levels lead to the excretion of glucose into the urine. The large amounts of glucose in the urine are accompanied by excessive amounts of water. The results are frequent urination and increased thirst. The loss of glucose calories in the urine can produce weight loss despite an increase in appetite. These cardinal early symptoms of diabetes are often referred to as the "polys":

- Polyuria: excessive amounts and frequency of urination
- Polydipsia: excessive thirst and intake of fluids; and
- Polyphagia: increased hunger

These symptoms can be severe enough to keep some people going to the bathroom frequently at night; in other people the symptoms may be nonexistent, or so subtle and so slowly progressive that they can go for many years in people with type 2 diabetes before it is recognized. Type 2 patients often develop one or more of the late complications of chronic hyperglycemia without ever recognizing or paying attention to these symptoms of hyperglycemia. In type 1 diabetes, symptoms of hyperglycemia begin more abruptly and are more prominent. In fact, type 1 diabetes is often first recognized when a patient is acutely ill and requires hospitalization for the potentially fatal complication known as diabetic ketoacidosis.

LABORATORY TESTS

Glucose control. Although diabetes can be suspected from the symptoms of high blood sugar or the development of acute ketoacidosis in type 1 diabetes, the diagnosis requires the finding of abnormal blood glucose levels. Diabetes is diagnosed either by a fasting (not eating for 12 hours) blood glucose of 126 milligrams per deciliter (mg/dL) or greater or by a nonfasting glucose of 200 mg/dL or greater in a person with the typical symptoms of diabetes. Fasting blood glucose levels between 110 and 125 mg/dL are defined as impaired fasting glucose. Less often, diabetes is diagnosed by measuring blood glucose levels over a two-hour period after administration of a standard amount of sugar by mouth (the oral glucose tolerance test).

Glucose in the blood attaches to the hemoglobin in red blood cells in varying amounts, depending on the concentration of glucose in the blood. Since this attachment is permanent and red cells survive an average of one hundred and twenty days, a measurement of the amount of glucose attached to hemoglobin, termed the glycohemoglobin or hemoglobin A1c, measures the average blood glucose level over the preceding three months. The American Diabetes Association has recommended that this test not be used for the initial diagnosis of diabetes, but this measure of average blood glucose levels is a valuable measure of diabetes control over the proceeding months.

When diabetic control is extremely poor, fat is rapidly broken down to form products known as ketone bodies. Detection of large amounts of ketone bodies in the blood or urine, particularly in a type 1 patient, is a danger signal.

Patients' monitoring of their diabetic control once relied on rough measurements of the amount of glucose in the urine. Now, patients with both types of diabetes can—and are expected to—monitor their blood glucose levels at regular intervals by using one of the many glucose-measuring devices (glucometers) to test a drop of blood obtained by pricking a finger. Home measurements of ketone bodies in the urine can be useful in determining when the diabetes is so out of control that a type 1 patient is at risk for developing ketoacidosis unless prompt countermeasures are taken.

Other important laboratory tests. When the type of diabetes is in doubt, the presence in the blood of antibodies to beta cells can confirm a type 1 diagnosis.

Additional blood tests obtained upon the initial diagnosis of diabetes, and at intervals during the follow-up, include a creatinine test to detect significant kidney abnormalities and a lipid profile (cholesterol, triglycerides, and HDL cholesterol) because of the increased frequency of elevated blood lipids and cardiovascular disease in people with diabetes. Detection of the earliest manifestation of diabetic kidney disease, the presence of small amounts of protein in the urine (microalbuminuria), is a routine test upon the diagnosis of type 2 diabetes and later in the course of type 1. Microalbumin is measured at intervals during subsequent physician visits to follow the progress of kidney disease.

PHYSICAL EXAMINATION

Regular blood pressure measurements are essential because elevated blood pressure speeds the development of cardiovascular disease, kidney disease, and damage to the eyes. The extremities are examined for any loss of sensation that indicates the presence of peripheral neuropathy (damage to the nerves in the extremities) and for the strength of pulses in the feet as a rough estimate of the adequacy of blood flow to the legs. A careful examination with an ophthalmoscope to look for the early signs of diabetic eye disease, after first diluting the pupils with eye drops, is a critical part of the initial evaluation of patients with type 2 diabetes. The first eye exam by an ophthalmologist in type 1 patients can be delayed for five years from initial diagnosis but annual follow-up exams are required. In patients with type 2 diabetes, an eye exam by an ophthalmologist is required at the time of diagnosis and then at least annually.

WHAT SHOULD YOU EXPECT?

Most often the symptoms of hyperglycemia are rather easily overcome by maintaining reasonable blood glucose levels. The major dangers of diabetes, however, are related to the acute emergencies and late complications of the disorder; these can be averted or delayed by excellent control of blood glucose and attention to the risk factors for cardiovascular disease.

ACUTE COMPLICATIONS OF DIABETES

Diabetic ketoacidosis and coma are associated with uncontrolled blood glucose levels and the accompanying symptoms of hyperglycemia: excessive thirst and increased urination. Ketoacidosis almost always occurs in patients with type 1 diabetes, but on rare occasions it can be a complication in patients with type 2 when they are under great physical stress, for example, after surgery or during a severe infection. By contrast, diabetic coma occurs only in patients with type 2 diabetes. Either ketoacidosis or diabetic coma can be the first manifestation of diabetes. Both are acute emergencies that require hospitalization and immediate treatment. Both must be distinguished from low blood sugar (hypoglycemia), which results from the treatment of diabetes rather than the diabetes itself. Severe hypoglycemia can also produce coma and require a trip to an emergency room, where it is treated with an intravenous infusion of glucose. All patients with diabetes should wear a medical alert bracelet so that the cause of any of these acute complications can be diagnosed and treated quickly.

Diabetic ketoacidosis. Ketoacidosis results when insulin levels are extremely low and the diabetes is totally out of control. Blood glucose levels can rise to as high as 1000 mg/dL because low insulin levels prevent the entry of glucose into cells. Unable to use glucose effectively as an energy source, the body turns to fat for its needs. Incomplete breakdown of fats leads to the formation of ketone bodies, which are strong acids that increase the acidity of the blood. As a result of the high blood glucose levels, large amounts of glucose are excreted in the urine, carrying with them excessive amounts of water.

Ketone bodies, along with minerals like potassium and magnesium bound to them, are also excreted in the urine. The combination of high blood glucose, dehydration from water lost in the urine, highly acidic blood, and depletion of minerals accounts for the manifestations of ketoacidosis.

Symptoms of ketoacidosis include:

- Deep sighing respirations with a fruity odor to the breath
- Loss of appetite
- Nausea
- Vomiting
- Abdominal pain
- Confusion
- Loss of consciousness

Patients may worsen the situation by stopping their insulin injections, thinking insulin is unnecessary because they are not eating. Ketoacidosis is treated with insulin, fluids, and replacement of lost minerals. Always fatal prior to the discovery of insulin in 1922, ketoacidosis can now be treated effectively but the outcome is still fatal in nearly 10% of episodes.

Coma. In people with this complication, blood glucose levels can exceed 1000 mg/dL. The disorder is termed "nonketotic" hyperosmolar coma because type 2 patients can make enough insulin to prevent the overproduction of ketone bodies seen in ketoacidosis.

Patients who develop this diabetic coma often have other severe underlying illnesses or they are bedridden and unable to obtain the fluids needed to overcome the dehydration resulting from their excessive output of urine. They become confused and drowsy and then can lapse into unconsciousness. Treatment with fluids and insulin may be effective, but the mortality rate is high because of the frequent presence of other major illnesses.

Hypoglycemia. Hypoglycemia (low blood sugar) is generally defined by a blood glucose level of less than 60 mg/dL. Most patients do not experience symptoms of hypoglycemia until their glucose level falls below 50 mg/dL. People with diabetes may have symptoms, however, when glucose levels fall rapidly over a short period of time, even though the blood glucose remains within normal limits. Hypoglycemia is a common occurrence when people with diabetes are treated with insulin or sulfonylureas, which increase the release of insulin from the pancreas in patients with type 2 diabetes. Symptoms of hypoglycemia result either from the release of epinephrine from the adrenal gland, triggered by a sharp drop in blood glucose levels, or from an inadequate supply of glucose to the brain, which absolutely requires glucose to function properly. Symptoms due to epinephrine release (adrenergic symptoms) include:

- Anxiety
- Tremor
- Hunger
- Numbness around the mouth
- Sweating
- Rapid heart beat

The poor supply of glucose to the brain can also cause neurological symptoms such as:

- Confusion
- Drowsiness
- Seizures
- Loss of consciousness
- Permanent brain damage

The adrenergic symptoms serve as an early warning to eat or drink something that contains sugar to raise blood glucose levels and prevent the more dangerous results of an inadequate supply of glucose to the brain. People with frequent episodes of hypoglycemia are at high risk for more severe episodes and neurological symptoms. Such patients often lose the adrenergic symptoms of hypoglycemia and develop serious neurological symptoms without warning, a condition referred to as unawareness of hypoglycemia. This unawareness may be overcome with a prolonged period (several months) without any hypoglycemic episodes, so it may be necessary to reduce the dose of insulin temporarily, even if average blood glucose levels rise as a consequence.

In addition, release of glucagon from the pancreas, to raise blood glucose levels, is a normal response to hypoglycemia that is gradually lost in people with long-standing diabetes.

People taking insulin or a sulfonylurea should always carry with them a rapidly absorbed source of sugar that can be taken at the earliest sign of hypoglycemia. Family members, friends, and coworkers should be told that the patient has diabetes and might develop hypoglycemia. The manifestations of hypoglycemia should be explained to these people so that they can alert the patient to its development in case the patient is unaware of unusual behavior.

Particularly dangerous is the possible occurrence of hypoglycemia while asleep or at a time of peak action of insulin, such as at the end of a workday when a patient may be starting a long drive home. A regular check on blood glucose levels may be warranted at bedtime and before beginning to drive a car.

COMPLICATIONS DURING PREGNANCY

Excellent control of blood glucose is essential throughout pregnancy to avoid the problems that can complicate both the early and late stages of pregnancy. During the first months of pregnancy, high blood glucose levels may cause a miscarriage and malformations or death of the fetus. Late in pregnancy persistent hyperglycemia can result in large-birth-weight newborns. Despite the difficulty of maintaining strict control, most women with diabetes are able to achieve the desired targets because they know the stakes are high and they can look forward to some relaxation of the intense treatment measures within a few months.

Women with known diabetes are urged to get their blood glucose under excellent control before becoming pregnant. In others, a glucose tolerance test is carried out in the twenty-eighth week of pregnancy to detect possible gestational diabetes in women over age 25 and in those at high risk for diabetes, for example in African Americans, obese women, and those with a family history of type 2 diabetes.

LATE COMPLICATIONS DUE TO HIGH BLOOD GLUCOSE

The late complications of diabetes resulting from poorly controlled blood glucose levels are damage to small blood vessels (microvascular disease), which affects the eyes (diabetic retinopathy) and kidneys (nephropathy), and to nerve injury (neuropathy).

Although it was long suspected that good control of diabetes would prevent or delay these complications, it was only in 1993 when publication of the Diabetes

Control and Complications Trial (DCCT) conclusively showed that intensive glucose control significantly reduced the incidence of these complications in patients with type 1 diabetes. Results from the United Kingdom Prospective Diabetes Study, published five years later, first showed similar benefits of better control in patients with type 2 diabetes. Unfortunately, some people first discover they have diabetes when they develop one of its complications.

Retinopathy. Diabetic retinopathy can damage the small blood vessels that supply blood to the retina (the nerve tissues at the back of the eye that transmit images to the brain). Diabetic retinopathy does not develop until people have had diabetes for at least five to ten years. In its initial stages the injured vessels develop bulges termed microaneurysms. The vessels can leak small amounts of blood and fluid. The resultant hemorrhages and leaks, along with the microaneurysms, which can all be seen in the retina during an eye exam, are referred to as background or nonproliferative retinopathy and are generally associated with no visual changes. In many people with diabetes, the retinopathy progresses no further.

A later, dangerous stage of diabetic retinopathy is the growth of small blood vessels on the retina and into the vitreous humor (a clear, gelatin-like substance) in the back of the eye. These fragile vessels may rupture and bleed into the vitreous, temporarily obscuring vision; the bleeding often stops eventually, but can leave behind scar tissue that pulls on and detaches a portion of the retina. Patients with diabetes are also more prone to macular edema—an accumulation of fluid under the macula, the part of the retina essential for fine-detail vision.

The United Kingdom Prospective Diabetes Study showed that a modest reduction in blood pressure significantly slowed the development of retinopathy in patients with type 2 diabetes. Early detection and treatment of proliferative retinopathy may prevent serious vision loss. Even with proper treatment, however, diabetic retinopathy can eventually lead to blindness. In fact, diabetic retinopathy is the leading cause of blindness in adults in the United States.

Nephropathy. Like retinopathy, kidney damage (nephropathy) only occurs after many years of diabetes mellitus—ten to fifteen years on average. The first evidence of kidney damage is the appearance of small amounts of protein in the urine. The damage can progress to larger losses of protein in the urine and to chronic kidney failure with the accumulation of waste products in the blood that may require either kidney dialysis or a kidney transplant. Significant nephropathy develops in about 40% of people with type 1 and 20% of those with type 2 diabetes. The progression of nephropathy can be slowed by controlling blood pressure and by treatment with an angiotensin-converting enzyme (ACE) inhibitor.

Neuropathy. More than half of the people with diabetes develop one of the several forms of nerve damage called diabetic neuropathy. The most common type is peripheral neuropathy, which affects the sensory nerves to the arms and legs. With the slow progression of peripheral neuropathy, all forms of sensation are gradually lost, beginning usually in the feet and moving progressively higher in the legs. Less often, sensation may be lost in the hands as well. The first symptoms are tingling and pain, which eventually change to numbness when the nerves are completely destroyed.

Another form of neuropathy, autonomic neuropathy, affects the nerves to the intestinal tract and other organs such as the heart. Autonomic neuropathy can interfere with emptying of the stomach, giving a feeling of fullness and causing nausea and vomiting, or produce diarrhea or constipation when it affects the nerves supplying the large bowel. Involvement of nerves to the heart can cause a rapid heartbeat. Erectile dysfunction (impotence), resulting from either autonomic neuropathy, diminished blood supply, or a combination of the two, affects a majority of men with diabetes.

Interference with the blood supply to a single nerve can produce loss of sensation or muscle strength in the area supplied by the affected nerve. These "mononeuropathies" tend to improve over a few months, whereas peripheral and autonomic neuropathies gradually worsen over time.

OTHER COMPLICATIONS

In addition to retinopathy, diabetes is associated with an increased incidence of other eye disorders, namely cataracts and glaucoma. Diabetes can decrease the formation of saliva, which leads to dry mouth and a greater number of cavities, with the loss of saliva's cleansing action and protection against mouth infections. Diabetes is associated with an increased frequency of gum diseases, gingivitis, and the more serious periodontitis, which can lead first to loosening and then loss of teeth. People with diabetes are more prone to all types of infections, such as vaginitis in women, urinary tract infections, skin infections, and even life-threatening infections such as tuberculosis. A rare complication of diabetes, particularly in young women, is a condition called necrobiosis lipoidica diabeticorum, a large area of thinned, purple-colored skin on the lower legs, which looks frightening but is not dangerous.

Cardiovascular disease. People with diabetes are at greatly increased risk for cardiovascular diseases resulting from atherosclerosis (hardening of the arteries). These cardiovascular diseases involve primarily the heart (coronary heart disease or CHD), central nervous system (cerebrovascular disease), and the legs (peripheral vascular disease). The major manifestations of CHD are chest pain (angina) on exertion or with stress and heart attacks. Cerebrovascular disease can cause a stroke or a mini-stroke, temporary episodes of blindness, or loss of strength in one leg, for example. The first symptom of peripheral vascular disease is pain in the thighs or calves of one or both legs that begins with walking and stops abruptly with rest (intermittent claudication).

Heart attacks are about two times more common in men with diabetes, and four times more common in women with diabetes, than in people who do not have diabetes. Strokes are nearly twice as common in diabetic patients when compared with nondiabetics. In fact, about 75% of people with diabetes die of cardiovascular disease—a quarter from a stroke, the remainder from CHD. Although people with diabetes are more likely than others to have hypertension and lipid abnormalities, the presence of these risk factors does not account fully for the greater incidence of cardiovascular disease in diabetes. Since studies have shown that better control of blood glucose has little or no effect on the prevention of cardiovascular disease, efforts must be directed to preventing or treating all of the other risk factors for CHD.

The diabetic foot. Foot problems are common in patients with diabetes because of the combination of peripheral neuropathy and peripheral vascular disease. As a result of insensitivity to pain, a patient may not be aware of the formation of blisters from shoes that fit poorly. Blisters may become infected and heal slowly because of the poor blood supply. The inadequate supply of blood to the legs can damage and even kill tissues, resulting in gangrene. An amputation may be necessary to remove gangrenous tissue or prevent the spread of chronic infections. In fact, diabetes is the most common cause of amputations not resulting from injury. Another complication of peripheral neuropathy is the destruction of a joint (called Charcot's joint), such as the ankle, when a patient does not notice repeated trauma to the joint.

HOW IS IT TREATED?

CONTROL OF BLOOD GLUCOSE

Blood glucose monitoring is an essential part of the treatment and control of diabetes. For the patient, monitoring is not only an educational tool but also makes it possible to make adjustments in meals, exercise, and insulin doses in response to glucose levels. The recorded glucose values brought to the doctor/diabetes team provide valuable information on the possible need to make adjustments in lifestyle habits or medications. The goal for all patients is to prevent complications by controlling glucose levels. The targets for good control are an average blood glucose under 150 mg/dL and a hemoglobin A1c of 7 or less. According to the results of the Diabetes Control and Complications Trial, these targets are a safe zone to delay or prevent the onset of complications.

LIFESTYLE MEASURES

The most effective way to treat (and prevent) type 2 diabetes is with weight control using a combination of dietary measures and exercise. Even a small amount of weight loss can have a major impact on blood glucose levels, as well as lowering blood pressure and improving blood lipid levels. Important in type 1 diabetes are consistency in the timing and content of meals as well as their timing with exercise.

Diet. Dietary concerns for those with diabetes center around the types of food to eat, caloric intake, and when to eat. The same types of food are recommended for both types of diabetes. Because of the high risk of cardiovascular disease in people with diabetes, the diet recommended by the American Diabetes Association is the same as the one advocated by the National Cholesterol Education Program. This diet restricts total fat to less than 30% of calories and saturated fat to less than 10% of calories. Dietary cholesterol is limited to less than 300 mg per day.

Also recommended are weight control and an increase in dietary fiber. If cholesterol levels remain too high, saturated fat is further limited to less than 7% of calories and cholesterol intake is reduced to less than 200 mg per day.

Saturated fat intake can be reduced by eating chicken, fish, margarine, and skim milk instead of red meats and dairy products (whole milk, cheese, and butter).

In addition, one can replace saturated fats with vegetable oils containing monounsaturated fats (olive or canola oils) or polyunsaturated fats (corn, soybean, or sunflower oils). Monounsaturated oils are now preferred because they are less likely to lower HDL cholesterol levels than polyunsaturated fats. In general, eating foods low in saturated fat also reduces the intake of cholesterol. The exceptions are eggs, which each contain an average of about 225 mg of cholesterol with only a small amount of saturated fat, and the shellfish crab, lobster, and shrimp, which have a high cholesterol content.

A study found that eating an egg a day had no harmful effect on CHD, except in people with diabetes. Another study showed that daily intake of a large amount of shrimp raised total and LDL cholesterol levels only modestly. Some experts question restrictions in total fat because the necessary increase in carbohydrate intake can raise blood triglyceride levels. They recommend instead a diet that contains about 40% of calories as fat, emphasizing foods rich in monounsaturated fats, such as canola or olive oil, avocados, and nuts.

While table sugar is not prohibited, its consumption should be limited. Sugar can produce an especially rapid rise in blood glucose and the calories in sugar can promote weight gain. In addition, sugar has no nutritive value, as opposed to the vitamin and mineral content of more complex carbohydrate-containing foods. There is no evidence, by the way, that eating a lot of sugar causes diabetes.

Studies have shown that water-soluble fiber, found in oats, barley, legumes, and many fruits, lowers cholesterol levels; and a recent study showed that an increase in total fiber intake from 24 to 50 grams per day also improved control of blood glucose levels in patients with diabetes. The American Diabetes Association recommends a fiber intake between 20 and 35 grams per day. (See "Get More Fiber in Your Diet" on p. 273.)

All patients taking insulin need to be consistent in the timing and content of their meals to avoid hypoglycemic episodes from skipping or being late for meals. Such patients may also need to have a regular snack in midafternoon or at bedtime.

Exercise. Regular exercise is an important health measure for people with diabetes. The usual recommendation is to get at least thirty minutes of aerobic exercise by walking, jogging, biking, or swimming or through household activities such as gardening or cutting the grass. Patients should choose a form of exercise that they will enjoy doing regularly. The exercise does not all have to be done at the same time; rather it can be broken up into three or more ten-minute sessions. Exercise not only helps to control weight but also improves glucose control and blood pressure independent of weight loss. Weight lifting is an acceptable alternative form of exercise.

The best approach for sedentary people who wish to begin exercising is to start walking, initially perhaps for only five minutes at a comfortable pace. The length and speed of the walk can gradually be increased as tolerated. Sedentary people with diabetes who decide to undertake more vigorous forms of exercise should first check with their doctor if they are over 35, particularly if they have a strong family history of CHD or other risk factors for CHD. The doctor may recommend an exercise stress test before starting such an exercise program.

The best time to exercise is one to two hours after a meal. Even then, some risks are associated with exercise. These include dehydration, hypoglycemia in patients taking insulin, and damage to the feet or eyes. Blood glucose levels should be checked before initiating intensive or prolonged exercise. The exercise should be postponed if blood glucose is greater than 300 mg/dL to avoid becoming dehydrated. If the glucose level is 100 mg/dL or less, have a snack containing 15 to 30 grams of carbohydrate. In addition, the dose of short-acting insulin should be reduced when planning to exercise. People with peripheral neuropathy should avoid high-impact exercise that may worsen foot problems, and those with proliferative retinopathy should not engage in activities, like weight lifting, that require sudden bursts of strength that may provoke bleeding into the eye.

ORAL MEDICATIONS

When lifestyle measures fail to control blood glucose levels in type 2 patients, many can be treated effectively with oral agents. These include agents that stimulate the secretion of insulin from the pancreas (sulfonylureas and repaglinide), drugs that increase the responsiveness to insulin (metformin and the thiazolidinediones), and those that slow the absorption of glucose from the intestine (acarbose and miglitol). Sulfonylureas and metformin are roughly equally effective in lowering blood glucose levels. Thiazolidinediones are slightly less effective when used alone. Because type 2 diabetes gradually worsens over time, control may require combinations of two or more oral agents and about 30% of type 2 patients require treatment with insulin.

Sulfonylureas

The sulfonylureas were the first oral medications found to lower blood glucose levels. The sulfonylureas initially available, such as tolbutamide (Orinase) and chlorpropamide (Diabinese), are relatively impotent and large doses are required. Though still effective, these drugs—referred to as the first generation sulfonylureas—have now largely been replaced by a second generation of more potent drugs. These include glimepiride (Amaryl), glipizide (Glucotrol), extended-release glipizide (Glucotrol XL), and glyburide (DiaBeta, Glynase, and Micronase).

More than 80% of people with type 2 diabetes will respond to a sulfonylurea if their initial blood glucose levels are less than 250 mg/dL. All of the sulfonylureas work in the same way and are generally well tolerated. Except for chlorpropamide, they all have the same potential side effects. The most common and serious adverse effect is hypoglycemia; some studies have shown that as many as 20% of patients taking a sulfonylurea have a significant hypoglycemic reaction each year. Hypoglycemia is more common in debilitated, malnourished, and elderly patients. Another problem is that most people who take sulfonylureas gain weight. Less frequent side effects are abdominal pain, heartburn, constipation, diarrhea, and water retention. The duration of action of chlorpropamide is so long that it can cause prolonged hypoglycemia. In addition, in some people who are taking chlorpropamide, alcohol can produce flushing, nausea, and headaches.

Repaglinide

Repaglinide (Prandin), although chemically quite distinct from the sulfonylureas, also stimulates insulin release from the pancreas. It acts on the pancreas more rapidly than the sulfonylureas and it only works for a short time. The result is a rapid, brief rise in insulin levels that peaks in thirty to sixty minutes and lasts for about two hours. Taken before each meal, repaglinide can reduce the rise in blood glucose levels that occurs after eating. Hypoglycemia, the most common side effect of repaglinide, occurs less often than with the sulfonylureas.

Metformin

Metformin (Glucophage) partly overcomes the insulin resistance of type 2 patients. It acts primarily to decrease the output of glucose by the liver, but also enhances the removal of glucose from the blood by muscles. Taken alone, metformin rarely produces hypoglycemia, and weight gain is less common than with sulfonylureas. The most common adverse effects—diarrhea, flatulence, bloating, and nausea—can usually be averted by taking the medication with meals and starting with a low dose that is gradually increased if needed. The danger of metformin is a rare accumulation of lactic acid in the blood, termed lactic acidosis, that is fatal in about half the people who develop this complication. Metformin should not be taken by anyone with an increased risk of developing lactic acidosis, including people with kidney or liver disease, heart failure, chronic lung diseases, or heavy alcohol intake. The most recent diabetic oral agent is Glucovance, a combination product containing glyburide and metformin.

Thiazolidinediones

The thiazolidinediones work to overcome insulin resistance primarily by increasing the uptake of glucose by muscles. These drugs are slightly less effective than sulfonylureas or metformin when used alone, but can be especially useful in combination with other oral agents or when given along with insulin in people with type 2 diabetes.

Troglitazone (Rezulin), the first drug in this class approved by the Food and Drug Administration (FDA), was associated with severe liver disease that required a liver transplant or was fatal in so many patients that the FDA removed it from the market.

More recently approved are pioglitazone (Actos) and rosiglitazone (Avandia). These agents are generally well tolerated; side effects include weight gain, fluid accumulation, and some danger of worsening heart failure. Like metformin, these thiazolidinediones do not cause hypoglycemia when used alone. In combination with sulfonylureas or insulin, however, hypoglycemia can occur unless the dose of sulfonylurea or insulin is decreased.

Because several months may elapse before these drugs reach their maximal effect on blood glucose levels, patients and physicians must allow enough time to learn whether the drugs are working and be alert for the possible development of hypoglycemia some time after the drugs are started. Because their chemical structure is similar to that of troglitazone, liver enzyme measurements are recommended before starting treatment with these drugs and periodically thereafter.

Acarbose and miglitol

Acarbose (Precose) and miglitol (Glyset) have a chemical resemblance to some of the complex carbohydrates in our diet. As a result, these drugs block the action of the intestinal enzymes required to convert these carbohydrates into the simple sugars that can be absorbed from the intestine. By slowing the breakdown and absorption of dietary carbohydrates, these drugs reduce the rise in blood glucose following a carbohydrate-containing meal. The agents are taken just before each meal.

The problem is that the carbohydrates not digested by intestinal enzymes enter the large bowel, which contains bacteria that break down these carbohydrates to form several different types of gases. Consequently, severe flatulence is so often a troublesome side effect of using these drugs that many people are unable to tolerate them. Taken alone, these drugs do not cause hypoglycemia. The hypoglycemia that may occur when they are used along with other medications cannot be treated with the usual forms of sugar, since their digestion and absorption are prevented by the drugs. In this situation, the hypoglycemia must be treated with pure glucose (not table sugar), fruit juices, or milk that contain sugars whose digestion is not blocked by the drugs.

Insulin

All type 1 patients must be treated with insulin, and many type 2 patients also require insulin.

Originally isolated from the pancreas of cows or pigs, all insulins now used in this country are biosynthetic products produced in bacteria from human DNA (all called Humulin insulins). The different types of insulin are characterized by their rapidity of onset and duration of action as rapid, intermediate and long-acting insulins. Rapid-acting (or regular) insulin begins to work in about thirty to sixty minutes, reaches a peak at about two hours and continues to work for about four to six hours. The onset and duration of insulin action are prolonged in the intermediate-acting insulins either by adding protamine (NPH insulin) or by forming large crystals of insulin with zinc (Lente insulin). The protamine or crystal formation delays the absorption of insulin from their subcutaneous injection sites.

Intermediate insulins begin to act in two to four hours, peak at eight to twelve hours, and continue to have some effect for about sixteen hours. Long-acting Ultralente insulin has even larger zinc crystals. Its action begins after four to six hours, peaks at eighteen to twenty-four hours, and may continue to work for as long as thirty-six hours.

An even more rapidly acting insulin, Humalog (Lispro), became available a few years ago and is widely used. Produced by altering the amino acid composition of insulin, Humalog begins to work in about fifteen minutes, peaks in two hours, and lasts for about four hours. A long-acting insulin, insulin glargine (Lantus), is also a modified form of human insulin. This form of insulin is given only once daily. It is slowly absorbed from the injection site and, after a few hours, is maintained at a relatively constant concentration in the blood, without the insulin peaks produced by the other forms of insulin. Early studies with Lantus show better control and less hypoglycemia than with NPH insulin.

Patients generally either take two injections of intermediate-acting insulin—before breakfast and before dinner or at bedtime—or, less often, a single injection of long-acting insulin. In addition, most patients add an injection of regular insulin thirty to forty-five minutes before one or more meals to cover the rise in blood sugar that follows the meal. Regular and intermediate-acting insulins can be mixed in the same syringe (drawing up the regular insulin first, and then the intermediate insulin) to give the two insulins with a single injection. Alternatively, patients can use prepared mixtures containing 70% NPH and 30% regular insulin (70/30 Humulin) or equal amounts of NPH and regular insulin (Humulin 50/50). A combination insulin, Humalog 75/25, contains 75% NPH and 25% Humalog to give a faster response after a meal.

Insulins are usually removed from a vial with needle and syringe and then injected. Some people find it more convenient to use an insulin pen injector that allows them to dial in the dose of insulin and eliminates the need to carry vials of insulin and syringes.

The most common and serious adverse effect of insulin is hypoglycemia. Blood glucose monitoring is recommended two to four times a day for people taking insulin to avoid hypoglycemia.

Problems at the sites of injection may include a local loss of fat tissue, overgrowth of fat, and allergic reactions. Insulin injections can be given in the upper arms, thighs, buttocks, or abdomen, which is the preferred location. The rate of insulin absorption from the arms or legs speeds up with physical activity. Injection sites should be rotated constantly to avoid a buildup of fat or fibrous tissue that can slow the absorption of insulin.

External insulin pumps. Improved blood glucose control can be obtained by the continuous infusion of rapid-acting insulin with a small pump that is usually hooked onto the belt. Insulin is delivered through a plastic tube that connects the insulin-containing pump to a needle placed under the skin of the abdomen. The device continuously delivers small amounts of insulin at rates that can be programmed to vary throughout a twenty-four-hour period to approximate the insulin needs. Patients also trigger the pump to inject additional amounts of insulin to account for the expected rise in blood glucose that follows each meal.

Insulin pumps are only used by type 1 patients who must have a stable personality and understand the possible dangers associated with the pump. Because the infusion connections may leak, the pump may fail, or the needle can become loose, patients using a pump must check blood glucose levels frequently to avoid a rapid fall in insulin levels that could provoke severe hyperglycemia and even an attack of ketoacidosis. Pump failure may produce ketoacidosis rapidly because there is no intermediate or long-acting insulin in the body. The cost of a pump, about five thousand dollars, is covered by many insurance companies.

PANCREATIC TRANSPLANTS

Successful transplantation and function of a normal pancreas could cure diabetes. Pancreatic transplants have been performed frequently for about twenty years. The problems with a pancreatic transplant are the need to drain the pancreatic secretions (which normally are released into the duodenal portion of the intestine) and to prevent rejection of the transplanted pancreas by the body's immune system.

The transplanted pancreas is surgically implanted into the lower abdomen and its secretions are most often drained into the bladder. More recent operations have drained these secretions into the intestine to avoid some of the problems associated with bladder drainage, including inflammation of the urethra, dehydration, and the need to replace sodium and bicarbonate lost through the bladder into the urine.

The most serious difficulty is overcoming the immune reaction that can cause rejection of the transplanted pancreas. Efforts to overcome transplant rejection involve the continuous use of immunosuppressive drugs.

Experience has shown that patients who have a pancreas transplant survive better when the surgery is combined with a kidney transplant. The American Diabetes Association recommends that a pancreas transplant should only be considered as an alternative to insulin treatment in patients with type 1 diabetes and end-stage renal disease. This recommendation is based on the better survival of the pancreas after the combined surgery and the fact that people who get a kidney transplant have to take immunosuppressant medication in any case. The most recent data indicates that the five-year survival rate after a combined pancreas-kidney transplant are 90% for the patient, 84% for the kidney, and 74% for a pancreas that produces normal blood glucose levels without any treatments for diabetes. Patients who have undergone a successful pancreatic transplant state that their quality of life is improved despite the fact that they have to continue to take immunosuppressants for the rest of their lives.

Retinopathy initially gets worse after a pancreatic transplant (as it does with any rapid improvement in blood glucose levels); overall it appears that retinopathy is not improved by a pancreas transplant. There is too little information to know how effectively pancreatic transplants prevent other late complications of diabetes. Additional problems with pancreatic transplants include a long waiting list to obtain a pancreas and the limited number of surgeons and centers that have extensive experience with the procedure.

PREVENTING AND TREATING LATE COMPLICATIONS OF DIABETES DUE TO POOR GLUCOSE CONTROL

Excellent control of blood glucose can delay or prevent these complications in patients with both type 1 and type 2 diabetes. The United Kingdom Prospective Diabetes Study in 1998 found that even modest improvements in diabetic control reduced the development of both retinopathy and nephropathy in patients with type 2 diabetes.

Retinopathy

Timely treatment of retinopathy with laser photocoagulation can stop or slow the progression of vision loss in most patients. For this reason it is crucial to detect the first manifestations of retinopathy with an eye exam by an ophthalmologist within five years of the diagnosis of type 1 diabetes and as soon as type 2 diabetes is recognized. After dilating the eye with drops, the ophthalmologist directs bursts of laser light to many spots in the periphery of the eye to form scar tissue that prevents bleeding from the overgrowth of small new blood vessels. Laser coagulation is carried out as an outpatient procedure, and may require more than one treatment. If the vitreous (the fluid within the eye) becomes too clouded with blood or scar tissue, removal of the vitreous and replacement with a solution of saline can often improve vision.

Nephropathy

Blood pressure control, ACE inhibitor drugs, and possibly a low-protein diet have been shown to delay the development of kidney disease. ACE inhibitors can lower blood pressure, but studies have shown that these drugs help to prevent the progress of renal disease even in those whose blood pressure is normal. There has been some difference of opinion concerning when to start treatment with ACE inhibitors. Most experts await the finding of protein in the kidney (microalbuminuria) as the first evidence of renal disease before starting an ACE inhibitor. Others start a low dose of an ACE inhibitor as soon as the diagnosis of type 2 diabetes is made. The progress of microalbuminuria is followed regularly so that the dose of the ACE inhibitor can be raised if necessary.

The Heart Outcomes Prevention Evaluation (HOPE) trial found that treatment with the ACE inhibitor ramipril (Altace) produced a very great reduction in coronary events in people with diabetes and one additional risk factor for coronary heart disease (microalbuminuria was considered a risk factor in this study). These findings suggest that an ACE inhibitor should be started upon diagnosis in almost all type 2 diabetics, since most of these patients have at least one risk factor in addition to diabetes. Some of the side effects of the ACE inhibitors can be managed with additional medications.

Progressive damage to the kidneys can lead to kidney failure with the accumulation of metabolic waste products in the blood. The symptoms of kidney failure can be reduced with a low-protein diet, antacids to bind phosphorus in the intestine and remove it in the stools, calcium supplements, and sodium bicarbonate pills. When kidney function is reduced to less than 10% of normal it is called end-stage renal disease, and dialysis or a kidney transplant are the only available treatments.

Neuropathy

Peripheral neuropathy. The pain associated with peripheral neuropathy is difficult to treat. Large doses of the antidepressants nortriptyline (Aventyl, Pamelor) or amitriptyline (Elavil) may help to relieve pain. Both drugs are given at night because they tend to cause sedation and can relieve the nighttime pain that can interfere with sleep. Small doses should be given initially and the treatment should not be discarded as ineffective until a patient gets no relief from gradually increasing to large doses. Another drug that may ease the pain of peripheral neuropathy is the anticonvulsant gabapentin (Neurontin). Though usually well tolerated, gabapentin can cause drowsiness and confusion.

Autonomic neuropathy. Poor gastric emptying (passage of food through the digestive system), with symptoms of fullness, nausea, and vomiting, may be avoided by substituting multiple small, low-fat meals for the usual three larger meals a day. High-calorie supplements and vitamins may be needed to maintain nutrition. Patients and caregivers should recognize that the unpredictable rate of gastric emptying may lead to erratic control of blood glucose levels. One of the drugs that may speed gastric emptying is metoclopramide (Reglan), which can be given by mouth thirty minutes before each meal and at bedtime. It can be given by subcutaneous or intravenous injection in patients with severe vomiting. The antibiotic erythromycin can also speed gastric emptying but is less effective when taken orally than when given intravenously. If nausea persists, phenothiazines or antihistamines may provide some relief.

If the diarrhea associated with autonomic neuropathy does not respond to the usual drugs for diarrhea, such as diphenoxylate (Lomotil), it may be due to an overgrowth of intestinal bacteria that can sometimes be cured with an antibiotic such as tetracycline.

Impotence may be delayed by good glucose control to slow the development of autonomic neuropathy. Smoking cessation and avoiding excessive alcohol intake can improve potency in some. As many as half of men with diabetes and erectile dysfunction may respond to Viagra. A larger percentage of men with diabetes can attain erections with injections of medications directly into the penis. If these measures fail, mechanical treatment with an external vacuum device, although awkward, is nearly always successful.

HYPERTENSION

The target for blood pressure in patients with diabetes is a systolic pressure less than 130 mm Hg and a diastolic pressure less than 85 mm Hg. Lifestyle measures to lower blood pressure include weight loss, exercise, and dietary measures—a reduced intake of sodium (especially salt) and an increase in dietary potassium. At least five classes of equally effective drugs are available to lower blood pressure: diuretics, beta-blockers, ACE inhibitors, calcium channel blockers, and alpha-antagonists. ACE inhibitors are the primary choice drug for the treatment of hypertension in patients with diabetes. Combinations of drugs from two or more classes are often needed to achieve acceptable control of blood pressure.

WHAT RESEARCH IS BEING DONE?

PREVENTION OF TYPE 1 DIABETES

The ongoing Diabetes Prevention Trial, Type 1 (DPT-1), is examining whether regular small injections or oral doses of insulin can delay or prevent the development of type 1 diabetes. The study, supported jointly by the National Institutes of Health, American Diabetes Association, and the Juvenile Diabetes Foundation International, is enrolling patients who have both a family history of type 1 diabetes and whose blood contains circulating antibodies against the beta cells of the pancreas.

A second large study (ENDIT) in Europe is examining whether oral nicotinamide will prevent or delay the onset of type 1 diabetes in subjects similar to those enrolled in DPT-1. Results will take time since subjects will be followed for five years in ENDIT and for six years in DPT-1.

PREVENTION OF TYPE 2 DIABETES

People with impaired fasting glucose are at increased risk for the development of type 2 diabetes. Another NIH multicenter trial, the Diabetes Prevention Program, has enrolled subjects with abnormal glucose tolerance based on an oral glucose tolerance test. The initial aim was to compare the effect of four different treatments in these subjects—intensive lifestyle modifications with diet and exercise counseling; standard care plus metformin; standard care plus troglitazone, or standard care alone—on the subsequent development of type 2 diabetes.

The troglitazone arm of the program was discontinued when one of the early subjects in the study died of liver disease while being treated with the drug. The possible effectiveness of metformin in preventing type 2 diabetes will become evident after the study is completed in 2002.

IMPLANTED INSULIN PUMPS

Several types of insulin pumps have been implanted beneath the skin. These pumps work in a manner similar to the external insulin pumps except that the catheter from the pump delivers insulin into the abdominal cavity rather than through a needle placed in the skin of the abdomen. Like an external pump, implanted pumps deliver insulin continuously in amounts programmed to vary appropriately throughout the day; the patient can trigger the delivery of an additional amount of insulin as needed for meals. The pump currently uses a concentrated form of insulin in a reservoir that must be refilled through a needle about every three months.

This type of device is called an open loop system because the patient must make decisions on the amount of insulin to inject.

Researchers are now trying to develop a closed loop system, in which continuous measurements of glucose levels would deliver a signal to the pump, which would stimulate the release of an appropriate amount of insulin. Technical issues related to the electronics used for signaling the pump, and the program to convert glucose levels into the amount of insulin to inject, can be solved with relative ease. The problem, however, has been an inability to create an implantable device that continues to measure glucose values reliably for more than a few days.

ISLET TRANSPLANTS

Many of the difficulties of a pancreas transplant could be overcome by transplanting beta cells instead of the whole pancreas. Islets containing the insulin-secreting beta cells can be isolated by treating a pancreas (obtained from a

NEWER GLUCOSE MONITORS

Many studies are under way to develop continuous and less invasive methods for home glucose monitoring.

Glucowatch

The glucowatch monitor is like a wristwatch that senses the glucose levels in tissues and displays the values on a screen. It is capable of frequent measurements but has several disadvantages. The values reflect blood glucose values some minutes earlier and the results can be greatly altered by sweating. The estimated cost for the device is about two hundred dollars; each sensor lasts for only twelve hours and must be replaced at a cost of about four dollars.

Continuous glucose sensors

These new devices record tissue glucose levels at five-minute intervals for up to three days. A tiny flexible sensor is inserted, generally into the skin of the abdominal wall (similar to the placement of a needle and catheter for an external insulin pump). The values obtained over a period of three days are downloaded into a computer. The patterns in glucose levels help the physician to make adjustments in therapy.

cadaver) with enzymes that cause it to fall apart. Because the islets, just like a whole pancreas, are "foreign" to their recipient, an immune response begins. Immunosuppressants must be given to prevent rejection of the islets. Possibly because of the ill effects of the immunosuppressants, the injected cells secrete insulin for only a short time, and then stop working. Since 1990, human islet transplants have been reported in two hundred sixty-seven type 1 patients, but in only 8% of them has the diabetes been "cured" for a year. The immunosuppressants include adrenal corticosteroids that tend to produce insulin resistance in the transplant recipients. Another difficulty is obtaining the large amounts of islets needed for the transplant.

An exciting report from Edmonton, Canada, in June 2000 described seven type 1 patients whose diabetes required no insulin for an average of about twelve months after receiving human islet transplants. The investigators used more powerful immunosuppressants that did not include corticosteroids and are less likely to damage the transplanted islets. All the patients required the infusion of islets into a vein supplying blood to the liver on at least two separate occasions. This procedure will be tested further in eight islet transplant centers with support from the NIH.

Another approach under investigation is the implantation of islets that are contained within a bag or tube of some form of material that will allow the entry of glucose, to provide the signal for how much insulin to secrete, and the outflow of insulin, but would prevent the entry of the cells or large proteins that destroy the islets as part of the immune response.

INHALED INSULIN

Insulin is rapidly absorbed into the blood from the tiny air sacs within the lungs. Several pharmaceutical companies are working on devices that will deliver various forms of insulin to the lungs in a way that will provide reliable and reproducible blood levels of insulin.

HOW CAN IT BE PREVENTED?

At the present time there are no known measures for the prevention of type 1 diabetes.

Type 2 diabetes can often be prevented with weight control through proper diet and exercise. Weight control is strongly recommended in people with a strong family history of type 2 diabetes. In the HOPE study, mentioned earlier, treatment of people with known coronary disease with the ACE inhibitor ramipril over a five-year period had the surprising effect of reducing the new onset of type 2 diabetes by 30%. These findings raise the question of whether ACE inhibitors should be used in all patients with coronary heart disease, or at least be considered the drug of choice for the treatment of hypertension. In a few years the results of the DPT-1 Trial will tell whether metformin prevents type 2 diabetes in high-risk people.

WHAT YOU CAN DO NOW

DIABETES EDUCATION PROGRAMS

Because diabetes is not really treated by doctors but by patients and their caregivers, one of the most important first steps is for both patients and caregivers to become thoroughly knowledgeable about the disorder. Although books, journal articles, and Web sites are valuable sources of information, patients and caregivers stand to learn best by attending one of the diabetes education programs widely available throughout the country.

It is advisable to have a spouse or other caregiver attend educational classes along with the patient. The information is valuable for the caregiver as well as the patient. Moreover, these programs often present large amounts of information and it is difficult for one person to retain all of it. A diabetes education program is most effective when a patient is prepared to learn and to make the necessary lifestyle and other changes. Patients are more likely to benefit from a program when they note symptoms or body changes that serve as a "wake-up call" to take better care of themselves. Others are motivated by recognizing the toll diabetes has taken on their family members or friends with diabetes.

An education program is less valuable in patients who are "denying" the disorder because diabetes was recently diagnosed or they have not yet accepted its consequences for other reasons. Caregivers should avoid initiating an education program when a patient is angry or bitter and unwilling to make changes. On the other hand, it is rewarding to both the educator and caregiver to see that an education program has made improvements in blood glucose control brought about by changes in a patient's attitude toward the disorder and willingness to make lifestyle changes.

HANDLING DEPRESSION

As a result of its impact on daily life and the threat of chronic complications, diabetes is often associated with symptoms of depression or anxiety. Depression is especially common in those with two or more chronic complications. It is important to recognize and deal with symptoms of depression and anxiety because, in addition to their discomfort for the patient, they can both result from and produce poor control of diabetes.

Caregivers must distinguish between transient bouts of "sadness" and the more prolonged and severe symptoms of clinical depression, which requires prompt professional help. Short-lived depressive symptoms may be alleviated by urging the patient to get out of bed at a regular hour, keep busy with their usual activities,

A CHECKLIST FOR DIABETICS AND THEIR CAREGIVERS

- Maintain a healthy diet
  - ✔ Be aware of which types of foods to eat or restrict
  - ✔ Maintain consistency in the timing and amount of food, especially in patients taking insulin, and the relationship of food intake to exercise
  - ✔ Remember to take recommended snacks
  - ✔ Low-fat diets help weight loss only if fat calories are not replaced with other calories and portion sizes are limited
  - ✔ Don't fall for the promotions for rapid weight loss. They either don't work or the weight is regained as soon as the program is stopped
- Exercise regularly
- Keep track of the timing of all medications
- Monitor insulin levels
  - ✔ Help young type 1 patients deal with their need to take insulin
  - ✔ Overcome the reluctance of type 2 patients to start taking insulin when it is needed
  - ✔ Decrease insulin doses to avoid hypoglycemia in patients with insulin insensitivity
  - ✔ Check blood glucose regularly and, in type 1 patients, check urine ketones
  - ✔ Measure glucose before meals at different times of the day on different days

- ✔ Keep a record and bring it to doctor's office
- ✔ Check glucose occasionally after meals in addition to before meals
- Be aware of the symptoms of hypoglycemia
- Avoid foot problems
  - ✔ Examine feet every day, and before and after exercise
  - ✔ Wear the right kind of shoes
  - ✔ Check the insides of shoes before putting them on
  - ✔ Do not wash feet in hot water
- Be aware that dietary supplements, like chromium picolinate, don't lower blood glucose (as some claim to do)
- Keep regular doctor visits
  - ✔ Schedule regular visits with an ophthalmologist
  - ✔ Make regular visits to a dentist
  - ✔ Arrange appointments with a podiatrist to cut toenails and examine feet, if necessary
  - ✔ Keep appointments with internist or endocrinologist
  - ✔ Bring all medications on some occasions, and always carry a list of them
  - ✔ Keep track of blood pressure, weight, and laboratory results (hemoglobin A1c, blood lipids)

and engage in exercise. Physicians and caregivers should remind patients that they can pursue their usual activities despite diabetes and that the extra demands of caring for diabetes have been proven to delay or prevent chronic complications. Patients may benefit from the interactions of a diabetes support group.

When patients appear especially anxious, caregivers should attempt to discover and deal with any specific cause(s) of worry. Anxiety may be reduced by reassurance that their diabetes can be controlled, good control will often prevent complications, and complications can be treated effectively if they occur. As with clinical depression, extreme anxiety requires professional treatment.

CARING FOR THE YOUNGER PATIENT: CHILDREN, ADOLESCENTS, AND TEENAGERS

When the diagnosis is first made, depression, apprehension, guilt, or anger are common in people of all ages, but especially in children and adolescents, whose refusal to take their insulin or even attend school can produce severe stress on parents and other family members. Teenagers with diabetes are also more prone to the eating disorders of anorexia nervosa and bulimia. The frustrations associated with diabetes management may be lessened by identifying them and allowing the patient a more active role in setting the goals for their own care. It is often difficult for teenagers to recognize that long-term consequences of diabetes do exist and that the hassle of diabetes management can prevent these complications. At the same time, youngsters must be encouraged to lead as nearly normal a life as possible. Young patients with diabetes may benefit from diabetes camps where they can interact and discuss common concerns with their peers. Information on summer camps and support groups can be obtained through local chapters of the American Diabetes Association and the Juvenile Diabetes Foundation.

ADDITIONAL RESOURCES

WEB SITES

American Diabetes Association

www.diabetes.org

Joslin Diabetes Center

www.joslin.harvard.edu

Juvenile Diabetes Foundation International

www.jdf.org

National Institute of Diabetes and Digestive and Kidney Diseases (NIDDK)

www.niddk.nih.gov

End-Stage Renal Disease

SIGNS & SYMPTOMS

- Change in urine volume
- Blood in the urine
- Foaming of urine
- Pain over the kidney
- Severe and troublesome itchiness
- Swollen ankles

In the last thirty to forty years, increasingly effective treatments to replace the kidney's function have been developed. These treatments include dialysis (where the blood is artificially cleaned of toxins) and the transplantation of a new kidney through surgery. In the United States alone, over three hundred and fifty thousand patients are alive today because of these interventions. These are all, however, imperfect therapies and require sweeping lifestyle changes for the patient. The changes include dietary modification, fluid restriction, compliance with numerous medications, and often attendance on a fixed schedule at a dialysis clinic. To maintain long-term compliance with these interventions, it is essential that the patient and those who care for him or her understand the need for these impositions. Compliance is especially important because noncompliance does not usually result in immediate consequences, but will lead silently to the development of future complications.

WHAT IS IT?

End-stage renal disease (ESRD) is the near-complete loss of normal kidney (renal) function. In the absence of effective treatment, this condition is rapidly fatal.

KIDNEY STRUCTURE AND DESIGN

Normal renal function is provided by two kidneys. Each kidney is about the size of a fist and both are situated deep within the abdomen, on either side of the spine. Each kidney is supplied by a large artery, which provides a very high rate of blood flow.

On arriving at the kidney, this large artery branches and divides repeatedly into a network of over a million tiny blood vessels. Each of these tiny vessels leads to a glomerulus, a filter-like structure. The pressure of the blood in the glomerulus pushes water and most small molecules through the filter; larger substances, such as cells and proteins, are too big to pass through the glomerular filter and so remain within the blood. One sign of kidney disease is when the glomerular filter becomes disrupted and allows the passage of large proteins into the filtrate. These proteins can subsequently be detected in the urine, a finding called proteinuria. Those substances that do pass through the filter (the filtrate) are collected on the far side within a tube (the renal tubule). The glomerulus and tubule collectively are called a nephron, a Greek word from which the medical term for the study of kidney disease, "nephrology," originates.

The healthy kidney creates a vast volume of filtrate (approximately 120 liters) each day. The tubule then reabsorbs substances that the body needs back into the blood. In this fashion the blood levels of numerous substances are maintained at the exact level required for optimal body function. The fluid and substances that are not wanted by the body remain within the tubule and travel through a system of collecting tubes, which eventually leads to the bladder. This material is removed from the body as urine upon voiding.

The rate at which this filtrate is generated is called the glomerular filtration rate or GFR. The GFR is used as a global measure of overall kidney function. Usually levels are greater than 120 milliliters per minute (mL/min). Dialysis is begun when this value is less than 10 to 15 mL/min, although the actual value in many patients when starting dialysis is only 5 to 6 mL/min. Thus, the normal kidney provides many times more than the minimal amount of function required for health. Indeed, some people are born with only one functioning kidney and never develop any problems with kidney failure.

FUNCTIONS OF THE KIDNEY

Excretion. We usually eat and drink without regard for the body's actual nutrient and fluid requirements. Nutrients along with other substances are absorbed from the bowel. The kidney plays an essential role in controlling the levels of these substances as well as removing the waste products, such as acid, that result from chemical reactions within the cells of our bodies. Although acid is normally present in the stomach, its level in the blood is kept at a very low level by the kidney. In the absence of kidney function the amount of acid and of many other toxins in the blood climbs dangerously high and causes symptoms, a state called uremia.

Metabolism. The kidney also plays an important role in modifying and deactivating, as well as excreting, many medications or chemicals. In the presence of kidney failure, many medications last far longer in the body and their blood level may climb dangerously high. Some common medications should be avoided altogether in the presence of kidney failure, such as the narcotic meperidine. On the other hand, some substances that are normally activated by the kidney require a much higher dose than usual in kidney failure. Vitamin D regulates the body's calcium level and keeps bones healthy and strong. It is widely present in diet and in most multivitamin pills but requires modification by the kidney before it can work effectively. Patients with kidney failure need to take supplements of a special form of the vitamin that is already activated.

Secretion. The kidney is also a secretory organ, manufacturing and releasing into the bloodstream the hormone erythropoietin. This hormone stimulates the bone marrow to produce red blood cells; with kidney failure there is usually inadequate erythropoietin production and as a result anemia develops.

WHO IS AT RISK?

The number of patients diagnosed and successfully treated with renal failure in the United States has increased dramatically over the last decade. The occurrence of renal failure increases with age and part of this increase relates to the increased proportion of older patients in the population. The risk of kidney failure is higher in many minorities, including Native Americans, African Americans, and Mexican Americans, than in persons of European ancestry. Much of this difference relates to socioeconomic differences in access to good medical care. Once the original damage occurs within the kidney, secondary processes, such as control of high blood pressure, often determine the speed and degree with which progressive kidney damage takes place; different ethnic groups appear to differ in the intensity of these secondary processes.

Medications may contribute to acute (usually temporary) renal failure, in which there is a good prospect for eventual recovery. Nonsteroidal anti-inflammatory agents, such as Advil or Motrin, may make pre-existing renal failure even worse and are best avoided, when possible, in patients with kidney disease. Some medications and herbal over-the-counter preparations have been associated with possible progressive kidney failure. These include the use of compound painkillers, which usually contain combinations of several different agents including acetaminophen and caffeine. In the absence of better data regarding the safety of these agents, long-term use of such compound painkillers, rather than single-agent products such as acetaminophen alone, should be avoided when possible

In addition, many different diseases may result in the development of chronic renal failure. As medicine has progressed many patients who previously may have died as a direct result of these illnesses are now surviving and are at an increased risk of developing renal complications because of their extended life spans. Some of these diseases associated with kidney failure are explained below.

"Sugar" diabetes (diabetes mellitus). Diabetes is the most common overall cause of kidney failure in the United States, currently accounting for 40% of new patients who develop kidney failure. In both type 1 (usually insulin dependent from an early age) and type 2 (adult-onset) diabetics, the leakage of protein and albumin into the urine is a marker of kidney involvement as well as a predictor of the course of the renal disease. In type 1 patients renal disease generally occurs fifteen to twenty years after the onset of diabetes and is often associated with the presence of diabetic changes in the back of the eye (diabetic retinopathy). Type 2 diabetes has a much less dramatic onset than type 1 diabetes and often goes undiagnosed. Thus, the average duration of type 2 diabetes before renal disease develops is less clear. Renal involvement with both forms is associated from an early stage with the presence of the protein albumin in the urine.

High blood pressure. High blood pressure (hypertension) is both a common cause and a common consequence of renal failure. Approximately 27% of new cases of end-stage renal failure in the United States are attributed primarily to the effects of high blood pressure. And almost all patients with renal failure from other causes eventually develop high blood pressure. If high blood pressure is not adequately controlled, it greatly increases the rate at which weakened kidneys progress to dead kidneys. Adequate control of blood pressure for someone with kidney disease is the lowest achievable blood pressure that does not cause symptoms or complications in that patient. The recommendation of the Joint National Committee on Prevention, Detection, Evaluation, and Treatment of High Blood Pressure for patients with kidney problems is for a systolic blood pressure of 130 mm Hg or lower and a diastolic blood pressure of 85 mm Hg or lower. If protein is present in the urine, clinical studies have shown that lowering blood pressure to 125/75 or less is both safe and effective in slowing loss of renal function.

Renal artery stenosis. Renal artery stenosis is a narrowing of the main artery to the kidney—the renal artery—and usually results from "hardening of the arteries" (atherosclerosis). It typically occurs in patients with symptoms of atherosclerosis elsewhere, such as angina. Other diseases, especially those associated with inflammation of the arteries, can also cause renal artery stenosis. The inadequate blood flow causes progressive damage to the kidney, often associated with very high blood pressure that is difficult to control. Both the blood pressure and renal function may improve after successful treatment of these blockages. Sometimes, however, these blockages occur in multiple small arteries within the kidney and it is not possible to remove or bypass them all.

Glomerulonephritis. A number of autoimmune diseases may affect the glomerulus, the filter-like structure in the kidney. These may occur in isolation (such as some forms of nephropathy), or be part of a more generalized disease, such as systemic lupus erythematosus or AIDS, which affects other organs as well as the kidneys. If the glomerulonephritis disrupts the glomerular filter, large amounts of protein enter the urine, giving rise to the nephrotic syndrome.

Heart or liver disease. Renal function often reflects a person's overall state of health and thus patients who develop severe problems, especially severe heart or liver function, often develop associated kidney problems. Sometimes these problems may also develop after a successful heart or liver transplant, in part as a result of some of the immunosuppressive medications used to keep the transplanted organ healthy.

Inherited kidney diseases. A wide range of inherited diseases may affect the kidney, the commonest of which is polycystic kidney disease. In this condition the kidneys develop numerous cysts, which increase in size and cause kidney dysfunction. The age at which the kidneys stop working varies greatly and some people never develop end-stage renal disease. Another often under-recognized inherited condition is the development of infections within the kidney from urine flowing from the bladder back up to the kidney (urinary reflux). Normally, valves at the bladder only allow urine to flow in the one direction, from the kidney to the bladder, but in predisposed patients these valves may not work, allowing urine and infections to travel up to the kidney. This often only occurs during the first few years of life, but may cause sufficient damage to result in kidney failure twenty or thirty years later.

HOW IS IT DIAGNOSED?

SYMPTOMS

The majority of patients are diagnosed with kidney problems before they have any obvious symptoms, although in many cases it is often late in the course of their kidney disease. When symptoms do develop, they usually do so gradually, over a period of months. As a result a patient frequently fails to realize how sick they have become and it is often a friend or caregiver who first notices this gradual deterioration.

Change in urine volume

The volume of urine produced each day is not a reliable indicator of kidney function. Although the prolonged absence of urine always suggests a problem with the kidney or urinary tract, this is a very late development in chronic kidney failure. More often patients continue to pass urine even when they have advanced kidney failure. This urine, however, is of poor quality and the kidney is not removing toxins from the body. In fact, a sign of renal disease is often an increased volume of urine due to inability of the damaged tubules to reabsorb water from the large volume of filtrate made by the kidney each day. Thus, the urine is very diluted. This increased volume results in the need to get up more frequently during the night to urinate, although many other conditions may also cause this symptom.

Pain over the kidney occurs rarely with kidney failure but may result from kidney stones or infections or when there is a sudden loss of blood to the kidney.

• Foaming of urine suggests that there is excess protein in the urine as a result of an impaired glomerular filter, a condition called the nephrotic syndrome.

• Blood in the urine (hematuria) makes the urine appear smoky or tea-colored. Blood in the urine that is visible to the naked eye may be due to some forms of glomerulonephritis, often in association with an upper respiratory tract infection. Overall, however, hematuria is a more common finding with bladder problems.

• Gastrointestinal symptoms. Often the first symptom of kidney failure a patient notices is loss of appetite and a slowly progressive weight loss. With more advanced failure, nausea and vomiting occur and are typically worse in the morning.

• Low energy levels result from anemia due to decreased erythropoietin levels. Because anemia develops slowly, patients often only recognize this symptom when anemia is advanced.

• Fluid overload is common with progressive kidney failure and may be especially severe in patients with nephrotic syndrome. It results in swelling; in non–bed-bound people, this is usually most noticeable around the ankles due to the effects of gravity. This accumulation of fluid (edema) can be demonstrated by pressing the skin with a fingertip against the bony prominence of the ankle. In the presence of edema, the skin indents, leaving a hollow, which gradually fills in slowly over about a minute. If fluid overload is severe it leads to excess fluid in the lungs (pulmonary edema), which causes shortness of breath. This symptom may be most obvious when lying flat and may awaken the patient from sleep.

• Heart problems. The accumulation of toxins with kidney failure eventually leads to pericarditis, an inflammation of the sac surrounding the heart. Symptoms include pain over the heart that gets worse on taking a deep breath. The heart also becomes increasingly irritable. In the setting of increased blood acid and potassium levels, it may start to beat either too fast or too slow, either of which can be fatal if not controlled.

• Itchiness. A severe and troublesome itch may result from a combination of reasons in ESRD, including uncontrolled uremia and a high parathyroid (PTH) level. The most common reason in dialysis patients, however, is a high blood phosphate level. The excess phosphate joins with calcium and is deposited in the skin.

• Easy bruising occurs because of the impaired ability of blood platelets.

• Headaches or visual disturbances may result from the development of very high blood pressure that often accompanies advanced kidney failure.

DIAGNOSTIC PROCEDURES

A wide range of tests are used to assess kidney function and diagnose the cause of kidney problems. In most cases we don't know the actual compounds that cause the various symptoms of kidney failure and are therefore unable to measure toxin levels directly. Instead we measure or estimate the GFR as a global measure of kidney function.

Blood tests

Blood tests, by themselves, are a very insensitive measurement of total kidney function. It is only after we lose over half of our kidney function that most of the commonly used blood tests give abnormal results. Thus any elevation in these blood tests above the normal range suggests the presence of substantial kidney problems. Two blood tests are used in this setting, serum creatinine and the serum urea level. For historical reasons, the latter is usually called the blood urea nitrogen or BUN. Neither of these substances is itself toxic. They are relatively easy and cheap to measure, however, and after a certain point their level tends to rise as the kidney function decreases.

Creatinine. Creatinine comes from muscle, so exactly how high levels climb with kidney failure depends on how well muscled a person is. (So an elderly lady with a low muscle mass will have a much lower serum creatinine than a well-muscled young man, even if they both have the same degree of kidney failure. Specific formulas are calculated to predict the actual GFR from the measured blood creatinine level

Blood urea nitrogen. BUN is largely a byproduct of protein intake in the diet; normal range is approximately 20 mg/dL; as levels climb toward 100 mg/dL complications become increasing likely and dialysis is usually started

Creatinine clearance. The traditional way to estimate the GFR is to calculate the creatinine clearance. Creatinine is filtered by the glomerulus and very little is secreted or reabsorbed by the tubule. The rate of filtration or "clearance" of creatinine is calculated by obtaining a complete collection of all the urine passed over a twenty-four-hour period and measuring the amount of creatinine in the sample and in the blood. A single missed urine void will lead to considerable inaccuracy.

Nuclear GFR. The GFR can be directly measured in clinical practice using the rate of excretion of a radiolabeled marker that is removed from the blood only through glomerular filtration. This test involves the injection of a very small amount of radioactive material, requires special equipment, and is expensive. It therefore tends to be used only in special circumstances, such as in research studies.

Immunological tests. Certain blood tests may be used as necessary to determine if various immunological and inflammatory diseases, such as lupus, hepatitis, and HIV, are responsible for or contributing to the renal disease.

Urine tests

As mentioned above, excessive protein in the urine, or proteinuria, is often a sign of renal disease, especially in patients with diabetes.

Urine dipstick. The dipstick is placed in a sample of urine and undergoes a color change in the presence of proteinuria. A disadvantage of this test is that the estimate of proteinuria depends on the concentration of urine. A special type of dipstick is used to detect the presence of albumin in the urine, which is the earliest clinical sign of diabetes involving the kidneys.

Twenty-four-hour urinary protein. This is traditionally assessed by measuring the total protein in a twenty-four-hour collection of urine, often at the same time as assessing the creatinine clearance. As with the creatinine clearance measurement, this test depends on an accurate and complete collection of urine.

Protein/creatinine ratio. This is the easiest way to accurately estimate the degree of proteinuria and can be done in either a random or a timed urine sample. In healthy persons this ratio is less than 0.15. A ratio of greater than 3 suggests dangerously high proteinuria.

Blood pressure

One of the most important tests to detect kidney problems is the measurement of blood pressure. Measurements may be made in the health provider's office, or at home by the patient or the patient's care provider.

Office measurements. Blood pressure should be measured after several minutes of resting using an appropriately sized blood pressure cuff and an accurate blood pressure machine.

Home measurement. Using a reliable automated device provides an important and underused opportunity for patients to monitor their blood pressure. The readings can be phoned into the care provider and trends reviewed at the next clinic visit. The home blood pressure monitor should be brought into the clinic periodically and checked against the office machine, to be sure the home monitor is working properly.

Radiology

Radiological tests are helpful in allowing the doctor to visualize abnormal size, shape, and function of the kidneys, which may indicate disease.

Kidney size. Size is usually examined using a sonogram (ultrasound). The sonogram is used to detect the presence of congenital abnormalities, such as a single kidney or polycystic kidney disease. It also helps rule out kidney obstruction due to a blockage of urine flow, in which case the kidney become dilated and balloons up. The sonogram can also give a sense of the patient's prognosis. In cases where the kidneys have become small and shrunken, there is usually little potential for recovery of renal function.

Kidney blood flow. Several different tests may be used for detecting blockages in blood supply to kidneys, including ultrasound, computed tomography, magnetic resonance imaging, and angiography. In the latter test, dye is actually injected into the blood vessel. Centers vary widely in their expertise and experience in using these different techniques and thus the most reliable test to use varies among different institutions.

Urinary reflux. To see if there is reflux between the bladder and kidney, a dye is placed in the bladder. The patient is then asked to urinate, and x-rays are taken to determine whether dye is forced up toward the kidneys.

Renal biopsy

In cases where there is unexplained progressive renal failure or proteinuria, the cause may be found by doing a kidney biopsy. In this procedure a small amount of kidney tissue, slightly bigger than the size of a match head, is removed from the kidney. This is normally performed on an outpatient basis or with an overnight hospital stay. The skin is anesthetized and a fine-needle biopsy needle is placed into the kidney with ultrasound guidance. Because the kidneys are several centimeters beneath the skin and can move with breathing, it can be a challenge to obtain a sufficient sample, especially in people who are overweight.

Renal biopsy is associated with a small amount of bleeding, similar to a nose bleed, from the site of the biopsy. This may lead to some mild discomfort in the area of the biopsy for a day or two. Having the patient remain on strict bed rest for twelve to eighteen hours after the procedure minimizes the risk of bleeding. It is essential that people undergoing biopsy have no risk factors for excessive bleeding, such as a congenital bleeding problem, and are not taking prescribed or over-the-counter medications that interfere with blood clotting, such as aspirin, Advil, or Motrin. These agents should be stopped approximately two weeks before the biopsy.

Renal biopsies are usually safe and well tolerated. In cases where a routine biopsy is not possible because of obesity or a bleeding tendency, a biopsy can usually be safely obtained using a laparoscopic procedure.

WHAT SHOULD YOU EXPECT?

The prognosis for patients with kidney failure varies a great deal and depends on a large number of factors. In general, patients who have a sudden onset of disease and who respond to treatment have a better outlook than those who have had a slow, gradual loss of kidney function. Many of the immunologically mediated forms of glomerulonephritis may respond completely to appropriate immunosuppressive therapy. While the ability to control renal disease varies, successful management always depends on the patient's ability to comply with the many required medical and lifestyle interventions.

Good kidney function is essential to live; we literally cannot live without it, because when toxins accumulate, symptoms of kidney failure develop, and, if untreated, lead inevitably to death. The treatment options for ESRD are hemodialysis, peritoneal dialysis, and renal transplantation. In suitable patients transplantation offers the best long-term solution to kidney failure. It is limited, however, by a lack of available donor organs. In addition, the transplanted kidney may deteriorate with time, forcing an eventual return to dialysis or the need for a repeat transplant. Fortunately the survival of renal transplant patients is continually improving because of improvements in management.

In the absence of transplantation, dialysis is life-saving. Unfortunately, it does not restore normal life expectancy, even in relatively healthy patients. Survival is heavily dependent in most cases on the degree and severity of the associated medical problems and frequently it is an exacerbation of these problems which leads to the patient's death rather than a problem with dialysis itself.

Development of chronic kidney failure can be overwhelming to the patient and the patient's family. Most people who require dialysis are over 60 years of age and often have cardiovascular disease, diabetes, impaired vision, and a host of other associated problems. Although less advanced kidney failure usually produces little in the way of symptoms, persons with end-stage disease, before starting dialysis therapy, often feel terrible. Superimposed on these symptoms is the urgent need to make decisions about which type of kidney replacement therapy to receive, which facility to choose, and many other important factors. Patients in this situation feel bombarded with information and ill-equipped to process it. Also, there is the realization that one's continued survival depends on faithfully visiting a dialysis facility several times a week or performing daily peritoneal exchanges. A supportive family or other social support system is crucial to help people with chronic renal disease adapt to the realities of treatment and to overcome the challenges imposed by the disease.

But take heart. After the first two or three months on dialysis, people often begin to feel much better, have more energy, and enjoy life again. People on dialysis can live long and live well. In fact, some persons have lived with end-stage disease for over thirty years. People who do well are those who take responsibility for their own health and medical care. It is important not only to be compliant with medications, dietary restrictions, and dialysis schedules but also to learn as much as possible about renal disease and its management. Dialysis is a highly technical therapy. Patients who become expert at this technique and partner with their care providers get the best results.

HOW IS IT TREATED?

Several options are available to patients with kidney failure, but all depend upon the speed of progression to kidney failure and the physical condition of the patient.

MEDICATION AND DIET

As kidney failure progresses many of the associated symptoms can be successfully managed with appropriate medications and changes in diet. Many of these dietary changes need to be continued even after starting dialysis, but they can usually be relaxed to some degree after successful kidney transplantation.

Phosphate control. Phosphate accumulates within the body with kidney failure. Unfortunately dialysis is not an efficient method of removing phosphate, thus patients have to use phosphate binders with each meal. These bind onto the phosphate and prevent their absorption by the gut. In the past aluminum-based binders were used, but these may cause bone problems and are now avoided. Several alternative preparations such as calcium acetate (Phoslo) and sevelamer (Renagel) are now available and in most cases it matters less which of these agents is used than that an effective dose is taken regularly with every meal or snack.

Parathyroid hormone level. In untreated kidney failure the combination of high phosphate, low calcium, and low activated-vitamin D levels in the blood result in stimulation of the parathyroid glands. These are four tiny glands, located in the neck, which secrete parathyroid hormone (PTH). In healthy subjects PTH helps to maintain normal calcium levels, by increasing absorption of dietary calcium and releasing calcium from bone. Excess levels, however, lead to the loss of too much calcium from bone. After prolonged periods of overstimulation, the parathyroid glands may begin oversecreting PTH in a completely uncontrolled fashion. If this happens, then the surgical removal of the parathyroid glands may be required. To prevent this problem and to maintain bone health, it is important to take activated vitamin D and to control phosphate levels through the use of binders. Activated vitamin D helps to increase absorption of calcium from the gut, to maintain a normal amount of calcium in bone, and to directly control the parathyroid glands. Oversuppression of PTH is also harmful to bone, because a certain degree of bone turnover is necessary to maintain bone health. The optimal PTH level for patients with kidney failure is higher than normal. The exact target, however, is uncertain and probably varies between patients. A good goal is a level in the 120 to 180 pg/mL range, as compared with a range of less than 54 pg/mL in patients with normal kidney function.

Potassium. Potassium is found in most foods, and fresh fruit and sodas are particularly rich sources. The level of potassium in the blood rises with the degree of kidney failure. Most kidney failure patients who are not malnourished tend to have high potassium levels. If such patients do not avoid potassium-rich foods, they may develop dangerously high levels resulting in potentially life-threatening heart problems. To avoid this, patients need to be aware of and avoid foods that are particularly rich in potassium. Most diuretics, medications that increase the volume of urine, also promote the excretion of potassium and are used for this purpose in persons with kidney failure who produce urine.

Hemoglobin. The decreased level of erythropoietin associated with kidney failure results in anemia. Anemia is quantitated by two measures that are related to the number of red cells in the blood, the hematocrit and the hemoglobin. Anemia is corrected by the administration of erythropoietin. The dose of erythropoietin is adjusted to keep the hemoglobin at approximately between 11 and 12 g/dL or the hematocrit between 33 and 36%.

Iron supplementation. Several complications may interfere with the adequate function of erythropoietin including infection, inflammation, and very high levels of PTH. The most common reason for a poor response to erythropoietin is iron deficiency. Iron is needed to make new red cells. Oral iron supplements are poorly absorbed and should not be taken at the same time as phosphate binders because the binders join to the iron rather than to phosphate and thus neither medication will work. Thus, neither the iron nor the binders can do their desired job. One solution is to administer iron supplements intravenously. This strategy is especially easy for patients who are being treated with hemodialysis. Although it's very effective, intravenous iron administration is associated with a small risk of reactions, so a small test dose is administered first. But with some newer iron preparations, the risk of reactions is lower than with traditional preparations. Patients with early renal failure and on peritoneal dialysis tend to have a lower requirement for iron.

Acidosis. The accumulation of acid within the body is especially a problem for patients who consume large amounts of animal protein. Severe acidosis can worsen the effect of high potassium levels, cause heart problems, lead to muscle loss, and weaken bones. Patients should avoid a high animal protein diet and take an alkali supplement, such as sodium bicarbonate or sodium citrate, to help neutralize the acid. With hemodialysis it may be necessary to continue alkali supplements, especially on nondialysis days.

HEMODIALYSIS

More than 63% of the American kidney failure population is treated by hemodialysis. In this treatment, blood is removed from the body a small quantity at a time and "cleansed" by a machine (a dialyzer). The dialyzer consists of two sets of tubes, running beside each other, separated by a filter. Blood runs in one set of tubes and in the other runs a water-based solution (the dialysate). Toxins and waste products move from one side of the filter to the other, from the blood to the dialysate. Calcium and alkali move in the opposite direction, from the dialysate into the blood. This process uses a large volume of dialysate, over 80 liters per treatment.

Duration of treatment

Most hemodialysis patients in the United States receive their dialysis in a dialysis outpatient clinic; a very small number undergo hemodialysis at home.

In-center dialysis. Hemodialysis is normally performed for four hours three times a week in a dialysis unit. This requires the rigorous attendance at a dialysis unit at the same fixed time each week. While on dialysis the patient is seated comfortably on a chair and is able to read, watch television, or sleep. Most dialysis units operate three shifts, 6 A.M. to 11 A.M., 11 A.M. to 2 P.M., and 2 P.M. to 6 P.M. It is possible to travel by receiving dialysis at other dialysis units but this requires a good deal of organization.

Home dialysis. Hemodialysis in the United States is normally conducted at a dialysis center but when resources and expertise allow, patients undergo dialysis in their own home. Most receive dialysis for the typical three- to five-hour treatment three times a week. Several centers, however, have experimented with providing a slower form of dialysis for much longer periods, such as for several hours a night, five or six nights a week. This method requires the use of specialized dialysis and monitoring equipment. Although highly selected patients have done very well with this treatment, this type of dialysis is still under study.

Types of vascular access

An essential requirement for hemodialysis is the ability to remove blood from the body and transfer it to the dialysis machine for several hours at a time on a regular basis, with minimal patient inconvenience or discomfort. This is achieved by creating a blood access, using one of several different techniques.

Arteriovenous fistula. Creation of an arteriovenous fistula is the preferred method of achieving access to the bloodstream for the purposes of dialysis. The fistula is created by a surgical procedure in which an artery is connected directly to a vein. The fistula is usually created in the upper part of the patient's nondominant arm (e.g., in the right arm of a person who is left-handed). Over the following several months the vein increases in size, until it is sufficient to allow for long-term dialysis. At the start of each dialysis session, two needles, one to take blood from the body and the other to return it, are placed in the large vessels leading from the fistula. The advantage of arteriovenous fistulas is that they tend to last a long time, often for many years, and that they have a much lower complication rate than other forms of access to the bloodstream. A limitation is that persons need to have good-quality blood vessels to successfully create the fistula. On rare occasions the access may result in inadequate blood flow to the hand beyond the level of the fistula, so that the fistula must be disconnected. A major limitation is the length of time required for a fistula to mature and be ready for use. A patient must therefore be referred for fistula placement several months in advance of the time when the access is needed.

Arteriovenous graft. An alternative method of obtaining access to the bloodstream is to join a vein to an artery using a piece of plastic tubing, called a graft. An advantage of this approach is that it can be successfully performed even in the presence of poor blood vessel quality. In addition, grafts take only two to three weeks to be ready for use. One problem, however, is that these accesses are more likely to "clot off" than fistulas and this recurrent clotting may result in the need for creation of multiple different grafts. In addition, the body's natural defenses are less effective within the graft and infection may tend to lodge there. Infection within a graft may be very dangerous and usually requires the removal of the graft.

Tunneled catheter. The least desirable long-term access option is to use an external catheter. These can, if necessary, be left in position for several months.

To reduce the risk of infection, the catheter travels (or "tunnels") for several centimeters within the skin after exiting the blood vessel, hence the name tunneled catheter. To secure the catheter in position, a cuff is situated within the skin tunnel. This cuff induces a fibrous reaction with the adjacent skin, causing the catheter to be held firmly in place. An advantage of these catheters is that they can be used immediately after their insertion, and thus provide an immediate and potentially life-saving access for dialysis. Disadvantages are that they become easily infected, tend to clot off frequently, provide a relatively low blood flow, and, consequently, a lesser amount of dialysis per hour of treatment.

Dialysis membranes

Several different types of dialysis filters are currently available for use in dialysis. As these filters have extensive contact with the patient's blood, there is a great potential for interactions between the dialysis filter and the blood. In a four-hour dialysis treatment, the equivalent of the patient's entire blood volume passes comes in contact with the filter approximately twenty-four times. There are two general types of membrane, cellulose and synthetic.

Cellulose membranes are made from naturally occurring fibers. These membranes, while effective, cause a range of reactions with blood and are associated with increased risks of infection, inflammation, and malnutrition. The basic cellulose structure can be modified to make these complications less likely.

Synthetic membranes are completely artificial and are much less likely to cause blood reactions. One type of synthetic membrane, however, made from polyacrylonitrile material, cannot be used at the same time as ACE inhibitors, a class of blood pressure medication widely used with dialysis.

Although synthetic membranes have many advantages over cellulose membranes, they are much more expensive to make. Their routine use is made feasible by the ability to use the same membrane multiple times. The membrane is always reused on the same subject. Following dialysis the membrane is carefully labeled with the patient's name and is cleaned and sterilized before the next use. Special tests are performed to ensure the membrane continues to meet certain minimal standards for on-going use. The benefits and risks of dialyzer reuse remain controversial. Dialyzer reuse has been associated with potential complications. However, the potential for such complication may be minimized by limiting the maximum number of reuses per membrane and by enforcing strict quality control of the reuse procedure. In such circumstances many nephrologists believe that the advantages of being able to use these synthetic membranes outweigh any potential disadvantages associated with the reuse process.

Fluid control

With in-center hemodialysis, fluid is only removed three times per week. In a patient with no residual renal function, all the fluid and fluid equivalents, such as ice, consumed between dialysis treatments accumulate in the body. If excessive, this accumulation leads to high blood pressure, fluid in the lungs, and associated shortness of breath and enlargement of the heart.

Goal weight. To determine how much fluid to remove with each treatment, the patient's goal body weight, also called their "dry weight," is estimated. Most weight gain in the two to three days between consecutive dialysis sessions results from accumulation of fluid. Thus, during each dialysis session, whatever fluid was gained since the previous treatment is removed. The goal weight is frequently adjusted as the patient's body weight increases or decreases over time. If the goal weight is set too low, excessive fluid will be removed from the patient, leading to a drop in blood pressure. This drop may be associated with additional symptoms, such as feeling lightheaded, sweating, cramps, nausea, and occasionally vomiting. If symptoms occur when the patient's fluid ingestion has not been excessive, it usually means that the patient is approaching their true dry weight. If symptoms persist the dry weight is usually increased by 0.5 kg (approximately 1 pound).

Rate of fluid removal. Symptoms of excess fluid removal depend not only on the absolute amount of fluid removed with dialysis, relative to the patient's goal weight, but also on the speed with which this volume is removed. Fluid in the body distributes itself between blood and the water that is situated inside the body's cells. Most of the water, about 60%, is inside our cells, and it takes time for this water to move from inside the cells back into the blood. Dialysis can only remove water that is within the blood vessels. As a result, especially during short dialysis treatments, an attempt to remove more than 5% of a person's predialysis body weight usually removes fluid from the blood quicker than the fluid inside cells is able to return to the bloodstream. Because this excess fluid is not readily accessible for removal during fast dialysis, blood pressure falls even though the patient may still be several kilograms above their true goal weight.

There is no good recourse for a patient on hemodialysis who does not watch his fluid restriction. If a 70-kg man drinks 3.5 liters of fluid on each day between dialysis sessions, equivalent to 10% of his body weight over two days, trying to remove this amount of fluid in a single dialysis session is almost always going to cause symptoms. However, if only 4 kg (4 liters) of fluid is removed from the patient in an attempt to avoid symptoms, the patient is left with 3 liters of excess fluid. This excess fluid contributes to high blood pressure and enlargement of the heart. If the patient continues to be careless about fluid control, then he will progressively gain more and more excess fluid, with eventually catastrophic results.

The best way to avoid these symptoms is by avoiding excess ingestion of fluid in the first place. With such compliance the increase in body weight between consecutive dialysis treatments is no more than 5% of the normal body weight. Another approach is to prolong the dialysis treatment to allow a slower rate of fluid removal per hour of dialysis but this can be impractical in a busy dialysis unit and many patients prefer not to spend additional time being dialyzed. Limiting fluid intake is often the most difficult aspect of change in lifestyle for patients on hemodialysis. It can be helped by avoiding all added salt and high-salt foods (such as canned foods), and by carefully monitoring the amount of fluid taken in each day. Such monitoring must become second nature for a hemodialysis patient. Checking the weight at the same time each morning and adjusting the fluid intake for the day in accordance with the amount already gained since the previous dialysis treatment also helps regulate intake.

Blood pressure control

The control of blood pressure in dialysis patients is directly related to the control of salt and water ingestion. As many forms of blood pressure ultimately depend on the amount of fluid in the blood vessels, dialysis, by regulating blood volume, provides an effective means of controlling blood pressure. If a patient is maintained close to his dry weight then the need for blood pressure medications can be much reduced. In some patients, however, an additional blood pressure agent may be necessary on nondialysis days to help control the blood pressures on these days.

Hemodialysis dose

Determining the quantity of dialysis required for a patient on dialysis to stay healthy is complicated. Because only a few of the many potential toxins that accumulate in kidney failure can be measured, we cannot rely on direct measurement of known toxins to determine the necessary amount of dialysis.

Global assessment. One important measure of dialysis adequacy is how the patient actually feels. In cases where the patient feels persistently unwell it is always wise to review whether the amount of dialysis is sufficient. However, because kidney toxins often only accumulate slowly with underdialysis, some patients may continue to feel reasonably well right up to the point where they develop a complication. Objective measures of the dialysis dose administered are thus required.

Urea reduction ratio (URR). The dose of dialysis is measured as the reduction in the blood urea levels between the start and finish of a single dialysis treatment, a test called the urea reduction ratio. The usual goal is to maintain a urea reduction ratio of greater than 65%.

Kt/V. In this measurement, "K" is the dialyzer clearance, expressed in milliliters per minute, and the "t" is time. So Kt, then, is clearance multiplied by time. This number is the volume of fluid completely cleared of urea during a single treatment. "V" is the volume of water a patient's body contains. The body is about 60% water by weight. If a patient weighs 70 kilograms, then V will be 42 liters. Kt/V compares the amount of fluid that passes through the dialyzer with the amount of fluid in the patient's body. This parameter should be maintained at greater than 1.2.

These measurements are only a guide in helping to establish minimal amounts of dialysis and the actual dialysis prescription must always be individualized to the particular patient. Levels significantly below these goals are likely to be insufficient for most patients. Reaching these goals, however, does not guarantee that the patient is receiving enough dialysis, especially if the dialysis is performed within a very short period of time (e.g., less than two hours). In the past, special types of equipment were used to permit very short dialysis times. In these circumstances, even though the URR or Kt/V may appear adequate, the patient may not do as well, on average, as one who receives the same dose of dialysis over a longer time period, such as three and a half to four hours or even longer.

These measures of dialysis dose are based on a single dialysis treatment. To validly reflect the adequacy of overall treatment during the month, the patient must receive a similar treatment three times a week, each week. If a patient misses treatment or intermittently stops dialysis early, then neither the URR nor the Kt/V will accurately estimate the long-term quality of dialysis.

Hepatitis B

Hepatitis B is a virus that damages the liver; it is an extremely infectious organism and readily transmissible by blood. In the early days of dialysis, before effective infection control measures were introduced, cross-infection with hepatitis B among both dialysis patients and staff was extremely common. With current practices this is much less of a risk, but all dialysis patients should receive the hepatitis B vaccine, preferably before they start dialysis, and have regular checks of their antibody status. Caregivers who are not regularly exposed to blood should not be at an increased risk of contracting hepatitis B.

PERITONEAL DIALYSIS

Approximately 9% of U. S. kidney failure patients are treated by peritoneal dialysis (PD). In PD, a special type of soft catheter is placed in the front of the abdomen, usually below the navel. This catheter leads into an internal space, the "peritoneal cavity," where the intestines and other abdominal organs lie. These organs are covered by a membrane, which has an extensive network of small blood vessels. Two to three liters of a special solution (dialysate) are introduced into the peritoneal cavity through the catheter. Toxic substances gradually move from the patient's blood into the dialysate. After several hours, when the fluid is saturated with toxins, the fluid is exchanged for fresh dialysate via the catheter.

In order to remove water, the dialysate is made hyperconcentrated by having a very high sugar content. Hyperconcentration results in water moving from the blood vessels into the dialysate. Therefore the volume of fluid drained out at the end of the exchange is greater than that instilled. The dialysate is manufactured with added calcium and alkali that the body needs, so that these substances travel from the dialysate into the blood vessels and can be used by the body.

Peritoneal dialysis can be performed in two different ways: continuous ambulatory peritoneal dialysis or automated peritoneal dialysis.

Continuous ambulatory peritoneal dialysis

Continuous ambulatory peritoneal dialysis (CAPD) is the original form of peritoneal dialysis and it is still widely practiced. Dialysate is exchanged after about six hours (thus four exchanges are made per day). It usually takes approximately half an hour for fluid to drain out and for fresh dialysate to be instilled into the peritoneum. Sometimes the number of manual exchanges is increased up to five per day, but it's hard for many patients to keep such a schedule.

Automated PD

This modality is also referred to as continuous cycler peritoneal dialysis (CCPD). It uses the same principles as CAPD except the catheter is connected to a special machine at night-time, which performs several automatic exchanges while the patient is asleep. This increases the delivered dialysis dose and enables many patients to get by with only one additional manual exchange during the day. Contrary to their expectations most patients rapidly get used to this and do not have significant sleep disturbance as a result of being connected to the cycler. On occasion, typical CAPD is performed with an additional single exchange in the middle of the night through the use of a simplified cycler. This approach achieves five exchanges per day with much less inconvenience for the patient.

Preparation and training

The PD catheter is placed approximately one month before it is expected to be required. The incision is allowed to heal for two to three weeks and then the patient undergoes one-on-one training with a PD nurse for about two weeks. Each PD nurse follows a relatively small group of PD patients and spends a great deal of time in assisting each patient individually. A wide range of accessories are available to help handicapped or visually impaired patients. After training, persons treated with PD are usually seen by the nurse at monthly intervals.

Peritoneal equilibrium test

Peritoneal dialysis depends on the diffusion of toxins across the peritoneum membrane. Patients vary, however, in the speed with which this occurs. This variability is measured by a test called the peritoneal equilibrium (PET) test. In this test, the patient performs a timed four-hour exchange and has blood tests measured at the start of and two and four hours after beginning the exchange. The dialysate fluid is also measured after four hours. The optimal duration and number of exchanges per day that the patient should use depends on the membrane transport type as determined by this test. The PET test is usually checked about a month after the start of dialysis and periodically thereafter. It should not be measured until at least three to four weeks have passed after an episode of peritonitis. Patients are then categorized as one of three types of "transporter": fast, slow, or intermediate.

Fast transporters. Transfer solutes quickly between the blood and the peritoneal dialysate. They are good candidates for multiple quick exchanges performed by a cycler at night-time.

Slow transporters. Better suited to using longer, slower exchanges of CAPD where usually the exchange is left in place for six hours.

Intermediate transporters. A large group of patients in between the fast and slow category. These patients are suited to either cycler or to traditional CAPD.

The decision as to which form of PD these patients use is largely determined by personal preference.

Dialysis dose

The rate of clearance of toxins is much less in PD than in hemodialysis. The lower clearance rate is compensated for by the continuous nature of peritoneal dialysis, which increases the effective, provided dose of dialysis. Nevertheless it may be difficult to achieve adequate dose of dialysis using traditional CAPD, especially in large patients. The development of automated PD has greatly improved our ability to provide a higher dialysis dose. Any remaining kidney function provides a substantial addition to the work done by dialysis. For this reason every effort should be made to preserve what remains of the native kidney function for as long as is possible.

Dialysis dose in peritoneal dialysis is measured by the Kt/V and by creatinine clearance. Recommendations for CAPD are to maintain a Kt/V of over 2.0 and a creatinine clearance of greater than 65 liters per week. Slightly higher targets are used for patients using cyclers. These recommendations assume that the patient complies with his dialysis prescription in a constant fashion. Noncompliance with PD may occur several ways. Patients may miss an entire exchange, fail to use the appropriate amount of fluid, or drain the dialysate too early. These habits are all easy to fall into and therefore must be strongly discouraged.

TRANSPLANTATION

The third strategy used in the treatment of end-stage renal disease is renal transplantation. Currently, about 28% of patients with kidney failure in the United States have a functioning kidney transplant (graft).

Cadaveric transplantation

Most transplanted kidneys are cadaveric grafts, meaning that they are removed after the donor's death, which is often the result of a motor vehicle accident. Transplantation is limited, however, by severe shortage of donor kidneys. This shortage is related to the failure of many people to consider or discuss with their families the possibilities of organ donation. Despite huge increases in the number of patients on dialysis over the last several years, the number of cadaveric organ donations has remained relatively static.

Living-related transplantation

A kidney may be also donated from a living donor, often a relative or a spouse. The potential donor undergoes extensive testing to see if his or her kidney is compatible with the recipient and to ensure that the donor has no evidence of active renal disease. Because one kidney provides adequate function, kidney donation is in itself does not create the risk of renal insufficiency for the donor.

The donated kidney may be removed using an open surgical or a laparoscopic approach. The advantages of the laparoscopic approach are the smaller wound, less abdominal discomfort, and quicker convalescence. The procedure is technically more difficult, however, and thus the success depends heavily on the experience of the surgeon.

Advantages of transplantation

Renal transplantation is the preferred method of treating renal failure because it restores native kidney function, including the hormonal activities of the kidney. Dialysis is no longer required after transplantation and dietary restrictions are much less severe than on dialysis. In addition, the option of a combined kidney-pancreas transplantation in diabetes offers the possibility of not only treating the kidney failure but also of correcting the underlying diabetes and preventing further diabetic complications.

Limitations of transplantation

Transplantation is not an easy solution nor indeed the right solution for all patients. Considerable lifestyle adjustments are still required. Most importantly the patient continues to require a large number of medications in order to maintain healthy graft function. Good compliance with these medications is essential if the graft is to survive. The chief problem with transplantation is the danger of rejection of the transplanted organ by the recipient's immune system. The immune system perceives the transplant as foreign tissue and tries to destroy it as it would an invading infection. To prevent this from happening, potent combinations of immunosuppressive medications are used. The downside of these medications is that they also decrease the ability of the immune system to destroy actual infections or abnormal growths such as tumors.

Transplant recipient evaluation

Each potential transplant recipient is evaluated by a team consisting of a transplant surgeon, a nephrologist, a medical social worker, and a nurse coordinator. The decision to list a patient for transplantation depends on the estimated risks and benefits of transplantation versus dialysis, as well as the patient's lifestyle preferences. Usual contraindications to transplantation are advanced age, a current or recent history of cancer, severe associated medical problems, or poor general health.

The pretransplant evaluation includes a detailed history, complete physical examination, and routine laboratory tests. Standard age- and gender-related screening is done to rule out the presence of any cancer. A cardiovascular assessment will usually include some form of cardiac exercise tolerance test or, in higher risk people, a dye study of the heart's blood vessels (coronary angiogram). Patients with some congenital problems or with long-standing diabetes will have a dye study of their bladder to ensure that it is working correctly. Additional specialized tests may be required depending on the individual.

PERITONEAL DIALYSIS: ADVANTAGES AND DISADVANTAGES

Advantages of peritoneal dialysis

- Treatment is continuous and requires less fluid restriction.
- Fluid shifts are less drastic than hemodialysis and patients with low blood pressure tolerate it better.
- Patients do not need to attend a particular dialysis unit at the same time each week.
- Greater ability to travel, though planning is still required for extensive trips.
- The patient or his caregiver is directly responsible for the dialysis. This help maintains a sense of independence and encourages rehabilitation.
- Is traditionally believed to be associated with better preservation of residual renal function.

Disadvantages of peritoneal dialysis

- The patient needs to be insightful and well motivated.
- There needs to be strict attention to aseptic techniques while performing exchanges.
- The patient needs stable living conditions with adequate storage space to store dialysate.
- The high glucose concentration in the dialysate may lead to weight gain and increased cholesterol levels. Diabetic patients may need to adjust their insulin regimen when the dialysate prescription is changed markedly.
- PD may remove excess potassium from the body and patients may even need to take potassium supplements.

Transplant donor evaluation

In cases of living donation the potential donor must be carefully assessed to limit any possibility of the donor having any current kidney problems. Such problems could result in both the donor and the transplant recipient having less than adequate kidney function. Patients with diabetes, high blood pressure, or with abnormal kidney function are thus excluded from donating. Special genetic testing may be required in cases of inherited kidney disease when the donor is a relation. Donation from young adults is also avoided. Patients undergo psychological evaluation to help ensure that they understand the implications of kidney donation and are in a position to make a suitable informed decision regarding donation.

Immunosuppressive therapy

Rejection of the transplanted kidney is prevented by using a combination of immunosuppressive medications. Higher doses are required in the initial period

Complications of peritoneal dialysis

Peritonitis. This infection within the peritoneum—the abdominal cavity—usually occurs due to a breakdown in aseptic technique during the performance of an exchange. This allows germs to enter the peritoneal cavity at the same time as the dialysate fluid. Recent developments in peritoneal dialysis equipment have helped to greatly reduce the chance that this occurs, so that many experienced PD patients may now go for over two years without a single episode of peritonitis. When peritonitis does occur it causes pain throughout the abdomen and cloudy dialysis fluid. It is treated by adding antibiotic directly to the dialysate, allowing for a very high concentration of antibiotic in the peritoneum. Such treatment is usually successful in quickly eradicating the infection. Most patients with peritonitis can be managed as outpatients and do not require hospitalization.

Exit site infections. These infections are treated with oral or intraperitoneal antibiotics but can sometimes be difficult to completely cure and may necessitate changing the catheter.

Failure to drain. Occasionally the dialysate is slow to drain out of the peritoneum, usually because of constipation, a condition that needs to be avoided. Occasionally it is because the catheter has become malpositioned or obstructed. Both situations can usually be corrected without having to actually remove the catheter, by changing its position under x-ray guidance.

Hernias. The pressure of the dialysate on the abdominal wall may cause hernia formation, which may require surgery to repair.

after transplant, lower doses are given later on. Combinations of agents allow lower doses of each agent to be used, with less potential for side effects. Many different treatment combinations exist. Most combinations consist of three agents, including steroids, either tacrolimus or cyclosporine, and either azathioprine or mycophenolate.

Steroids. Steroids, such as prednisone, are the most widely used form of immunosuppressive agent. Although effective, they are associated with potential side effects at high doses, including worsening of diabetes, hypertension, osteoporosis, and cosmetic changes. To avoid these effects the steroid dose is usually rapidly decreased over the first three months post-transplantation to a low maintenance dose, which is much less likely to cause problems. Once treated with steroids for a while, the body temporarily loses its ability to make its own in response to illness or stress. Thus, it is important that steroid tablets not be stopped suddenly, especially if the patient is ill.

Cyclosporine and tacrolimus (also called FK506). These two drugs are related agents. Patients take one of these drugs twice a day, about twelve hours apart. It is important to take them at about the same time each morning and night. The dose is adjusted in accordance with blood levels. Cyclosporine and tacrolimus have a relatively narrow range of blood levels in which they exert their protective effects. If the blood level climbs above this range they can cause a rapid, though usually reversible, decrease in kidney function. For this reason blood levels are monitored closely. Levels are checked twelve hours after the previous dose and before the next dose is taken. These drugs may cause a mild increase in unwanted hair growth and in gum hyperplasia; the latter can be prevented with regular oral hygiene. Both agents may exacerbate existing or cause new onset hypertension and diabetes and may cause neurological side effects including tremors and headaches.

Azathioprine (Imuran) or mycophenolate (CellCept). These drugs are also often used in addition to steroids and either cyclosporine or tacrolimus to prevent transplant rejection. Blood levels of these agents are not routinely measured. Excess doses cause potentially dangerous low white blood cell counts and infections. Mycophenolate is less likely to cause a low white cell count, although it may predispose to some viral infections such as cytomegalovirus infections. It may cause gastric upset, nausea, vomiting, and abdominal pain. Administering the medicine three times a day rather than twice a day, so that the doses are smaller, can reduce these gastrointestinal side effects.

Complications of kidney transplantation surgery

Early kidney dysfunction. Loss of kidney function soon after transplantation may result from mechanical obstruction to the flow of urine, high blood pressure, a toxic blood level of the immunosuppressive agents cyclosporine or tacrolimus, infection, or acute rejection. Acute rejection occurs when the body's immune system overwhelms the immunosuppressive drugs and starts to destroy the transplanted kidney. A decrease in renal graft function may therefore be due to either immunosuppressive levels being too low, with associated rejection, or alternatively too high, with a resultant toxic effect on the kidney. The first step in management is usually to check the blood level of cyclosporine or tacrolimus, whichever is being used, and to adjust the dose as necessary. Renal ultrasound and urine cultures are also often performed to rule out obstruction or kidney infection. In many cases, however, a transplant biopsy is required to establish the cause of the problem. As the transplanted kidney is relatively close to the skin in the lower abdomen, it is much easier to biopsy than a native kidney. Most transplant recipients will undergo several biopsies in the course of follow-up.

If rejection is confirmed, treatment depends on the degree of dysfunction and the current immunosuppressive regimen. Options include using a large dose of steroids, changing the immunosuppressive regimen to include an agent not previously used, or, in advanced cases, using a special antibody preparation to alter the immune response.

If caught early enough, the result of treating an episode of rejection is good. Frequent blood tests are therefore performed, especially in the first few months post-transplant to detect early rejection and adjust the dose of immunosuppressive medications.

Late graft dysfunction. A different set of problems called chronic rejection may damage the kidney at a later stage. These injuries are characterized by damage to the blood vessels in the kidney and their cause remains a mystery. A major contributing cause is probably a long-term side effect of the same medications, cyclosporine, and tacrolimus, which have made such a dramatic improvement in short-term graft survival by preventing transplant rejection. High blood pressure or high cholesterol levels may contribute to late graft dysfunction in some patients, so it is critically important to treat these medical problems.

Infections. To help prevent infection in the initial period post-transplantation, antibiotics are used (Bactrim, Septra) to prevent infection with *Pneumocystis* pneumonia, as well as an antiviral agent to protect against cytomegalovirus infection (acyclovir [Zovirax] or ganciclovir [Cytovene]). While they are on immunosuppressive medications, patients don't develop the usual signs and symptoms of an infection, such as a fever. Patients and their caregivers, therefore, need to be on the lookout for any suggestion of an infection, and to alert the doctor at the first sign so that appropriate tests can be done.

WHAT RESEARCH IS BEING DONE?

Dialysis and transplantation are areas of intense, ongoing research.

DIALYSIS RESEARCH

Cardiovascular disease. Cardiovascular disease remains the most common cause of death for dialysis patients. Some of this increased risk results from the usual cardiac risk factors such as smoking, diabetes, and high blood pressure, which are commonly present in patients with kidney failure. Much research is also being conducted into additional risk factors for cardiovascular disease that may be associated directly with kidney failure or with its treatment.

Vascular access survival. A main goal of hemodialysis research is to find ways to prolong the life of vascular access and to screen for early problems before the access stops working.

Hemodialysis dose and membrane type. The influence of dialysis dose and hemodialysis membrane type on treatment outcome is currently being investigated by a large NIH-sponsored randomized controlled trial. Likewise, the benefits and risks of daily and night-time hemodialysis compared with the thrice-weekly dialysis schedule are being evaluated.

Peritoneal dialysis solutions. New and improved PD solutions that may cause fewer side effects are being developed. Some of these solutions are already available in Europe but have not yet been approved for use in the United States.

TRANSPLANTATION RESEARCH

Immunosuppression. Extensive research is under way to establish newer and better antirejection agents and combinations of agents with fewer side effects. The ultimate goal of transplantation research is to find a way to maintain a graft without the need for immunosuppressive medications.

Alternative sources for kidney donation. Because of limited organ availability, research is investigating ways of using less than ideal kidneys for transplantation and for transplanting kidneys where the match is less than optimal. One option for solving this lack of availability—xenotransplantation or transplantation of kidneys from a nonhuman source—is still a long way from being a realistic solution.

HOW CAN IT BE PREVENTED?

The best way for healthy people to avoid developing kidney disease is to follow routine health advice: control high blood pressure, maintain good control over diabetes, avoid becoming obese, and stop smoking and stay quit. An alarming number of people have undiagnosed high blood pressure and a high proportion of those diagnosed have their blood pressure inadequately controlled. Patients with underlying diseases at high risk for developing kidney disease, such as diabetic persons, should be regularly monitored. If kidney disease is detected, they should be referred promptly to a kidney specialist—a nephrologist—for evaluation.

EARLY KIDNEY FAILURE

If a patient already has a specific disease, then specific intervention may be available to slow or stop early kidney failure. For example, in both type 1 and type 2 diabetes, the maintenance of good blood sugar control has been shown to retard disease progression. And no matter the type of renal disease, high blood pressure increases the rate of progression to end-stage disease, so control of high blood pressure is therefore essential.

Blood pressure control. Control of blood pressure is essential for managing kidney disease, regardless of the original cause. For blood pressure control to be adequate, patients must follow a salt-restricted diet. The use of a particular class of blood pressure agents, angiotensin-converting enzyme (ACE) inhibitors, delays disease progression in both diabetic and in many other forms of kidney disease. A related group of blood pressure agents, angiotensin II receptor blockers, are believed to have similar protective benefits, but this is not as clearly proven yet. A difficulty with both of these classes of drugs is that they may provoke a sudden deterioration in kidney function in patients with a blockage in their renal artery (renal artery stenosis) or if the patient becomes dehydrated. They also tend to increase levels of potassium, a problem that is especially dangerous in advanced kidney disease. Therefore close patient monitoring is essential when these agents are first started. In general, however, the advantages of these agents outweigh their potential problems and ACE inhibitors are now the cornerstone of treatment for an increasing number of different kidney diseases.

Dietary protein restriction. Restricting dietary protein to retard the progression of renal failure is controversial. Several studies support the role of protein restriction in delaying kidney failure. One large study, however, funded by the NIH, proved inconclusive. Some nephrologists strongly believe in the benefits of protein restriction. It is widely agreed, however, that if protein restriction is to be attempted, it is essential to guard against malnutrition. This requires the close supervision of the patient by a trained renal dietitian. This sort of supervision is not currently reimbursed by insurance, so it may not be a feasible option. One easy and safe option is for patients to avoid an excessive protein intake, without actually attempting to follow a formal, very low protein diet.

Lipid control. Abnormalities in blood lipid levels, including increased cholesterol levels, commonly occur with renal failure and are particularly severe in patients with a nephrotic syndrome. These abnormalities continue to be a problem even on dialysis or with a kidney transplant. These abnormalities predispose to the development of vascular damage, including heart problems. There is also evidence to suggest that they may accelerate the progression of kidney failure. For both these reasons abnormal blood cholesterol levels should be controlled. Effective medications are readily available to help patients keep their cholesterol in check.

ADVANCED KIDNEY FAILURE

Once kidney function deteriorates to a certain level, it becomes likely that complete or almost complete loss of kidney function will eventually occur. At this point, appropriate treatment may slow down progression, but it is unlikely to prevent total kidney failure. In this case, it is essential for the patient to become educated regarding the options of renal replacement therapy. This educational process is a team undertaking, involving input from the nephrologist, primary care provider, nurse educator, dietitian, and medical social worker, as well as from the patient and his family. It may take several months and many discussions for a patient to adequately understand what the treatment options are for end-stage kidney failure and to decide which option may best suit his lifestyle. Several months of preparation may be necessary to develop a functioning hemodialysis access or to complete the transplant evaluation process. The usual goal is to start dialysis before the patient develops symptoms or complications from kidney failure.

WHAT YOU CAN DO NOW

For patients with moderate kidney failure:

- Be evaluated by a nephrologist
- Measure and record blood pressure regularly
- Get advice and follow-up from a trained renal dietitian
- Avoid all added salt and salt-rich foods
- Make sure the patient takes medications regularly and on time
- Discuss options of dialysis long before it is necessary to start actual treatment
- Start process of transplantation evaluation and hemodialysis access creation well in advance of anticipated need to start dialysis
- Understand blood tests and follow the results over time
- Understand that the time to start dialysis is when the blood tests indicate that the kidney has all but failed, but before the symptoms associated with kidney failure occur

For patients with end-stage renal disease:

- Attend hemodialysis on time and avoid signing off early
- Use the prescribed number of PD exchanges and the correct fill volume
- Carry an updated list of medications with you (including the ones that are regularly given in the dialysis unit)
- Know what the patient's goal ("dry") weight is
- Understand and know how patient's levels of dialysis dose, anemia, nutrition, blood pressure, calcium, phosphate, PTH, and vascular access type compare with national recommendations, available from The National Kidney Foundation.
- Follow the appropriate diet
- The patient should be weighed each morning and their fluid intake adjusted to avoid excess weight gain
- Learn to recognize the signs and symptoms of dialysis access infection or peritonitis

ADDITIONAL RESOURCES

WEB SITES

American Association of Kidney Patients

www.aakp.org

American Diabetes Association

www.diabetes.org

American Heart Association

www.americanheart.org

American Kidney Fund

www.akfinc.org

Kidney Directions

www.kidneydirections.com

Life Options Rehabilitation Program

www.lifeoptions.org

National Heart, Lung, and Blood Institute

www.nhlbi.nih.gov

National Kidney Foundation

www.kidney.org

TransWeb.org (University of Michigan)

www.transweb.org

United Network for Organ Sharing

www.unos.org

Fecal Incontinence

- Inability to retain fecal matter at will

Fecal continence requires four things:

1. The ability to sense the need to defecate, to know when a bowel movement is imminent.
2. The ability to sense the difference between gas, liquid, and solid stool.
3. Intact nerves and muscles to the rectum and anus, and muscle tone in the pelvic floor.
4. The desire to maintain continence.

For many people, fecal incontinence is the ultimate indignity. It is involuntary—passing flatulence, stool, or diarrhea against your will, being unable to hold it until you get to the bathroom. Fecal incontinence carries such a stigma in our society that many people suffer from it in silence, too embarrassed to see a doctor for help. The social ramifications of fecal incontinence can be cruel and devastating, and may contribute to shame and isolation. Although more common in women and people with poor general health, it is most prevalent in the elderly, affecting between 13 and 47% of elderly people who are hospitalized, and as many as two-thirds of all nursing home residents. In fact, fecal incontinence is often the deciding factor in nursing home admissions. It is a hidden disease, affecting up to 5% of Americans with varying degrees of severity, and with a multitude of causes.

Fecal incontinence is a grossly undertreated problem, in large part because of sufferers' reluctance to seek help, but also because not all physicians understand that effective treatment exists. The good news is that as many as 80% of people with fecal incontinence can be helped and can have a reduction of symptoms, and more than half can be cured.

WHAT IS IT?

The first thing to say here is that an occasional episode of fecal incontinence can happen to anyone. Projectile diarrhea resulting from a bout of food poisoning,

253

for example, may be so severe that it overrides the body's normal mechanisms to control defecation. This is usually a very temporary problem—like a "blip" on a radar screen—that resolves on its own.

Chronic fecal incontinence is another story, and the first step to finding an effective treatment is to figure out what's causing the problem—which nerves or muscles are not working as they should, and whether any other disease is at least partly to blame.

WHAT'S SUPPOSED TO HAPPEN

In the normal digestive process, the food we eat—which, as it's being digested, spends most of its time in our bodies as a liquid—is mixed with various food—dissolving juices, kneaded like bread dough and pushed through the intestines, squeezed along through hundreds of muscle contractions like toothpaste through a tube. In the colon (the large intestine; many doctors use the words large bowel and colon interchangeably), the average person's daily intake of food—originally about two quarts of material, now concentrated to a liquid cupful—begins to resemble stool, or feces. Excess water is removed and absorbed, and the mass, now in solid form, is slowly propelled by muscles in the sigmoid (the tail, or distal, end of the colon, named for its "S" shape) into the rectum—the first of a series of anatomic barriers designed to keep stool inside the body until it can be expelled at an appropriate time. The rectum, basically, is a storehouse, a reservoir that relaxes and distends to hold stool. During a normal bowel movement, muscles in the rectum flex and shrink like rubber bands to push the stool into the anal canal, and then out through the anus—a powerful, muscular valve. The anus is made up of two rings of muscle—called the internal sphincter and the external sphincter—which act as doors to control the passage of stool and gas. We only have control over half of the anus—the external sphincter, which is ultimately responsible for keeping feces and gas contained inside the body. The other part, the internal sphincter, is involuntary; when it senses the presence of stool, it automatically relaxes. Wrapped around both of these sphincters is yet another muscle—this one shaped like a sling—called the puborectalis. When the puborectalis contracts, it works like a purse string, pinching off the colon and further preventing defecation.

Gas, too, is present in the gut. Some of it is created there—methane, for instance, is a normal byproduct of intestinal fermentation; so are hydrogen and carbon dioxide. The body makes gas when it processes carbohydrates and amino acids. People who have trouble digesting lactose (found in dairy products) or other forms of sugar produce large amounts of hydrogen. Excess hydrogen also is generated as the intestine grapples with high-fiber fruits and vegetables. (Because these are not entirely digestible, the part that is not absorbed by the body passes as "bulk" in the stool.) Some people naturally are prone to make more methane than others; in fact, this tendency can be inherited, and runs in many families. But gas also enters our bodies with every sip of drink and swallow of food. We tend to swallow more air when we are nervous; also, certain conditions (such as peptic ulcer disease) that involve excessive salivation can cause more air to be swallowed. Although much of it never winds up in the bowel—it goes out the way it came in, through the mouth, in belches (particularly when we drink carbonated beverages)—some of it is passed out of the body through flatulence. Most people pass gas many times a day—often without realizing it—usually in tiny, unnoticeable amounts.

There is great variability in the definition of "normal" bowel movement and activity. For example, some people defecate several times a day, others only a few times a week. However, a normal bowel movement is solid but not hard, is not painful to pass, and should not contain any blood. Solid stool is easiest to sense, and to control; for most people with fecal incontinence, the biggest challenge is diarrhea.

Liquid stool is not only harder to retain, it's more difficult to sense, and often gives less notice of its arrival—a shorter "warning time" to get to the toilet. Diarrhea in addition to another problem (loss of rectal sensation, for example) can push someone over the edge from being "borderline incontinent"—able to make it to the bathroom in time, even if it's just barely—to having full-fledged incontinence. Although involuntary flatulence—however embarrassing it may be—is not generally considered a medical problem, excessive flatulence may be a symptom of another condition, such as irritable bowel syndrome or food intolerance (improper digestion of nutrients), both characterized by explosive stool.

Fecal incontinence is largely a mechanical problem, resulting from failure of the body's checkpoints to control involuntary passage of feces and gas. (Note: The exception to this is fecal incontinence as a result of mental illness or cognitive impairment—the kind of incontinence most difficult to treat.) But many underlying conditions can exacerbate the problem. Any disorder that leads to chronic diarrhea, severe gas, explosive stool or constipation can stack the deck against someone prone to incontinence who, under ordinary circumstances, might manage to be continent most of the time. About 80% of people with fecal incontinence are able to regain continence of solid stool, but it is harder to regain continence of diarrhea. Therefore, managing fecal incontinence, a complicated problem, usually requires a combined treatment plan: First, dealing with any underlying illness—and, whenever possible, turning diarrhea into solid stool, through diet, supplements, and medication—as well as strengthening the body's defenses against incontinence.

WHAT CAN GO WRONG?

Here are the most common reasons for fecal incontinence.

Anal sphincter dysfunction

This is damage to the external sphincter or the puborectalis muscles, and it's usually caused by trauma—childbirth, for example (especially one or more difficult deliveries requiring forceps or other assistance, or resulting in a large episiotomy), abdominal surgery, or anal intercourse (which can injure the sphincter and diminish muscle tone).

Nerve damage

Injury to the spinal cord or nerves—caused by trauma, surgery, or neuromuscular diseases such as spina bifida, multiple sclerosis, or myasthenia gravis—can lead to a loss of rectal sensation, diminished reflexes or muscle tone in the rectum, anus, and pelvic floor, and also may hinder the ability of the colon's muscles to move stool into the rectum. Diabetes also can contribute to long-term damage to the peripheral or autonomic nerves, and as a result, up to 20% of people with diabetes have fecal incontinence. Uncontrolled diabetes also can be associated with diarrhea caused by bacterial overgrowth (which is treatable with antibiotics—see below).

Impaired reservoir function of the rectum

This can be caused by scarring or nerve and tissue damage from inflammatory bowel diseases, such as ulcerative colitis or Crohn's disease; by radiation to the rectum (from treatment of prostate cancer, for instance); by surgery; or by rectal ischemia—poor blood flow to the rectum, which can happen when someone has arteriosclerosis, or "hardening" of the arteries. The result is that the rectum simply cannot hold very much stool at a time.

Severe constipation and fecal impaction

Most common in elderly, disabled, or bedridden patients, it also may be caused, or compounded, by the constipating side effect of many medications. Impacted stool is literally stuck—rock-hard and lodged in the rectum or anus—and diarrhea may leak around it. Proper diagnosis is essential, because a fecal impaction can be life-threatening, and may lead to bleeding, ulcers, or even perforation of the colon.

Impaired cognitive function

Dementia, severe stroke, or even severe depression can lead to a situation where incontinence occurs either because of lack of control or lack of concern over its presence. This cause of incontinence is the least likely to be treatable unless the underlying cause can be treated (as is the case with depression).

HOW IS IT DIAGNOSED?

A careful, detailed medical history and physical exam are essential, not only to pinpoint the exact cause but also to determine the right treatment. Here are some questions the doctor will likely ask the patient.

How often does the incontinence occur? If episodes are very rare—once or twice a month, for example—no treatment may be needed.

Under what circumstances does it happen? It may be that the situation is not medical, but logistical—if, for example, the patient can't walk down the hall or climb the flight of stairs to the toilet in time, or needs to be helped up and into a walker. Many people with mild dementia, if given the opportunity, encouragement, and help, know when they need to go to the bathroom, and would prefer to defecate in the toilet than in a diaper. Unfortunately, at many understaffed nursing homes, it is easier, or more efficient, to change adult diapers on a regular schedule rather than help patients to the bathroom whenever they need to go. In consequence, patients lose precious independence and dignity.

What is the stool like? Is it often loose? Explosive stools or excessive gas may signal an underlying problem (trouble digesting certain types of food, for example, or irritable bowel syndrome), which also should be treated. The other extreme is constipation, which can lead to bowel and rectal irritation, and diarrhea in addition to (and sometimes, oozing around) hard stool.

When did the incontinence start? Was it brought on by the start of a new medication? Certain drugs are known to cause diarrhea; for other medications (particularly opiates, which are also constipating), the side effect may be drowsiness—which may affect someone's ability to sense the need to get to the bathroom, or the desire to get there in time. Or, did incontinence happen after the onset of another condition, such as a stroke?

Does it happen mainly when you're awake, or when you're asleep or drowsy? If it does not happen during sleep, it may be more likely to respond to a bowel regimen or biofeedback.

How much warning do you get? Obviously, doctors don't expect patients to carry a stopwatch. The real issue here is, can the patient hold it in at all? If so, for how long? Long enough, for example, if he's in the car on the way back from the grocery store, to make it home, or even to the first public restroom he sees?

If you are not incontinent all the time, do you often strain when you're having a bowel movement? This could cause trauma or nerve damage to the rectum and anus.

Have you had previous surgery in the rectal area—for hemorrhoids, for example—or infections there? During the physical examination, the doctor will check for scars (from difficult childbirth—particularly if forceps are used—or from infection), irregularities (changes in the shape of the anus, from childbirth trauma, or previous surgery), rectal prolapse (when the rectum droops, or pushes out through the anus, impeding the sphincter), and sphincter tone (the patient will be asked to "bear down" on the doctor's gloved finger). The doctor may also check anal reflexes (similar to the test for knee reflexes during a routine physical exam) with a pinprick test. The normal anus is very sensitive, and responds immediately when it is touched—especially when the stimulus is sharp—by closing up. This reflex is descriptively called the anal "wink." A rectal exam also may detect the presence of hard stool.

DIAGNOSTIC TESTS

Fecal incontinence can also be diagnosed using one or more diagnostic tests.

Flexible sigmoidoscopy. This test takes less than thirty minutes and is generally performed as an outpatient procedure. The sigmoidoscope is a small, lighted, flexible tube, about two feet long, and equipped with a video camera, which is inserted through the rectum. It allows the doctor—family doctor, internist, or a gastroenterologist—to check for any abnormalities in the rectum and sigmoid colon.

Anorectal manometry. This test, usually performed by a gastroenterologist, uses balloons to measure pressure, and can detect a loss of muscle tone, sensation, and motor function in the rectum and anal sphincters. The manometer measures the contractions of the external anal sphincter, and gives readouts, or "tracings"—much like that of a seismograph as it registers earthquakes. Many women compensate for a loss of muscle tone in the sphincters and pelvic floor by contracting certain muscles instead of relaxing them.

Electromyography. This test measures the nerve supply and muscle responses of the puborectalis and external anal sphincter by checking for electrical responses in the muscles nerves (similar to an electrocardiogram), and is usually performed by a gastroenterologist. Sometimes (after radiation therapy, for example), the rectum is not able to sense that it is full, or is unable to expand when stool is present.

Defecography. This is an x-ray test of the rectal anatomy, and it shows how the rectum and anus work together during defecation. It can show a loss of pelvic floor muscle function and tone, or show pelvic floor prolapse (when the pelvic floor muscles are damaged, and the rectum is shifted downward).

Rectal retention and defecation studies. These measure the muscles' ability to retain and push out solids and liquids.

Tests to determine food intolerance. By itself, food intolerance does not cause fecal incontinence. But again, its symptoms—painful bloating, flatulence, and diarrhea—can magnify the problem in someone with weakened sphincter muscle tone. Several tests can help identify intolerance to lactose, the sugar in cow's milk. One of these is a hydrogen breath test after drinking lactose. Hydrogen is not usually detectable in the breath. But when the body has trouble digesting sugars such as lactose, gut bacteria react by producing hydrogen and other gases, which are absorbed into the bloodstream, carried to the lungs, and breathed out. There is also a blood test to diagnose lactose tolerance, which is given on an empty stomach. The test involves taking several blood samples over the course of two hours. The first measures the "fasting" blood glucose level; then, the patient is asked to drink a lactose-containing beverage, and further blood samples will be taken to determine whether the glucose level rises (as it should, normally). People who are lactose-intolerant are missing a key enzyme called lactase. This is made by cells lining the bowel, and its job is to break down milk sugar into simpler, easier-to-digest forms. If there's no lactase, the lactose will not be absorbed, and the glucose level should remain the same.

Tests to determine bacterial overgrowth. Bacterial overgrowth can be diagnosed by a breath test, or by the presence of undigested fat in a stool sample, or by treatment with antibiotics.

HOW IS IT TREATED?

Because fecal incontinence is rarely a simple problem, treatment can vary greatly, depending on the particular kind of incontinence (solid, liquid, gas, or a combination), and whether other health or digestive problems are making everything worse. Thus, an important first strategy is to find and treat any underlying conditions.

IF INCONTINENCE ALTERNATES WITH CHRONIC CONSTIPATION

Chronic constipation (including impaction) can cause "overflow" incontinence—when liquid stool oozes around solid stool that's rock-hard, dry, rough, difficult to pass, or is moving at a glacial pace through a sluggish bowel. What's causing the constipation? Sometimes it is simply an artifact of age. Often, however, something else is happening, as well: For example, many medications, including general anesthesia, can slow down bowel "motility," or activity and movement. Opiates (painkillers like codeine, hydrocodone [Vicodin, Lortab], and morphine), tranquilizers, antidepressants, sedatives, anticholinergic drugs (like the antihistamine Benadryl), even having too much iron in the diet or taking vitamins with extra iron can be constipating. Being bedridden, or very sedentary, adds to the problem, as do some illnesses such as Parkinson's disease, thyroid disease, or ulcerative colitis; and other factors such as stress, lack of exercise, poor diet (with too little fiber, fruits and vegetables, and water), and chronic pain.

The first objective is to promote "complete" defecation—ridding the rectum of everything that's in it. Because not everyone responds to every form of treatment in the same way, there may be some trial and error involved in finding the best way to do this. Some physicians start with fiber, using natural "bulking" agents—psyllium or polycarbophil supplements such as Metamucil, FiberCon, Citrucel, or

Konsyl. Other physicians start with a "low-residue" diet, which has much less fiber. Your doctor may also prescribe an initial course of laxatives. A stool softener—such as docusate (DSS, Colace) or mineral oil—may help, by breaking down stool as it sits in the colon, allowing it to absorb more water and become softer, and better able to move to the rectum. Your doctor may recommend giving several enemas containing phosphate solutions (such as Fleet) until the colon is free of stool, or may suggest mineral-oil enemas, which lubricate the stool. If there is an impaction, several mineral-oil enemas may be enough to dislodge it; if this does not work, the next step is a simple procedure called "digital removal" (which can be done in a doctor's office), in which the doctor's gloved finger is used to remove the impacted stool. Although not terribly pleasant, this procedure should not be painful, and does not require anesthesia.

For many people, the best long-term strategy is to establish a "bowel regimen." This may mean sitting on the toilet at regular intervals—two or three or more times—every day. It also may mean a regular schedule of enemas once or twice a day (and then, like clockwork, sitting on the toilet at the same time every day) to keep the colon and rectum free of feces.

IF CONSTIPATION IS SEVERE, OR IS COMBINED WITH SENSORY LOSS

This is most common in people who are disabled, bedridden, or paralyzed; injury to the spinal cord can not only cause a loss of sensation of the lower colon and rectum, it also may hinder the colon's ability to contract and propel stool into the rectum. Again, the most important thing is to avoid any buildup of stool, and keep the flow of stool moving with regular defecation. If there is sensory loss below the colon, defecation must be stimulated, either with digital stimulation (by a gloved finger in the anal canal) or with use of a glycerin suppository (a fast-acting lubricant that works within an hour). Some patients require an aggressive approach, which should be planned with your own doctor or one who has expertise in treating spinal cord injuries.

IF INCONTINENCE IS ASSOCIATED WITH DEPRESSION

Finding the right antidepressant medication—a process that may take some time, may involve trial and error, and often requires patience—may be of great benefit in two ways. First, simply relieving the burden of depression may promote the desire to maintain continence. Second, some antidepressants are in the class of anticholinergic drugs, whose known side effects include dampening, or slowing down, bowel activity—in effect, they're mildly constipating. In some cases, combining antidepressants with a bowel regimen may be enough to stop the incontinence.

IF INCONTINENCE IS ASSOCIATED WITH MILD, CHRONIC DIARRHEA OR SOFT STOOLS

If your doctor can't pinpoint any specific cause (the most likely ones are listed below), treating the diarrhea with medication may solve or greatly reduce the problem. The idea is to cause mild constipation—and to give the patient enough control to reach the bathroom in time. This also may be combined with a daily bowel regimen of going to the bathroom at the same times every day. Several drugs are very effective at slowing down the bowel movement—again, anticholinergic drugs, or specific antidiarrheal medications such as diphenoxylate and atropine (Lomotil) and loperamide (Imodium). Or a mildly constipating antacid, such as Amphogel, available over the counter, might be helpful.

Another approach to treating mild chronic diarrhea is adding soluble fiber—"bulking" agents (psyllium or polycarbophil supplements such as Citrucel, Metamucil, FiberCon, or Konsyl) to the diet. When adding fiber to any diet, it's best to do it slowly. Too much fiber can cause crampiness, flatulence, and distension. Also, as with treating constipation, this is a process of trial and error. For some patients, the added bulk may be counterproductive, and may lead to even more incontinence.

IF THE DIARRHEA HAS A TREATABLE CAUSE

Many people with diarrhea-related incontinence are helped simply by treating the underlying illness that's causing the liquid stool. Some of the most common causes of diarrhea are listed below.

Chronic infections. The two most common are *Giardia* (in the small intestine), which can result from drinking water infected with parasites, and *C. difficile* (in the large intestine), which can result from a course of antibiotics. Both may be treated by metronidazole (Flagyl).

Food intolerance. Lactose intolerance (inability to digest the sugar found in milk, diagnosed by tests described above) affects an estimated 50 million American adults. It's most common in Asian Americans, but is also prevalent in Jewish, African-American, Native-American, and Mexican-American families. Intolerance to fructose (the sugar found in grapes, apple and pear juice, honey, dates, nuts, figs, and the sweetener in many soft drinks) is less common, but an estimated 70% of healthy people cannot completely absorb heavy amounts of fructose (the amount contained in a pound of grapes, for instance). Less common still is intolerance to sucrose, found in table sugar, candy bars, and many fruits. All of these sugars are also found in many prescription drugs, vitamins, and over-the-counter medicines, especially oral liquid preparations of medications.

For fructose and sucrose, the only treatment is avoidance, which can be managed largely by reading the labels of packaged foods before buying them. If you need extra help, ask your doctor for a list of foods to avoid.

Many people with mild lactose intolerance are helped by taking an enzyme-replacement supplement (LactAid, Dairy Ease) before they eat dairy products. This supplement contains the enzyme lactase. Special milk, from which 70% of lactose is removed, also is easier to digest. But if lactose intolerance is severe, your best bet here, too, is avoidance—a challenge in the American diet, where nonfat dry milk is added to improve the taste of many foods (particularly those labeled "low fat" or "fat-free"), including cakes, cookies, and other snack items, hot dogs, lunch meats, salad dressings, margarine, soups, and instant potatoes, to name a few. Because any milk product can produce symptoms, watch out for these words on food labels: whey, dry milk solids, sodium caseinate, and curds.

Irritable bowel syndrome ("spastic colon"). Because irritable bowel syndrome can mimic other conditions, it is often a "diagnosis of exclusion"—making sure nothing else is causing the symptoms that include diarrhea and/or constipation, abdominal pain, and excessive flatulence. Here, the problem is a hypersensitive bowel that overreacts to any form of stimulation (including the presence of gas or stool in the colon or rectum) by going into spasms. Stress, medications, and certain foods may trigger symptoms. Some people are helped by changing the diet—particularly by avoiding dairy products and high-fat foods, cruciferous vegetables (cabbage, Brussels sprouts, cauliflower, and broccoli), fruit sugars, and coffee. Bulking agents can be helpful, as well, preventing spasms, but also by keeping the stool soft. Medications also can ease symptoms: One form of treatment is an anti-spasmodic drug such as hyoscyamine (Levsin) or dicyclomine (Bentyl); another approach is a tricyclic antidepressant.

IF INCONTINENCE MAY BE RELATED TO DIABETES

Among the many complications of diabetes is bacterial overgrowth (which can be detected by tests described above). In this condition, bacteria colonize and accumulate on the lining of the small intestine—which normally is sterile—like algae on the inside of a fish tank. The bacteria soon start breaking down bile salts, and generally having a detergent effect—similar to what would happen if you drank soap—causing diarrhea, distension, and flatulence. Bacterial overgrowth may result from other, less common conditions, but whatever its cause, treating the underlying illness will help; in turn, treating the bacterial overgrowth may help ease fecal incontinence. The initial treatment is to knock out the bacteria with a short course—one to two weeks—of an antibiotic such as ampicillin or ciprofloxacin. This may produce several months of freedom from symptoms. If diabetes is the cause, the next step is to keep the overgrowth from coming back, by keeping blood sugar under control.

IF INCONTINENCE IS ASSOCIATED WITH EXCESSIVE FLATULENCE

The first strategy is to investigate the diet, and—largely by trial and error—identify (and stop eating) foods that produce more gas. Fiber supplements can cause gas, as can a diet that's naturally high in fiber. Coffee causes flatulence in some people, as do fruits, legumes, and vegetables—particularly the cruciferous kind (cauliflower, cabbage, Brussels sprouts, and broccoli). Excess sugars in dried beans can be removed before they're cooked, either with the traditional method of soaking the beans overnight, or with an over-the-counter product such as Beano, which breaks down these sugars. Simethicone (Mylicon, GAS-X), a drug that reduces gas bubbles, may be beneficial, as may some antispasmodic drugs, such as dicyclomine.

BIOFEEDBACK

The next step, a simple technique called biofeedback (a form of therapy that is paid for by most insurance companies and health plans), is extremely helpful in more than 70% of people who are able to contract their external anal sphincter or gluteal muscles (the muscles in the buttocks), and those who are able to feel when stool enters the rectum. Not everyone is a candidate for biofeedback, a process of muscle strengthening. It takes determination, persistence, and hard work.

Biofeedback uses a small balloon probe, which is inserted in the rectum. The idea is to teach patients to recognize when they're having a contraction, to coordinate what they're feeling with the contractions that appear on the machine, to connect this feeling with rectal distension, and to learn to do it on their own. Once patients have mastered the external sphincter contraction, the next step is "homework"—to practice contractions often, at least three times a day, and then to contract the sphincter at the least sensation of rectal urgency or distension.

This special training, called Kegel exercises, can be practiced anywhere—while sitting (even while urinating), standing, or lying down—and can help delay flatulence, as well as stool. It may be easier to practice them while lying face-up on the bed, with knees bent, and feet about twelve inches apart; it may be easier for patients to hold their feet up in the air rather than flat on the bed. As tightly as they can, patients are to clench the muscles around the anus—the ones used when trying not to pass gas—and hold for five seconds, eventually working up to twenty seconds. They can then relax slowly, let the muscles go, and then repeat. This comes easier to some people than others, and setbacks are common—but patients shouldn't be discouraged if results don't come immediately.

Some hospitals offer home monitors, with a rectal probe that monitors contractions, that allow patients to measure how much they're pushing or relaxing, and do repetitions to tone up the muscles in the anal sphincter pelvis and rectum, just as they would tone up their legs or abdominal muscles in the gym. For most people, biofeedback takes about six to ten sessions (after the initial evaluation) with the nurse or therapist (and lots of practice in between) to master.

SURGERY

For some people who are not able to tighten their anal sphincter muscles through exercises and biofeedback, surgery can help. There are many variations to this operation, depending on the exact nature of the problem—for example, someone with large hemorrhoids may simply need to have the hemorrhoids removed—but it is possible to tighten the anal canal and change the angle of the anal muscles. With this surgery, there is always the risk of scar tissue, and of further damage to the anorectal muscles and nerves. Thus, it is essential that you find a surgeon who specializes in this kind of procedure. Even at its best, the operation is not for everybody because even a surgically tightened sphincter can't always hold back diarrhea.

Another surgical procedure, colostomy, is a last-resort operation. An ostomy is a surgically made opening in the abdominal wall that creates a new exit route for stool, which then collects in a small plastic bag, firmly affixed to the skin. Before undergoing this procedure, patients should discuss all of their concerns—many patients take a list of questions to the doctor, so they won't forget anything—with their doctor and enterostomal therapist (a nurse who is specially trained to help people face quality-of-life issues with ostomies). The doctor should be able to supply the names of other patients who have gone through this procedure, and should provide information about local support groups. After surgery, if at all possible, a home nurse should visit, to help the patient learn to care for the ostomy. (Many insurance companies will pay for a home health nurse.)

After a colostomy, meticulous cleanliness and maintenance are as important as ever. The colostomy bag does not adhere well to irritated skin; in turn, leakage of stool may aggravate this irritation. Some people have an allergic reaction to the bag, which results in skin irritation (changing brands should fix this problem); hair follicles can also cause irritation (shaving the area with an electric razor or clipping with scissors can help). Some people develop a skin infection, which usually gets better with a thin layer of nystatin powder, applied each time the bag is changed. If constipation was a problem before the colostomy, it may be afterward, as well. Bulk fiber (or other medicine or dietary supplements) may help regulate bowel movements. Complications include problems with blood flow (the colon, in general, has a less well developed blood supply than the small intestine); some people develop scar tissue that may eventually need treatment.

WHAT RESEARCH IS BEING DONE?

Much exciting research is under way to expand the options and improve quality of life for people with fecal incontinence. Some of the most promising areas of investigation include:

- Use of electrical stimulation of the pelvic and anorectal nerves to improve function and continence.
- Creation of an artificial anal sphincter.
- Development of better imaging tests to evaluate the sphincter and surrounding anatomy, including early evaluation of obstetrical trauma using ultrasound.

- Creation of new topical (applied externally) medications to improve sphincter tone.
- Refinement of surgical approaches, using muscle flaps and chronic electrical stimulation, to improve muscle tone.

WHAT YOU CAN DO NOW

There is a good chance that if you have fecal incontinence, or are caring for someone who does, the material in this chapter can help change your life. But the problem won't stop today, or even tomorrow; diagnosing the cause, determining the right treatment, and implementing it usually takes time—weeks to months. So until the incontinence improves, or goes away entirely, there are some issues that need to be addressed now.

The first is getting past the emotions that make fecal incontinence such a difficult problem. It's safe to say that nobody wants stool leakage—and, to make matters worse, it's usually not a secret when it occurs. There is no privacy with fecal incontinence; patients with this problem are acutely aware of the smell, for instance, and it's often easier to start avoiding people and social settings than to deal with the embarrassment and anger that comes from "having an accident" in public—even if "public" is your own spouse. Fecal incontinence in men often happens at night, during sleep, when the anal sphincter is at its most relaxed, because they are unable to sense the buildup of pressure that signals the presence of stool in the rectum. For women—especially women who have had many children, and who have little muscle tone in the anal sphincter or pelvic floor muscles, fecal (and urinary) incontinence often has a hair-trigger onset. A stimulus as slight as a cough or sneeze, or even laughter, can bring it on.

Most people with fecal incontinence desperately want help. They might not be able to ask for it, but if you are persistent, tactful, and respectful, they may allow you to give it to them. This may be as simple as providing transportation to keep appointments with the doctor (or nurse, if regular biofeedback sessions are scheduled). Or providing some help to get to the bathroom, and making sure necessary items—the appropriate diaper or pad for the job required, and special cleansing agents—are available and easy to reach. Large adult diapers, such as Poise (which has a gel that wicks moisture away from the skin), are best for large amounts of liquid stool. But for smaller amounts—for someone who has mild incontinence—a small, thin pad (Depends makes one) is adequate.

Until a long-term solution is found (medicine, lifestyle changes, or surgery, all described in this chapter), your short-term goal should be to avoid infection and other complications. If you are a caregiver and you must change diapers, do it often. Ideally, check the diaper every hour, change it whenever it's wet, and apply a "moisture barrier" such as Keri-Cleans or Carrington Moisture Barrier after every bowel movement. Many skin products specifically made for the anal area are available over the counter; they come in sprays, oils, wipes, and foams. (Avoid products that contain alcohol, which can burn the skin. Also, avoid products for babies, particularly ointments that contain zinc oxide. This is fine for occasional diaper rash in infants, but zinc oxide can burn or irritate the skin when it's used daily.) People with fecal incontinence who are not kept meticulously clean run the serious risk of infection and skin breakdown. Similar to bedsores, these wounds, called decubitus ulcers, can penetrate deep in tissue, sometimes reaching all the way to bone. At best, they are uncomfortable; at worst, they are agonizing. Some people with mild irritation are helped by sitting on a "donut" cushion, which takes the pressure off the perirectal area.

ADDITIONAL RESOURCES

ORGANIZATIONS

About Incontinence, International Foundation for Functional Gastrointestinal Disorders

www.aboutincontinence.org

International Foundation for Functional Gastrointestinal Disorders

www.iffgd.org

BOOKS

Schuster, Marvin M., and Jacqueline Wehmueller. *Keeping Control: Understanding and Overcoming Fecal Incontinence.* Baltimore: Johns Hopkins University Press, 1994.

Gastrointestinal Disorders

The National Institutes of Health has estimated that one in thirteen Americans has a chronic digestive problem. The costs of this are staggering. Digestive conditions are responsible for about thirty-five million annual doctor visits and forty billion dollars a year in medical costs.

The scope of gastrointestinal disorders is less surprising when you consider how complex this system is. From mouth to anus, the digestive tract is roughly thirty feet long and has about a dozen different parts. At every stage there's a complex interplay of hormones, nerve signals, muscular contractions, and digestive enzymes. As you get older, the risk that one or more of these elements will go out of balance gradually—then more sharply—rises.

The gastrointestinal system has two basic jobs: to extract nutrients from foods and pass them into the bloodstream for use by the body's cells, and to eliminate wastes once the nutrients have been absorbed.

Entire textbooks have been written about chronic gastrointestinal diseases, but the most common ones can be counted on one hand—constipation, diverticular disease, gastroesophageal reflux disease, irritable bowel syndrome, and ulcers.

It's very likely that any person, old or young, who is ill enough or dependent enough to require the assistance of a caregiver will suffer one or several of these gastrointestinal conditions at some point in their illness. Responses to surgery or medications, inherent side effects of other illnesses, or even a change in diet may set the stage for any one of these conditions to develop. Each of these conditions can make life difficult. A few of them may be life threatening in some cases. But they can all be controlled with medical treatments or simple lifestyle changes.

Constipation

- Hard stools that are difficult or painful to pass
- Uncomfortable "fullness" feeling
- Straining for a bowel movement
- Still feeling "full" in the bowels after a bowel movement

Constipation may be the most common digestive problem in the United States, and it's certainly the most misunderstood. People often assume they're constipated when they don't have a daily bowel movement, but the digestive system is rarely this predictable, even under normal circumstances.

Some people have two or more bowel movements daily, while others have one every other day. In addition, it's normal for bowel habits to change over time.

Doctors usually define constipation as having fewer than three bowel movements a week. Bowel movements that are difficult or painful are also a sign of constipation, as is any sudden change in your normal bowel habits.

To understand constipation, it's helpful to know how the large intestine, or colon, works. The colon is never entirely empty. Stools may remain there for twelve to twenty-four hours, giving the body time to reclaim fluids.

The stools are propelled though the colon by a series of muscular contractions. This process, called peristalsis, occurs throughout digestion. Constipation may occur when peristalsis doesn't occur as often or as vigorously as it should. This may be due to side effects from medications, not getting enough fiber or fluids in the diet, or health problems such as low levels of thyroid hormone (hypothyroidism) or Parkinson's disease.

Constipation is rarely serious, but it's important to talk to your doctor if you notice any change in your normal bowel habits, or if you find yourself straining or experiencing pain when you have bowel movements. This is especially true if you're suddenly constipated but never were before. Constipation that comes on rapidly may mean there's an obstruction that's preventing the normal passage of stools.

WHO IS AT RISK?

About 4% of Americans report having fewer than three bowel movements a week. Constipation is most common in the elderly. The intestinal muscles get weaker with age, and older people are more likely to be taking medications that have con-

THE GASTROINTESTINAL PATHWAY

Imagine that you've just chewed and swallowed a bit of food. Here's what happens next:

The esophagus is the first destination. This 10-inch muscular tube carries food from the mouth to the stomach. That's basically all it does. There aren't a lot of disorders that affect the esophagus. The main risk is that the lower portion will get "burned" with stomach acids, which causes heartburn. The esophagus also can develop cancers.

The stomach is the next stop. This organ—approximately 12 inches long, and 6 inches wide—is capable of holding more than a quart of food at a time. It isn't merely a storage depot. It's more like a cement mixer. The stomach pulverizes food, bathes it in acids, and prepares it for the next stage of digestion. Stomach acids are so strong that they can damage the body's tissues—which is precisely what happens when you get an ulcer.

The small intestine receives food from the stomach. This is where most of the nutrients get absorbed. The small intestine is about 21 feet long. The inner surface is densely studded with microvilli—microscopic projections that transport nutrients through the intestinal wall and into the blood. As with the esophagus, the biggest threat to the small intestine is in the high-acid environment nearest the stomach.

The last stop is the large intestine, or colon. By the time food reaches the large intestine it has very little nutritional value. The large intestine—approximately 5 feet long and 2 inches wide—does absorb liquids and minerals, but its main job is to store and consolidate wastes, then expel them from the body as feces. This thick, muscular organ is always contracting and relaxing. Many digestive problems result in intestinal cramps—the internal equivalent of a charley horse.

stipation as a side effect. Among those 65 years and older, 6.8% take laxatives three to ten times weekly.

Constipation is more common among nonwhites, possibly because of dietary factors. Women have a higher risk for constipation than men, although the reason for this isn't clear. People who don't get a lot of fiber or fluids in their diets also have a higher risk for constipation.

HOW IS IT DIAGNOSED?

Constipation can be caused by a variety of medical problems, so your doctor will want to take a complete health history and do a physical exam. He may order laboratory tests to rule out conditions such as diabetes or hypothyroidism. In addition, he may do one or more of the following:

Abdominal exam. The doctor will feels the abdomen to check for the presence of hard stools in the colon and to determine if there's bloating (distension) caused by an accumulation of stools.

Digital exam. The doctor inserts a gloved, lubricated finger into the anus to see if the rectum is full or if there's a "plug" of hardened stool that's interfering with normal bowel movements. He may ask the patient to squeeze the anal (sphincter) muscle to make sure the muscular strength is normal.

Barium enema. This test is used to check for polyps or tumors in the colon. The patient is asked to hold the enema fluid inside the intestine while x-rays are taken. Any abnormalities in the colon will appear on the x-rays as dark silhouettes. The enema is somewhat uncomfortable, but it isn't painful.

Sigmoidoscopy or colonoscopy. These are procedures in which a lighted, flexible tube (a sigmoidoscope or colonoscope) is inserted into the large intestine through the anus. They allow the doctor to examine the inside of the colon for abnormalities that may be hindering the normal passage of stools. Sigmoidoscopy is used to examine the rectum and the lower third of the colon. It can be done without anesthetic. Some patients may experience cramping as the tube moves through the lower colon. Colonoscopy is used to examine the entire length of the colon. The patient is sedated but awake before the procedure begins.

Transit measurements. In unusual cases it may be necessary to measure how rapidly stools move through the colon. The patient swallows a capsule that contains particles that are visible on x-rays. Several days after taking the capsule, the doctor will take x-rays of the colon in order to determine how far the particles have moved. This test helps determine whether the peristaltic activity of the colon is normal.

WHAT SHOULD YOU EXPECT?

Constipation is uncomfortable, but it's rarely serious. The standard treatments include getting more fiber and water in the diet and perhaps the occasional use of laxatives. Once the initial problem is resolved, constipation can usually be prevented by making simple lifestyle changes.

GET MORE FIBER IN YOUR DIET

Fruits and vegetables are excellent sources of dietary fiber. Eat two to four servings of fruits and three to five servings of vegetables a day. If you find it's difficult to eat this much produce with meals, try eating more fruits and vegetables as snacks. For example, cut carrots, celery, and other vegetables into bite-size pieces and keep them in the refrigerator. Stock up on bananas, apples, and other fruits. One avocado, although high in fat, contains almost 7 grams of fiber, nearly 25% of the recommended daily amount. Half a cup of prunes has more than 4 grams of fiber. Artichokes, though very expensive, are very high in fiber, with more than 6 grams per artichoke.

Eat whole grains. They have at least twice as much fiber as refined grains such as white rice or white bread. Whole-grain hot cereals are superb sources of fiber. A serving of cooked oatmeal, for example, has more than 4 grams of fiber. A serving of bulgur (a type of wheat germ) also has more than 4 grams of fiber.

Include bran in your diet. Oat, wheat, and corn bran are exceptionally high in fiber. They aren't particularly appetizing when eaten on their own, but you can add a few tablespoons to other foods, such as cereal, muffins, or biscuits.

Eat high-fiber breakfast cereals. As long as you avoid the sugary brands, breakfast cereals can be an important source of fiber. A serving of raisin bran, for example, may contain more than 7 grams of fiber.

Eat more beans. All legumes, including canned beans, are very high in fiber. Split peas, for example, supply more than 8 grams of fiber per serving. Half a cup of black beans provides more than 6 grams of fiber. Kidney beans are even better, with almost 7 grams in ½ cup.

HOW IS IT TREATED?

In many cases no treatment is necessary. Your doctor may explain that a daily bowel movement isn't essential for health, despite the claims from laxative manufacturers.

Sometimes, however, constipation is a persistent problem. The goals of treatment are twofold: To remove any hardened stools that may have accumulated in the colon, and to help reestablish normal bowel movements.

Your doctor can provide information lifestyle changes and may prescribe a laxative. In addition, he may recommend one or more of the following actions.

Changing medications. Many over-the-counter and prescription drugs may cause constipation. Common offenders include calcium supplements, some antacids, and drugs used to treat depression. Be sure to bring a list of all the medications the patient is taking when you visit the doctor. He may recommend replacing some of the drugs with other, nonconstipating medications.

Finger extraction. This is a procedure in which the doctor uses a gloved finger to break up and remove stools that have accumulated in the rectum, a condition called impaction. If the constipation came on suddenly or there's a "leakage" of diarrhea, there may be impaction. Finger extraction is unpleasant, but not painful. It can be done in the doctor's office and usually takes about five or ten minutes.

LAXATIVES

There are several kinds of laxatives, each of which should be used only under your doctor's supervision. They include:

Stimulant laxatives such as castor oil or bisacodyl (Dulcolax). These irritate the intestinal wall and stimulate the intestinal contractions needed for bowel movements.

Saline laxatives such as milk of magnesia. They draw water into the colon, which promotes a bowel movement.

Stool softeners such as docusate (Colace). These soften the stools so they pass more easily.

The laxatives that are recommended for home use are called bulking laxatives. Their main job is to hold water. Some bulking laxatives, in fact, can hold sixty to one hundred times their weight in water. The extra water makes the stools larger, softer, and easier to pass. The bulking laxatives include:

Concentrated wheat fiber. It comes as a tasteless powder that's about 80% fiber. It's similar to the dietary fiber found in foods and can be taken several times a day.

Psyllium. Available in liquid, granule, and powder forms, psyllium absorbs water and also promotes the growth of helpful bacteria in the colon.

Methylcellulose. Like other bulking laxatives, it holds a tremendous amount of water. Studies have shown that people who use methylcellulose may have an increase in bowel frequency from two to four stools weekly.

Bulking laxatives are relatively safe, but they should still be used only with the approval of your doctor.

Enemas. These may be used to soften and remove hardened stools from the colon. An enema may be given in your doctor's office, but usually he'll give instructions on using them at home. There are several types of enemas. Enemas containing a phosphate solution (such as Fleets) soften stools while at the same time drawing additional water into the colon.

Surgery. This is very rarely necessary except in cases when constipation is caused by a structural abnormality in the colon.

WHAT RESEARCH IS BEING DONE?

Doctors have a good understanding of the underlying causes of constipation. The current treatments—primarily changes in diet and the occasional use of laxatives—are very effective. Researchers hope to learn more details about how the colon works, but the treatment options are unlikely to change for most people.

A possible exception is when constipation is caused by nerve conditions (neuropathies). When the nerves aren't working properly, the colon may not contract with enough force to remove stools from the body. A condition called Hirschsprung's disease, for example, is believed to be caused by a dysfunction of nerve networks in the colon. Doctors suspect that nerve problems may be responsible for some types of constipation where there isn't a known cause. Sometimes overuse of laxatives can damage the nerves of the colon and cause constipation.

HOW IS IT PREVENTED?

Get more fiber. The best preventive strategy for constipation is to increase the amount of fiber and water in your diet. Dietary fiber is simply the tough, structural parts of fruits, vegetables, and other plant foods. It isn't absorbed by the body. Rather, it stays in the intestine and absorbs tremendous amounts of water. This makes stools softer and easier to pass. You may temporarily experience increased gas and bloating when adding additional fiber to your diet; this will decrease as your body adjusts to the dietary change.

Fiber helps in other ways, as well. As it absorbs water it causes the stools to get larger. This triggers the muscular contractions needed to propel them through the colon. Fiber also encourages the proliferation of intestinal bacteria (the flora), which are about 80% water. Studies have shown that when people eat coarse forms of fiber such as bran, the stools move through the colon about 33% faster. The faster transit time means the stools hold onto more moisture, which is important for regularity.

Dietary fiber is only one part of an overall prevention plan. Several other strategies are helpful in preventing constipation.

Drink more water. Drink at least 64 ounces (two quarts) of water a day. It will make the stools softer and easier to pass. It's fine to substitute juices for water, although some juices have hidden calories you may not want. Don't depend on coffee, tea, or caffeinated soft drinks to provide extra fluids. These beverages act as diuretics, which means they remove water from the body.

Exercise. Get at least twenty to thirty minutes of exercise a day. Researchers aren't sure why, but regular exercise appears to help stimulate the intestinal contractions needed for regular bowel movements. Exercise also stimulates thirst, which encourages drinking more water.

Establish regular bowel habits. When you feel the urge to go, go—don't put it off. It's also good to get in the habit of going to the bathroom right after meals, especially after breakfast. That's when the urge to have a bowel movement is often strongest. Allow up to thirty minutes of toilet time. Be sure to avoid excessive straining.

WHAT YOU CAN DO NOW

The fastest solution for constipation is to use a laxative, but it's rarely the best solution. The regular use of laxatives can make the colon "lazy" and less likely to work properly on its own. For those times when quick relief is needed, however, laxatives can be very effective.

Diverticular Disease

Diverticular disease is extremely common. By age 60, nearly half of Americans will have it. Among those 85 and older, the rate is 66%.

SIGNS & SYMPTOMS

- Rectal bleeding
- Severe abdominal cramping
- Fever, nausea, and general weakness

WHAT IS IT?

Diverticular disease is more of an anatomical curiosity than a genuine health problem for most people. For reasons that still aren't clear, the muscular bands that encase the colon sometimes contract simultaneously rather than in the proper alternating rhythm. This allows some of the contents of the colon—a mixture of fluids, gas, and solid wastes—to stay in one place rather than moving downward toward the anus. Over time this material begins pressing against the colon wall, causing it to stretch and bulge. The bulges are called diverticula.

Diverticula can form anywhere in the colon, but are most common in the sigmoid colon just above the rectum. Most diverticula are smaller than a dime. Many are the size of pinheads. It's not uncommon for people to have dozens or even hundreds of diverticula.

About 80% of those with diverticular disease will have no symptoms beyond occasional flatulence or mild abdominal pain. In many cases, in fact, diverticular disease is discovered accidently during an examination for some other unrelated health problem.

In about 20% of cases, however, diverticular disease does cause symptoms. This usually occurs when the diverticula get infected or damaged. You may notice one or more of the following:

Rectal bleeding. This is the most common symptom of diverticular disease. Because the colon contains a lot of blood vessels, the bleeding may be profuse.

Severe abdominal tenderness or cramping. This may occur when a hard piece of stool (a fecalith) abrades a diverticulum, causing inflammation or infection. This condition, called diverticulitis, is much more serious than simple diverticular disease.

Fever, nausea, and overall weakness. The tissue covering the diverticula is thin and fragile. If the tissue ruptures (perforates), bacteria from the colon will escape into the abdominal cavity. This may cause a life-threatening infection called peritonitis.

Once "uncomplicated" diverticular disease makes the transition to diverticulitis, the potential complications are quite serious. These include:

Fistula. This is an abnormal connection between parts of the body that aren't usually connected. When a diverticulum perforates, the damage may spread to the vagina, ureter (the tube leading from the kidneys to the bladder), the skin, or to other diverticula. Tissue in the body may form a "bridge" between the different locations, which will have to be surgically removed. Between 12 and 25% of those with known diverticular disease will develop a fistula at some point.

Obstructions. Tissue damage from diverticulitis can result in the buildup of scar tissue, which may narrow or even block the colon. Obstructions are rare, occurring in about 2% of cases.

Perforation. This is the most serious complication of diverticulitis. It's fairly rare, but the mortality rate is high, ranging from 6.1 to 25.7%. Perforation always requires hospitalization and treatment with antibiotics. In addition, surgery will be needed to remove the region of the colon that has perforated.

WHO IS AT RISK?

The elderly have the highest risk for diverticular disease, although first-time attacks may occur when you're in your 40s or 50s. The risk is much higher in industrialized countries, probably due to low dietary fiber. Genetics also appears to be involved. Studies have shown, for example, that 90% of diverticular disease in Western countries occurs in the sigmoid colon, the portion nearest the rectum. In the East, it's more likely to occur higher in the colon, in the cecum or ascending colon.

HOW IS IT DIAGNOSED?

The first (and sometimes the only) sign of diverticular disease is sometimes rectal bleeding. It's important to call your doctor any time you notice blood in the stools. Since many conditions besides diverticular disease can cause rectal bleeding, your doctor may need to perform a variety of tests to identify the source of the problem.

Abdominal exam. The doctor will press on the left side of the abdomen to check for tenderness. This may be a sign that one or more diverticula are inflamed or infected. In addition, the doctor will check for "rebound" tenderness—pain that occurs after he removes his hand. Rebound tenderness usually means the damage is more widespread, usually because a diverticula has begun to perforate.

Laboratory tests. The doctor will want to check the patient's blood count (the hematocrit). Reduced levels of red blood cells may indicate bleeding. High levels of white blood cells may indicate infection.

Barium enema. This is a procedure that helps define the inside of the colon. You'll be given an enema containing barium, and x-rays will be taken while you hold the fluid inside. Diverticula in the colon will appear on the x-rays as dark silhouettes. The enema is somewhat uncomfortable, but not painful.

Colonoscopy. In this procedure, a flexible lighted tube (a colonoscope) is inserted into the anus. It allows the doctor to view the entire length of the colon. The test isn't as effective as the barium enema for detecting diverticular disease, but it may be necessary to ensure that symptoms aren't caused by polyps (growths) or cancer in the colon. Colonoscopy takes about an hour and can be done in the doctor's office or in the ambulatory suite of a hospital. Patients are lightly sedated before the test.

Ultrasound or CT scans. Each of these tests is used to visualize the colon wall. They will reveal if the colon wall is thickened or inflamed in places. They also detect diverticula or pockets of infection (abscesses).

Angiography. This is a procedure in which a dye is injected into the arteries and viewed with x-rays. Angiography is usually done to help your doctor identify the source of serious rectal bleeding. If the radiologist does discover damaged blood vessels, he can often stop the bleeding during the test.

Radionuclide scanning. This is another x-ray technique for identifying the source of bleeding. a small amount of a radioactive chemical called a "tag" is injected into the patient. The tag emits gamma rays (similar to x-rays), which are detected by a gamma camera and analyzed on a computer. This is a very accurate test, especially when bleeding is too slight to be detected with angiography.

WHAT SHOULD YOU EXPECT?

The prognosis for those with diverticular disease depends on the severity of the symptoms. In the mildest cases, the patient probably won't experience anything worse than intermittent bouts of gas, abdominal discomfort, or changes in bowel habits, possibly followed by years with no symptoms at all. Rectal bleeding caused by diverticular disease usually clears up on its own, although about 25% of people will have a recurrence. Diverticulitis is often the most serious complication. The infection can be treated with antibiotics, but surgery may be needed at the time of the attack of diverticulitis, or later, if it does not resolve with antibiotics.

HOW IS IT TREATED?

As long as diverticular disease is "silent," no treatment is necessary. When there's serious rectal bleeding or infection, however, several treatments are available.

Vasoconstriction. If there is a lot of rectal bleeding, the doctor may inject a drug that causes the damaged blood vessels to shut down (constrict). Another option is to "spray" the area with a gel that seals blood vessels and stops bleeding. (See "Angiography," above.)

Electrocoagulation. This is another technique to stop bleeding. While the patient is undergoing colonoscopy, the doctor may use an electrical probe (a cautery) to seal damaged blood vessels.

Antibiotics. If diverticulitis develops, antibiotics are essential for stopping infection. Minor infections can often be treated with oral antibiotics. For more serious infections, the antibiotics will be given intravenously, usually in the hospital.

Surgery. Surgery may be required when the colon has been severely damaged by diverticulitis or when antibiotics can't control the infection. There are several forms of surgery for diverticular disease. The most common procedure is called "resection and primary anastomosis." The damaged part of the colon is removed ("resected"), then the two healthy ends are reunited. Less often, it may be necessary for the doctor to perform a two-part procedure. The first part involves a temporary colostomy, in which the body's wastes are rerouted into an external bag. This is done in order to give the colon time to heal. After several weeks or months, the colostomy is removed and the colon is reconnected.

Temporary fast. It may be necessary to give up food entirely if symptoms are severe. In this situation, the patient is admitted to the hospital, and given fluids and antibiotics intravenously. This treatment may last for several days up to two weeks, depending on how long it takes the colon to heal.

WHAT RESEARCH IS BEING DONE?

Diverticular disease is a relatively simple condition. Most people won't have serious symptoms, and the current treatments are very effective. As a result, research has focused on managing the more unusual cases, especially those involving perforation and abdominal infection (peritonitis).

A frightening trend in recent years has been the emergence of bacteria that don't respond to antibiotics. Researchers are working hard to develop new drugs that will target antibiotic-resistant organisms.

HOW IS IT PREVENTED?

A great deal of evidence has linked diverticular disease to diets low in fiber. There are several reasons that the fiber in foods is protective. Dietary fiber makes the stools larger and easier to pass. This means that there's less pressure in the colon.

All plant foods—fruits, vegetables, legumes, and whole grains—contain dietary fiber. Doctors recommend getting 25 to 30 g of dietary fiber daily. The best way to get enough fiber in your diet is to follow the advice of nutritionists and eat two to four servings of fruits, three to five servings of vegetables, six to eleven servings of whole grains, and up to two to three servings of beans daily. (See "Get More Fiber in Your Diet" on p. 273.)

Supplemental forms of fiber may be helpful if it's difficult to eat enough fruit, vegetables, and other high-fiber foods. One of the best "bulking agents" is psyllium, available in pharmacies and natural food stores. In addition, wheat, corn, and oat bran are very concentrated sources of fiber.

WHAT YOU CAN DO NOW

Diverticular disease always needs to be managed by a physician. It's essential to call the doctor if there is rectal bleeding, abdominal tenderness, or other symptoms. In addition:

Immediately reduce the amount of fiber in the diet if the patient is experiencing symptoms. Even though dietary fiber helps prevent diverticular disease, it worsen symptoms during flare-ups.

Avoid popcorn, sunflower seeds, or other hard-to-digest foods. They may get lodged in the colon and increase the risk of infection.

Your doctor may recommend a "clear diet" during flare-ups. This means having nothing but liquids, juices, or broth for several days or longer. Going without solid foods will give the colon a chance to heal. Liquid diets must be carefully balanced in order to be healthy, however, so don't do this on your own without talking to your doctor.

SIGNS & SYMPTOMS

- A burning sensation in the upper abdomen (heartburn)
- Discomfort after eating high-fat or large meals
- Frequent belching
- Acidic taste in the mouth

Gastroesophageal Reflux Disease

Nearly everyone gets heartburn occasionally. For about seventeen million Americans, however, it happens almost every day. And it's more serious than most people imagine.

WHAT IS IT?

Heartburn is the main symptom of a condition called gastroesophageal reflux disease (GERD). This is a digestive disorder in which digestive juices, rather than staying in the stomach, flow backward (reflux) into the esophagus.

Digestive juices consist of hydrochloric acid and pepsin. They're highly corrosive. The stomach is insulated with a thick layer of mucus, but the esophagus—a 10-inch muscular tube that carries food to the stomach—isn't similarly protected. The acids literally burn the surface layer of cells (the esophageal epithelium).

In addition to heartburn, GERD may result in frequent belching. The belches may be accompanied by an acidic or sour-tasting fluid in the mouth. Some people may develop hoarseness or have difficulty swallowing. In addition, up to 80% of those with asthma also have GERD. It's believed that some of the refluxed acids are breathed (aspirated) into the airways, causing them to narrow or go into spasm (bronchospasms).

The esophagus is normally protected from stomach acid by a muscular ring of tissue called the lower esophageal sphincter (LES). This muscle is designed to open when you swallow, then snap shut afterward. If you have GERD, the muscle is either weaker than it should be or it relaxes at the wrong times, permitting the upsurge of acids.

Don't ignore heartburn and other symptoms of GERD. Over time the acids may cause chronic inflammation of the esophagus (esophagitis). Scar tissue may form and narrow the esophageal opening. A condition called Barrett's esophagus may also develop. This occurs when the normal cells lining the esophagus are replaced with acid-resistant cells. The risk of esophageal cancer in those with Barrett's esophagus is thirty to one hundred twenty-five times higher than in people without this condition.

GERD can almost always be controlled with lifestyle changes and medications. If you or your loved one are having symptoms frequently, or are using antacids or other medications more than twice a week, it's essential to see your doctor.

WHO IS AT RISK?

More than 36% of Americans suffer from heartburn at least once a month. Heartburn and other symptoms of GERD are most common in the elderly and women during pregnancy. However, men with GERD are two to four times more likely than women to develop Barrett's esophagus.

HOW IS IT DIAGNOSED?

The doctor will probably be able to diagnose GERD just from hearing about the symptoms. For example, heartburn and belching tend to get worse at night and after meals because the "holding power" of the LES is lower at these times. Tight clothes and bending over may increase symptoms. So will eating large meals or high-fat meals.

Rather than ordering expensive tests, the doctor may simply prescribe acid-reducing medications and recommend following antireflux precautions. These may include not eating for several hours before bedtime, elevating the head of the bed, and avoiding caffeine, alcohol, and fatty or spicy foods.

If symptoms clear up within several weeks, nothing needs to be done beyond choosing the right drugs and continuing to follow anti-reflux precautions. If this doesn't help, other tests will probably be needed.

Endoscopy. This test involves inserting a lighted, flexible tube though the mouth and into the esophagus. The doctor examines the esophagus for signs of inflammation or tissue damage. He may take a tissue sample (a biopsy), which will be sent to a laboratory for analysis.

Barium swallow. This is an x-ray procedure that outlines the inside of the esophagus. The patient swallows a chalky solution, then x-rays are taken. Any anatomical abnormalities in the esophagus will show up as silhouettes on the x-ray.

Ambulatory pH monitoring. This test uses a probe to measure the acid level (pH) in the esophagus and the frequency of reflux episodes. The probe is inserted through the nose and into the esophagus, and attached to a small portable monitor. It sounds uncomfortable, but the probe is very thin and the monitor is unobtrusive. The measurements will probably be taken over a twenty-four-hour period to determine if acid levels in the esophagus are unusually high.

Esophageal manometry. This is a test that measures pressure in the esophagus and the sphincter muscle. This test may be done if a motility disorder is suspected as the case of pain. GERD cannot be confirmed by manometry alone.

WHAT SHOULD YOU EXPECT?

Most people with GERD wait one to three years before seeing a doctor. This is unfortunate because the prognosis is excellent for those who receive medical care. When GERD isn't accompanied by tissue damage or inflammation, the success rate of treatment is approximately 80%. Even when inflammation (esophagitis) is present, therapy with acid-reducing medications and behavior modification for changes in lifestyle can significantly relieve the discomfort. Some patients take the medications and make mild changes in their behavior for the rest of their lives.

Studies have shown that heartburn and other symptoms invariably return when people quit using medications and do not comply with the recommendations to modify their behavior.

HOW IS IT TREATED?

The goal of treatment is to prevent stomach acids from damaging the esophagus, to heal damaged mucosa, and to prevent complications. This can be achieved by drug therapy to reduce the amount of acid in the stomach and strengthen LES pressure. Medications alone won't change the course of refluxed acids. Behavior modification is necessary to reduce reflux flow. (See "How Is It Prevented?" below.). Antireflux surgery is sometimes recommended when severe symptoms don't respond to medications and behavior modification.

Over-the-counter and prescription drugs are generally very effective for treating this condition. The doctor will likely recommend one or more of the following medications.

H2-blockers. These are the most frequently prescribed drugs for GERD. Available over the counter and by prescription, H2-blockers such as cimetidine or famotidine and ranitidine inhibit the action of histamine, a natural chemical that controls acid secretion in the stomach. Up to 85% of people who take H2-blockers will get partial or total relief from their symptoms. These drugs are usually recommended when symptoms are mild or moderate.

Proton pump inhibitors. These are the most powerful acid-blocking drugs. They're often recommended for those with esophagitis or for people who don't improve after taking H2-blockers. Prescription drugs such as omeprazole, lansoprazole, and rabeprazole work by blocking the pumping mechanism inside acid-producing cells in the stomach.

Most people with GERD will improve dramatically when they start taking medications and follow anti-reflux precautions. In rare cases, additional treatments may be required. These include:

Mechanical dilation. This procedure may be necessary when acid damage has resulted in an obstruction (stricture) that narrows the esophagus and makes swallowing difficult. A mercury-filled balloon is inserted into the esophagus and then inflated. This helps enlarge (dilate) the esophageal opening.

Fundoplication. This is a surgical procedure that increases the tension in the LES. It involves tightly wrapping a portion of the stomach around the lower section of the esophagus. This technique is successful in about 80% of cases, and it usually requires spending a few days in the hospital. It can usually be done through a laparoscope.

Esophagectomy. This is an extensive surgical procedure that may be necessary for those with advanced Barrett's esophagus, or for those who have already developed cancer of the esophagus. The esophagus is removed entirely and "replaced" by pulling the stomach upward into the chest.

There are several other possible treatments for Barrett's esophagus. These include photodynamic therapy, in which the damaged cells lining the esophagus are coated with a light-sensitive drug and then destroyed; laser therapy, in which the cells are burned away with a laser; and multipolar electrocautery, in which the cells are burned away with an electrical wire.

WHAT RESEARCH IS BEING DONE?

The drugs used for treating GERD aren't ideal because most of them target acid secretion rather than the underlying problem—the weakened "holding power" of the LES. Researchers hope to develop medications that will specifically target the LES without affecting other muscles. In addition, the ideal drugs would more closely mimic the natural constriction-relaxation cycles of the LES.

HOW IS IT PREVENTED?

GERD is almost always a lifelong problem. It can't be prevented, but there are ways to significantly reduce the symptoms by following daily antireflux precautions. These measures may be all that is needed to treat mild cases of GERD. For example:

Elevate the head of the bed at least six inches. Sleeping with the torso slightly upright makes it more difficult for stomach acids to splash into the esophagus.

Avoid certain foods. Chocolate, coffee, onions, peppermint, and fried or fatty foods can temporarily weaken the LES, causing heartburn and other symptoms. Everyone reacts to foods differently, however. You may want to make a note of everything the patient eats for several weeks. This will help identify foods that appear to make the symptoms worse.

Eat smaller meals. Putting a lot of food in the stomach causes acid levels to rise. The closer acids come to the esophageal opening, the more likely they are to cause symptoms. It's better to eat several small meals throughout the day rather than one or two large meals.

Don't eat within three hours of going to bed. Acid levels increase after meals, and lying down after eating causes gravity to work against you.

Quit smoking. Cigarette smoke weakens the LES. Smoking also increases air swallowing, which can induce frequent belching.

Lose weight if necessary. People who are overweight are more likely to have GERD than those who are leaner.

Avoid tight-fitting clothes, such as girdles or tight jeans. They may increase pressure on the LES, especially when you bend over.

WHAT YOU CAN DO NOW

The symptoms of GERD usually come on quickly. One way to get relief is to swallow several times. Saliva neutralizes acids and also helps wash them back into the stomach.

Over-the-counter antacids are often helpful. Medications such as Mylanta, Rolaids, and Maalox contain minerals that neutralize stomach acids. Antacids are very safe, although those containing magnesium may cause diarrhea, and those with aluminum may cause constipation. Your doctor may recommend alternating the different kinds of antacids to minimize side effects.

One thing antacids won't do is heal inflammation in the esophagus. Be sure to talk to your doctor if you or your loved one are depending on antacids for long-term relief. He may recommend taking H2-blockers or other acid-blocking medications on a daily basis, while saving the antacids for short-term relief.

- Change in stool frequency
- Changes in stool consistency
- Changes in how bowel movements feel
- Bowel movements accompanied by clear or white mucus
- A "bloated" feeling

Irritable Bowel Syndrome

Irritable bowel syndrome (IBS) is second only to colds as a cause of lost work days. It's responsible for about three million doctor visits and two billion dollars' worth of medications annually. It's not uncommon for people with IBS to spend hours a day in the bathroom—or to restrict their social activities because they're afraid of losing control.

WHAT IS IT?

Despite its profound impact, doctors aren't even sure if IBS is a "real" disease. No one knows what causes it. The symptoms can't be explained by medical tests. As a result, doctors classify IBS as a "functional disorder"—a constellation of symptoms without a known cause.

For a long time doctors thought that IBS was caused by stress, which is why it went by such inaccurate names as "nervous colon" or "spastic colitis." Emotional stress undeniably plays a role in IBS, but it doesn't cause it.

Here's what is known. People with IBS appear to have unusual contractions (peristalsis) in the colon. The colon normally contracts six to eight times in a twenty-four-hour period. But it behaves differently in people with IBS, depending on their symptoms. In those who mainly have constipation, there may be few or no contractions in a day. For those with diarrhea, there may be twenty-five contractions a day.

It's not known whether these contractions play a direct role in causing IBS. It's possible that people with IBS simply have a lower threshold for intestinal pressure. Contractions that would normally go unnoticed might be painful for those with IBS.

For women with IBS, the symptoms tend to flare at the beginning of the menstrual cycle, which suggests that hormones may be involved. Research has shown that two chemicals (prostaglandin E2 and F2) are elevated during the first day of menstruation. It's possible that some cases of IBS are linked to these chemicals.

WHO IS AT RISK?

IBS occurs three times as often in women as in men. The onset of IBS usually occurs in late adolescence or early adulthood; it rarely makes its first appearance after age 50. There's some evidence that the risk of IBS is higher in those with a history of depression or panic or anxiety disorders. Doctors aren't sure, however, if people with these psychological issues actually have more IBS, or if they're simply more likely to report symptoms to their doctors.

HOW IS IT DIAGNOSED?

SYMPTOMS

The symptoms of IBS vary widely from person to person, but nearly everyone with this condition will have frequent abdominal pain, a bloated feeling, flatulence, and diarrhea or constipation—or alternating cycles of diarrhea and constipation.

When you see your doctor, he'll ask a lot of questions about your bowel habits. A frequent feature of IBS is abdominal pain or discomfort that's relieved when you have a bowel movement.

In addition, the diagnosis of IBS requires that you have two or more of the following symptoms about 25% of the time:

Altered stool frequency. This means that the frequency of your bowel movements has either increased (three or more bowel movements a day) or decreased (fewer than three a week).

Changes in stool consistency. The stools might be lumpy and hard, or loose and watery.

Changes in how bowel movements feel. Perhaps you've begun straining to have bowel movements. Or you could be having a sense of urgency before bowel movements. Many people with IBS feel like their bowel movements aren't "complete."

Bowel movements are accompanied by clear or white mucus.

A feeling of bloating or abdominal distension.

TESTS

Because there aren't specific medical tests for IBS, it's often called a "disease of exclusion." This means that your doctor will have to make sure that the symptoms aren't caused by something else. He'll probably recommend one or more of the following tests.

Lactose-free diet. The symptoms of IBS are very similar to symptoms caused by an unrelated condition called lactose intolerance. Many Americans don't produce enough of an enzyme (lactase) that's needed to digest a sugar (lactose) found in milk, cheese, and other dairy foods. Eating these foods may cause diarrhea, cramping, and other types of digestive discomfort. Before doing any other tests, the doctor may recommend a lactose-free diet for several weeks. If symptoms don't improve, other tests will be scheduled.

Abdominal exam. The doctor will check for tenderness over the area of the sigmoid colon, to the left and below the belly button. People with IBS are often tender in this area.

Sigmoidoscopy or colonoscopy. This is a procedure in which a lighted, flexible tube (a sigmoidoscope) is inserted into the anus. It allows the doctor to examine the lower third of the colon (sigmoidoscopy) or the entire colon (colonoscopy) for abnormalities, such as an unusual narrowing (a stricture), ulcers, areas of inflammation, or tumors.

Most people will experience only mild discomfort during sigmoidoscopy or colonoscopy. For those with IBS, however, the procedure may trigger painful spasms. Regardless of what the test reveals, excessive discomfort during the procedure may be a sign of IBS.

Barium enema. The patient is instructed to hold the enema fluid inside the intestine while x-rays are taken. Any abnormalities in the colon will appear on the x-rays as dark silhouettes. This procedure also allows the doctor to see if there are unusual intestinal contractions, especially in a part of the colon called the descending colon.

Depending on the symptoms, the doctor may need to examine the inside of the esophagus, stomach, and a portion of the small intestine (upper endoscopy), or he may suggest barium x-rays of the small intestine (a small bowel series). In addition, he may order a variety of lab tests, including blood tests, to determine if there's bleeding, inflammation, or infection in the intestine.

WHAT SHOULD YOU EXPECT?

People with IBS typically experience intermittent symptoms for years or even decades. However, IBS tends to "burn out" over time. It's relatively rare in those 50 years and older. The symptoms can be significantly reduced with a combination of diet, lifestyle changes, and medication.

HOW IS IT TREATED?

The symptoms of IBS vary widely. Treatments that work for one person may not work for another. Many of the treatments for IBS, including dietary changes and stress reduction, can be done at home. In addition, a number of prescription medications can significantly reduce the symptoms.

Anticholinergic drugs. Also called antispasmodics, these prescription medications help prevent a chemical in the body (acetylcholine) from stimulating the smooth muscles of the intestine. A drug called dicyclomine, for example, works very quickly. It can be taken at the onset of pain or just before meals as a preventive measure. Another drug, hyoscyamine, can be taken under the tongue (sublingually) for very fast relief. These drugs are mainly used to relieve abdominal cramps, although they may reduce bloating (distension) in some people.

Antidepressants. These medications can help relieve IBS symptoms even in those who aren't depressed. Antidepressants help in a variety of ways. Some medications (tricyclic antidepressants) help reduce painful contractions in the colon. Other drugs (serotonin reuptake inhibitors) increase brain levels of a chemical called serotonin, which has calming effects and indirectly reduces pain. People with IBS are often very sensitive to the side effects of antidepressants. One new drug that targets serotonin receptors is tegaserod (Zelmac) for constipation-predominant IBS. Your doctor may have to try several drugs to find the one that works best for your or your loved one.

Prokinetic drugs. Also called promotility drugs, these medications reduce the activity (motility) of the colon. There's some evidence that they can help reduce cramps and bloating and also promote normal bowel movements. These medications haven't been well studied for IBS, however, so they probably won't be your doctor's first choice.

Narcotics. Sedating medications such as loperamide and diphenoxylate help control diarrhea and also reduce painful contractions in the colon. Because of the risk of addiction, however, these drugs are rarely used for IBS.

WHAT RESEARCH IS BEING DONE?

IBS has caused untold frustration for patients as well as doctors. The symptoms are well known, but no one's been able to find a physical mechanism to explain them. In recent years, however, researchers have finally identified some potential physical causes.

Studies have shown, for example, that people with IBS may have colonic activity that's more "disorganized" and forceful than those without this condition. In addition, people with IBS appear to have a lower pain threshold in response to pressure in the colon.

The next step for researchers is to identify the mechanisms in the colon (or elsewhere in the body) that trigger this increased sensitivity. At that point it may be possible to design drugs or other treatments that will help raise the pain threshold to normal levels.

HOW IS IT PREVENTED?

Until doctors have a better understanding of what causes IBS, prevention will remain elusive. There's some evidence, however, that lifestyle factors such as reducing emotional stress and eating a healthy diet may be helpful for some people.

WHAT YOU CAN DO NOW

IBS is a long-term problem, and everyone controls the discomfort in different ways. Here are a few strategies that may help:

Keep a "food diary" to help you identify foods that make symptoms worse. Doctors aren't sure why, but foods that are high in fat often aggravate IBS. Beans and other foods that cause gas may also be a problem. Caffeine, alcohol, and some dairy producs can often aggravate IBS, as can the artificial sweetner Sorbitol, found in many sugar-free items.

Get more fiber into the diet. Fiber makes stools larger and softer, so the colon doesn't have to contract as hard to move them along. Fiber also helps relieve diarrhea and constipation, two of the most common symptoms of IBS. The doctor may recommend getting up to 30 grams of fiber a day in the form of fruits, vegetables, and whole grains. (See "Get More Fiber in Your Diet" on p. 273.)

It's normal to have an increase in gas when first adding more fiber to the diet. The discomfort can be minimized, though, by adding fiber gradually over a period of weeks or months. In addition, use a fiber supplement containing psyllium. It tends to produce less gas than other forms of fiber. Remember to drink plenty of water (two quarts per day) when adding fiber to help equalize the pressure inside the colon, add moisture to stools, and decrease the need to strain during defecation.

Fiber doesn't work for everyone. Between 15 and 25% of those with IBS will feel worse when they eat more fiber. The best advice is to increase fiber intake over several weeks and see if symptoms improve. If they don't, talk to your doctor about other dietary options.

Reduce stress. Even though emotional stress doesn't cause IBS, it invariably makes the symptoms worse. Try breathing exercises or techniques such as meditation or biofeedback. In addition, getting regular exercise has been shown to help reduce stress. It doesn't have to be vigorous exercise. Taking a walk around the block once or twice a day may be enough.

Talk to a therapist. There's some evidence that psychotherapy may be helpful for those with IBS, including people who haven't responded to medical treatments.

In one study, people with IBS were divided into two groups. Those in one group received the standard medical treatments only. Those in the second group received medical treatments along with psychotherapy and relaxation therapy. The people in the psychotherapy group had a significant reduction in discomfort. They also had less stress and took less time off from work than those in the medicine-only group.

| SIGNS & SYMPTOMS

- Gnawing or burning in the abdomen between the belly button and the breastbone
- Pain that worsens at night or between meals
- Nausea
- Weight loss
- Blood in the stools

Ulcers

The stomach contains the harshest environment in the digestive tract. It has an acid level (pH) of 2, which is similar to the pH of battery acid. Stomach acids are so corrosive, in fact, that they would digest the stomach itself if it weren't coated with a protective layer of mucus and cells (the mucosa).

In millions of Americans, however, the mucosal layer weakens or breaks down. This allows digestive juices to come into contact with the unprotected tissues underneath. This can result in peptic ulcers, small sores that form in the lining of the stomach or the duodenum (the part of the small intestine nearest the stomach).

WHAT IS IT?

Most ulcers are smaller than a pencil eraser. But because the sores are constantly bathed in acids, they're painful and slow to heal. Most people with ulcers will experience a gnawing or burning pain in the area between the belly button and the breastbone. The pain tends to flare at night or between meals. Other symptoms may include nausea, unexplained weight loss, or blood in the stools.

Most ulcers only damage the superficial layers of tissue. In some cases, however, an ulcer may break through (perforate) the outer wall of the stomach or duodenum. This allows intestinal bacteria to pour into the abdominal cavity. The result may be a life-threatening infection called peritonitis.

As recently as the 1980s, experts believed that most ulcers were caused by stress. Emotional stress does raise acid levels and may contribute to ulcers, but it doesn't cause them.

Most ulcers are caused by one of two things: a bacterium called *Helicobacter pylori* (or *H. pylori*) or the regular use of aspirin, ibuprofen, or other nonsteroidal anti-inflammatory drugs (NSAIDs). A third type of ulcer, called a stress ulcer, is common in those who have had a serious illness or have undergone extensive surgery. Stress ulcers are potentially serious, but they usually resolve on their own or with medical treatment.

H. pylori and NSAIDs cause ulcers in very different ways, so it's worth taking a separate look at each one.

ULCERS FROM *H. PYLORI*

Most ulcers occur in the duodenum (duodenal ulcers), and about 80% of these have been linked to infection with *H. pylori*. Worldwide, this is the most common gastrointestinal infection. It causes inflammation and weakens the mucosal lining. It also appears to cause a slight increase in acid secretions and a reduction in acid-neutralizing compounds such as bicarbonate.

There are still some unanswered questions about *H. pylori*. Most people with ulcers are infected with the organism. But millions of people without ulcers are also infected. Only about 10 to 20% of those infected with *H. pylori* develop an ulcer. It may be that certain subtypes of *H. pylori* are more likely to cause ulcers than others. It's also possible that it takes a combination of factors—for example, exposure to the bacterium plus a genetic tendency—for ulcers to form.

H. pylori thrives in parts of the world where there's overcrowding and poor sanitation. In the United States, the rate of infection has been declining by about 25% every ten years. This may be partly due to the widespread use of antibiotics in children. The drugs used to treat ear infections, for example, may do "double duty" by killing ulcer-causing bacteria.

ULCERS FROM NSAIDS

The second leading cause of ulcers is the use of aspirin and other NSAIDs. People who use these medications regularly are ten to twenty times more likely to get ulcers than those who don't use them.

Unlike the ulcers caused by *H. pylori*, which generally occur in the duodenum, ulcers caused by NSAIDs are more likely to form in the stomach (gastric ulcers). Gastric ulcers tend to be the most serious. Studies have shown, for example, that people who take 1000 mg (about three regular tablets) of aspirin daily are nine to ten times more likely to be hospitalized for ulcers than those who don't use the drugs.

NSAIDs stop pain and inflammation by disrupting the body's production of hormone-like substances called prostaglandins. But there's an unfortunate side effect. The body uses prostaglandins to maintain the stomach's protective lining. When prostaglandin levels drop, the risk for ulcers rises.

WHO IS AT RISK?

About 4 million Americans have ulcers, and approximately three hundred and fifty thousand new cases are diagnosed each year. Ulcers are twice as common in Hispanics and African Americans as they are among whites. Overall, about 12% of American men and 9% of American women will get an ulcer at some point in their lives.

Duodenal ulcers are four times more common than gastric ulcers. The risk for duodenal ulcers peaks between the ages of 22 and 55. The risk for gastric ulcers is highest between the ages of 40 and 70. People in this age group are more likely to be taking NSAIDs regularly, often for relieving arthritis or other inflammatory conditions.

Your risk for getting an ulcer is higher if you have a close relative who also has them. Smoking and drinking alcohol also increase the risk of getting an ulcer.

HOW IS IT DIAGNOSED?

If a patient has never had an ulcer before and is in good health generally, the doctor may decide it's not worth doing tests. Rather, he'll initiate a treatment plan without making a firm diagnosis.

The doctor will likely prescribe acid-reducing drugs for several weeks. If the ulcer symptoms disappear, no further testing may be needed. If the symptoms don't get better—or if the patient improves initially but gets another ulcer later— then additional tests will be needed. These may include some of the following:

Blood test. The doctor will take a blood sample and send it to a laboratory for analysis. The presence of *H. pylori* antibodies indicates infection with the bacterium.

Breath test. This is another test for *H. pylori*. The patient exhales into a plastic bag. *H. pylori* produces large amounts of a substance called urease, which can be detected in the breath sample.

Endoscopy. This test allows the doctor to look at the inside of the stomach and duodenum. He'll insert a flexible, lighted tube (an endoscope) through the mouth and down into the stomach and duodenum. If he sees an ulcer, he may take a tissue sample (biopsy), which will be analyzed in a laboratory. Endoscopy is mainly used when symptoms are severe or to rule out other conditions such as stomach cancer. Patients are lightly sedated before having the test, and the throat is numbed with a topical anesthetic.

Upper GI series. Also called a barium swallow, this is an x-ray test that outlines the structure of the stomach and small intestine. The liquid will pool inside the ulcer craters, making them easier to detect. The upper GI series is also used to detect structural abnormalities such as a unusual narrowing (a stricture) or a tumor in the intestine.

WHAT SHOULD YOU EXPECT?

As recently as twenty years ago, long-term cures for ulcers were rare. People who got one ulcer invariably had recurrences. Today, cures are commonplace. Even when a cure isn't possible, medications are very effective at reducing or even eliminating symptoms.

The treatments for gastric ulcers, however, have remained problematic. These ulcers usually occur in people who are taking NSAIDs for arthritis or other long-term conditions. Giving up the medications allows the ulcers to heal, but at the expense of more pain from the "original" condition.

An exciting new breakthrough has been the development of drugs called COX-2 inhibitors. These medications are just as effective as older NSAIDs for relieving pain and inflammation, but they appear to be less likely to damage the stomach's protective lining.

HOW IS IT TREATED?

There are many potential treatments for ulcers. This makes it possible for the doctor to tailor the therapy to the patient's symptoms and circumstances. Below are the main treatments used today.

H2-receptor antagonists. Also called H2-blockers, these medications reduce the amount of acid in the stomach and duodenum. They work by inhibiting the action of a chemical (histamine) that controls acid secretion. The H2-blockers may be used for all types of ulcers, including those caused by *H. pylori*. They relieve discomfort and help ulcers heal more quickly. Taking these drugs for several weeks may be the only therapy needed. They rarely cause side effects, so they're also safe for long-term use.

Proton pump inhibitors. Like the H2-blockers, these drugs reduce the amount of acid secreted in the stomach. They're the most effective acid-blocking (antisecretory) drugs available. Because of their high cost, however, they're usually recommended only when symptoms are severe or when H2-blockers aren't effective.

Synthetic prostaglandins. A prescription drug called misoprostol is commonly recommended for those with gastric ulcers. It helps maintain the stomach's protective lining by "replacing" prostaglandins in the body. Misoprostol is usually used in combination with acid-blocking medications.

Antibiotic therapy. This is the treatment of choice for infection with *H. pylori*. The doctor will prescribe a "cocktail" that consists of several antibiotics along with bismuth subsalicylate, the active ingredient in Pepto-Bismol. Doctors hope to develop a single drug that will eradicate *H. pylori*. The current treatment includes taking one or more antibiotics; a common combination is clarithromycin and an antiacid medication such as omeprazole. The medications are usually taken for fourteen days. Treatment with antibiotics will often eliminate the bacterium (and the ulcer) for good.

Because most ulcers are caused by *H. pylori*, the doctor may recommend antibiotics even if the patient hasn't been tested for the bacterium. In fact, patients may be given antibiotics even if they test negative. The current tests for *H. pylori* have a high rate of "false negatives." That is, they may fail to detect the bacterium even when it's present.

Reducing NSAID use. This is essential when stomach ulcers are caused by one or more of these medications. Once the drugs are discontinued, most ulcers heal fairly quickly. But giving up NSAIDs doesn't mean giving up pain relief. It's often possible to get the same results with safer medications. Acetaminophen, for example, doesn't damage the stomach mucosa, but is just as effective as NSAIDs at relieving pain that's caused by noninflammatory conditions. In addition, the doctor may recommend one of the COX-2 inhibitors such as celecoxib (Celebrex) or rofecoxib (Vioxx). These are NSAIDs that reduce pain and inflammation without apparently increasing the risk for ulcers.

Surgery. The standard medical treatments for ulcers are so effective that surgery is rarely needed. However, should an ulcer perforate the stomach or intestinal wall, the damaged area may need to be "patched" with tissue taken from another part of the intestine. For bleeding ulcers, it may be necessary to seal the damaged blood vessels. When acid levels can't be controlled in any other way, it may be necessary to cut the nerves that trigger the release of stomach acids.

WHAT RESEARCH IS BEING DONE?

The *H. pylori* bacterium is so prevalent that researchers have begun to investigate therapies that don't involve antibiotics. Studies are currently being conducted to develop a vaccine, which could prevent infections before ulcers have a chance to develop.

This research is especially important because *H. pylori* is rapidly becoming resistant to antibiotics. An effective vaccine would circumvent this problem, as well as the side effects that may occur with antibiotic therapy.

HOW IS IT PREVENTED?

Because the majority of ulcers are caused by infection, the preventive strategies are limited. However, several lifestyle factors have been found to make a difference.

Use "enteric-coated" aspirin. It dissolves in the intestine rather than in the stomach. A small chance exists that ulcers may develop in the duodenum rather than in the stomach if the patient is taking enteric-coated aspirin. Always take aspirin or other NSAIDs with meals.

Try acetaminophen instead of aspirin or other NSAIDs.

Always take the lowest possible dose to relieve symptoms.

Try to quit smoking cigarettes. Smoking slows the healing time of ulcers and also increases the risk of recurrences.

Drink alcohol in moderation. Alcohol may increase ulcer symptoms and it also slows the time it takes them to heal.

Don't take potassium or iron substances without talking to the doctor. Both of these minerals may irritate the stomach and increase the risk of ulcers.

WHAT YOU CAN DO NOW

Doctors have a saying about ulcers: "No acid, no ulcer." Reducing the amount (or the concentration) of acid in the stomach is the fastest way to relieve discomfort and help the ulcer heal. Ulcers are potentially serious, so it's essential to talk to the doctor as soon as you notice symptoms. In the meantime, here are a few ways to minimize the discomfort:

Eat something. Ulcer symptoms generally flare at night or between meals when the stomach is empty. Eat small, frequent meals and don't skip meals. Having something to eat right away—crackers, a slice of bread, or a piece of fruit—will help buffer the acid and reduce the intensity of the "burn."

Avoid caffeine. Coffee, tea, and soft drinks with caffeine temporarily increase levels of stomach acid.

Avoid alcohol, another stomach irritant.

Take an antacid or H2-blocker, especially at bedtime. Both are very effective. Antacids help neutralize acid that's already in the stomach. They're a good choice for fast relief. H2-blockers reduce the output of acid-secreting cells in the stomach. They're good for long-term protection, but won't provide quick relief once a flare-up has started.

Don't drink milk to soothe an ulcer. This traditional home "remedy" for ulcers can actually make them worse. Milk increases levels of stomach acid.

ADDITIONAL RESOURCES

WEB SITES

National Institute of Diabetes and Digestive and Kidney Diseases

www.niddk.nih.gov

Hearing Disorders in Older Adults

earing impairment is the most common chronic disability in North America. More than 28 million Americans—about 10% of the population—suffer from some type of hearing difficulty, and older persons are more likely to have problems than any other group. By age 70, about 60% of all people have lost enough hearing to be candidates for hearing aids.

The debilitating effects of hearing loss are not visible to others as is the case with many health problems, but hearing impairment nonetheless exacts a high toll. Hearing loss can lead to isolation, social embarrassment and depression, and create a communicatively less active lifestyle in advanced age. Some research has shown that people with hearing loss are more likely to suffer from diminished function and memory failure. All told, treatment, education programs and lost productivity from hearing disorders cost the nation about $56 billion each year.

The good news about hearing loss is that it is usually treatable. Most people with hearing impairment can benefit from hearing aids or other approaches. Indeed, rehabilitation through hearing aids, assistive devices and surgeries has shown great advances in the past ten years, and can provide immense improvements in quality of life. People can prevent further hearing loss with a combination of treatment and lifestyle changes designed to reduce everyday noise. Caregivers can play a dual role in caring for the elderly with hearing impairment. Caregivers can encourage their hearing-impaired loved ones to experiment with treatments and hearing devices, so that they can remain socially engaged and maintain their independence. And caregivers themselves can learn a number of techniques to ensure greater communication and engagement with the elderly.

WHAT IS IT?

HOW WE HEAR NORMALLY

The hearing pathway is composed of the external, middle, and inner ear, which are connected to the center of hearing within the brain by a hearing nerve. The external ear consists of the pinna, or auricle, and the external auditory canal directs sound to the tympanic membrane or drum.

Sound perception is the end result of a series of events that begins within the outer ear and external auditory canal. Although these structures are passive in the human, together they intensify sound and help direct it from the environment to the eardrum. Small bones (ossicles) in the inner ear work together to transmit the vibratory energy to the inner ear. This is accomplished by the vibrating motion of the middle-ear bones that create a fluid wave within the fluid-filled compartments of the cochlea.

The cochlea is lined by the basilar membrane, on which sits the delicate organ of Corti that houses the specialized transducers of sound: the hair cells. Sounds that enter the ear cause vibrations in a series of bones that connect with the

THE PATH TO HEARING LOSS

Dozens of underlying causes can lead to hearing loss. Medications, childhood illnesses, noise exposure, and structural problems in the ear all can play a role. Hearing disorders are generally divided into two broad categories, depending on where the damage or dysfunction occurs in the ear.

Sensorineural hearing loss. This is caused by damage to the structures of the inner ear, namely the cochlea; the auditory nerve, which sends impulses to the brain for interpretation; or the brain itself. Most hearing losses that occur at birth and are acquired in adulthood are sensorineural.

Conductive hearing loss. The conduction of sound waves from the outer ear to the inner ear is damaged somehow. This could be due to a buildup of earwax, a torn eardrum, fluid in the ear, malfunction of the sound-transmitting bones of the middle ear, or tumors in the auditory canal. Most hearing losses that occur in childhood are conductive in nature.

cochlea. When the cochlea receives the vibrations, the fluids stimulate the hair cells. Each ear contains approximately sixteen thousand hair cells. Movement of tufts of hairs on the top of these cells stimulate trains of neuroelectric impulses in the hearing nerve, relaying information contained in the sounds of speech and the environment to the brain.

COMMON HEARING DISORDERS AMONG THE ELDERLY

Presbycusis. Also called age-related hearing loss, presbycusis is the most prevalent hearing problem facing older adults, and is one of the most common disorders of general health overall. It occurs gradually as people age, and usually affects both ears to roughly the same degree.

Presbycusis arises from damage to specialized transducer cells within the cochlear portion of the inner ear. Over the course of years, the number of hair cells on the Corti diminishes and people begin to suffer partial hearing loss, typically beginning with the higher pitches, thus reducing the ability to appreciate consonant speech sounds. Though this is a process linked to normal aging, it is often accentuated by prior exposure to loud and constant noise. A number of health conditions, including high blood pressure, diabetes, and circulatory or vascular diseases can cause the hearing levels to worsen as well. In some instances, long-term use of medications—including aspirin, diuretics, antibiotics, and chemotherapeutic agents—can worsen a hearing loss.

Structures of the middle ear can play a role in conductive hearing loss. These include the three small bones that make up the ossicular chain: the malleus (hammer), incus (anvil), and stapes (stirrup). When the mobility of the chain of middle ear bones is reduced by a buildup of abnormal bone, a conductive hearing loss results. This is called otosclerosis, which also occurs in the elderly population.

In most cases of presbycusis, the symptoms are similar. For example, presbycusis usually begins by affecting a man's ability to hear higher-frequency female voices. Human speech usually occurs within a range of 500 to 4000 Hertz (Hz) (cycles per second), which is a measure of how fast sound waves are being generated. People with presbycusis usually lose the ability to hear sounds above 1000 Hz, which includes the sounds made by pronouncing consonants like S, F, and combination sounds like "th." This often leads to complaints from an elderly person that other people's speech sounds mumbled or slurred, as speech signals lose their distinguishing characteristics and the ability to discriminate speech sounds is diminished. Conversations are more difficult to follow when background noise is present, be it other speech, music, or sound reverberations. Women's voices, which usually have higher frequencies, are more difficult to hear than men's. Music may become less enjoyable because some notes or instruments are too high to hear. On the other hand, certain sounds can be annoying or excessively loud to a person with presbycusis. Finally, there may be phantom sounds, or tinnitus, that produces a ringing or hissing sound in the ears.

Because presbycusis comes on gradually, people often don't notice the symptoms for years. Most people only seek help when everyday conversations become difficult to follow.

Tinnitus. This term comes from the Latin word *tinnire*, which means to ring or tinkle. It is the sensation of sound perceived in the head or ears without any apparent external stimulus. Most commonly, it manifests as a ringing in the ears.

Tinnitus is a widespread problem. Nearly everyone has experienced the condition occasionally, although it is usually short-lived and little more than a minor nuisance. About 50 million Americans face the problem on a frequent basis, and many have chronic, persistent tinnitus, defined as lasting more than three months with no sign of resolving. Many problems can trigger tinnitus. An accumulation of earwax in the outer ear canal is a frequent culprit. In the middle ear, a perforated eardrum or fluid accumulation can cause tinnitus. Infections, allergic reactions, or injury to the delicate bones of the middle ear also can be to blame. In many of these cases, correction of the underlying problem can remedy the tinnitus. Certain medications have been linked to tinnitus, notably aspirin and similar drugs, and a few antibiotics. Discontinuing these drugs usually resolves the tinnitus.

When the tinnitus is centered in the inner ear, it is more difficult to address. The disorder often accompanies presbycusis, noise-induced hearing loss, Ménière's disease, and other inner-ear conditions. In these cases, although little can be done to cure the tinnitus, there are options for managing the severity of the symptom. For some, tinnitus also appears to have a strong psychological connection. Many people suffering from stress, depression, or other emotional difficulties find it difficult to cope with the condition. Treatment of the psychological aspects of one's difficulties may be extremely helpful.

Many people learn to tolerate chronic tinnitus, adjusting to the noise level and maintaining a good quality of life. Others, however, require counseling and training to lower the impact on their lifestyle. In some cases, devices that help mask the tinnitus prove effective in treating the condition. It's important for patients to understand that tinnitus does not cause hearing loss and will not shorten one's life.

NOISE-INDUCED HEARING LOSS

This form of sensorineural hearing loss affects people of all ages. It is caused by excessive exposure to loud noises—machines, police sirens, amplified music, firearms, power tools, and even toys. It's the leading cause of hearing impairment in younger Americans, and often deepens the hearing loss of older adults.

Noise-induced hearing loss follows a path similar to the sensorineural hearing loss of presbycusis. The noise can overwhelm structures in the inner ear, especially the hair cells that make up the Corti inside the cochlea. These become brittle and damaged and are rendered inoperable in transmitting impulses to the brain. In effect, noise causes hearing loss due to wear and tear of the inner ear. Although most older people are already losing hearing due to presbycusis, excess noise can speed up the process; presbycusis does not protect one from the damaging effects of noise.

Like presbycusis, noise-induced hearing loss first affects a person's ability to hear higher-frequency sounds. Over time, the hearing impairment can spread to mid-tone and lower frequencies, causing more profound and complete hearing loss. Experts have discovered that prolonged or repeated exposure to noise over 90 decibels can cause gradual hearing loss; this is the equivalent of the noise from a lawnmower or motorcycle engine. A typical conversation is held at a 60-decibel level; guns, firecrackers, and most power tools operate at more than 100 decibels. Hearing loss can occur after as little as fifteen minutes of exposure to 100-decibel noise. A single exposure to extremely loud noise can cause immediate and permanent hearing loss.

WHO IS AT RISK?

Age is the biggest risk factor for hearing disorders among the elderly. The prevalence and severity of presbycusis grows with increasing age. This is also true of tinnitus; people over the age of 50 are twice as likely to develop the condition as those who are younger. Several other risk factors can lead to early hearing loss.

Smoking. A recent study of 3753 people found that smokers are about 70% more likely to suffer from hearing loss than nonsmokers. Nonsmokers who were exposed to secondhand smoke also seem to be at increased risk

Family history. This connection has been controversial. But data from the famous Framingham Heart Study and a follow-up study of the study subjects' offspring has found a significant link. The likelihood of developing presbycusis appears to be higher in the children of those who also have the disease. The link appears to be much stronger for females than males.

Use of certain medications. Sensorineural hearing loss and tinnitus have been linked to the use of aspirin and other salicylates and, rarely, to ibuprofen and other nonsteroidal antiinflammatory drugs (NSAIDs). Antibiotics that contain chemical compounds known as aminoglycosides also may cause hearing impairment. These include gentamicin, tobramycin, streptomycin, and others that are typically given intravenously, in a hospital setting. Quinine, prescribed as an antimalarial drug, can cause hearing damage if used at high doses over a long period of time. Some loop diuretics such as furosemide (Lasix) also can cause tinnitus, especially if large doses are administered intravenously too rapidly. Other drugs that may occasionally cause hearing problems include cisplatin and intravenous erythromycin. Drug-induced tinnitus and hearing loss are often only reversible by discontinuing the medication if the medication has been taken by mouth.

Underlying disease. People with diabetes tend to have a higher than normal occurrence of hearing loss, as do those with high blood pressure, atherosclerosis, and other circulatory disorders, and people with neurological diseases, including multiple sclerosis, stroke, Parkinson's disease and Alzheimer's disease

HOW IS IT DIAGNOSED?

PHYSICAL EXAM

When a person begins to complain hearing impairment or hearing loss, the first stop is usually the primary care physician. The doctor may be able to discover the underlying cause if it is readily apparent, such as earwax blockage in the ear canal. The visit generally begins with a simple interview, to define the type and severity of the symptoms and discover possible underlying causes. Typically, the doctor will want the patient to describe the hearing loss (*Is there a ringing sensation in one or both ears? Do you feel any pain in the ears? What kind of medications are you taking, and how large is the dosage?*)

This question-and-answer session usually is followed by an examination with an otoscope, a simple, hand-held device that includes a magnifying lens and a light. The doctor uses the otoscope to look inside the auditory canal. A cone-shaped plastic piece, called the speculum, slips into the ear and focuses the light beam. The doctor will move the speculum gently in all directions to examine the entire visible area. The procedure usually is painless, although the patient may feel some discomfort if the ear is infected.

Otoscopic examination can reveal a number of potential problems. Earwax can build up on the walls of the canal or against the eardrum, blocking sounds before the middle and inner ear have a chance to detect them. The eardrum may be discolored; while it's usually off-white or light gray, a reddish or yellow tint may indicate infection. Small bubbles may be visible behind the eardrum, a sign of fluid buildup in the middle ear. Perforations in the eardrum may be detectable. The auditory canal itself may have fluid in it, or the walls of the canal may show signs of infection. In rare cases, an unusual growth in the canal may block sound transmission.

The general physician also may conduct an informal hearing examination to check for the degree of hearing impairment. These tests may include using a tuning fork to check whether a person can hear the vibrations. The fork is struck and placed near one ear at a time, and is sometimes placed against the base of the skull. This helps determine whether the hearing loss is caused by conductive loss in the outer ear, or by problems in the middle or inner ear. The doctor also may ask the patient to listen as he whispers in one ear or places a ticking watch near the ear.

HEARING TESTS

If the doctor is able to identify and treat the underlying cause of hearing impairment, no further diagnosis may be necessary. But if he is unable to find a cause, or has additional questions or concerns, the doctor may refer the patient to an ear specialist. These include otolaryngologists, also known as ear, nose, and throat doctors, or otologists, who specialize in diseases of the ear and skull base. These doctors will conduct a more thorough examination, and could order additional tests, including blood work, x-rays and even computer-assisted tomography (CAT) scans or similar procedures to check for structural problems or growths that may be affecting hearing. An electroencephalogram (EEG) test may also be performed to test the brain's response to sound stimuli. This can help pinpoint causes of hearing loss that initiate in the brain.

The most common tests are usually performed by a trained hearing care provider known as an audiologist. The audiologist is usually asked to measure the extent of hearing impairment and search for possible causes in the inner and middle ear.

Audiogram. The main test for hearing is called an audiogram. It's a common procedure that's often used to screen for hearing loss in school children, and is frequently indicated for older persons as well. The patient sits in a chair and wears a pair of headphones. The headphones deliver a precise series of pure tones at various volumes and frequencies. The tests include sounds in the normal useful range of human hearing, from about 250 Hz to 8000 Hz. The patient is asked to raise her hand or push a button when she hears the tones. Sounds may be placed in one ear at a time or in both ears simultaneously. As with the tuning fork test, a device is placed against the base of the skull to see if hearing levels are affected by conductive problems in the ear canal or middle ear.

Results from the test are placed on a chart called an audiogram. This gives the audiologist a precise, graphic picture of the nature of a person's hearing loss. The patient's chart is then compared to the normal levels of hearing for a person of his or her age. A loss of hearing up to about 20 decibels is considered to fall within the normal range. Anything more than that is considered hearing impairment.

Tympanogram. The audiologist also can conduct a tympanogram, which tests for middle ear problems that could be leading to hearing loss. This painless procedure tests how well the eardrum is vibrating, which can in turn affect how well sound is transmitted to the bones of the middle ear and then to the cochlea. The audiologist places a small device similar to an ear plug against the outside of the auditory canal; the device then changes air pressure in the ear to see how well the eardrum vibrates at different settings. Normally, the pressure inside the ear equals the outside air pressure. A higher than normal reading can indicate fluid presence in the middle ear or other problems. As with audiography, the test is painless and takes just a few minutes to complete.

Auditory brain stem response. The auditory brain stem response (ABR) test checks for the normal transmission of electrical impulses along the auditory nerve. Usually, a small speaker is placed near the ear and a clicking sound is produced. Electrodes placed on the head track the nerve signal as it travels to the brain. The electrodes can detect where the nerve impulse breaks down or grows weaker. The ABR test usually is conducted when a doctor suspects the presence of a tumor that is impinging on the auditory nerve. This test is frequently requested when the patient shows signs of sensorineural hearing loss in one ear. In typical cases of age-related hearing loss, the impairment affects each ear to about the same degree.

HOW IS IT TREATED?

Many types of conductive hearing loss can be treated quickly, easily, and painlessly. Excessive earwax in the auditory canal, for instance, can be removed by the doctor with little more than warm water and a swab. It's not recommended that patients or caregivers try to remove significant earwax deposits, as this can lead to damage to the eardrum or parts of the middle ear. Most perforated eardrums are simply cleaned and allowed to heal by themselves. The patient may be given a mild painkiller until healing is complete. Minor ear infections usually respond well to antibiotics or other treatments, and fluid buildup usually disappears as a result. In cases where fluid is more resistant, the doctor may drain the middle ear with the help of tubes inserted through the eardrum. This process is called a myringotomy.

In cases of tinnitus, identification of the underlying cause is key to treatment. If a doctor can find the cause, such as allergy, he or she can usually work to cure the problem and allow the tinnitus to disappear of its own accord. If a medication is suspected of causing the problem, the doctor may stop the prescription or switch to another medicine to see if the tinnitus dissipates. Unfortunately, most of the time doctors are unable to find the cause of tinnitus. Many times, the condition will resolve on its own. But when it does not, the doctor may take a multidisciplinary approach to address the patient's suffering.

This approach can include counseling designed to assure the patient that tinnitus does not threaten hearing and may simply disappear. In severe cases, the doctor may prescribe a short-term regimen of antidepressants or nighttime sedatives to help the patient cope with the condition. When a patient with chronic tinnitus shows an inability to function with the condition, the doctor may recommend evaluation for an amplification device similar to a hearing aid. These devices are designed to produce white noise that helps mask the ringing sensation and allows the patient to focus on other sounds. The patient is able to adjust the level of the masking sound to make best use of the device. Presbycusis, noise-induced hearing loss, and other sensorineural forms of hearing loss cannot be cured. Treatment options thus focus on allowing the patient to regain as much functional use of his or her residual hearing as possible. This usually involves recommending a hearing aid. While these devices are not perfect, they can restore at least partial hearing to most people with presbycusis. Recent technological advances have enabled more and more people to enjoy sound more fully. Other treatment options include counseling to help deal with the emotional stress of hearing loss; therapy that teaches the person how to make better use of her remaining hearing—like speech-reading, which involves using visual cues to help understand what another person is saying, and strategies to conserve remaining hearing by reducing exposure to noise.

When hearing has deteriorated to the point of deafness or near-deafness, and when a hearing aid cannot help, the patient may be a candidate for a cochlear implant. This is an electronic device that fits inside the inner ear and simulates the work of the damaged hearing organs in the cochlea. The procedure has been available for more than fifteen years, but remains relatively rare. About 35,000 procedures have been performed, half of them on children. The average adult who receives the implant requires from three months to a year to understand speech without lip reading.

Because most people who "lose their hearing" do, in fact, retain nerve function in the ear, they can benefit from a cochlear implant. The retained nerve fibers remain responsive to the electrical signals from the implanted receive and trains of impulses that reflect a sound code reach the brain via the auditory nerve. People with cognitive dysfunction or dementia also do not make good candidates, as much training is required to learn how to use the device. Because of the rigorous training involved, candidates and their families must show great commitment to the procedure.

WHAT YOU CAN DO NOW

As stated earlier, presbycusis and noise-induced hearing loss cannot be cured. But as many as 95% of people who have these conditions can benefit from the use of a hearing aid. Preventative measures are usually successful in stopping further hearing loss for those with noise-induced hearing loss. These same measures often can slow down the progression of presbycusis as well.

Patients who receive cochlear implants now show very positive results on the average. One survey, however, found that 75% of patients who received the implants said their quality of life had improved greatly within nine months after the surgery.

In most tinnitus cases, the underlying cause for the ringing sensation is never found. When caused by medication, earwax blockage or other discoverable conditions, tinnitus is often reversible. Most people who do not show spontaneous improvement, however, learn to live with the condition. Those who have difficulty often are referred to tinnitus clinics for further examination, counseling and training. Research shows that about 80% of people who are treated at these clinics show improved ability to cope with the condition.

Devices that mask tinnitus are not especially successful unless they are used as part of an overall behavioral training program that serves to change one's perception of tinnitus. Only about 10% of patients say they experience periods when the tinnitus seems to disappear. Others receive partial benefit. For this reason, doctors often downplay these devices when discussing treatment options.

HOW IS IT PREVENTED?

Presbycusis is age-related and largely unavoidable. Most cases of tinnitus are idiopathic in nature, and as such are difficult to prevent. But noise-induced hearing loss is completely preventable, provided the proper steps are taken. The loss that has already occurred will not reverse itself, but further loss can be avoided. Earplugs and muff-type headsets are the standard tools. They can be purchased at drugstores and other locations, and can reduce noise exposure to acceptable levels. Some gel-filled models are especially good at blocking noise, and can be purchased through an audiologist or at a specialty store or pharmacy. Simply placing cotton balls in the ear will not significantly block noise.

Earplugs should be used any time a person anticipates being exposed to noise above about 90 decibels. This level commonly occurs with exposure to machine noise, at concerts where amplified music is played, on airplanes, when power tools are in use, or when riding on a motorcycle or snowmobile. In general, caregivers should make sure the person wears ear protection in situations when one must raise his voice to be heard or when you can't hear a person standing less than two feet away. Make note of occasions when the person has complained about pain or ringing in the ears, or when he or she has mentioned that speech seems dull or muffled. Anticipate these exposures, and make certain the person—as well as the caregiver—is wearing proper protection.

Regular hearing exams are a good way to track presbycusis and monitor any other hearing disorders. The patient's primary care physician or hearing specialist should be able to recommend a testing schedule.

WHAT RESEARCH IS BEING DONE?

As computer technology continues to advance, improvements in hearing aids, cochlear implants, and other devices are likely. Complete hearing aid implants are about five years away; these should offer greater hearing assistance and more convenience to the user. Cochlear implants should get progressively smaller, and no longer will require the insertion of a separate electronics package under the skin near the ear.

Researchers have identified a number of genetic markers for hearing disorders. One genetic mutation apparently predisposes people to deafness caused by aminoglycoside antibiotic use. This and other findings could some day help screen people for hearing loss risk, and help them avoid triggers like certain drugs or noise that could lead to problems later.

WHAT YOU CAN DO NOW

CHOOSING A HEARING AID

Hearing aids have grown more complex, more effective, and more expensive in recent years. Choosing the right one can be key to helping a person with hearing impairment return to a normal, productive lifestyle. The audiologist who helps select the model, the caregiver, and the patient must all work together to find a suitable choice.

Cost is certainly an issue. The newest "smart" models, which use digital technology and fit inside the ear canal, cost anywhere from $900 to $3000. Many of the more expensive models are self-adjusting; they are able to amplify the sounds important for the wearer to hear, like speech or music, while filtering out the kind of background noise that frequently plagues people who wear older models. Others require only a single touch to adjust to different situations, and still others have remote-control devices that are much more convenient to operate. The newer aids also have the advantage of being inconspicuous, but are not appropriate for all hearing losses, particularly those that are more severe. This can help convince reluctant patients to try a hearing aid, which is a large part of the battle in coping with hearing loss. About 50% of all people who could benefit from a hearing aid simply won't try them, partially because they're afraid of the stigma that accompanies a visible hearing aid.

Older analog models are larger and more obviously seen, but have the advantage of costing a fraction of their digital counterparts. They also usually have larger controls that are easier to adjust then the smaller knobs and buttons on many newer models.

It's also important to explain to a person with hearing impairment that a hearing aid will not be perfect. Despite advances in technology, they still cannot help everyone understand spoken words perfectly. Background noise is still an issue. And they still are not as easy to operate as some would like. But they represent the best hope for millions of people with hearing loss to overcome feelings of isolation and other social problems.

Over the years, the hearing aid industry has been plagued by unscrupulous dealers and high-pressure tactics. To avoid these problems, try to get a referral

SUCCESSFUL COMMUNICATION

When communicating with a person who is hard of hearing, try to observe the following guidelines:

• When holding a conversation, turn off televisions, radios, and other sources of background noise.

• Be sure to face the person to whom you are speaking. This helps them see your face and make out what you are trying to say.

• For the same reason, make sure the lights in the room are bright and that the light source is in front of you. Backlighting makes it more difficult for the person to see your face.

• Do not speak when eating or chewing gum.

• Use facial expression to help convey mood. Maintain eye contact when speaking.

• Speak somewhat louder than normal, but do not shout. Shouting can reinforce a person's feelings of inadequacy. It also can raise the pitch of your voice and make it harder for the person to hear you.

• If a person fails to understand you, try rephrasing your thoughts. Certain words may be harder to detect than others.

• Have the person repeat what was heard, particularly if it requires their action.

• Reinforce your communications by writing down important phrases and items.

• When dining in restaurants, try to sit in a quiet corner of the room. This will help eliminate background noise.

• Remain patient, positive, and sympathetic.

• When a group, be sure to include the hearing-impaired person in the conversation. Do not speak *about* the person, speak *to* her. This helps avoid frustration and feelings of isolation.

It's also important to tell people with hearing troubles to speak up for themselves. Encourage them to tell others that they have trouble hearing, and have them ask people to speak slowly and not shout. Although this may be embarrassing at first, it is beneficial in the long run. The person will learn that it's possible to communicate with others, and they will benefit from the interaction.

to a qualified audiologist from a physician familiar with ear pathology. If you go to an audiologist without such a recommendation, be sure to ask whether he has any financial ties to hearing aid manufacturers. This will help ensure that the aid the audiologist selects will best meet the patient's needs. It's also a good idea to insist on at least a thirty-day trial with a money-back guarantee. This will help ease the patient's fears about spending so much money for an aid that may not work.

LIVING WITH HEARING IMPAIRMENT

Of all perceptual impairments—including loss of eyesight—hearing loss is considered by many experts to have the greatest impact on function. Successful aging requires that one maintain the social connectivity that serves to maintain physical and mental health. Caregivers must be sensitive to the special needs of the hearing impaired, and must take steps to make the person able to participate in everyday activities to the highest degree possible. Many difficulties center on the person's relationship with family, friends and caregivers. People with hearing impairments often feel a decrease in energy and an increase in overall fatigue. Because of this, they may limit personal interaction. This, in turn, can lead to social withdrawal and feelings of isolation and depression. It's vital, therefore, to make an effort to include the person in as many social and family activities as possible.

People with severe hearing loss can benefit from a variety of household appliances designed for their needs. Telephones with adjustable volume controls can make it easier to hear both the ring and the words being spoken by the caller. For those who are completely deaf, special telephone systems called Telecommunications Devices for the Deaf (TDD) or Teletypewriters (TTY) allow people to communicate by typing words and having the incoming words placed in video form. Lights on the unit alert people when the phone is ringing. Most new television sets are equipped with closed-caption capability, and most shows now feature captions along with the video broadcast.

People with mild cases of tinnitus sometimes can create sufficient background noise to distract them from the ringing sensation. Some suggestions:

- Buy a loud-ticking clock.
- Try tuning the radio static to or in-between FM stations. FM bands carry a brighter signal and serve to better mask tinnitus.
- Purchase a commercial white-noise generator.

People with tinnitus are usually advised to avoid stressful situations, and to try to avoid excessive fatigue or the use of stimulants like coffee or tea.

ADDITIONAL RESOURCES

WEB SITES

**American Speech-Language-Hearing Association
ASHA Action Center**

800-498-2071, available 8:30 A.M. - 5:00 P.M. Eastern

TTY 301-571-0457

www.asha.org

Better Hearing Institute

800-EAR-WELL

www.betterhearing.org

National Institute on Deafness and Other Communication Disorders

www.nidcd.nih.gov

Hypertension (High Blood Pressure)

SIGNS & SYMPTOMS

- Hypertension is often called "the silent killer" because there are no outward signs or symptoms to indicate that something is wrong. There is no way to tell that a person has high blood pressure except by measuring it.

High blood pressure, also called hypertension, is very common. In the United States, about one of every four persons is hypertensive. Hypertension is important because it often results in stroke, heart attack, and kidney failure. The good news, however, is that treatment is effective and can prevent these complications. The tragedy is that many people with high blood pressure don't even know they have it. High blood pressure causes few if any symptoms so hypertension is often undiscovered until blood pressure is measured or organ damage results. Unfortunately, even those who know they have hypertension often have blood pressure that remains too high. This occurs because people make treatments such as lifestyle changes and medication a low priority. A common question heard in the clinic is "Why should I take medication if I feel well?" The answer is to prevent the life-threatening complications that can occur if blood pressure remains too high. Therefore, the support and understanding of caregivers and family members is essential to ensure that people with hypertension modify their lifestyle and take their medications.

WHAT IS IT?

Hypertension is often misunderstood to mean nervous tension, anxiety, or stress. Instead, hypertension is simply the condition of high blood pressure. Blood pressure is the pressure of blood in a medium-sized artery, typically the brachial artery in the upper arm. Blood pressure is often described with two measures: systolic

317

pressure and diastolic pressure. The systolic pressure is the higher number and represents the peak pressure generated by the heart during its contraction. The diastolic pressure is the lowest pressure and represents the blood pressure when the heart is relaxed. Hypertension is defined as:

- having systolic blood pressure of 140 mm Hg or greater;
- having diastolic pressure of 90 mm Hg or greater; or
- being on antihypertensive medication for an elevated blood pressure, even if the blood pressure is now in the normal range.

Another point of confusion concerns the term "low blood." This term is occasionally used as a synonym for anemia, the state of having too little hemoglobin, the blood's oxygen-carrying component. Some people believe that if they have "low blood" or anemia, they cannot have high blood pressure or hypertension. This is not true. Many people with anemia, a common condition especially among menstruating women, have hypertension.

WHO IS AT RISK?

In most people, blood pressure level and their personal risk of hypertension result from an interaction of genes and lifestyle. Genes control the regulatory system that maintains the essential balance between low and high blood pressure. These genes evolved over many thousands of years when salt and food were limited. During this stage in human development, high levels of physical activity and maximum exercise capacity were necessary for survival. These conditions are still present in some preindustrial societies and, in such societies, average blood pressure is low and does not increase with age. In industrial societies, however, average blood pressure is higher and rises with age. This higher blood pressure is due to changes in lifestyle, such as:

- higher sodium and alcohol intake;
- lower potassium intake due to a decreased consumption of fruits and vegetables; and
- higher rates of obesity due to increased calorie intake and decreased physical activity.

In environments that lead to high blood pressure, people's genes may predispose them to the harmful effects of these environmental factors. In most cases, however, genes alone are not enough to cause high blood pressure. Although blood pressure and hypertension tend to run in families, even people with strong family histories of high blood pressure can modify their risk of developing hypertension by improving their lifestyle.

So, who, then is at risk? Everyone. Almost one in every four people living in the United States has high blood pressure. In fact, most people will develop high blood pressure during their lifetime. This is true because blood pressure rises as we age, eventually reaching damaging levels in most people. Some people are at especially high risk. For example, African Americans have higher blood pressure than other ethnic groups. Other factors that influence blood pressure include weight, exercise, alcohol intake, diet, and a family history of hypertension. Therefore, people who are overweight, exercise less, drink more alcohol, or eat more salt tend to have high blood pressure. However, *all* people are at risk. Even people who are active, lean, and salt conscious develop hypertension. This is the reason why everyone should have regular blood pressure checks.

Most people in the United States would benefit from a lower blood pressure even though their pressure is not above 140/90 mm Hg. Blood pressure is a measure of one of the characteristics of your body, similar to height and weight. And like with height and weight, people have a range of blood pressure values. People with a higher blood pressure are considered hypertensive, just like people who weigh more are considered obese. However, there is no level of blood pressure above which a person is at risk of blood pressure complications and below which he or she is not. In fact, the risk of organ damage increases as blood pressure increases. Therefore, most people would benefit from having a lower blood pressure, even if they are not considered "hypertensive." The same is true for weight. While you may not be obese, your future health would probably benefit from a small weight reduction. For this reason, most people should adopt the lifestyle modifications discussed below, not just people who are "hypertensive." In addition, changing your lifestyle now may prevent you from developing hypertension later.

SPECIAL POPULATIONS AT RISK

Ethnic minorities. As populations move to the United States from less industrialized settings, their blood pressure tends to rise and hypertension tends to become more common. Among population groups in the United States, Native Americans have about the same hypertension rate as whites. Hispanic Americans tend to have blood pressure the same as or lower than the general population. African Americans, however, have one of the highest rates of hypertension in the world. In fact, hypertension occurs earlier and is more severe in African Americans than other groups. This epidemic has resulted in a very high occurrence of stroke, heart disease, and kidney failure. Therefore, treatment of hypertension among African Americans is vitally important.

Women. Hypertension occurs in many situations unique to women. Oral contraceptives ("the pill") can raise blood pressure a small amount. Occasionally, a woman on oral contraceptives will develop hypertension. If hypertension develops, the contraceptive should be stopped in most cases and the blood pressure allowed to normalize. If hypertension continues, then antihypertensive therapy should be started.

Pregnant women often have hypertension that was present before they became pregnant and is not due to the pregnancy itself. In these cases, the goal of treatment is to prevent the short-term risks of hypertension to the mother, while avoiding treatment that threatens the baby. If hypertension begins during pregnancy, methyldopa is the treatment of choice. If a woman is already on medication before becoming pregnant, then in most cases the medication can be continued—with the notable exception of ACE inhibitors and angiotensin II receptor blockers. ACE inhibitors and angiotensin II receptor blockers should be avoided because of their potential to damage the fetus. (See Drug Therapy, below, for a further discussion.)

Preeclampsia refers to hypertension in pregnant women and is characterized by high blood pressure, protein in the urine, edema or swelling of the face or hands, and, occasionally, abnormalities of kidney and liver function. Preeclampsia can be life-threatening and women with this condition require close monitoring by their physician.

Older persons. In industrialized countries, blood pressure rises as we age. Both diastolic and systolic blood pressure increase until mid-life, when diastolic pressure begins to fall, while systolic pressure continues to rise. The fall in the diastolic blood pressure and continued rise in systolic blood pressure after mid-life is due to the stiffening of blood vessels. Eventually, the diastolic blood pressure will fall until it is no longer elevated. This condition is called isolated systolic hypertension. Hypertension in older persons will respond to lifestyle modifications such as salt reduction and weight loss. Treatment of isolated systolic hypertension with thiazide diuretics, beta-blockers, and calcium channel blockers has been shown to lower risk of stroke, heart attacks, and death.

HOW IS IT DIAGNOSED?

Hypertension is often called "the silent killer." It earned this name because people seldom know they have high blood pressure until organ damage has occurred. There is no way to tell that a person has high blood pressure except by measuring it.

While blood pressure is easy to measure, determining if a person has high blood pressure is more difficult. Blood pressure is constantly changing in response to the body's needs, but must be maintained within a narrow range. If the blood pressure falls too low, the organs are starved of oxygen and nutrients. If blood pressure rises too high, then the blood vessels, and the organs they supply, are damaged. It is higher during the day, especially with exercise, and lower at night. The normal daily variations in blood pressure can make it hard to obtain a reading that reflects a person's average blood pressure. Therefore, medical decisions regarding blood pressure are usually based on several measurements taken on different days. If the blood pressure is especially high, however, immediate attention is required.

The care of people with high blood pressure begins with good blood pressure measurement. Given the high level of blood pressure variability, good measurement depends upon using an approach that remains the same at each assessment. The patient should avoid tobacco and caffeine for at least thirty minutes and should sit quietly for at least five minutes before the measurement is taken.

The diagnosis of hypertension is rarely made based on only one or two blood pressure readings. Due to blood pressure's natural variability, several measurements should be made at each visit and averaged. On the initial visit, the blood pressure should be measured in both arms and in the arm with the higher pressure subsequently. Hypertension is diagnosed when the blood pressure remains high over the course of several measurements separated in time by at least a day. Hav-

AMBULATORY BLOOD PRESSURE MONITORS

A device called an ambulatory blood pressure monitor is gaining wider acceptance. This small, unobtrusive device has a blood pressure cuff that is worn by the patient. It can be programmed to inflate and take blood pressure readings every fifteen to thirty minutes throughout the day and night while the person goes about his or her normal activities. There are many advantages to this type of assessment.

• The person or caregiver becomes more aware of the blood pressure. Therefore, he or she is better able to take an active role in its treatment.

• A person's blood pressure may not be well controlled during the entire period between medication doses. The ambulatory blood pressure monitor measures blood pressure throughout the day and may alert the patient, caregiver, or care provider that a change in medication dose is needed.

• Blood pressure may be abnormally high when it is measured in the clinic but normal outside the doctor's office. This is often referred to as "white coat hypertension." Many believe that this is caused by the patient's anxiety at being in the clinic. In this case, the ambulatory measurements are a better approximation of the typical blood pressure. A caveat is that blood pressure measured at home is almost always lower than that measured in a doctor's office.

• Ambulatory blood pressure measurements are a good way to evaluate someone whose blood pressure remains too high despite treatment but who has symptoms of low blood pressure at other times. Oftentimes, it is caregivers who raise this concern. These persons may have normal blood pressure at home but a high blood pressure in the clinic.

• Lastly, the major advantage of ambulatory monitors is they simply provide more data, 50 readings, for example, compared to two or three in an office setting. Given the variability in blood pressure, more readings yield a more precise estimate

Ambulatory blood pressure monitors are not covered by most insurance providers. A less expensive alternative is a home blood pressure device that is not worn. These devices are less expensive (usually less than $100) and are effective. The only disadvantage is that the person must stop his or her usual activities to take readings The most important consideration in choosing a device is how accurate it is. Periodically, independent evaluations of instruments are published. The device should be checked periodically by comparing readings with those obtained by a mercury sphygmomanometer.

ing the patient or their caregiver checking his or her blood pressure outside the office can improve the estimate of a person's blood pressure level and, probably, adherence with medications.

Table 1 lists the classification of blood pressure for adults 18 years of age or older and recommended follow-up according to the Sixth Report of the Joint National Committee on Detection, Evaluation, and Treatment of Hypertension (JNC-VI). This classification gives the optimal levels of blood pressure (in persons

TABLE 1

Classification of blood pressure for adults age 18 and older*

Category	Systolic (mm Hg)		Diastolic (mm Hg)
Optimal†	less than 120	and	less than 80
Normal	less than 130	and	less than 85
High-normal	130 - 139		85–89
Hypertension‡			
Stage 1	140–159	or	90–99
Stage 2	160–179	or	100–109
Stage 3	more than 180	or	more than 110

*Adults age 18 and older who are not taking antihypertensive drugs and are not acutely ill. When systolic and diastolic blood pressure fall into different categories, the higher category should be selected to classify the individual's blood pressure status. For example, 160/92 mm Hg should be classified as stage 2 hypertension, and 174/120 mm Hg should be classified as stage 3 hypertension. Isolated systolic hypertension is defined as systolic blood pressure of 140 mm Hg or greater and diastolic blood pressure below 90 mm Hg and staged appropriately (e.g., 170/82 mm Hg is defined as stage 2 isolated systolic hypertension). In addition to classifying stages of hypertension on the basis of average blood pressure levels, clinicians should specify presence or absence of target organ disease and additional risk factors. This specificity is important for risk classification and treatment.

†Optimal blood pressure with respect to cardiovascular risk is below 120/80 mm Hg. However, unusually low readings should be evaluated for clinical significance.

‡Based on the average of two or more readings taken at each of two or more visits after an initial screening.

Source: Reprinted from the Sixth Report of the Joint National Committee on Prevention, Detection, Evaluation, and Treatment of High Blood Pressure. National Heart, Lung, and Blood Institute, National High Blood Pressure Education Program. Washington DC: NIH Publication No. 98-4080, November 1997.

not taking medications to lower blood pressure) and makes several important points:

- Risk of organ damage increases as blood pressure increases.
- A person can be hypertensive because of a high diastolic blood pressure, a high systolic blood pressure, or both. For example, if the systolic blood pressure is 145 mm Hg and the diastolic blood pressure is 75 mm Hg, a patient is considered to have stage 1 hypertension based on the high systolic blood pressure.
- A "normal" blood pressure may not be the best blood pressure. Perhaps the best blood pressure in healthy people is a systolic blood pressure below 120 mm Hg and a diastolic blood pressure below 80 mm Hg.

EVALUATING THE PATIENT WITH HIGH BLOOD PRESSURE

Once a patient has been diagnosed with hypertension, the doctor will have three issues to consider:

- Does the person have organ damage from blood pressure or other causes?
- Is the person at high risk of future organ damage because of risk factors other than high blood pressure?
- Is there evidence of a potentially curable cause of high blood pressure? "Curable" hypertension is rare and is called "secondary" hypertension because the hypertension is secondary to an identifiable disease.

These goals are detailed below.

Determining existing organ damage. The doctor will try to determine whether the patient has suffered organ damage, since organ damage is obviously serious and calls for aggressive treatment. The doctor will take a medical history to see if there is a history of vascular disease including heart disease, stroke, kidney disease, and poor circulation to the legs should be sought. The patient's eyes will be examined for signs of bleeding or leakage of proteins due to the effect of hypertension on the blood vessels in the retina. A neurological exam will likely be performed to determine if there is evidence of past stroke. An electrocardiogram (ECG) will also likely be given to determine if there is evidence of cardiac enlargement or previous damage from known or silent heart attacks. The urine will be examined for protein and microalbumin, since their presence indicates hypertensive kidney damage, and blood levels of serum creatinine and potassium will also be measured.

Determining risk of future organ damage. The doctor will look for the risk of future organ damage by uncovering other cardiovascular risk factors, such as diabetes, tobacco use, elevated cholesterol, sedentary lifestyle, and family history of cardiovascular disease in first-degree relatives, among others. This is important for several reasons. First, risk factors tend to cluster together. In other words, a person with hypertension is more likely to have diabetes than a person without hypertension. Second, these other risk factors should be treated as well. Risk factors tend to work together to damage organs. Perhaps the best illustration of this is the combination of diabetes and hypertension. Diabetes is the presence of high blood sugar. People with diabetes are at high risk of developing heart, kidney, and nerve disease. We have recently learned that one of the best ways to reduce the risk of complications in people with diabetes is to reduce the blood pressure. The converse is true in people with high blood pressure. The effect of hypertension on organs can be reduced by treating other risk factors such as elevated cholesterol or diabetes, and by stopping smoking. Finally, people with other risk factors should begin blood pressure treatment at lower levels of blood pressure because of their increased risk of organ damage. For example, a person who has no evidence of organ damage and no other risk factors may not need treatment unless the systolic blood pressure is greater than 140 mm Hg or the diastolic is greater than 90 mm Hg. In contrast, someone with kidney disease should start blood pressure treatment if their systolic blood pressure is greater than 130 mm Hg or the diastolic is greater than 85 mm Hg. In fact, many doctors believe that persons with diabetes should be treated with a particular type of blood pressure medication called an ACE inhibitor regardless of their blood pressure.

Determining secondary hypertension. The third and final issue is to determine whether there is evidence of a disease that causes hypertension, usually called secondary hypertension. Fewer than 5% of people with established hypertension have a secondary form of hypertension—that is, an underlying disease that causes high blood pressure. Lifestyle factors, which are not usually included under secondary causes of high blood pressure, account for a large proportion of high blood pressure. Correction of the underlying abnormality in secondary hypertension may, but does not always, lead to a normal blood pressure. Because secondary hypertension is rare, evaluating all people with high blood pressure would lead to unnecessary anxiety and risks. Therefore, doctors do not look for secondary causes of hypertension unless there is a sign, symptom, or lab test result that suggests a secondary cause may exist.

WHAT CAN CAUSE SECONDARY HYPERTENSION?

Secondary hypertension is high blood pressure that is caused by some underlying disease. Sometimes—but not always—it is possible to control this hypertension by controlling the underlying disease. Some of the common conditions that cause secondary hypertension are listed here.

• Narrowing of the artery to the kidney, also called renal artery stenosis, is the cause of about 1% of hypertension. A recent onset or worsening of hypertension in older persons suggests a diagnosis of kidney artery narrowing as the result of hardening of the arteries (i.e., atherosclerosis), especially if there is evidence of atherosclerosis elsewhere. Causes of hypertension secondary to causes other than kidney artery narrowing are much less common.

• A history of dizziness on standing after lying down, or experiencing palpitations, and high blood pressure that is highly variable raises the suspicion of a rare tumor of the adrenal gland called a pheochromocytoma. (Please note, however, that many people, especially older people, experience lightheadedness or dizziness when standing. In almost all cases this is not due to a pheochromocytoma but rather a type of nervous system abnormality called orthostatic hypotension.)

• Increasing ring and shoe size, headaches, and a history of diabetes suggest an endocrine abnormality called acromegaly.

• Temperature intolerance, changes in hair and skin, changes in bowel habits, and other symptoms raise the possibility of an overactive thyroid gland contributing to hypertension.

• Several hormone-related illness also contribute to secondary hypertension, including Cushing's syndrome, and hyperadrenalism and hyperparathyroidism, which are disorders of the adrenal and thyroid glands, respectively.

Several factors in the patient's medical history suggest the possibility of secondary hypertension: severe hypertension in a young person, especially given no family history of high blood pressure; a poor response to therapy, as indicated by very high blood pressure (systolic higher than 180 mm Hg or diastolic higher than 110 mm Hg) on three or more blood pressure measurements; accelerated or malignant hypertension; and, in an older person, sudden onset of severe hypertension or a worsening of blood pressure control in otherwise well-controlled hypertension. Accelerated hypertension is blood pressure that is so high that it must be reduced immediately to prevent organ damage. When accelerated hypertension is accompanied by evidence of brain swelling, it is called malignant hypertension because it was universally fatal before antihypertensive medications were developed. Accelerated hypertension is a medical emergency.

WHAT SHOULD YOU EXPECT?

High blood pressure is important because it damages the body's organs. The organs at greatest risk include the heart, brain, and kidneys. In fact, high blood pressure is one of the most common causes of stroke, heart attack, heart failure, and kidney failure. Research is ongoing regarding its possible role in dementia and other conditions. People who have high blood pressure that remains too high may experience these complications as they age. The good news is that the risk of developing these complications can be lowered with proper management of blood pressure and other risk factors. Proper management is discussed below and relies on a good relationship between patient and health care provider. Two foundations of this relationship are the periodic blood pressure measurement and the repeated reinforcement of lifestyle modifications and adherence to drug therapy.

HOW IS IT TREATED?

Once the diagnosis of hypertension is made and the evaluation complete, two questions must then be asked: When should elevated blood pressure be treated, and with which therapy? Of course the answers to both questions are related and depend on the patient's circumstances. As for when therapy should begin, an argument can be made that everyone—regardless of blood pressure—should adopt a healthy lifestyle designed to lower their blood pressure and other risk factors to avoid the rise in blood pressure, and the attendant risk, that occurs as we age. These lifestyle changes can be both population-based (for example, decreasing the salt content of processed foods), or individual-based (for example, a prescription for a healthy lifestyle tailored to each person).

Table 2 describes treatment recommendations developed by the Joint National Committee on Prevention, Detection, Evaluation, and Treatment of High Blood Pressure. The time to begin treatment depends upon blood pressure level, presence of organ damage, and presence of other risk factors.

Specific treatment options are discussed below.

LIFESTYLE CHANGES

Nearly everyone should adopt a lifestyle designed to reduce blood pressure and other cardiovascular risk factors. (The rare exception is someone who is unlikely to experience cardiovascular disease due to the presence of another disease such as a malignancy. In addition, some of these lifestyle changes should not be made in a person with cardiovascular disease without a doctor's evaluation - for example, an exercise regimen.)

People with high-normal levels of blood pressure especially should implement lifestyle changes because they are at higher risk of developing hypertension. In people with blood pressure above the optimal range, lifestyle modifications may be all that is required to produce the desired fall in blood pressure. In those requiring medical treatment, lifestyle modification will improve other cardiovascular risk factors, enhance the blood pressure- lowering effect of the drug therapy, and may even allow the patient to be taken off drug therapy.

Several principles are helpful in achieving success with lifestyle interventions. Reasonable, attainable short-term goals should be established. Over time, short-term successes can build incrementally toward the overall goal. Persons with high blood pressure should be seen frequently for short visits to provide feedback pertinent to the intervention (e.g., weight, urine sodium concentration) as well as positive reinforcement and problem solving. The family, especially the food preparer, should be

TABLE 2

Categories of risk for high blood pressure, and recommended treatment*

Blood pressure stages (mm Hg)	Risk group A (no risk factors, no TOD/CCD†)	Risk group B (At least 1 risk factor, not including diabetes; no TOD/CCD)	Risk group C (TOD/CCD and/or diabetes, with or without other risk factors)
High-normal (130 - 139/85 - 89)	Lifestyle modification	Lifestyle modification	Drug therapy
Stage 1 (140 - 159/90 - 99)	Lifestyle modification (up to 12 months)	Lifestyle modification‡ (up to 6 months)	Drug therapy§
Stages 2 (at or above 160) and 3 (at or above 100)	Drug therapy	Drug therapy	Drug therapy

*All patients recommended for drug therapy should also be encouraged to attempt lifestyle modifications.

†TOD/CCD means target organ disease or clinical cardiovascular disease.

‡For patients with multiple risk factors, drugs should be considered as initial therapy, plus lifestyle modifications.

§For those with heart failure, renal insufficiency, or diabetes.

Source: Reprinted, with changes, from the *Sixth Report of the Joint National Committee on Prevention, Detection, Evaluation, and Treatment of High Blood Pressure.* National Heart, Lung, and Blood Institute, National High Blood Pressure Education Program. Washington DC: NIH Publication No. 98-4080, November 1997.

involved, and other health professionals, particularly nutritionists and nurses, or community resources such as weight loss centers, can play a part. Remember, successful lifestyle interventions take time. But the wait, and the effort, is worth it.

The JNC-VI recommends the following therapies for blood pressure reduction:

- A healthy diet
- decreased salt intake

- weight loss
- increased physical activity
- limited alcohol intake
- increased potassium intake

These lifestyle interventions, plus a few others, are detailed below.

Healthy diet. A large clinical trial—Dietary Approaches to Stop Hypertension (DASH)—tested the effect of the change of whole dietary patterns on blood pressure. This approach differs from the traditional emphasis on the effect of one dietary component. The DASH diet is rich in fruits, vegetables, and low-fat dairy foods, and is reduced in saturated fat, total fat, and cholesterol. It emphasizes whole grains, poultry, fish, and nuts and is reduced in red meats, sweets, and sugar-containing beverages. The DASH diet reduced systolic blood pressure by 11.5 mm Hg in the study participants who had high blood pressure and by 3.5 mm Hg among the participants with normal blood pressure. These amounts are similar to the amounts of blood pressure reduction achieved with medications.

Limited salt. *"The lower the amount of salt in the diet, the lower the blood pressure, for both those with and without hypertension."* This statement by the National Heart, Lung, and Blood Institute summarizes the findings of the DASH-sodium trial. This trial was designed to test the short-term blood pressure-lowering effect of sodium reduction to levels below the recommended daily intake. Compared to those eating a typical American diet, the DASH diet, combined with a daily intake of 1.5 grams of sodium, lowered the systolic blood pressure of all participants by an impressive 8.9 mm Hg, a reduction comparable to the blood pressure-lowering effect of drugs. Those with hypertension experienced an even greater reduction in systolic blood pressure of 11.7 mm Hg. This evidence confirms the blood pressure-lowering effect of salt reduction seen in other studies and clinical trials. People with high blood pressure are currently advised to reduce sodium intake to 2.4 grams per day. Given the new data, this recommendation may change to 1.5 grams of sodium per day (3.75 grams of sodium chloride or table salt).

Weight loss. Losing weight is a highly effective way to reduce blood pressure in hypertensive people who are overweight. Virtually every clinical trial that has examined the influence of weight loss on blood pressure has documented a substantial fall in blood pressure with even modest weight loss. It is estimated that a 10-pound weight loss will result in an average fall in systolic blood pressure of 7.5 mm Hg.

Increased physical activity. Regular aerobic physical activity can lower pressure, according to many observational studies and a few clinical trials. Brisk walking for thirty-five minutes, running 1.5 miles in fifteen minutes, or stair walking for fifteen minutes, performed four or more days per week have all been shown to reduce blood pressure.

Limited alcohol intake. Drinking more than two alcoholic beverages a day is one of the most common reversible causes of high blood pressure, accounting for 6 to 11% of hypertension in men. The JNC-VI recommends limiting alcohol intake to no more than 1 ounce (30 mL) of ethanol per day—that is, 24 ounces of beer, 10 ounces of wine, or 2 ounces of 100-proof liquor. Women and lighter-weight men should further reduce their alcohol intake to no more than 0.5 ounce of ethanol per day. A word of warning: those who drink heavily and stop drinking abruptly can experience alcohol withdrawal, which may be life-threatening and will raise blood pressure markedly for a few days. People who drink heavily should consult their doctor for advice regarding alcohol cessation.

Potassium supplements. In contrast to sodium, higher potassium intakes are associated with lower blood pressure. Therefore, an adequate intake of potassium (90 mmol/day) can lower blood pressure, especially in the setting of excess sodium intake. This amount of potassium is easily achieved with a diet rich in fresh fruits and vegetables. Persons with kidney disease or on some antihypertensive medications can have difficulty excreting potassium, so patients should seek the advice of their doctor before increasing potassium intake.

DRUG TREATMENT

The availability of effective, well-tolerated drugs for hypertension is a medical success story. Death from high blood pressure and cardiovascular diseases has fallen in the United States over the last twenty years. Antihypertensive drug therapy in patients with mild and mild to moderate hypertension prevents death. Antihypertensive drug treatment of accelerated hypertension prevents both blood pressure-related organ disease or damage (stroke, kidney disease, and heart failure) and cardiovascular events due to hardening of the arteries (heart attacks, strokes due to hardening of arteries). Many studies have shown that that lowering blood pressure with medications reduces stroke risk by over 40% and coronary heart disease by over 20%.

Most of the studies used diuretics and beta-blockers, but more recent clinical trials have also demonstrated benefit from newer types of medication, such as ACE inhibitors and calcium channel blockers. Each type of medication, or class, works in a different way and, therefore, may have particular advantages and disadvantages. We know little about the relative effect of various classes on the prevention of organ damage. The Antihypertensive and Lipid- Lowering Treatment to Prevent Heart Attack Trial (ALLHAT) is a large clinical trial involving 42,448 hypertensive people that is designed to compare the efficacy of different types of antihypertensive drugs in the prevention of cardiovascular disease. Although this study will not end until 2002, we have already learned important information about the effect of an alpha-adrenergic blocker doxazosin (Cardura) compared to a thiazide diuretic. (Hydrochlorothiazide is the most common thiazide diuretic and people usually take the generic form. Dyazide and Maxzide are popular combination drugs that include a thiazide.) Those taking doxazosin experienced a higher rate of heart failure than those taking the diuretic. Therefore, the doxazosin arm of the study was stopped. Thus, doxazosin and medicines like it—terazosin (Hytrin) and prazosin (Minipress)—should not be used alone to treat high blood pressure. Such clinical trials are necessary to determine whether these new, usually more expensive, classes of drugs provide greater protection from organ damage.

When to start medications

The time to begin medications to lower blood pressure depends upon the presence, extent, and future risk of organ damage (see Table 2). In fact, patients with some types of end-organ disease benefit from treatment with antihypertensive medications regardless of their blood pressure, and probably through mechanisms in addition to blood pressure-lowering. ACE inhibitors reduce risk of future disease, including the risk of dying, in people who have suffered a heart attack or who have congestive heart failure. Therapy with spironolactone (Aldactone), a type of diuretic or "water pill," adds additional benefit in people with congestive heart failure. ACE inhibitors also prevent progression of renal disease in people with kidney damage, especially if they have diabetes. Finally, a large clinical study, the

Heart Outcome Prevention Evaluation (HOPE) trial, demonstrated that treatment with the ACE inhibitor ramipril (Altace) prevented cardiovascular disease in those with, or at high risk of developing, atherosclerosis. People included in this study were older than 55 and had had a heart attack or other vascular event or had diabetes with at least one other cardiovascular risk factor.

For patients who do not fit any of the above criteria, the time to begin treatment depends on how high the blood pressure is and the associated risk factors. As indicated previously, people with a systolic blood pressure of 130 mm Hg or greater or a diastolic of 85 mm Hg or greater should adopt lifestyle modifications. Drug therapy should be added if the blood pressure stays above 140 mm Hg systolic or 90 mm Hg diastolic despite lifestyle modification. Any elevation beyond a systolic blood pressure of 135 mm Hg or a diastolic blood pressure of 85 mm Hg should be treated if the patient has organ damage or diabetes.

Another issue is the target blood pressure, i.e., the treatment goals, for antihypertensive therapy. Doctors have been concerned that, although blood pressure treatment is good, overtreatment could be hazardous and could increase the risk of heart attack. Persons who have kidney disease with a substantial amount of protein in the urine (more than 1 gram a day) should have their blood pressure lowered to less than 125 mm Hg systolic and 75 mm Hg diastolic. This strategy has been shown to prevent progression of kidney disease and to be safe.

The current consensus on target blood pressure in patients without this degree of kidney disease is based in large part on a recent clinical trial, the Hypertension Optimal Treatment (HOT) trial, which assigned patients randomly to three groups with different treatment goals. All three groups enjoyed much lower rates of cardiovascular disease than expected. In addition, there was a rise in participants' sense of well-being, which was most dramatic in those with the lowest blood pressure. We can conclude from the HOT trial that it is safe to lower the diastolic blood pressure to around 82 mm Hg in most patients with hypertension, and physicians have adopted these more stringent treatment goals. We also learned that most patients need more than one antihypertensive medication to meet these goals.

Drugs commonly used to control hypertension

The several classes of medications are used to control high blood pressure work through different mechanisms. There are so many classes of medications because there are many different systems controlling blood pressure. Many people need medications from several different classes to achieve a normal or optimal blood pressure. For example, it is not uncommon for a person to take both a diuretic and an ACE inhibitor (examples include Lotensin, Capoten, Vasotec, Prinivil, Monopril, Accupril, and Altace). In addition, even when one drug may be sufficient to control blood pressure, the provider may choose to prescribe several drugs. This is done to reduce side effects that may occur when a drug is used at high doses. When a second drug is added, the dose of the first drug can often be reduced, minimizing its side effects. Multiple drugs are often used to provide the patient benefit from several classes of medications. For example, a person with heart disease may take a diuretic, an ACE inhibitor, and a beta-blocker, even though he or she only needs one of these drugs for high blood pressure. This is often done in the above situation because each of these medications has been shown to extend life expectancy in certain people with heart disease.

Ideally, the choice of a particular drug should be based on the drug's proven ability of the agent to prevent future organ damage and cardiovascular disease. The JNC-VI report recommended thiazide diuretics (hydrochlorothiazide, chlorthalidone) and beta-blockers (propanolol, atenolol, metoprolol) as the first drugs of choice because such evidence was only available for these classes at the time of its writing. Currently, similar data is available for other classes of medications such as calcium channel blockers and ACE inhibitors. Once-a-day dosage, a limited side effects, and lower cost are all factors that encourage people to take the medication and should influence the choice of agent. Now that we know that most patients will need more than one drug, less emphasis is being placed on treatment with one single agent.

Thiazide diuretics. Thiazide diuretics (hydrochlorothiazide, chlorthalidone) were the first available effective drugs for hypertension. Diuretics can be used in almost any patient with hypertension, and they are often considered the treatment of choice for patients with isolated systolic hypertension, for older people, and for those who have trouble paying for their medications. (A year's supply of thiazide diuretics costs less than $10.) Thiazide diuretics are particularly effective in lowering blood pressure among older persons and African Americans. Another advantage of these drugs is that they help maintain body stores of calcium, an important consideration in postmenopausal women, who are prone to osteoporosis. A disadvantage of these drugs is their potential for decreasing the body's level of potassium and magnesium. Physicians may counteract this by adjusting the dose or recommending that the patient take potassium supplements. Other side effects include elevation of uric acid and total and very low-density lipoprotein (VLDL) cholesterol levels. Again, physicians can minimize these effects by adjusting the dosage and/or recommending that patients follow a diet recommended by the American Heart Association. For those rare patients who are allergic to thiazide diuretics or require more effective elimination of excess body salt and water, several other types of diuretics that can be used.

Beta-blockers. Beta-blockers lower blood pressure in most patients but are somewhat less effective than diuretics in the elderly and in African Americans. Beta-blockers are effective in preventing a second heart attack and should be used in hypertensive patients with a previous heart attack unless there is a reason not to. Beta-blockers are effective in the treatment of chest pain due to heart disease and the prevention of migraine headaches. Recent studies have demonstrated that particular beta-blockers benefit people with heart failure as well. Generic beta-blockers are available at a monthly cost of less than $20. Examples of common beta-blockers include metoprolol, atenolol, and propranolol.

Because they can cause reversible narrowing of the airways, only certain types of beta-blockers designed to have minimal effect on airways should be used with caution in persons with asthma or chronic obstructive pulmonary disease. Despite their effectiveness in preventing a second heart attack, most beta-blockers tend to lower high-density lipoprotein (HDL) (often referred to as "good") cholesterol. Beta-blockers may decrease the amount of blood pumped by the heart, decrease the diameter of blood vessels, and, therefore, may worsen symptoms of peripheral vascular disease. Beta-blockers increase the risk of developing diabetes but only by a small degree. They may also mask symptoms of low blood glucose in people with poorly controlled diabetes.

Angiotensin-converting enzyme (ACE) inhibitors. ACE inhibitors prevent the formation of angiotensin-II, a powerful blood vessel constrictor. They are the treatment of choice in hypertensive patients with diabetes, heart failure, and most types of kidney disease. ACE inhibitors reduce the death rate in patients with heart failure and in those who have had a heart attack, especially if heart failure is present.

ACE inhibitors slow the progression of kidney disease, regardless of cause, but are especially effective in diabetics. There is evidence from two studies that ACE inhibitors may actually prevent the onset of diabetes.

One of the most common adverse effects of these drugs is cough, occurring in up to 20% of patients. The cough is usually dry and not bothersome but can necessitate stopping the medication. ACE inhibitors are absolutely contraindicated during pregnancy, because they can damage or even kill the fetus. Unlike the thiazide diuretics, ACE inhibitors can raise potassium levels, so potassium supplements and other medications that raise potassium are usually discontinued. Over nine ACE inhibitors are available in the United States at this time. Commonly prescribed ACE inhibitors include enalapril (Vasotec), lisinopril (Prinivil and Zestril), benazepril (Lotensin), and captopril (Capoten).

Angiotensin receptor blockers. This class of medications works by blocking the receptor that angiotensin-II occupies. Their side effects are similar to those of ACE inhibitors but their effect on long-term outcomes is not as well studied. Cough is less a problem than with ACE inhibitors, so that patients who develop cough on ACE inhibitors are often switched to this class. Studies testing the effectiveness of angiotensin receptor blockers in reducing organ damage are ongoing. Agents in this class include losartan (Cozaar) and valsartan (Diovan).

Calcium channel blockers. Like thiazide diuretics, calcium channel blockers are especially effective in lowering blood pressure in elderly persons and in African Americans. The three types of calcium channel blockers are dihydropyridines (nifedipine [Procardia and Adalat], felodipine [Plendil], isradipine [DynaCirc], amlodipine [Norvasc], among others), diltiazem (Cardizem), and verapamil (Calan, Covera).

Verapamil is better at reducing heart hypertrophy, or thickness, than beta-blockers and other calcium channel blockers in patients with hypertensive heart hypertrophy. Like beta-blockers, these drugs are effective in the treatment of chest pain (angina) and migraine headaches. They do not worsen peripheral vascular disease. A dihydropyridine has been shown to decrease the death rate in older persons with isolated systolic hypertension. Perhaps the greatest advantage to calcium channel blockers is the small number of side effects.

In the past, dihydropyridine have been used to treat persons with heart failure, but these drugs don't have the beneficial effect of ACE inhibitor or beta-blockers.

In fact, some types of calcium channel blockers may actually increase the death rate in patients with heart failure.

Alpha-1-blockers. Alpha-1-blockers have many beneficial effects in addition to their blood pressure-lowering effect. For example, alpha-1-blockers lower cholesterol levels and improve symptoms of bladder outlet obstruction in men with enlarge prostates. However, the large ALLHAT study demonstrated an increased rate of heart failure in participants on the alpha-1-blocker doxazosin (Cardura) compared to those on a thiazide diuretic. This is not evidence that doxazosin is harmful, just that it is not as effective as the diuretic in reducing cardiovascular disease. People currently taking an alpha-1-blocker should discuss the advantages and disadvantages of continuing the drug with their doctor. They should not stop it without first talking with their doctor. If a person is starting drug therapy for hypertension, an alpha-1-blocker is not the best choice for initial therapy. In addition to doxazosin other drugs in this class include terazosin (Hytrin) and prazosin (Minipres).

A major problem with alpha-1-blockers is the occurrence of lightheadedness on arising, especially after taking the first dose. Low blood pressure with standing is less common when the initial dose is small and when longer-acting preparations are used.

Central sympatholytics. Central sympatholytics are very effective agents and were the mainstay of antihypertensive therapy for many years. They block some of the symptoms of opiate withdrawal and are effective in reducing heart excess thickness of the heart wall. However, they have worse side effects than other classes of drug therapy. Because these drugs may impair cognition, they should not be the first choice of drug for elderly patients. They also tend to lose their effectiveness when used alone. These drugs are inexpensive and available in generic form. The most commonly prescribed drug in this class is clonidine, which is also the only hypertension medication available as a patch, applied to the skin just once a week.

Dosage and follow-up

In most cases drug treatment should begin with the lowest effective dose. If blood pressure remains elevated after one to two months, the dose should be increased or a new medication added. Blood pressure should be measured at different times of the day to ensure maintenance of normotension throughout the day.

Adherence to medical therapy

The most common reason for poor control of hypertension is that patients don't take their prescribed medications. Patients who miss follow-up appointments or who drop out of care are most likely to be skip or stop taking their medications. But there are several steps physicians can take to improve this.

- Frequent visits between the patient and physician to assess adherence and to check on side effects.
- Once-a-day-dosing is more convenient for many patients, especially the elderly. For patients who take two or more medications, pills or tablets that combine both drugs are available.
- Improving the patient's access to medications by minimizing costs and maximizing insurance coverage.

WHAT RESEARCH IS BEING DONE?

High blood pressure is an active area of research. Scientists are investigating the causes, prevention, and treatment of hypertension.

Genetics. The genetics of hypertension is an active area of research. High blood pressure runs in families and has a strong genetic component. If we knew the genetic causes of hypertension, we could better predict who was at risk of developing hypertension and its complications. We could then intervene while the person's blood pressure was normal to prevent high blood pressure from developing. Understanding the genetics of hypertension will also lead to better treatments of hypertension. New drugs will be developed based on identified genes and old drugs will be better matched with appropriate patients based on their genes. The genes themselves may someday be manipulated to change blood pressure physiology.

Physiology. Despite twenty-five years of dedicated research we still don't fully understand the physiology of blood pressure regulation. As mentioned before, blood pressure is controlled by many interacting systems. Given this complexity, scientists tend to focus on one aspect of blood pressure regulation. But so far, no one has assembled all of the pieces of knowledge into one complete understanding of blood pressure. Gene-based research is offering a whole new level of inquiry into the physiology of human hypertension.

Lifestyle modification treatment. The nonpharmacologic treatment of high blood pressure is an area of exciting discoveries. Trial after trial has shown that high blood pressure can be effectively treated with lifestyle modifications. The next phase of research will concern the translation of these encouraging results into patient care. In particular, maintaining a healthy lifestyle is difficult and many studies are currently investigating ways to help people succeed in lifestyle modification.

Drug treatment. The pharmacologic treatment of hypertension is also an area of active research. Most research concerns the development of new drugs that work in ways similar to old drugs. The advantages of the new drugs often include fewer side effects and less frequent dosing requirements. Not only new drugs, but whole new classes of drugs are also being developed. Some newer drugs in the pipeline appear to be more effective in reducing systolic blood pressure than our currently available medications. These drugs work in new ways and may offer new benefits not previously obtained with blood pressure medication. But the effect of new drugs on preventing organ damage and death must be evaluated before they are recommended for general use.

HOW CAN IT BE PREVENTED?

The prevention of hypertension is a major concern for the individual and for society. Since most people eventually develop high blood pressure, most of us should be practicing prevention. While few prevention trials have been performed, many believe that lifestyle modifications prescribed for those with hypertension will also work to prevent its occurrence (see "Lifestyle Changes" on p. 328). While we do not diagnose hypertension until a person has a sustained blood pressure above a given cutoff, people below this cutoff are also at risk. In fact, the relationship between blood pressure and organ damage is continuous throughout the range of blood pressure. Therefore, a person with a systolic blood pressure of 130 has a greater risk of organ damage than a person with a systolic blood pressure of 120, even though both blood pressures are "normal." For this reason, many argue that everyone should modify their lifestyle in such a way to lower blood pressure. If we were able to decrease the average blood pressure of Americans, for example, the decrease in strokes, heart attacks, and kidney disease would be dramatic.

While people with the highest blood pressure are at greatest risk, most people have blood pressure that is not high enough to justify medical treatment but is high enough to damage blood vessels after many years. Therefore, measures designed to lower the blood pressure of the general population can significantly reduce the burden of organ damage.

WHAT YOU CAN DO NOW

Everyone's blood pressure should be check regularly (at least once every two years). This is all the more true for persons over 60 since blood pressure typically rises with age and the risks of heart disease and stroke rise accordingly. If blood pressure is consistently above the optimal range, then lifestyle changes and, possibly, medication are recommended. People who have high blood pressure that is being treated by medication need to have their blood pressure checked periodically as well. Starting medication is not enough. Blood pressure must be monitored to be sure the treatment is effective. In addition, certain medications require that other health norms be monitored, such as the blood potassium level. Therefore, maintaining a regular relationship one's health care provider is essential.

There is hope for those who have suffered organ damage because of high blood pressure or other factors. Effective treatment will often allow healing of past damage. In most cases, treatment will also prevent or minimize future damage as well. Therefore, for those who do have organ damage, a relationship with a health care provider is even more essential.

Finally, many good sources of additional information concerning high blood pressure and associated diseases are available. A few of these sources are listed below.

ADDITIONAL RESOURCES

WEB SOURCES

American Heart Association. *High Blood Pressure*. Internet on-line. Available from www.americanheart.org/presenter.jhtml?identifier=2114. [Accessed July 1, 2002].

National Institutes of Health, National Heart, Lung, and Blood Institute.

Facts about the DASH Diet. Internet on-line. Available from http://www.nhlbi.nih.gov/health/public/heart/hbp/dash/new_dash.pdf. [Accessed July 1, 2002]

National Institutes of Health, National Heart, Lung, and Blood Institute. *The Sixth Report of the Joint National Committee on Prevention, Detection, Evaluation, and Treatment of High Blood Pressure*. Available from http://www.nhlbi.nih.gov/guidelines/hypertension/jncintro.htm [Accessed July 1, 2002].

National Institutes of Health, National Heart, Lung, and Blood Institute. *Your Guide to Lowering High Blood Pressure*. Available from http://www.nhlbi.nih.gov/hbp/. [Accessed July 1, 2002].

Human Immunodeficiency Virus and AIDS

The last twenty years of the twentieth century witnessed the birth of one of the craftiest diseases ever to threaten the human race. Infection with the human immunodeficiency virus (HIV) spreads quietly in its host for the first eight to ten years before striking with the first signs of illness. Since infected individuals are seldom ill initially, they can spread it to many others without knowing it. Those who die tend to be in the prime of their lives, robbing family and society of unfulfilled love, aspirations, and economic worth. Despite this great tragedy, social stigma and lack of coordinated efforts have abetted the spread of HIV. As has been typical with other epidemics in human history such as the plague or typhus, society's initial reflex is to seek the defensive shield of denial, or to ostracize those infected, either physically or emotionally.

In less than twenty years, HIV has infected more than 47 million people. When the epidemic appeared to start in the early 1980s, HIV was originally confined to North America, Western Europe, and sub-Saharan Africa. Now, the disease is present worldwide. The highest levels of new infections are currently found in Africa, India, and Southeast Asia. At the beginning of the year 2000, an estimated

SIGNS & SYMPTOMS

HIV INFECTION
- Generalized swelling of lymph glands
- Meningitis
- Peripheral neuropathy (numbness in hands and feet)
- Chronic or unexplained fever
- Chronic diarrhea
- Unexplained dementia
- Unusual weight loss
- Mild-to-severe cold or flu-like illness
- Fever, muscle aches, headache
- Nausea, vomiting, diarrhea
- (Sometimes) sore throat, fever, mild rash, and swollen glands, especially of the neck

FULL-BLOWN AIDS
- *Pneumocystis carinii* infection (a fungal pneumonia)
- HIV-related wasting syndrome (unintentional weight loss of more than 10% of body weight)
- *Cytomegalovirus* infection
- Tuberculosis
- Kaposi's sarcoma
- *Mycobacterium avium* infection
- Chronic herpes simplex
- HIV-related dementia
- Toxoplasmosis (a parasitic infection usually of the brain)

343

33.6 million people were living with HIV infection as determined by the United Nations program on HIV/AIDS. As many as sixteen million have perished because of this viral infection, with more than 90% of cases now occurring in developing countries. An astonishing 16,000 people are newly infected each day.

The disease called the acquired immunodeficiency syndrome (AIDS) was described in the early 1980s by physicians in New York and San Francisco who saw previously healthy, young gay men fall ill with bizarre infections usually seen only in individuals with severely weakened immune systems. The discovery of HIV as the cause of AIDS in 1984 by French and American scientists was quickly hailed as the key to halting the blight.

WHAT IS IT?

The HIV virus appears to weaken the immune system of the body, leaving it defenseless against disease and infections that are normally resisted. The human immune system is a complex and still incompletely understood process wherein white blood cells and antibodies work much like a defending army that can be quickly organized to destroy invading germs and foreign organisms. Helper T-cell lymphocytes (also known as CD4 cells) are the critical coordinators of the immune response. HIV infects and destroys these CD4 cells over time, leaving the immune system with a deficiency of its defense mechanism. Some scientists promote views claiming that HIV does not cause AIDS. This discredited theory receives enough attention to distract and undercut efforts to stop the spread of the virus.

An unusual coalition including activists, scientists, physicians, the pharmaceutical industry, and politicians tackled the emerging AIDS epidemic, but more than ten years elapsed before an effective treatment was discovered. By the 1990s, tremendous gains in both basic science research and clinical treatment made HIV the most well-studied virus known to date. Despite these considerable efforts, there remains no cure for HIV and no effective vaccine for prevention. Though infection with HIV is less bleak than just five years ago because of promising therapies, the infection is most successfully fought by individuals who not only muster the courage to fight this disease but who are also aided by family and friends to deal with its daunting challenges. Living with HIV has become extraordinarily complex for patient, health care provider, and family caregiver alike. A primer illustrating the workings of HIV and how it causes disease becomes essential for understanding all the issues of caring for someone infected with the virus.

RETROVIRUSES

Viruses cause many familiar diseases such as influenza, chicken pox, cold sores, measles, and colds. Viruses are the smallest of parasites, and they can only exist by depending on a host cell to perform essential functions for viral growth and replication. In humans, the host cell for the AIDS virus is primarily the CD4 cell and, to a lesser extent, other members of the white blood cell family. HIV belongs to a family of viruses called retroviruses. The "retro" is derived from this virus's reversal of the normal flow of genetic information from DNA to RNA. A specific HIV enzyme protein, called reverse transcriptase (RT), converts viral RNA into DNA that may then replicate or insert itself into the host cell DNA. HIV embeds itself into host cells. This one characteristic may make the infection nearly impossible to cure, since the virus becomes part of the host cell's own genetic material.

MEANS OF INFECTION

Exposure to HIV is typically acquired by direct injection of contaminated blood, as in intravenous drug use or by infected bodily fluids such as semen. Once HIV penetrates skin or mucous membrane barriers lining the anus or vagina, it can spread and infect a great number of different cell types within the body. The cell most at risk from HIV infection is also the cell most critical for coordinating the immune response to an infection: the CD4 cell.

The attack upon these CD4 cells allows HIV to incorporate its viral genes into the host cells. The virus then freely replicates within these cells. As the virus breaks out of cells, HIV can infect more and more CD4 cells, thereby continuing the cycle. More than a billion CD4 cells are destroyed each day. HIV also infects immature immune cells in the bone marrow and thymus gland.

Over time, these tendencies exhaust the ability of the immune system to manufacture these essential lymphocytes. While the entire process remains incompletely understood, the effects of HIV killing CD4 cells, coupled with the immune system's inability to sufficiently manufacture new lymphocytes over time, appear to cause the weakened immune system of AIDS.

HIV is a chronic infection. Like most chronic infections, this retrovirus has somehow developed the ability to prevent the infection from being removed ("cleared") by the immune system. For most people, the virus quietly progresses over many years with little evidence of illness until the immune system is sufficiently weakened to allow life-threatening infections or cancers. A person only develops AIDS in the later stages of HIV infection when his immune system is so damaged that he can no longer fight off infections or tumors that are normally routine events in healthy individuals.

PROGRESSION OF HIV/AIDS

The natural history of the HIV/AIDS disease can be divided into several understandable stages.

Initial infection. Once exposure to HIV has occurred, it binds to CD4 cells and then spreads throughout the lymph system with evidence of the virus in blood circulation within five to seven days. This initial infection, called "acute HIV infection" or "acute seroconversion syndrome," produces symptoms in up to 80 to 90% of people. Typical symptoms may include fever, swollen lymph glands, sore throat, rash, muscle aches, headache, or diarrhea. The illness is often not recognized by patients or health care providers, who usually dismiss the symptoms as due to a routine cold or flu-like syndrome. The first symptoms typically start about two weeks after acquiring the infection, but in rare circumstances have taken up to ten months to occur. After the initial immune response, all symptoms subside within two to four weeks, after which HIV lives on, silently, for many years.

Established infection. Once infection is established, there appears to be an individual equilibrium between the virus and the host immune system. Normal numbers of CD4 cells average between 500 and 1400 cells per milliliter (cells/mL) of blood. Initial HIV infection often lowers this amount by one-third six months after infection. Then, for an average patient, the CD4 numbers decrease by 50 to 100 cells per year. The average amount of HIV virus detected within the blood stream is between 30 copies/mL and 50,000 copies/mL, although the range can be between less than 50 copies/mL to more than 750,000 copies/mL. This amount of HIV virus is often referred to as the viral load, a measure of newly produced viruses in the body. Some (2 to 13%)

infected with HIV have stable CD4 counts with little evidence of disease. So-called "long-term nonprogressors," their CD4 counts remain above 600 cells/mL with no antiviral therapy for more than seven years.

Immune system decline. Most individuals see a steady decline in their immune system function from HIV. Early symptomatic HIV infection may include thrush (a yeast infection of the mouth and throat), pulmonary tuberculosis (TB), shingles, or abnormal Pap smear of the cervix, and also can include serious disorders such as cervical cancer or lymphoma.

Before 1993, AIDS was defined when the immune system became weak enough to allow for odd infections or cancer. These so-called AIDS-defining conditions include in rank order:

- *Pneumocystis carinii* (a fungal pneumonia)
- HIV-related wasting syndrome (unintentional weight loss of more than 10% of body weight)
- *Cytomegalovirus* infection (usually of the eyes)
- TB
- Kaposi's sarcoma
- Disseminated *Mycobacterium avium* infection (a less virulent cousin of TB)
- Chronic herpes simplex
- HIV-related dementia
- Toxoplasmosis (a parasitic infection usually of the brain)

The Centers for Disease Control (CDC) revised the definition of AIDS in 1993 to include the sole distinction of a CD4 cell count of less than 200 cells/mL. This revision allowed identification of people at high risk of developing an AIDS-defining infection or illness within the next twelve to eighteen months.

Advanced HIV infection. Advanced HIV infection applies to individuals who have CD4 cell counts of less than 50 cells/mL. These individuals have a limited life expectancy of less than twelve to eighteen months unless HIV-related antiviral therapy is used. Causes of death typically may include one of the conditions listed above, and/or problems such as cryptococcal meningitis (due to a fungus), progressive multifocal leukoencephalopathy (chronic brain infection due to the JC virus [see below]), lymphoma, or other cancers.

WHO IS AT RISK?

HIV is not spread by casual contact or even close, nonsexual contact that would normally occur at work, in school, or at the home. Infection requires transmission of bodily fluids containing infected cells or virus such as blood, semen, or vaginal secretions. Sexual transmission and intravenous drug use remain the predominant means of acquiring HIV since the blood bank supply is now well screened.

Infection from a spouse or other sexual partner. What are the chances of becoming HIV infected from a spouse? Precise numbers are difficult to come by, but available data suggests that transmission is eight times more likely from man to woman than vice versa. If sexually transmitted diseases such as herpes or syphilis are present, this risk may be higher because these ulcer-producing infections may make HIV infection easier to acquire through tissue breaches, but regular condom use lowers the likelihood. Rates of infection in wives of HIV-infected hemophiliacs were between 20 and 25% when analyzed in reports from the mid-1980s.

Injection drug users. Injection drug use accounts for about one third of all newly reported HIV cases. Some cities have very high rates of infection in the drug-using population: In New York City it's 34 to 61% and in Baltimore, 26 to 31%, but there are fairly low rates in New Orleans (1%) and Miami (5%). The chance of becoming infected by using intravenous drugs appears to range between 3 and 4% per year. Studies have suggested that by staying in drug-treatment or needle-exchange programs, individuals may lower their risk.

Blood transfusion. Hemophiliacs were formerly at high risk of HIV infection because of a heavy reliance upon donated blood products; however, there have been very few cases since the blood bank supply began screening for HIV in 1985. The current odds of acquiring HIV from donated blood are estimated to be between 1 per 450,000 units and 1 per 600,000 units because of falsely negative blood donor screening.

Mother-to-infant transmission. Another form of transmission is from mother to infant. This perinatal transmission accounts for only a tiny percentage (less than 2%) of HIV infection in the United States, but it is vastly more common in developing countries.

Occupational exposure. Occupational exposure of health care workers has been a legitimate fear since the recognition of the epidemic. There have been surprisingly few cases of HIV infection acquired from patients. To date there have been less than 100 documented infections due to occupational exposure with an additional 200 or so cases that are "possible" but less well confirmed. Through 1999, of 56 cases confirmed by the CDC, 23 involved nurses, 19 laboratory technicians, 6 physicians, 2 surgical technicians, 1 dialysis technician, 1 respiratory therapist, 1 health aide, 1 embalmer, and 2 housekeeping or maintenance workers. Most cases involved blood exposures by accidental needle-sticks.

Household members. A frequently asked question by partners, friends, and families is whether a household member infected by HIV poses a risk to anybody living at home. To date, household transmission had been identified in only eight people, five of whom had clear exposure to bloody material from infected patients. As long as care is taken with any bloodied material, there is no risk of acquiring HIV by merely living in the same household. Even saliva from an HIV infected person does not pose a risk, so sharing of unclean glasses or utensils, while perhaps not prudent, seems to pose no unusual risk. There has only been one identified potential episode of HIV spread by kissing, and that case involved a woman deep kissing her HIV-infected male partner who had bleeding gums.

COMMON FEARS AND MISPERCEPTIONS

Some fears or misconceptions about how one contracts HIV/AIDS are shared by many. Scientific investigation has proven many untrue. These include the transmission of HIV by mosquitoes or other insects. One cannot "catch" HIV by sharing toilet seats or eating food prepared by HIV-infected individuals. This virus cannot survive for any period on inanimate surfaces, so routinely used objects about the house such as sofas, remote controls, linens, eating utensils, and telephones do not have to be disinfected or handled separately. If HIV could be transmitted in casual fashion then many more people would be currently infected.

HOW IS HIV DIAGNOSED?

Often the person who has fearfully delayed testing suspects the diagnosis of HIV. Others are blissfully unaware they have the infection until they develop AIDS.

Regardless, testing is imperative for anyone with lifestyle or occupational exposure placing him or her at risk of contracting HIV. Friends and family members should urge initial and then regular testing of anybody at risk. Since HIV is now a treatable infection, putting off the diagnosis not only is dangerous to the person, but also places society at risk for others becoming infected.

Many individuals in the United States with HIV/AIDS are not receiving medical care. Up to one third of individuals with HIV receive their diagnosis within two months of an AIDS-defining illness. There are many barriers to receiving care, including lack of insurance or chaotic lifestyles among the mentally ill or homeless. Unlike most other medical diseases, once HIV is diagnosed, homeless or financially limited patients may usually obtain government sponsored care and HIV medications without charge.

Initial HIV infection. Unfortunately, diagnosis of the acute HIV syndrome is rarely made, even though up to 90% of individuals have identifiable symptoms. The symptoms of the initial HIV infection are often no different than that of a mild-to-severe cold or flu-like illness with fever, muscle aches, headache, nausea, vomiting, diarrhea, or abdominal pain. At times, the illness may resemble infectious mononucleosis with sore throat, fever, mild rash, and swollen glands, especially of the neck.

Health care providers are increasingly recognizing this syndrome, but still, most diagnoses are suggested by the patient, who may have had a high-risk exposure. Therefore, individuals who may be at risk of acquiring HIV should not disregard viral illnesses without considering whether they may be due to HIV. Standard HIV tests are often negative in this early stage of infection, so the diagnosis is best established by using HIV RNA or HIV DNA testing using polymerase chain reactions (PCR) that specifically check for the presence of the virus. This test is often the same viral load test (quantitative RT-PCR) used to monitor people with known HIV infection.

Many AIDS experts are calling for better recognition and treatment of acute HIV infection. Early use of the right antiviral medication appears to limit further damage to the immune system, and best allows for the suppression of HIV and effective, long-lasting response to medications. For now, the earlier the diagnosis, the better the outcome.

Early or asymptomatic HIV infection. Many people who are diagnosed with HIV tend to be symptom-free. They likely acquired HIV years ago, but their immune system has not yet weakened enough to cause any of the typical problems that would point toward AIDS.

The cornerstone of HIV diagnosis is the detection of antibodies the body makes in response to the viral infection. Antibodies are specific proteins that are produced by the immune system to fight off infection. Unfortunately, antibodies made against HIV appear ineffective in the body's fight against the virus. However, these antibodies form the foundation of the current screening test, called an enzyme immunoassay (EIA), that detects these unique antibodies as indirect evidence of HIV infection. If the EIA test is positive, a confirmatory test called the Western blot is performed. This Western blot has a greater than 99.9% accuracy in detecting HIV infection. The Western blot relies upon a technique that identifies individual HIV-specific antibodies, allowing for precise identification.

False-positive tests, including the Western blot, are extremely rare, but false-negative tests may occur. The most common exception is in newly acquired HIV infection. Falsely negative tests often occur within two to four weeks of initial infection before the HIV-specific antibodies are made that result in a positive EIA. Health care providers who wish to detect HIV infection at this stage (acute HIV infection) employ one of several tests based on the PCR that specifically check for the presence of the actual human immunodeficiency virus.

HIV-2 (the sister virus of HIV-1) may remain undetected by standard HIV EIA or Western blot. HIV-2 is far more commonly found in Africa, and causes problems similar to HIV-1-related AIDS, but with a slower rate of progression. Only seventy-eight individuals in the United States were known to be infected with HIV-2 in 1998, and fifty-two of those were born in West Africa. Specialized tests are available to check these possibilities, and especially should be considered if the virus may have been acquired from a person native to Africa or Southeast Asia.

Symptomatic HIV infection. As HIV weakens the immune system, some problems may arise that do not fall into the typical AIDS classification. Most individuals do not develop any symptoms until their CD4 cell counts fall below 100 or 200. However, women with CD4 cell counts greater than 500 cells/mL may be predisposed

WHO SHOULD BE TESTED?

Who should be checked for HIV infection? If you have any doubts, this is reason alone to ask your health care provider for a test. The CDC has issued guidelines for testing based on populations at higher risk of acquiring HIV. These include:

- Persons with sexually transmitted diseases
- Persons in high-risk categories: injection drug users, gay and bisexual men, hemophiliacs, regular sex partners of persons in these categories or persons with known HIV
- Prostitutes, persons who received blood products from 1977 through May 1985, and heterosexual persons with more than one sex partner in the past twelve months or lacking regular use of protective condoms
- Persons who consider themselves at risk or request the test
- Pregnant women
- Individuals with active TB

- Both recipient and source of any occupational exposures (including any blood or internal body fluid)
- Patients aged 15 to 54 years admitted to a hospital in which more than 1% of patients have HIV infection
- Health care workers who perform exposure-prone invasive procedures
- Blood and tissue organ donors
- Anybody who has clinical symptoms or laboratory findings that suggest HIV infection

Issues of confidentiality

Confidentiality remains an important issue to many people. Informed consent for HIV testing is required in forty-one states. With the widespread dissemination of medical information for insurance and employer payment purposes, HIV testing is often not confidential. Many hospitals, laboratories and public health offices have established a truly confidential testing process whereby samples are

to recurrent or severe bouts of vaginal infections due to the yeast *Candida*. Both sexes may note swollen, nontender lymph glands in areas about the neck, under the arms, or in the groin, a condition called progressive, generalized lymphadenopathy.

When CD4 cell counts fall to 200 to 500 cells/mL, infectious problems may include recurrent bacterial pneumonia, pulmonary TB, shingles (herpes zoster), thrush (*Candida* infection of the mouth or throat), *Candida* esophagitis, oral hairy leukoplakia (white, furry coating of the tongue due to the Epstein-Barr virus) or

identified by a code only known to the person tested, rather than the sample linked by identification of name or Social Security number. If confidential testing is important to you, be certain to inquire about testing procedures so that anonymous testing is performed.

Home testing

HIV testing in the privacy of one's home is possible. There are a number of different HIV home collection test systems and kits that have appeared on the market, available through the Internet and through magazine or newspaper promotions. However, only one HIV-1 Home Collection Test System is currently approved by the United States Food and Drug Administration (FDA), the Home Access Express HIV-1 Test System manufactured by Home Access Health Corporation.

Because the Home Access test consists of multiple components, including materials for specimen collection, a mailing envelope to send the specimen to a laboratory for analysis, and includes pre- and posttest counseling, it is considered a testing system.

This approved system uses a simple finger prick process for home blood collection which results in dried blood spots on special paper. The dried blood spots are mailed to a laboratory with a confidential and anonymous personal identification number (PIN), and analyzed by trained clinicians in a certified medical laboratory using the same procedures that are used for samples taken in a doctor's office. The results are obtained by the purchaser through a toll free telephone number using the PIN, and posttest counseling is provided by telephone when results are obtained. (Information from the U. S. Food and Drug Administration Web site [http://www.fda.gov/cber/infosheets/hiv-home2.htm], accessed June 30, 2002.)

Kaposi's sarcoma (a malignancy due to human herpes virus 8, HHV-8). Noninfectious complications possible during this stage include abnormal Pap smears or cervical cancer in women. Hodgkin's or non-Hodgkin's lymphoma occur more frequently than in non-HIV-infected individuals. Anemia and certain blood disorders are also more prevalent.

Any of these problems diagnosed by a health care provider should prompt HIV testing, especially if no alternative cause is obvious.

HOW IS AIDS DIAGNOSED?

A person is only diagnosed with AIDS when the immune system has weakened sufficiently to cause a characteristic opportunistic infection or problem, or the CD4 cell count has fallen below 200 cells/mL. As the CD4 count continues to fall, any of the problems listed above become more likely. Because the immune system is so critical for the body's balance with its environment, just about any problem can develop, and physicians identify new problems almost every year. Additionally, a severely weakened immune system often predisposes people with AIDS to more than just one infection or problem at a time. For example, bacterial pneumonia and fungal infection may be present simultaneously.

An opportunistic infection is so termed because the infection would not become established in a person with a normal, healthy immune system. Typically, these infections are commonplace microbes found in air, water, food, or soil that rarely cause trouble for most people. Certain frequent opportunistic infections are prevented by the use of medications prescribed when the CD4 counts are appropriately low. Besides the problems listed below, people with AIDS can also have any of the problems listed in the Symptomatic HIV Infection section (see p. 351).

Pneumonia. *Pneumocystis carinii* pneumonia (PCP) remains a common problem, often the first illness in individuals who do not know they have AIDS. This fungus causes a dry, hacking cough along with fever and shortness of breath as the infection spreads within the lungs. Bacterial pneumonias (especially with *Streptococcus pneumoniae*) are more common in people symptomatic from HIV.

Fungal infections. Several other fungal infections may strike individuals with AIDS. Cryptococcosis often causes a chronic meningitis or lung infection. Residents of California or the Southwestern United States with AIDS may be exposed to coccidioidomycosis, a fungus present in sand and soil that can cause infections, especially of the bone, skin, muscle, brain, or joints. Individuals with AIDS living in the Mississippi or Ohio River valleys may succumb to histoplasmosis, a bacterial infection from a common resident of water and soil that in immunosuppressed humans may cause meningitis, lung infections, or infection that spreads widely throughout the body.

Cytomegalovirus (CMV). A member of the herpesvirus family, cytomegalovirus (CMV), is a common infection that can cause vision loss when it reactivates in the retina because of a waning immune response. This eye disease is diagnosed by an ophthalmologist looking for characteristic damage to the retina. CMV retinitis may cause blindness if not treated promptly. CMV may also infect almost any organ in the body, including the intestines, the esophagus, the brain, the bone marrow, or the liver. Diagnosis of CMV infection in these organs usually requires a biopsy of tissue.

JC virus. A less commonly encountered viral infection causes progressive multifocal leukoencephalopathy. Individuals with this disorder suffer from seizures, dementia, delirium, and neurological weakness, caused by the JC virus, which may progress with frightening speed. Existing therapies are poor at halting this brain infection.

Parasitic infections. Parasites are single-celled animals capable of living within an agreeable host. Unfortunately, the weakened immune system of individuals with AIDS makes them ideal hosts for many parasites. Toxoplasmosis most commonly causes a brain infection that can cause seizures, weakness, or behavioral changes. Though usually ascribed to handling cat feces or kitty litter, toxoplasmosis is acquired most often by eating the parasitic cysts in undercooked meats such as beef.

The most common parasitic infections in AIDS patients are found in the gut, where they can cause chronic, loose, or watery bowel movements, and abdominal cramping. Malabsorption, or faulty absorption of nutritive material from the intestine, is a frequent problem that may foster progressive weight loss and weakness. A number of parasites can cause these intestinal problems but the most common are cryptosporidia and microsporidia, both of which are fiendishly difficult to treat. These parasites are most commonly acquired by drinking contaminated water.

Tuberculosis and *Mycobacterium avium* complex. Tuberculosis threatens many AIDS patients, and may be frequently found in organs other than the lung. When CD4 counts fall to less than 50 cells/mL, a cousin of TB called *Mycobacterium avium* complex infection often causes fever, weight loss, abdominal pain, diarrhea, and anemia.

Neurological complications and HIV dementia. For reasons not completely understood, neurological complications are frequent in AIDS patients, but only some are directly attributable to actions of the human immunodeficiency virus. Other neurological complications include development of numbness or tingling in the feet and possibly weakness. Medically termed peripheral neuropathy, this can occur in the setting of AIDS, although many drugs used to treat HIV infection also cause this problem. One of the most devastating illnesses is HIV dementia. Up to 10 to 15% of AIDS patients experience this problem, which may cause impairment of memory or concentration along with inattentiveness and confusion. As HIV dementia worsens over months, muscle weakness, speech impairments, inability to eat, and even coma may develop.

Other complications. Various other problems that can arise include congestive heart failure from HIV directly weakening the heart muscle in the setting of AIDS. The most common cancer is lymphoma, although in AIDS, the lymphoma may affect the brain more frequently and aggressively.

Up to 18% of AIDS patients experience HIV-related wasting syndrome. This is defined as involuntary weight loss of more than 10% of baseline body mass, along with chronic diarrhea, weakness, and fever not attributable to any other identifiable cause such as an infection. Underweight HIV patients may find some benefit with a number of prescription drugs such as anabolic steroids, like Megace (megestrol acetate), that may stimulate the appetite and increase body mass.

Because advanced HIV infection may cause so many different symptoms, problems that should prompt HIV testing include:

- Generalized swelling of lymph glands
- Unexplained dementia
- Meningitis
- Peripheral neuropathy
- Chronic or unexplained fever
- Chronic diarrhea
- Unusual weight loss

Some routine laboratory tests that may prompt testing for HIV include:

- Findings of anemia
- Low platelet count
- Low white blood cell count (especially low lymphocyte counts)
- Elevated amounts of antibodies

WHAT SHOULD YOU EXPECT?

Once HIV becomes an established infection, it remains life-long since no cure is yet known. For an average patient without any specific treatment for HIV, ten to twelve years elapse from initial infection until death. There appear to be no clearly defining differences in this timeline according to race, gender, or ethnicity. For approximately 20% of HIV-infected individuals, AIDS develops more quickly, in as little as five years. This life expectancy was typical before the use of newer drugs that can halt or slow HIV's assault on the immune system.

If HIV is diagnosed during the acute phase of infection (acute HIV syndrome) or within six months of initial infection, early antiviral treatment should be strongly considered, because much scientific evidence suggests this is the best possible strategy to arrest damage from HIV.

SPEED OF PROGRESSION

Two factors that portend faster progression to AIDS include an illness of more than fourteen days during the acute infection as well as the presence of thrush or prolonged fever. Findings published in 1997 showed that viral loads of greater than 30,000 viral copies/mL greatly predicted fast progression to AIDS. HIV-infected individuals with high viral loads had a median survival of only 4.4 years until an AIDS-related death, while viral loads of less than 10,000 viral copies/mL meant reduced risks of developing AIDS, with median survival of more than ten years.

From studies done on people who do not progress to full-blown AIDS for many years (called "long-term nonprogressors"), HIV-specific CD4 cells that are able to fight the HIV virus appear to be much higher than in individuals at the same stage of infection who ultimately progress to AIDS. This finding may not be so surprising, since the CD4 cells coordinate immune responses. Preliminary studies indicate that aggressive antiretroviral therapy very early into HIV infection protects activated HIV-specific CD4 cells from damaging effects of HIV infection. This may preserve immune responsiveness to naturally fight the HIV infection, as in nonprogressor populations.

For those outside the initial six-month window of treatment, important treatments will be detailed below. The development of highly active antiretroviral therapy has revolutionized the treatment of HIV/AIDS and stemmed what had been a terminal disease. Starting with the use of highly active antiretroviral therapy in 1996, there has been a 23% decline in deaths attributed to AIDS and an additional 47% decline by 1997. The incidence of opportunistic infections has declined by 60 to 80%. For individuals with HIV who have access to these advanced therapies, fear of imminent death has been replaced by the potential for long, productive lives.

PROVEN INTERVENTIONS

Four therapeutic interventions have been proven to prolong survival:

- Highly active antiretroviral therapy
- Prevention of *Pneumocystis carinii* pneumonia for CD4 cell counts less than 200 cells/mL, by using sulfa (or similar) drugs
- Prevention of *Mycobacterium avium* infection in individuals with CD4 counts less than 50 cells/mL, by using the antibiotics clarithromycin or azithromycin
- A health care provider with significant HIV-care experience (defined as experience in the care of more than fifty patients with HIV/AIDS)

HIV infection is still often handled by both patients and health care providers as an infectious disease or purely medical problem. There is growing recognition that how one deals emotionally with HIV is the single most important factor in predicting successful treatment. For example, effective counseling of HIV-infected patients and anybody in their support system in some studies is a better predictor of improvement in quality of life than any purely medical parameter such as CD4 counts or HIV viral load determinations. Mental health problems such as depression are especially common following diagnosis with HIV, occurring in up to 20% of HIV-infected individuals. It is significantly associated with perceived poor health and interference with activities of daily living. Every effort should be made to educate the HIV-infected to important aspects of their disease, and to provide counseling or mental health treatment if necessary. Many partners, family, and friends find that caring for someone with HIV/AIDS can strengthen bonds with that person.

HOW IS IT TREATED?

AZT. The first drug used to treat HIV infection, zidovudine (AZT, Retrovir), was originally developed in 1964 as a potential cancer treatment but was shelved when proven to be less than effective. Scientists found that this nearly forgotten drug was highly effective against an enzyme critical in the early stage of HIV replication called reverse transcriptase. Drugs similar to AZT were soon developed that also targeted this enzyme. Called nucleoside analogs (NRTI's or "nukes"), this group includes didanosine (ddI, Videx), zalcitabine (ddC, Hivid), stavudine (d4T, Zerit), lamivudine (3TC, Epivir), and abacavir (Ziagen).

Although potent in the test tube, these drugs did not cause durable suppression of HIV in the body. The virus was able to mutate even in the face of two or three of these drugs with uncanny speed.

HAART: The AIDS cocktail. When a new class of drugs was developed against a different target within the HIV virus, called the viral protease, the new era of "AIDS cocktail" or highly active antiretroviral treatment (HAART) arrived. First released in 1996, these new drugs called protease inhibitors proved especially potent when combined with nucleoside analogs such as AZT or 3TC. Available protease inhibitors include amprenavir (Agenerase), indinavir (Crixivan), nelfinavir (Viracept), ritonavir (Norvir) and saquinavir (Fortovase or Invirase).

Other drugs, called nonnucleoside reverse transcriptase inhibitors (NNRTIs or "non-nukes") also joined the parade that now totals fourteen medications available for HIV infection. These NNRTI's include nevirapine (Viramune), delavirdine (Rescriptor), and efavirenz (Sustiva); this last drug has become quickly popular because of its once-daily dosing.

HAART has become a miracle for many individuals with AIDS who had been facing near-certain death. HAART is a combination of antiretroviral drugs, most commonly combining three or more anti-HIV drugs. They are highly successful because the nucleoside analogs and nonnucleoside reverse transcriptase inhibitors stop HIV from replicating in an early phase of viral replication while the protease inhibitors work at a later step. There are over two hundred and fifty potential combinations of drugs using three of the available anti-HIV medication classes, although some are more commonly used than others.

Several groups have published recommendations regarding appropriate combinations of drugs for HAART. The International AIDS Society, USA (www.iasusa.org) and The Department of Health and Human Services/Kaiser Family Foundation (DHHS/KFF) (www.hivatis.org) publish recommendations on their Web sites. The DHHS/KFF is updated monthly. DHHS/KFF uses an expert panel to recommend specific drug combinations that in well-designed studies appear to work against HIV with acceptable side effect profiles.

TAKING MEDICATIONS

Both guideline groups freely admit that there are many acceptable regimens. Often HIV health care providers must factor many aspects before deciding on a specific combination. One especially important factor is the development of drug resistance. Greatly feared by treating health care providers, since entire classes of drugs become less potent, this especially happens when the antiretroviral drug doses are missed on a regular basis. Any decision to enter drug therapy should not then be done casually. Often the initial therapeutic regimen of drugs works the best.

Successful response to treatment is closely tied to strict adherence (taking all medications without missing doses). One study showed that if adherence to HAART therapy was greater than 95%, then there was a greater than 81% chance of achieving low HIV viral loads. If there is a less than 70% daily adherence to HAART then there is a less than 6% chance of successfully achieving a low viral load. When resistance does develop, subsequent trials of drug combinations always carry a higher risk of treatment failure.

REMINDER SYSTEMS

The single most important act for HIV-infected patients to perform is to make taking their medication the top priority. Many individuals develop a reminder system to prompt pill popping to occur on schedule. Digital wristwatches with alarms are favored by many, while several manufacturers have made pillboxes with alarm systems. Taking HAART is seldom easy, because the burden of pills can be as high as between twenty and thirty pills daily—often with some taken on empty stomachs while others need to be taken with meals. Research is under way to simplify regimens so that the pill burden can be reduced. Even now, some HAART regimens may be taken with as few as five pills a day.

GOALS OF HAART THERAPY

Goals of HIV therapy should both improve the quality of life while prolonging it. Realistically, the current HAART therapy achieves this goal by reducing the viral load to low or undetectable levels (viral suppression) for as long as possible. This maneuver appears to halt progression to AIDS, and lessens the chances of the emergence of resistant viral mutants. Ideally, the drugs used should have minimal side effects and allow someone to realistically comply with the directed pill burden. The primary numerical goal of HAART therapy is to reduce the HIV viral load to low (fewer than 50 copies/mL) or undetectable levels. This goal should be achieved by week 24 after initiation of HAART.

For many, this goal is not obtainable since only 15 to 30% of patients achieve this sustained level. However, other studies suggest that keeping viral load less than 5000 copies/mL correlates with a less than 5% chance of developing AIDS-defining complications. For individuals who sustain viral suppression, there is an average rise of 100 to 200 CD4 cells/mL in the first year. Subsequent increases then occur, but are lower and more gradual.

WHEN TO START THERAPY

When to start HIV therapy remains one of the more divisive issues in HIV management. Assuming the person is ready and responsible for HIV treatment, most experts and guideline committees try to divide HIV-infected individuals into groups that have either a low likelihood of progression to AIDS (the "nonprogressors") or groups with assured rapid evolution into AIDS. For example, it is highly recommended that treatment begin for individuals with HIV viral loads of greater than 20,000 or 30,000 copies/mL, regardless of CD4 count, since high viral load measurement is the best single predictor for progression to AIDS. Conversely, if the viral load is less than 5,000 and the CD4 cell count is greater than 500 cells/mL, then this person may well be an HIV nonprogressor, so close observation is recommended, but treatment held off. Individuals that fall in between these two groups are generally advocated to start therapy, or at least give it strong consideration.

WHEN MEDICATIONS DO NOT WORK

HAART regimens may fail to achieve low viral loads for a number of reasons but most commonly this is due to patients not taking their antiretroviral medications.

Other reasons include inadequate potency of the drug combination, insufficient drug absorption, and viral resistance to the prescribed medications. Medicines may be changed if viral loads rise consistently during therapy, or do not fall sufficiently low. Failure of the CD4 count to increase, or even development of opportunistic infections in the setting of low viral load measurements, do not necessarily mean that the medications should be changed.

Drug regimens that are devised after the failure of a HAART treatment are often called salvage or rescue therapy. Some experts use the patient's previous drug history to guide them as to what new drugs to chose and which to avoid. Assessment of an individual patient's viral resistance is now possible using either HIV genotyping or phenotyping methods, but many experts criticize these costly techniques because they often do not identify up to 20% or more of the resistant virus types. Laboratory assessment of HIV resistance may be a better indicator of which medications to avoid, rather than which to use. Some HIV health care providers prefer not to use any viral resistance testing, and merely see if an individual's response to the medication adequately lowers viral burden since this is what truly matters.

ALTERNATIVE TREATMENTS

When HAART medications fail to reverse the progressive damage of the HIV virus and health begins to fail, some individuals turn to alternative health methods in desperation. Unfortunately, there are many remedies hawked by well-meaning as well as mercenary groups that promise to boost the immune system or fight the progressive ills of AIDS. The U. S. Food and Drug Administration has a dedicated AIDS Health Fraud Task Force that has investigated suspicious, unapproved therapies such as heavy water, ozone, and hydrogen peroxide therapies. Still, many HIV patients use megadose vitamin and nutritional supplements, herbs, chelation, and heat-shock treatments in the belief that they may "boost" the immune system. These are just a few of the costly therapies that have failed to provide their purported benefit. The federal government has gone so far as to prosecute individuals in Maryland and Virginia on charges of fraud related to their promotion of aloe vera injections for the treatment of AIDS and cancer. Any treatments that fall outside of the mainstream should be scrutinized closely, and discussed with the treating health care provider.

MEDICATION SIDE EFFECTS

A comprehensive listing of HAART side effects is beyond the scope of this chapter. Common side effects of any medication may be found in information provided by a qualified pharmacist, health care provider, or several of the Web-based groups listed in the resource section at the end of this chapter.

All HAART regimens may cause gastrointestinal side effects including nausea, vomiting, diarrhea, or loss of appetite. Often these symptoms may moderate after the first few weeks of therapy. Medications such as ddI, d4T, and ddC have a higher incidence of causing peripheral neuropathy, which may result in burning pains or numbness of the feet and occasionally weakness. AZT may produce mild anemia. Rash may occur when taking any NNRTI. Approximately 5% of patients have a severe rash, and some fatalities have been noted, especially with use of abacavir. Inflammation of the pancreas may be a consequence of ddI, ritonavir, or 3TC (in children). Individuals using these drugs may suffer from severe abdominal pain, nausea, and vomiting (also known as pancreatitis). In some cases, patients have died from these side effects.

A peculiar set of problems can occur in populations taking protease inhibitors. By no means universal, some patients taking protease inhibitors develop diabetes with elevated blood sugars, or elevated blood cholesterol, or an odd fat redistribution syndrome. This change in body fat distribution is sometimes also called the "lipodystrophy syndrome" or "pseudo-Cushing's syndrome." Fat may accumulate on the upper back (the so-called "buffalo hump") or around the abdomen. Wasting of both muscle and fat occurs in the arms and legs. Similar changes have also been described in HIV-infected individuals who are not receiving protease inhibitors, so whether these drugs are affecting a single process or multiple aspects is unclear.

These potential protease inhibitor-induced changes may occur singly or in combination. At this time, it is unclear exactly how often these changes occur and when in the time course of taking protease inhibitor medications. There are also no universal recommendations for monitoring but some authorities recommend blood glucose screening two or three times a year with periodic assessments of blood cholesterol and triglyceride levels. Treatment of elevated cholesterol can be tricky as medications used to lower cholesterol may interact with the protease inhibitors. For either elevated cholesterol or body fat redistribution, these difficulties may reverse with cessation of protease inhibitor use. However, this decision requires careful analysis by both patient and health care provider given the effectiveness of protease inhibitors in prevention of AIDS.

Medication side effects that even include potential fatalities can add a daunting feature to an already challenging set of problems that make treating HIV more complicated than diabetes or cancer. Though not perfect, these medications do have the capability of stanching the relentless advance of HIV. An optimistic rather than fretful approach to HIV treatment will better one's odds of doing well with treatment.

LABORATORY TESTS

HIV-infected individuals who are starting HAART should expect to have HIV viral load measured immediately before and at two to eight weeks after starting therapy and periodically (three to four months) thereafter, to monitor the effectiveness of therapy. If the viral load is not undetectable (meaning below the limits of the test) or less than 50 copies/mL, the medications may be changed. CD4 counts do not need to be checked frequently, but are rather a more important component of staging the disease so that decisions regarding prophylaxis of opportunistic infections can be made. Other tests that a health care provider may order include complete blood counts (CBC), since abnormalities of blood cells are very common in HIV infection and can be affected by medications, and chemistry panels to assess kidney and liver function.

Patients with HIV often are at risk of other infections that can be spread by intravenous drug abuse or sexual transmission. Blood tests are recommended for assessing exposure to hepatitis A, B, or C viruses, and syphilis. A skin test (Mantoux, PPD) is mandatory for determining prior exposure to TB. HIV-infected women need regular gynecological examinations and Pap smears because of their high rates of venereal diseases, pelvic inflammatory disease, atypical Pap smears and cervical cancer.

PREVENTING OPPORTUNISTIC INFECTIONS

For patients with AIDS, meaning CD4 counts less than 200 cells/mL, medications are prescribed to prevent some common opportunistic infections. Taking sulfa drugs such as trimethoprim-sulfamethoxazole (Bactrim, Septra) daily can significantly lessen risk for the most common opportunistic infection, *P. carinii* pneumonia. Alternatives such as dapsone daily or aerosolized pentamidine monthly may be used in cases of sulfa intolerance.

Evidence of past exposure to TB is based on the Mantoux skin test. Purified, sterile proteins of the TB bacteria are injected just under the top layer of skin on the forearm. Within two or three days, if sufficient swelling develops, then the test is positive, meaning that either active or dormant TB exists. A chest x-ray or other tests may be needed to determine whether active TB is present. To prevent dormant TB from reactivating, isoniazid (INH) taken with pyridoxine (vitamin B6) is given for nine months.

The parasite *Toxoplasma gondii* can cause devastating brain infections in AIDS patients. If an antibody test for *Toxoplasma* is positive and CD4 counts are less than 100 cells/mL then daily sulfa drugs such as trimethoprim-sulfamethoxazole, or dapsone plus pyrimethamine and leucovorin, are recommended for prevention. Individuals with HIV/AIDS are urged not to handle cat feces or kitty litter, which may contain toxoplasma cysts. Thorough cooking of meats is also recommended since ingestion of rare meat is a leading cause of acquiring the parasite.

A relative of TB, *Mycobacterium avium* complex (MAC), occurs in up to 50% of AIDS patients with CD4 counts less than 50 cells/mL. This infection may cause severe wasting, fevers, abdominal pain, diarrhea, and anemia. Preferred medications that reduce the risk of developing MAC include erythromycin-like drugs—either clarithromycin daily or azithromycin weekly.

Many AIDS patients who take HAART experience increases in CD4 counts as the HIV viral load is suppressed. The rebuilding of the immune system depends upon maintaining a healthy lifestyle. That means eating well, performing regular exercise and not smoking, drinking, or using illicit drugs. This immune reconstitution does not happen in every individual; however, those who have CD4 counts greater than 100 cells/mL for six months may discontinue treatment for MAC and toxoplasma. As counts rise above 200 cells/mL for six months then even PCP treatment can be discontinued. These heartening events were not even imaginable five years ago.

Because of the success of HAART, many HIV-infected people formerly facing death are now living normal lives. HIV health care providers have been increasingly directing routine health care for issues that would be the same as for non-

HIV-infected people of the same age—for example, screening for cholesterol, diabetes, and breast, colon, and prostate cancers.

Some vaccines are routinely recommended for HIV-infected individuals. For gay men and individuals who use intravenous drugs, hepatitis B immunization should be given to everybody who does not have evidence of prior infection. Immunization against hepatitis A is advocated especially for gay men, injection drug users, and individuals infected with hepatitis C. Many health care providers recommend annual influenza immunization.

WHAT RESEARCH IS BEING DONE?

Despite the great progress in recognition and treatment of HIV infection, it is not yet time to declare victory over HIV and AIDS. Many questions remain regarding the long-term effectiveness and safety of HAART drug regimens. Critical to any future gains over the virus, basic science investigation remains fundamental to better understanding of HIV and the human immune response to this infection. The National Institutes of Health plans to asked the U. S. Congress for $2.7 billion directed toward HIV research for fiscal year 2003.

Vaccine development. The goal for prevention of any infectious disease is a vaccine. This strategy has worked fabulously well to vanquish maladies such as polio, measles, and mumps from industrialized societies. The need for an HIV vaccine has become ever more dire, as the frightening dimensions and staggering costs of the global AIDS epidemic grow. Few countries can afford the costs of HAART regimens that can cost as much as $15,000 a year for a single patient. Unfortunately, vaccines tested to date have failed to either protect from HIV infection or even boost the immune system response against the virus. Several vaccines are in early human clinical trials, although none have generated particularly high expectations. For the moment, the highest priority is to arrest the alarming spread of the disease in the developing world.

New medications. Pharmaceutical research efforts are under way both to develop new medications to overcome the problem of drug-resistant strains and to simplify drug regimens so individuals can take fewer pills daily. One investigational medication that may soon come to market (the manufacturer plans to submit it to the FDA for approval in Fall 2002) is emtricitabine, a drug that is similar to the nucleoside analog 3TC, and tenofovir, which was approved by the FDA in October 2001, is closely related to adefovir, a nucleotide analog. These two drugs may represent an improvement over existing drugs because of their once-daily dosing. Several new protease inhibitors that have been designed to be dosed once a day are in the early stages of development. A number of novel drugs are in development that target other stages in the HIV life cycle that may prove to be especially useful as resistance problems grow with wider use of antiretroviral medications.

By seeking to improve on the existing HIV antiretroviral medications, many studies have been published and more are under way that ask whether these medications can be taken on a simplified schedule. Some evidence already exists that supports the use of either ddI or 3TC once daily, but adoption of this dosing schedule has not become widespread yet, and is likely to remain this way until more trials are performed.

Clinical trials. The AIDS Clinical Trial Group helps coordinate many trials relevant to HIV/AIDS. Many studies are ongoing that either study specific combinations of antiretroviral medications or their use in specific situations, such as recent HIV infection or salvage therapy. Given the many potential combinations, all drug regimens cannot be studied. Moreover, as HIV has become a treatable disease with HAART, recruitment of study patients has become more difficult.

In perhaps no other area of medicine today is treatment changing as rapidly as in the area of HIV care. Not infrequently, practices are adopted that may be based on only theory or limited experimental data. Trends in HIV care are often faddish and quick to change. One such strategy that has received attention is called structured treatment interruption. Though based on skimpy data, this approach is based on an observation that for some individuals who stop taking their HAART medications, resistant HIV viral strains tended to decrease while original drug susceptible viruses reemerged to dominate. This virus appeared to be more easily suppressed when HAART was restarted. Another potential benefit is that the HIV-specific immune responses may be boosted by repeated exposure to high levels of the virus. This maneuver may assist controlling the virus, whereas HIV-specific immune responses wane when there is prolonged or complete viral suppression. Trials presented to date are not large enough to draw any conclusions yet, but unfortunately many well-read HIV-infected patients or adventuresome health care practitioners have already seized upon this data to embrace structured treatment interruption.

HOW CAN IT BE PREVENTED?

Condoms and spermicides. Unprotected sexual intercourse (either heterosexual or homosexual) is the predominant mode of HIV transmission throughout the world. Consistent use of male latex condoms has been effective in the prevention of HIV. However, condoms may break or slippage may occur, reducing their effectiveness. The female condom (an intravaginal pouch) can be as effective as the male condom in stopping HIV transmission as well as other venereal diseases. For reasons not well understood, the female condom has a contraceptive failure rate of up to 26%. The contraceptive failure rate has therefore limited the role of the female condom. An active area of research centers on vaginally applied microbicide preparations as a prevention of HIV and other sexually transmitted diseases.

Despite well-demonstrated benefits, many studies have shown low rates of condom use among sexually active homosexual and heterosexual men. Use of alcohol or drugs is routinely associated with even lower condom use. In San Francisco, a study found that oral sex provided the route of HIV transmission in 8% of men who had sex with men. Oral sex may be safer than anal or vaginal sex, but it is not safe sex. Condom use during oral sex can lower the risk of infection.

Abstinence and monogamy. Although abstinence is the most effective method to prevent sexual transmission of HIV, monogamous couples have low rates of HIV infection, and generally adopt safe sex practices more often than those who have multiple sex partners. Partner notification is another mechanism that may lower the rate of sexual transmission of HIV.

Injection drug use. Injection drug users have lower rates of drug use and HIV infection if they are enrolled in drug-treatment programs. However, an estimated 80% of active drug users in the United States are not in programs either because of choice or lack of availability. Many drug users are asked to bleach their needles and syringes in order to sterilize any HIV present. However, studies in Baltimore and New York City did not find this practice effective. Some municipalities have established needle-exchange programs or allow purchase of needles and injection equipment without prescription by a health care provider.

Blood transfusion. Acquiring HIV by blood transfusion or organ transplantation is now an extremely rare event in the United States since high-risk populations are no longer allowed to donate, and all blood products and organ tissues are screened for HIV. Predonation of blood for planned surgical procedures, if feasible, would logically reduce any risk of acquiring HIV.

PREGNANT WOMEN

All pregnant women are recommended to undergo HIV testing. For HIV-positive women, use of intravenous AZT during labor lowers by 66% the chances of the baby becoming infected by HIV. For women already on HAART who conceive, there are no formal recommendations regarding their therapy, but generally they should continue drug treatment according to standard guidelines throughout the pregnancy, although this decision must be individualized with each women and her health care provider. To date, fetal registries have not shown higher rates of congenital defects from mothers who used HAART during their pregnancy.

Some health care providers recommend a delay or interruption of therapy during the first trimester of pregnancy. If the pregnant woman's HAART regimen does not include AZT, this drug should be added. Efavirenz and hydroxyurea should be avoided during the pregnancy because of known problems with fetal malformations. Breast-feeding may cause transmission of HIV to the baby, so use of formula is recommended.

UNIVERSAL PRECAUTIONS

For health care workers, universal precautions have been adopted, since the risks of HIV and other infections cannot be known for every patient. Therefore, every patient should be treated as if he or she might have HIV. This strategy depends on using gloves in all situations that may cause exposure to body fluids, as well as following safe work practices regarding disposal of needles and other sharp or surgical instruments.

In case of accidental exposure, especially by needlestick, the United States Public lic Health Service recommends that every wound be thoroughly washed with soap and water, or mucous membranes be flushed vigorously. If their HIV status is not

CARING FOR HIV-INFECTED PERSONS

Although HIV has been transmitted between family members in the household setting, this type of transmission is extraordinarily rare. To prevent even such rare occurrences, the CDC has published a set of recommendations to prevent exposures to blood from persons who are HIV infected or at risk for HIV infection:

• Gloves should be worn during contact with blood or other body fluids that could contain blood, such as urine, feces, or vomit.

• Cuts, sores, or breaks on caregiver and patients' exposed skin should be covered with bandages.

• Hands and other parts of the body should be washed immediately after contact with blood or other body fluids. Surfaces soiled with blood should be disinfected appropriately.

• Practices that increase the likelihood of blood contact, such as sharing of razors and tooth-brushes, should be avoided.

• Needles and other sharp instruments should be used only when medically necessary and handled according to recommendations for health care settings. (Do not put caps back on needles by hand or remove needles from syringes. Dispose of needles in puncture-proof containers.)

known, every patient who is the source of an exposure should be tested for HIV as well as hepatitis viruses.

Depending on the likelihood of the source being HIV-infected and the kind of exposure, postexposure treatment may be recommended. For most high-risk exposures, the Centers for Disease Control suggest using AZT and 3TC. Other drugs such as protease inhibitors may be added, if the source patient is HIV-infected or he was already taking HAART or had done so in the recent past.

Some investigators have tried to address whether antiretroviral drugs are useful in situations other than occupational exposures that may lead to high risk of acquiring HIV, e.g., following unprotected sex or sharing of needles. Use of AZT and 3TC has been proposed to lessen the chances of becoming HIV infected in such settings. However, data to support this practice are not available. Use of postexposure treatment in these settings must be considered an unproven intervention that should be discussed by patient and physician.

WHAT YOU CAN DO NOW

The first step for many individuals is acknowledging that they either have a risk of acquiring HIV or may already have it. Individuals should be tested routinely if they use intravenous drugs or do not practice safe sex. Testing can be performed by a health care practitioner or by the local public health department.

If a person tests positive for HIV, they can seek care from health care providers or practices that have experience caring for individuals infected with HIV. Local county medical societies usually maintain lists of physicians who specialize in HIV care. Physicians with expertise in the subspecialty of infectious diseases may have active HIV practices, or can refer you to one. Hospitals in cities or academic medical institutions may maintain HIV clinics that practice high-quality care. If a health care practitioner currently is caring for 50 or more HIV-infected patients, this correlates with better outcomes. The AIDS Clinical Trials Group Web site (www.actis.org) lists trials and locations of many investigational studies. The medical practices and the medical schools participating in these trials have high levels of HIV care, and may be excellent resources for second opinions if needed.

As important as medical care is, it is equally important that people with HIV/AIDS have both informational and emotional support to fight HIV infection. Ignorance is no friend, especially when dealing with a foe as crafty and complex as the human immunodeficiency virus. Partners, family, and friends can participate in smoothing out the emotional roller coaster ride that comes with a positive HIV diagnosis. Organizations listed in the Additional Resources section have excellent information, hotlines, and/or counseling services.

ADDITIONAL RESOURCES

ORGANIZATIONS

Centers for Disease Control and Prevention (CDC)
AIDS Hotline: 800-342-AIDS (2437)
In Spanish: 800-344-7432
TTY 800-243-7889

www.cdc.gov/hiv
Popular 24-hour hotline and Web pages feature comprehensive information about HIV/AIDS treatment, prevention, and other services.

Gay Men's Health Crisis Hotline

212-87-6655 or 800-AIDS-NYC (243-7692)

www.gmhc.org

The Gay Men's Health Crisis has a hotline offering information about medical treatments, supportive care health insurance, housing, and estate planning for individuals in all stages of the illness. Mental health services are provided for individuals with HIV as well as their partners, family, and friends, including free individual psychotherapy and support groups.

HIV/AIDS Treatment Information Service (ATIS)

800-HIV-0440 (800-448-0440)

www.hivatis.org

Frequently updated, federally approved guidelines for the treatment of HIV and AIDS-related infections.

The National Women's Health Information Center (NWHIC)

800-994-WOMAN

www.4women.gov

General women's health information also provides links to publications and other organizations by using their search engine: enter AIDS, under topics.

AIDS Clinical Trials Information Service (ACTIS)

800-TRIALS-A (800-874-2572)

www.actis.org

Site lists federally and privately funded HIV-related clinical trials.

The National Association of People With AIDS (NAPWA)

202-898-0414

www.napwa.org

Group provides educational programs and reading material for many aspects of HIV care.

National Institute of Allergy and Infectious Diseases, National Institutes of Health (NIAID) 301-496-5717

www.niaid.nih.gov/publications/aids.htm

Site offers up-to-date treatment information on infectious, allergic, and immunologic diseases, including AIDS and hepatitis.

HIV InSite

www.hivinsite.ucsf.edu

A project of the University of California San Francisco (UCSF) Positive Health Program at San Francisco General Hospital Medical Center and the UCSF Center for AIDS Prevention Studies, which are programs of the UCSF AIDS Research Institute.

BOOKS

Bartlett, John G. *Medical Management of HIV Infection*. Baltimore: Port City Press, 1999. (Full text can be found online at http://hopkins-aids.edu/publications/index_pub.html.)

Updated annually, this comprehensive but practical guide has become indispensable for many HIV health care providers.

Multiple Sclerosis

Multiple sclerosis (MS), a chronic disease of the central nervous system, is one of the leading causes of disability in young people. Unlike many neurologic diseases, which are more likely to strike as a person grows older, MS initially occurs most often in people between the ages of 20 and 40. It is a disease of alternating flare-ups and remissions with an unpredictable course that can severely impair a person's functioning—or have minimal impact on someone's life. Because of the variable but often progressive nature of MS, it places a unique burden on caregivers, whose hands-on services may not always be needed, especially in earlier stages of the disease, but who may find themselves called upon to assist in the most basic of activities of daily living later in the course of this illness.

Until the past decade, doctors could offer people with MS little more than treatment for symptoms and supportive care. In the past seven years, however, four different medications have been approved to treat the disease itself, offering hope for slowing the progression of MS and minimizing the damage it causes.

SIGNS & SYMPTOMS

Early symptoms of MS may be confined to one side of the body, but are likely to spread to both sides as the disease progresses.

- Overall lack of energy, sleepiness, or lethargy, or easy fatigability during physical tasks such as walking or other moderate exercise.
- Legs may feel weak and heavy
- Weak or heavy feelings, progressing to difficulty walking, with frequent trips or falls
- Pain around or behind the eye, blurry vision, or loss of vision
- Numbness or feelings of "pins and needles"; perhaps feelings of pressure or burning in the chest
- Frequent and strong need to urinate
- Bowel dysfunction, either constipation or involuntary bowel action
- Depression
- Less common: tremor, lack of coordination, slurred speech, sudden paralysis, or decline in cognitive function

WHAT CAUSES IT?

Multiple sclerosis is caused by destruction of the outermost coating of a nerve, an insulating membrane called the myelin sheath. Nerve transmissions travel in the form of electric impulses down the length of the elongated portion of a nerve, the axon. The axon is surrounded by the myelin sheath, a fatty material. When our nerves are healthy, impulses are transmitted quickly, smoothly, and efficiently from the brain to the spinal cord and the rest of the body. The signals translate to lifting a foot, moving a leg, swinging an arm, and all the other motions of our body that are usually so effortless we are barely conscious of them. However, if the myelin breaks down, the electrical impulses can no longer travel unimpeded. Deterioration of the myelin sheath results in short-circuiting of the nerve impulses, which may prevent the impulse from reaching its destination. This can affect vision, movement, sensory feelings, and cognitive abilities.

Myelin is produced by a type of cell called an oligodendrocyte, or simply oligo. In people with MS, the myelin sheath and the oligos are injured in some way. The deterioration is usually preceded by inflammation. Sometimes there is also damage to the underlying axon, and it is probably the injury to the axon that causes permanent neurologic impairment. Myelin is injured in multiple sites around the brain and spinal cord, and its breakdown results in scarred, or sclerotic, areas—thus the name, multiple sclerosis. The sclerotic areas harden into sections of plaque. The multiple locations of myelin breakdown are responsible for the variability of symptoms in people with MS.

The cause of MS is unknown. It is believed that it is an autoimmune disease in which the body's immune system attacks normal tissue, in this case, the oligo cells and the myelin. It may be triggered by a virus—other demyelinating diseases are known to be caused by certain viruses. Magnetic resonance imaging (MRI) shows inflammation at the site of deteriorating myelin at the time of flare-ups, and subsiding inflammation during remission.

One of the most distinctive features of MS is the way its symptoms come and go. It is classified into four categories by the patterns of remission and relapse:

Relapsing-remitting. In most people with MS, the disease begins with an acute episode, a clearly defined flare-up of symptoms. The time when symptoms are evident is referred to as a flare, an attack, or a relapse, and usually lasts from days to

374

weeks. This is followed by remission, with partial or full recovery. The period of remission is variable, and may range from months to years.

Primary progressive. In about 15% of patients, MS progresses from the onset, with only occasional plateaus and brief temporary improvement of symptoms. There are no exacerbations or relapses in primary progressive MS.

Secondary progressive. After beginning with a relapsing-remitting period that can last for decades, symptoms persist and worsen, with only infrequent relapses and progressive neurologic debilitation. A majority of MS patients eventually move from the relapsing-remitting to the secondary progressive stage.

Progressive relapsing. Seen most often in people who develop MS after the age of 40, there is progression of disease from the onset as well as clear-cut acute flare-ups. There may be brief periods of recovery or remission. This is the rarest form of MS.

WHO IS AT RISK?

More than 350,000 people in the United States have MS. Two hundred new cases are diagnosed each week in the United States. More than half of all cases are first diagnosed in people between the ages of 20 and 40 and less than 10% in people over 50.

While specific risk factors for multiple sclerosis are unclear, it is known to strike more women than men, more Caucasians than people of color, and more often in cooler climates in the higher latitudes away from the equator than close to the equator. Looking at ethnicity, highest rates of MS are in northern European Caucasians and lowest rates in African-Americans and Asians. It is virtually unknown in Eskimos. Looking at geography, in the United States, the rate of MS is nearly twice as high in the region above the 37th parallel as below. For example, in Boston (latitude 41 degrees N) the prevalence of MS is 120 cases in 100,000 population; in New Orleans (latitude 30 degrees N) it is 50 per 100,000.

It was once hypothesized that MS was caused by trauma, but recent studies have found that there is no relation between trauma and onset or exacerbation of MS. Conversely, people with MS are at higher risk than the general population for trauma because of their vision problems, impaired balance, and lack of coordination. As the ethnicity data indicate, it is likely that there are genetic factors involved in the development of MS. No one has yet pinpointed a multiple sclerosis gene or genes; however, there is some evidence pointing to the role of at least an inherited tendency to the disease. In identical twins, if one twin gets MS, the other has about a 30% chance of also getting it. A child with a parent with MS has a 4% chance of getting the disease, compared with a 0.1% average risk (one chance in one thousand) for the general population. However, more than 80% of people with MS do not have a first-degree relative with the disease.

Research on the genetics of MS indicate that it is probably caused by alterations in a number of genes, not just one, and this genetic pattern may only predispose a person to the disease if certain environment factors (e.g., a virus) are in place. Researchers are studying the genetics of families with a number of cases of MS to try to pin down the genes involved in MS.

MS AND PREGNANCY

MS strikes people in their 20s and 30s, the childbearing years, and more often women than men. Women with MS will have to consider the impact of their condition when they make decisions about pregnancy. In fact, the disease is often in remission during pregnancy, but is likely to flare in the first three to six months after childbirth. This may affect the care a woman can give to her newborn, and a caregiver for mother and child can play an essential role. There is no evidence that pregnancy or breast-feeding has a negative effect on the long-term course of MS, and MS does not appear to negatively influence pregnancy or childbirth. However, the drugs used to treat MS (see "How Is It Treated?," below) have not been tested for safety in pregnancy, and women who accidentally become pregnant while taking interferon-beta or other anti-MS drugs should discontinue their medication during pregnancy.

HOW IS IT DIAGNOSED?

There is no definitive diagnostic test for MS, neither from clinical symptoms, laboratory findings, nor imaging. However, a combination of all of these methods of assessment can establish a fairly certain diagnosis. Often a person is diagnosed with *probable* MS upon first evaluation, with a more definitive diagnosis deferred until symptoms recur.

In general, MS is diagnosed when:

- Two attacks or more have occurred, at least 24 hours in duration each and at least a month apart.
- An MRI shows more than one area of myelin sheath damage, with the damage having occurred at more than one period of time.

Either of these findings alone can point to other diseases. Also, a negative MRI does not definitely rule out the presence of MS, since about 5% of cases are not detected by MRI. Other diagnostic tools include examination of the cerebrospinal fluid and evoked potential tests. The cerebrospinal fluid is obtained through a lumbar puncture (spinal tap); in a person with MS it will usually contain certain markers of immune abnormalities called oligoclonal bands. However, these bands may also be indicators of other diseases. Evoked potential tests measure electrical response in the brain to visual, auditory, and sensory stimuli and can reveal subtleties not detected in other neurologic exams. Again, these tests are not specific for MS and may indicate other diseases, so all of the findings must be considered together.

Since MS strikes different areas of the brain or spinal cord, the symptoms are variable in intensity and duration from one person to the next. They can be mild or severe, short or long-lasting. While early symptoms may be confined to one side of the body, they are likely to spread to both sides as the disease progresses. Symptoms experienced most frequently are listed below.

Fatigue. This is the most commonly reported MS symptom, felt by 90% of patients, and can be the most disabling. It may be experienced as overall lack of energy, sleepiness, or lethargy, or it may be felt as easy fatigability while walking or during other moderate exercise. A person's legs may feel weak and heavy.

Motor impairment. This may begin as weak or heavy feelings and progress, sometimes rapidly, to difficulty walking with frequent trips or falls.

Visual impairment. Pain around or behind the eye, blurry vision, or loss of vision result from inflammation of the optic nerve, a condition known as optic neuritis. It is often the symptoms of optic neuritis that prompt a person with MS to first see a doctor.

Other sensory impairment. Numbness or feelings of "pins and needles" are common. Some people with MS report feelings of pressure or burning in their chest.

Bowel and bladder impairment. Frequent and strong need to urinate is often an early symptom of MS. Many patients also experience bowel dysfunction, either constipation or, less often, involuntary bowel action.

Depression. Depression is very common. As many as 70% of people with MS report symptoms of depression at some time.

Other symptoms. Less commonly, symptoms can include tremor, lack of coordination, slurred speech, sudden paralysis, or decline in cognitive function. Because these symptoms can indicate a number of diseases, it is important to get a thorough medical work-up if you experience any of them.

WHAT SHOULD YOU EXPECT?

Multiple sclerosis can take its toll on the central nervous system (brain and spinal cord), but it does not affect other organs, except secondarily. However, there is no cure. But most people with MS have a normal life expectancy. And even though a popular concept of this disease envisions an infirm patient in a wheelchair, two-thirds of people with MS are walking on their own 20 years after diagnosis. Often MS is mild, resulting in inconvenience rather than impairment. But in the worst cases, MS can rob an individual of the ability to walk, to speak, to write. Most patients can anticipate at least moderate disability within 15 years of getting MS, although the latest treatments available may be changing that prognosis.

A recent study found that the fatigue that is a hallmark of MS also contributes to cognitive dysfunction. People with MS had decreased visual memory, verbal memory, and verbal fluency in the course of a four-hour cognitive testing session, compared with healthy subjects who showed improvements in those areas by the end of the session.

Primary progressive and progressive relapsing disease are associated with the worst outcomes. Patients usually move from relapsing-remitting MS to secondary progressive within five to fifteen years. In general, patients who do best are females, those with a younger age at onset, and those who have complete recoveries from symptoms after an attack and do not develop disability early in the course of the disease. Other factors associated with an unfavorable prognosis (and which may, therefore, call for more aggressive therapy) include weakness and lack of coordination at onset, a short interval between initial and second attack, and a high relapse rate in early years.

Historically, one of the biggest problems in the management of MS has been predicting its course. The increasing role of MRI in diagnosing MS is also being applied to measure the progression of the disease and the effect of medications. As newer techniques and refinements become more widely available, health professionals will be able to apply them to gain greater insights into the progression of MS. Much of today's research is directed at studying the natural history of the disease and searching for markers that may assist neurologists in making better predictions about an individual's disease course.

HOW IS IT TREATED?

Multiple sclerosis is a disease that has been with us since antiquity, and was accurately described in the late 1800s. But it is only in the past decade that scientists have had sufficient understanding of the mechanisms of MS to come up with effective treatments. Until the 1990s, treatment was limited to trying to alleviate symptoms. With new discoveries, treatment is now aimed at the immune system—turning off the autoimmune reaction as early as possible in the course of the disease to prevent permanent nerve damage and disability. There are many disagreements about the best way to treat MS—which drugs to use, at what doses, and for how long—but there is consensus that it is important to treat as soon as possible, especially in persons predicted to have an unfavorable prognosis, to prevent harm to the central nervous system. The National Multiple Sclerosis Society has recommended initiation of therapy as soon as possible following a definite diagnosis of relapsing MS.

For many years, the main drugs used to treat MS were corticosteroids such as prednisone, which are anti-inflammatories and suppress the immune system. These drugs are only moderately effective at relieving symptoms temporarily and shortening the duration of attacks, and do little to halt the progress of the disease. From 1993 to 2000, the Food and Drug Administration approved four drugs specifically to treat multiple sclerosis. Two (interferon beta-1b [Betaseron] and interferon beta-1a [Avonex] are interferons, and work to modulate the immune system. A third (glatiramer acetate [Copaxone]) is a mixture of four amino acids that has some similarities to myelin basic protein, a major component of myelin. The fourth (mitoxantrone [Novantrone]) is a chemotherapy agent that suppresses and modulates parts of the immune system. While all have been shown to be effective for reducing attacks and slowing progression of relapsing MS, they have potential side effects and are expensive—$10,000 a year or more, with the need for continuing long-term treatment. And none can be considered a cure—modern medicine has not yet come up with a cure to offer people with MS.

Ultimately, the best weapon against MS may turn out to be a cocktail, a combination of some of the different drugs now used, along with the medicines of the future that are still being devised and studied in today's laboratories. Because this disease follows such different courses in individuals, each treatment plan must be tailored to the individual patient. It is likely that treatments will be long-term—maybe even life-long, since nothing now available actually cures MS—so long-term toxicity will have to be assessed.

THE BETA-INTERFERONS

Interferons are proteins that the body produces naturally in response to a foreign stimulus, such as a virus. They have been reproduced in synthetic form in the laboratory for more than ten years and their therapeutic use has been investigated for a number of diseases, including cancer. There are three categories of interferons, labeled alpha, beta, and gamma, depending on the types of cells that produce them.

In MS, beta-interferons have a modulating effect on the immune system and have been shown to increase the time between attacks, lessen the severity of attacks, and decrease the amount of cumulative damage from demyelination seen on MRIs. In the mid-1990s, as the data about the effectiveness of these drugs grew, a group of MS researchers concluded, "This treatment may alter the fundamental course of relapsing multiple sclerosis." Two years later researchers reported "interferon beta-1a treatment is associated with robust, clinically important beneficial effects on disability progression." And the latest studies show that interferon beta-1a treatment, until now used primarily to treat well-established MS, is also useful in the very early stages of the disease.

Beta-interferon clearly has an important role in treating many people with MS, but health care professionals are still working out when it should be begun, which drug works best for which patients, what the best doses are, when the treatment should be stopped, and long-term effects of treatment. Interferon beta-1b (Betaseron) is given via a subcutaneous (under the skin) injection every other day. Interferon beta-1a (Avonex) is administered in a weekly intramuscular injection, usually in the thigh, upper arm, or hip. Potential side effects of both drugs are flu-like symptoms such as chills and fever, malaise and sweating, and muscle aches, especially when a person first starts taking them. To prevent this, the doctor may prescribe a slowly increasing dose that increases to the full dose after a few weeks, or even months. Depression, including suicidal thoughts, is a symptom of MS that may sometimes be aggravated by interferon. Increased sensitivity to sunlight may occur and protective measures are recommended. People taking these drugs also must deal with having injections given at home and related issues such as injection technique and rotation of sites. The caregiver is an important part of the injection regimen, either as a partner to gather supplies and monitor or to actually give the injections. Some patients prefer injecting themselves, others would rather someone else do the injecting—it is a matter of personal preference.

GLATIRAMER ACETATE

Glatiramer acetate (Copaxone) was approved for treatment of relapsing-remitting MS in 1996. Extensive research on this agent has shown a significant reduction in relapses, a reduction in new and enhancing MRI lesions, and a positive effect on disease progression. The original Phase III trial of Copaxone conducted in North America was extended as an open-label study—meaning that all patients in the study went on the active drug—and continues to demonstrate a sustained effect on relapse reduction and disease progression.

Copaxone is injected daily in the subcutaneous tissue. Side effects include injection site redness, itching, and mild discomfort. In addition, a small percentage of patients experience a postinjection reaction. Usually occurring only once or infrequently, this is described as a flushed feeling, with rapid heartbeat, sweating, and shortness of breath. It occurs immediately after the medication is injected and persists for five to fifteen minutes.

381

MITOXANTRONE

The newest approach to fighting MS is a chemotherapy agent used against cancer. Chemo drugs kill the fastest growing and dividing cells—among them, cancer cells, hair follicle cells, red blood cells, and the white blood cells that make up the immune system. Mitoxantrone (Novantrone) is used to treat types of leukemia and prostate cancer, but when cancer researchers observed its effects on the immune system, they realized that it might be effective against MS. In ten years of MS studies, it has been shown to slow the progression of neurologic impairment and reduce new lesions in the brain. In the autumn of 2000 it was approved for treatment of MS.

Novantrone is given through intravenous infusion once every three months. It has the side effects of many chemo drugs: nausea and hair loss, increased risk of urinary tract infections, and menstrual problems and infertility for women. Nausea and vomiting are treated preventively along with the administration of chemo, so chemotherapy is not the sentence of misery it once was. Patients may also notice that there is a blue-green discoloration in their urine and in the whites of their eyes for twenty-four hours after the drug infusion. But another side effect of Novantrone is a potentially dangerous weakening of the heart muscle, which can lead to heart failure. The risk is cumulative—the more you get of the drug, the more dangerous it is. Therefore, Novantrone is only given to patients with healthy hearts and only for two to three years or eight to twelve doses. Patients taking this should have their heart and blood monitored regularly.

OTHER DISEASE TREATMENTS

Immunosuppressive drugs that have been used include azathioprine (Imuran) and methotrexate, but with minimal efficacy by themselves.

TREATING SYMPTOMS

Corticosteroids are still an important part of MS treatment. A severe attack will probably be treated with intravenous steroids. The drug used most often is a form of prednisone.

A variety of other drugs are used to treat different symptoms of MS. Effective medications are available to treat the many varying manifestations of this disease—fatigue, spasticity, tremor, bladder problems, bowel dysfunction, depression, sexual dysfunction. Although treatment may not completely relieve symptoms, often it can make them more tolerable.

Physical and occupational therapy are useful for some patients, and an aerobic exercise program can contribute to cardiovascular health and improved bladder and bowel function, and help alleviate fatigue and depression. Sometimes assistive devices (for example, canes, walkers, or ankle-foot braces) are helpful. One of the most important things to remember in seeking treatment is the need for health care providers who are experienced with treating MS, who have seen it in its many different forms. No two cases are exactly alike, and a clinician needs to see dozens of cases before patterns of the disease are evident. In addition, team of specialists will need to be part of long-term care.

WHAT RESEARCH IS BEING DONE?

Basic questions about MS remain unanswered, and researchers are looking for the causes of this disease, whether they lie in the immune system, infectious agents, genetics, or—most likely—a combination of the three. Magnetic resonance imaging and MR spectroscopy are providing new insights into what multiple sclerosis does to the brain, and these images are playing an increasing role in determining treatment and monitoring outcomes. Another focus of MS research, aided by MRI, is to determine the relationship between inflammation and degeneration of the myelin sheath and axon.

A number of clinical trials are under way to assess the effects of medications and combinations of drugs. It is important that drugs for MS be tested in rigorously controlled studies because some studies have found a very high percent of placebo responses in people with MS; that is, patients taking a sugar pill respond to it as if it were an effective medication. This may be partly because this is a disease of spontaneous remissions. The study of MS can also be complicated because it can vary so much from one person to another. Researchers designing studies must take these unique qualities of MS into account.

Scientists are investigating several ways of repairing damaged myelin. One approach is to give growth factors that awaken what are called neural stem cells. These cells are the precursors to all of our normal brain cells, including the cells that make myelin (called the oligodendrocytes). Deep in our brains, there lies a reserve population of neural stem cells, which may exist to help repair brain damage. The challenge is to find a way to activate these cells and get them to where they are needed. A second approach would be to transplant neural stem cells or the actual myelin-producing cells from another person or animal donor. This would require a transplantation procedure and suppression of the immune system to prevent rejection of the foreign cells.

Neural stem cells should not be confused with bone marrow stem cells, which are the cells that make up our blood, including the white blood cells that constitute our immune system. Growth factors have been identified that can force the bone marrow stem cells into the blood, where they can be harvested and saved for transplantation, either into the same patient or a closely matched recipient. Bone marrow stem cells are used to reconstitute the immune system after strong chemotherapy has been used to kill the "bad" immune cells that are causing the attack on the myelin. This approach is being used in MS, but is very risky and several patients have died from infections.

Fatigue is one of the most disabling features of MS, and researchers are looking for new drugs to combat it. One that shows promise in early studies is modafinil (Provigil), a drug that is used to treat narcolepsy.

In looking for new drugs to use against MS, several small studies and patient anecdotes have suggested that marijuana or its active ingredient tetrahydrocannabinol (Dronabinol, Marinol) can alleviate MS symptoms, particularly spasticity. One study of the use of tetrahydrocannabinol in mice with an MS-like disease found that the drug controlled spasticity and tremor in the mice, and the researchers recommended further study of cannabinoids and MS. However, sedating drugs may further impair memory and other thinking problems associated with MS.

HOW CAN IT BE PREVENTED?

There is no known way to prevent MS. However, a combination of the new treatments available and the ongoing refinement of MRI and related imaging techniques points the way to possible preventive efforts in the future, and at least secondary prevention right now. That means the disease itself may not be preventable, but if it is detected early, progression and damage to the nerves can be slowed down. A recent study confirmed this hypothesis. In the CHAMPS study, begun in 1996 and designed to last five years, patients who had experienced just one demyelinating attack of MS were treated with interferon beta-1a (Avonex). Others were treated with a placebo. Investigators ended the study early because one group was doing so much better than the other, with 44% fewer MS attacks or evidence of attacks showing up on the MRI. This turned out to be the group being treated with Avonex. This result was good news for anyone in the early stages of MS, and this and other drugs will have a growing role in further treatment and secondary prevention.

WHAT YOU CAN DO NOW

Being diagnosed with MS can be stressful and cause uncertainty. No one can predict the course this disease will take, the amount of disability to expect. Becoming informed with up-to-date findings can help both patients and caregivers. The National Multiple Sclerosis Society sponsors a "Knowledge Is Power" program, a free, at-home, six-week educational series that can be a good way to start.

Even with disease progression, many measures can be taken to make things easier for a person with MS. These include:

- Avoid excessive stress when possible
- Avoid exposure to infections
- Treat yourself to massages and relaxing baths
- Talk to your doctor or physical therapist about different types of exercises you can use to maintain muscle tone and joint mobility
- Avoid heat (i.e., non-air-conditioned rooms in summer, hot tubs). Soaking your feet and ankles in cool water can relieve fatigue and re-energize you

Striving to maintain independence is important for most people, but allowing yourself the use of assistive devices can help prevent fatigue and make you more functional than you are without them.

Redesign your home to meet your physical needs. The National MS Society publishes a pamphlet with many practical tips as to how to do this.

Look for local support groups for both patients and caregivers. Some of the best tips for people with MS and their caregivers come from Inside MS, a quarterly publication of the MS Society. This magazine offers practical suggestions from people living with MS and those caring for them.

ADDITIONAL RESOURCES

ORGANIZATIONS AND WEB SITES

Consortium on Multiple Sclerosis Centers

Timothy L. Vollmer, MD, program director

Yale University Neuroimmunology Program

P.O. Box 208018

New Haven, CT 06520-8018

203-764-4289

www.mscare.org

Multiple Sclerosis Association of America

706 Haddonfield Road

Cherry Hill, NJ 08002

800-532-7667

www.msaa.com

Multiple Sclerosis Foundation

6350 North Andrews Avenue

Fort Lauderdale, FL 33309

800-441-7055

www.msfacts.org

National Multiple Sclerosis Society

733 Third Avenue

New York, NY 10017-3288

800-344-4867

www.nmss.org

National Rehabilitation Information Center

1010 Wayne Avenue

Silver Spring, MD 20910-5633

800-346-2742

www.naric.com

National Institute of Neurological Disorders and Stroke

www.ninds.nih.gov

U.S. Food and Drug Administration

FDA Approves Novantrone for Treating Advanced Multiple Sclerosis, FDA Talk Paper

Internet on-line. October 13, 2000.

http://www.fda.gov/bbs/topics/ANSWERS/ANS01046.html

BOOKS

Books have been written about MS by professionals and by patients and their family members. Following is just a small sampling of recent publications. Check your local library or bookstore for a more complete list.

Cohen, Marion Deutsche, and Marty Wyngaarden Krauss. *Dirty Details: The Days and Nights of a Well Spouse.* Philadelphia: Temple University Press, 1996.

Compston, Alastair, et al. *Mcalpine's Multiple Sclerosis.* New York: Harcourt Brace, 1998.

Kraft, George H., Marci Catanzaro, and Nancy J. Holland. *Living with Multiple Sclerosis: A Wellness Approach.* New York: Demos Vermande, 2000.

Lander, David L. *Fall Down, Laughing: How Squiggy Caught Multiple Sclerosis and Didn't Tell Nobody.* Los Angeles: J.B. Tarcher, 2000.

MacKie, Carole, et al. *Me and My Shadow: Learning to Live With Multiple Sclerosis.* London: Aurum Press Ltd. 1999.

Nichols, Judith Lynn. *Living Beyond Multiple Sclerosis: A Woman's Guide.* Hunter House, 2000.

Schapiro, Randall T. *Symptom Management in Multiple Sclerosis.* New York: Demos Medical Publishing Co., 1998.

Schwarz, Shelly, and Shelley Peterman Schwarz. *300 Tips for Making Life with Multiple Sclerosis Easier.* New York: Demos Vermande, 1999.

Shatzky, Dorothy, and Joel Shatzky. *Facing Multiple Sclerosis: Our Longest Journey.* Roseville, Calif.: Dry Bones Press, 1999.

Osteoarthritis

Osteoarthritis is not an inevitable part of aging, but it becomes harder and harder to avoid as the years go by. More than half of all people age 65 or older show signs of osteoarthritis, and four out of every five people who reach age 75 will develop it in at least one joint. All told, the condition affects nearly 21 million Americans. That makes osteoarthritis the most common of all joint disorders, and the leading cause of musculoskeletal disability in the country.

Osteoarthritis (OA) affects mainly the knees, hips, fingers, feet, neck, and lower back. Also known as degenerative joint disease, the disease is marked primarily by the deterioration of cartilage. Without cartilage, bones lose their shock-absorbing buffers and begin to rub against each other. This causes pain, joint stiffness and, in advanced cases, inflammation. Unlike other forms of arthritis, osteoarthritis is usually asymmetrical; one knee or hip may be affected while the other remains healthy. Nonetheless, osteoarthritis can be a debilitating disease, robbing people of their ability to walk or even move their hands without tremendous pain.

WHAT IS IT?

Despite years of focused research, scientists still don't know the exact cause or causes of osteoarthritis, and have found no way to reverse its effects. But new treatments are making it easier for people to live with the disease. Modern medications can ease pain with far fewer side effects than their predecessors. Surgery can improve motion in some joints, especially the knees. Joint replacement surgery is a proven option that can restore mobility for many people who have advanced osteoarthritis in their knees and hips. And new treatments, though still far from proven, at least offer hope that doctors one day will be able to reverse the disease by rebuilding cartilage in damaged joints.

THE ROLE OF CARTILAGE

Though there's still much debate over exactly how osteoarthritis begins in a joint, the most obvious early sign is cartilage breakdown. Cartilage is a dense, rubbery substance that serves a number of important functions throughout the body. It gives shape to ear lobes and noses, provides structure for the larynx, trachea and bronchi and helps stabilize and cushion the spine. All human bones begin as cartilage; it forms the template for the entire skeletal system that replaces cartilage as embryos grow in the womb.

There are three main types of cartilage in humans:

Fibrocartilage. Found mainly in the disks that act as cushions between vertebrae in the spine.

Elastic cartilage. Appears in the outer portion of the ear.

Hyaline cartilage. Found in a great number of places, including joints like the hips, knees and fingers. The specific type of hyaline cartilage found in joints is known as articular cartilage, a bluish-white or gray, semi-opaque material that's extremely tough and somewhat elastic.

In humans, articular cartilage forms a cap on bones that meet in joints—such as the femur thigh bone (femur) and the shin bone (tibia) in the knee. The cartilage serves two important functions. First, it provides shock absorption for bones in the joint. When humans walk, for instance, the articular cartilage in the knee eases the stress from the weight of the body. Articular cartilage also is very slippery, allowing the joints to slide back and forth with a minimum of friction. Articular cartilage is made of a complex matrix of materials that give it these important properties.

When performing properly, articular cartilage provides valuable service to the body. Humans, for example, place a great deal of pressure on the bones in the legs when walking. Cartilage responds to this pressure by releasing much of the fluid stored in its matrix. This cushions the load on the ends of the bones, keeping them from rubbing against each other. When weight is lifted from one leg, the cartilage quickly reabsorbs the fluids it just expelled—preparing the hips and knees for the next step. In fingers and other joints, the slippery nature of cartilage allows for continuous, smooth movements.

Articular cartilage appears to be designed to last a lifetime. Under normal circumstances, the complex matrix of material in articular cartilage can regenerate new tissue to replace worn tissue. Unfortunately, many factors—some known and some unknown—destroy this delicate balance and lead to osteoarthritis.

OA appears to have both a biomechanical and biological basis. Physical trauma clearly plays a role. Sudden injury to a joint can predispose it to osteoarthritis—including broken bones, torn cartilage, or similar problems. Long-term repeated trauma to the joints also leads to OA. Joints that are badly aligned or that move improperly can create abnormal stress that takes a toll over a period of years. Normal motion is good for cartilage; because it's not fed directly by blood vessels, cartilage relies on nutrients from the fluid it squeezes in and out to regenerate. But repeated improper motions, caused by features like bowlegs, legs of differing lengths, or an unusual spine shape, can eventually overwhelm the joint's ability to repair itself. This feature of osteoarthritis once led to its reputation as a "wear and tear" disease. Researchers now know that this is an inaccurate description. Not everyone who suffers trauma to a joint develops OA, and not everyone with OA shows signs of trauma.

There also appears to be a biochemical basis for the disease that is at least as important as the mechanical one. Researchers know that enzymes that cause cartilage breakdown—called matrix metalloproteinases—are found in unusually high levels in the cartilage of people with osteoarthritis. These enzymes are produced by cells called chondrocytes located within the cartilage. Proteins called cytokines appear to instruct the chondrocytes to create the enzymes. Other chemicals in the body can stimulate the production of new cartilage tissue. Among these are insulin-like growth factor-1 (IGF-1) and transforming growth factor-beta (TGF-b). But scientists have not found a connection between the levels of IGF-1 or TGF-b and osteoarthritis in human joints. Some people with OA have high levels of the growth factors in their affected joints, while others have normal or low levels. Researchers are still looking into the exact biochemical mechanisms that contribute to the disease.

Most experts recognize two separate subsets of OA. The first is called primary, or idiopathic, osteoarthritis. This is the classic, slow-onset form of the disease that strikes men and women after the age of 45 and has no readily apparent cause. In the other form, called secondary osteoarthritis, the cause can be more easily determined. It usually involves previous injury to a joint, congenital joint deformities, certain diseases that cause skeletal abnormalities, and other conditions that predispose people to OA, such as rheumatoid arthritis or Paget's disease.

Whatever the true cause or causes, once cartilage production falls out of balance, the tissue begins to soften and weaken. The surface of the cartilage becomes uneven and ragged, and sometimes cracks or fissures appear in the tissue. At this early stage, people usually feel little or no pain in the affected joint. When cartilage wears away more completely, the bones in the joint begin to rub against each other and pain develops. The bone underneath the cartilage, called subchondral bone, becomes thickened and hardened from the increased pressure. The bones may develop spurs that make motion in the joint even more difficult. In addition to these spurs, some people may develop subchondral cysts, fluid-filled sacs located in the bone just under the cartilage. These occur when watery synovial fluid from the joint is forced by pressure into the bone itself. Eventually, these cysts can collapse, further damaging the joint.

Researchers are beginning to focus more on these bone changes as a cause, rather than a byproduct, of osteoarthritis. There's some evidence that repeated tiny fractures in the ends of bones might impede cartilage's ability to function and regenerate normally. People with osteoarthritis usually have higher than normal bone density in their affected joints—perhaps because of repeated micro-fractures and repairs. This stiffer, less flexible bone may make cartilage more prone to breakdown. Animal studies have shown that changes in bone structure may indeed occur before cartilage starts to erode. It's interesting to note that people with osteoarthritis often have higher bone density throughout their bodies, which is why they are less likely to suffer from osteoporosis and other diseases linked to low bone density.

OA affects joints in different ways. Knees and hips commonly develop spurs, subchondral cysts, and other pressure-related problems. In the hands, bony knobs called Heberden's nodes can develop on the finger joints closest to the nails. Bouchard's nodes are similar and appear on the middle joints of fingers. Both types of nodes can interfere with a joint's ability to move freely, making it difficult and sometimes painful to perform fine tasks with the hands. In the neck and spine, spurs on the vertebrae are common. They are usually not painful, unless they begin to press on nerves that run through the backbone.

Stiffness also becomes a common feature in joints afflicted with osteoarthritis. Early in its progression, OA causes temporary stiffness, particularly in the morning or after long periods of inactivity. This usually disappears within thirty minutes of waking, and can be aided by stretching or walking. But stiffness becomes more severe as OA progresses. In later stages, stiffness becomes a permanent feature, as the joint loses part of its range of motion.

In its early and middle stages, osteoarthritis rarely causes inflammation in a joint. In fact, doctors sometimes use the term osteoarthr*osis* instead of osteoarthr*itis* because the suffix "-itis" literally means "with inflammation." But if OA continues to develop in a joint, inflammation eventually may occur. This often happens when the joint lining, called the synovium, becomes irritated and the body tries to soothe and heal it by flooding the joint with fluid. While this may work for a while, the excess fluid can ultimately make the joint even more unstable and painful. Inflammation may even lead to additional cartilage destruction, since it may release more chemicals that break down healthy cartilage tissue. Pain from osteoarthritis can come and go. Sometimes, bones in a joint rub together for so long that they actually smooth each other's ends—a process called eburnation. This allows the joint to move more freely, at least temporarily. Unfortunately, the bones are still in contact with each other and usually will begin to degenerate again in time. As the disease progresses, joint breakdown and pain may reach the point where the patient has great difficulty moving without significant and constant pain. At this stage, joint replacement may become a viable option—perhaps the only way a person can regain use of the joint.

WHO IS AT RISK?

Osteoarthritis pain leads to more than seven million visits to doctors' offices each year in America, and accounts for more than thirty-six million lost work days. Almost everyone who lives long enough will develop signs of OA that could be seen on an x-ray. Between 10 and 15% of all Americans over age 45 suffer with pain and loss of mobility in the knee alone. But just why these degenerative changes and accompanying symptoms become more pronounced in some people than others remains mysterious. Though the picture still isn't clear, certain factors (described in detail below) seem to put some people at greater risk of developing the more painful and debilitating aspects of osteoarthritis:

- Age
- Body weight
- Gender
- Hormone replacement therapy
- Race or ethnicity
- Heredity
- Previous injury to a joint
- Occupational and recreational activity
- Nitrate use
- Smoking

Age. About one in every three white Americans between the ages of 25 and 74 has clinically detectable signs of osteoarthritis. The risk rises noticeably with increased age; by the time a person reaches 75, he or she has about a four in five chance of showing signs of OA. The risk seems to plateau as people reach their 70s. Those who reach this point without symptoms of the disease are unlikely to develop it later in life. The link between age and OA would appear to confirm its reputation as an inevitable part of getting older. But doctors do not believe this is necessarily the case. There's still no clear biological link between normal aging processes and the type of cartilage degeneration found in osteoarthritis.

Body weight. Obesity is a major risk factor for osteoarthritis. Obese women are nine times more likely to develop the disease than women of normal weight, and obese men are four times more likely than men of average weight. Researchers believe that increased weight puts extra burden on weight-bearing joints like hips and knees, making them more likely to break down in people susceptible to osteoarthritis.

A national survey of nearly 17,000 Americans aged 25 and older shows that the connection between OA and body weight grows stronger as people become more obese. The study used six weight classifications: underweight, normal weight, overweight, and then three increasing levels of obesity. Researchers used the Body Mass Index—an equation that uses a person's height and weight—to determine the different levels.

Only 2.59% of normal-weight men in the study had osteoarthritis, while 4.4% of overweight men had the disease. The figures jumped to 4.7%, 5.5%, and 10% among men in the three classes of obesity. For comparison, a 5-foot 10-inch man was considered normal weight if he weighed 129 to 173 pounds; overweight if he weighed 174 to 208 pounds; and at the highest level of obesity if he weighed more than 277 pounds.

Among women, 5.2% of those in the normal weight category had osteoarthritis. This compared to 8.5% of those deemed overweight, and 9.9%, 10.4%, and 17.2% for the three obese classes. The normal weight range for a 5-foot-5-inch woman was 111 to 149 pounds, while women of the same height were considered overweight if they weighed 150 to 179 pounds. Those who weighed more than 240 pounds were placed in the highest obese category.

Interestingly, underweight women are at slightly greater risk of developing osteoarthritis than women of average weight. Researchers have not figured out why, or even if, there's a firm connection between being underweight and getting OA. Underweight men, by comparison, were at far less risk for osteoarthritis than men of normal weight.

Gender. Women are about twice as likely as men to develop osteoarthritis. Before age 45, men show symptoms of OA more frequently. But between 45 and 55, the gap disappears, and after 55, women are far more likely to develop the disease, especially in finger joints. Osteoarthritis is often more severe in older women than in older men. In fact, OA is the leading cause of activity limitation among women. These statistics indicate a possible link between osteoarthritis and menopause in women. Sex hormones such as estrogen, in fact, are known to affect the production and destruction of cartilage. Many researchers speculate that the loss of these hormones after menopause takes away the protection younger women seem to enjoy from OA. Unfortunately, researchers have not been able to identify which women are more likely to develop the disease based on factors like the age menstruation began or ceased, or whether or not a woman had a hysterectomy. There's some evidence that having children gives women some protection from osteoarthritis.

A recent study also points to a connection between the higher incidence of osteoarthritis in women and the shoes they wear. Researchers compared the force that women's knee and hip joints had to handle when they were barefoot with the force they endured while wearing high-heeled shoes. The steep foot angle in the shoes greatly increased the force, enough to make the joints of a woman of normal weight endure the pressure of a woman who was overweight. While this study was preliminary, some researchers believe it can help explain part of the difference between OA rates in women and men.

Hormone replacement therapy. Since estrogen appears to aid in cartilage growth and maintenance, it seems logical that starting hormone replacement therapy after menopause would help prevent osteoarthritis. A 1996 study of more than 4000 white women over the age of 65, for instance, found that taking oral estrogen reduced the chances of developing OA in the hip. Women taking the hormones were only 62% as likely to get osteoarthritis as the women who were not. Those who took estrogen continuously for ten years or more seemed to get even more protection; they were only 54% as likely to develop the disease in their hips.

Other studies have found a similar connection in the knees. But it's important to note that women who stop taking the hormone treatments appear to lose their protection soon after. And women who had osteoarthritis before starting the treatment usually did not see a slowing or reversal of their conditions. In addition, some studies have found that hormone replacement may have no effect on OA, or might even increase the chances of developing the disease. Researchers believe that hormone therapy may hurt some women because it increases their bone density. While this helps fight against osteoporosis, harder bones may lead some people to develop OA. Because of these mixed findings and the fact that hormone replacement therapy itself poses certain risks and side effects, most doctors cannot recommend hormone replacement therapy as a way to prevent osteoarthritis.

Race or ethnicity. People of all races and ethnic backgrounds in the United States appear to get osteoarthritis at similar rates, with two possible exceptions. People of Hispanic and Asian/Pacific Islander backgrounds both report having fewer cases of all types of arthritis. No one is sure why these groups may have lower rates. Some researchers speculate that the groups may simply report having less arthritis for cultural or socioeconomic reasons.

Heredity. Research points strongly toward a genetic component in osteoarthritis. In addition to inheriting physical characteristics that can foster OA—unusual structure in joints, bow legs, knock knees, etc.—people are likely to inherit family genes for the production of chemicals that impair cartilage and bone functions.

Scientists have long known about the link between family and Heberden's nodes, a type of osteoarthritis that causes knobby bone enlargements in the finger joints. The disease clusters in families, and appears to grow worse in succeeding generations. Women are affected more than men. One study looked at parents and offspring who both had Heberden's nodes, and found that 50% of the children had symptoms that were worse than their parents.' In addition, the children developed the disease at a much earlier age on average—43 years old, compared to 61 years old in the parents.

Recent research with female twins also shows a strong link between genetics and osteoarthritis in the hips and knees and led researchers to state that genetics played a role in anywhere from 39 to 65% of all cases of osteoarthritis in the hands and knees.

No one has identified specific genes responsible for osteoarthritis; it's likely that more than one set of genes play a role. Researchers are focusing on several genetic mutations, such as those that alter the production of type II collagen, a main structural component in cartilage. People with mutations in this gene set seem more likely to suffer osteoarthritis in a number of different joints in their bodies. Changes in the gene for IGF-1 might also have an effect. This growth factor stimulates the body to tear down and rebuild cartilage; an imbalance in this process could result in the destruction of articular cartilage.

Previous injury to a joint. People who seriously injure a joint are much more likely to develop OA in the affected area. The injury usually involves damage to the cartilage, and is especially common in the knees. Those who have surgery to repair torn cartilage or other damage in the joint are even more likely to get OA. This is a leading cause of secondary osteoarthritis, OA that has a known cause.

Occupational and recreational activity. Researchers have found an apparent link between certain occupations and the onset of osteoarthritis in the knees and hips. The jobs typically involve prolonged or repeated kneeling, squatting, heavy lifting, or stair climbing. Farmers, who often perform all these physical tasks, are known to suffer OA at higher rates than people in other occupations. But while these activities may increase the incidence of OA, they don't necessarily affect the progression of the disease. While the jobs may increase the chances of developing early osteoarthritic changes in a joint, other factors—obesity, joint structure, heredity—play a major role in determining whether a person eventually suffers pain and loss of mobility. The same seems to hold for sports and other recreational activities. Exercise is usually good for weight-bearing joints; it strengthens surrounding muscles, and the compression/release effect on a joint actually keeps cartilage healthy. But exercise can be harmful for people who are predisposed to osteoarthritis. These include men and women with unstable or mechanically unsound joints, previous history of damage to a joint, family history of osteoarthritis, and other risk factors. One study of three hundred and fifty-four men and women aged 55 and older found that those with a history of regular sports participation were up to 3.2 times more likely to develop osteoarthritis in the hips and knees than those who did not exercise regularly. Studies of women found that those who were highly active in recreational activities as teen-agers were about twice as likely to eventually develop OA of the hip than those who were less active.

Experts stress that people should not avoid exercise for fear of developing osteoarthritis. Most top athletes, including long-distance runners, never develop symptoms of OA. Overall, the benefits of moderate exercise usually outweigh the risks to joints. Selecting a low-impact form of exercise, such as swimming or walking, can provide hips and knees with enough work while not endangering the cartilage.

Diet. There is some evidence that intake of certain vitamins may help slow the progression of osteoarthritis. Two studies have found that low intake of vitamin D can increase the speed with which OA develops in a joint. However, one study of the hip found vitamin D prevented the development of hip OA, while the other study found low levels of vitamin B increased the progression of knee OA.

Other vitamins, notably A, C, and E, may also help fight the progression of OA. Researchers believe that sufficient levels of these vitamins may lessen oxidative damage in cartilage tissue and other parts of the joint. It's not possible at this point to make specific recommendations about diet and osteoarthritis, other than to make sure intake of all vitamins meets recommended daily allowances.

Nitrate usage. People who take nitrates daily to control angina and other heart conditions may be at higher risk for developing osteoarthritis. A study of elderly women found that those taking nitrates every day were about twice as likely to have OA of the hip. Those taking nitrates occasionally did not face the same risk. The reason for this possible connection is not entirely clear. But nitric acid has been shown to stop the development of cartilage in live test subjects. People using nitrates should talk to their doctors before discontinuing use of nitrates.

Smoking. Several studies have found a strange, inverse link between cigarette smoking and osteoarthritis. People who smoke are actually at slightly lower risk of developing the disease. Scientists have not figured out why this occurs and they stress that the dangers of smoking greatly outweigh any small reduction in the risk of osteoarthritis.

HOW IS IT DIAGNOSED?

Pain drives most people with OA to the doctor for the first time. In its early stages, osteoarthritis does not produce any noticeable symptoms. But as the disease progresses, people notice changes in joints that begin to affect their lifestyles. People with OA in one or both hips, for example, have trouble walking properly, and feel dull and/or sharp pains across the groin and sometimes into the buttocks. Those with OA in the knees often complain that the joint is unstable and prone to buckling. People with osteoarthritis of the hands may have trouble completing everyday tasks like writing without pain or stiffness. And those with degeneration in the spine sometimes complain of pain shooting outward from the spine across the upper body—the result of spurs compressing nerves in the backbone. These patients may also notice other symptoms, such as numbness or weakness in the extremities or difficulty controlling bowel or bladder movements.

Diagnosing osteoarthritis is a vital first step in treating the disease. There are more than one hundred and twenty different types of arthritis and dozens more conditions that can mimic osteoarthritis. OA often co-exists with rheumatoid arthritis, gout or other forms of arthritis. Making the right diagnosis allows the doctor to choose an efficient course of treatment without aggravating the other conditions.

The doctor will first ask if the patient or his family has a history of arthritis and, if so, which type or types. Some forms of osteoarthritis are hereditary—most notably the formation of Heberden's and Bouchard's nodes on the joints of the fingers. After this, the doctor will probably perform a physical examination to check for the telltale signs of osteoarthritis.

Crepitus. This is the crackling that joints make when their cartilage is worn, cracked. or fraying. The doctor will move the joint gently, listening and feeling for the crackling or popping. Crepitus can occur in a joint before the patient notices any pain.

Limited range of motion. The doctor will manipulate the joint in question to see if it can move freely within its normal range. Cartilage breakdown and osteophytes often restrict how far a joint can move.

Pain on passive motion. In moderate to advanced cases of osteoarthritis, the joint may be painful even when not bearing weight or using muscles to move. The doctor will check to see if the joint hurts when he moves it without help from the patient.

Morning stiffness. This usually lasts thirty minutes or less in cases of osteoarthritis. After that, the joint returns to its typical state. Prolonged stiffness is more often a feature of other types of arthritis, such as rheumatoid arthritis.

Lack of swelling. Inflammation is not typical in mild to moderate cases of osteoarthritis. If these are present, it may indicate other forms of arthritis, such as rheumatoid arthritis. Swollen joints also are typical in cases of bursitis. Swelling in the bursa sacs in a joint, which are designed to pad the connections between ligaments, tendons, and bones, causes this condition. Housemaid's knee, technically known as prepatellar bursitis, and anserine bursitis (knee pain while climbing stairs) are treated in part with rest and heat, which rarely help in osteoarthritis.

Joints with mild to moderate osteoarthritis are generally not red, tender, or warm to the touch. This may change in advanced cases, but these symptoms are much more often associated with other types of arthritis—including rheumatoid arthritis, gout, or pseudogout.

After finishing his physical examination, the doctor may opt for x-rays and laboratory tests to confirm the diagnosis. X-rays look for the most obvious sign of osteoarthritis: narrowing of the space between two bones in a joint. Cartilage does not appear on x-ray pictures. But healthy cartilage is thick enough to create distance between the ends of the bones. If the space appears smaller than usual, or uneven, it's usually a sign that osteoarthritic changes are taking place in the joint. This space varies from joint to joint, and from person to person, depending on the individual's size and other factors.

X-rays also show other changes in the joint, most notably, the presence of spurs, subchondral cysts, and rough edges on the ends of bones. It's important to note, however, that the degree of osteoarthritic changes that show up on an x-ray often does not correlate with the pain and symptoms a patient may feel. In some cases, drastic changes shown on the x-ray do not cause pain in a patient; in others, relatively minor changes can cause significant pain and stiffness.

In some cases, x-rays can indicate the presence of other conditions. If the bones in a joint appear to be demineralized—that is, lacking in density because they've lost calcium—a diagnosis may lean toward rheumatoid arthritis. Rheumatoid arthritis can lead to bone loss, whereas this is not typically the case in osteoarthritis.

Blood tests are not standard in cases of osteoarthritis, although they can be used to rule out other types of arthritis or other diseases. Common blood tests for arthritis include red blood cell counts, white blood cell counts, and tests for the level of rheumatoid factor in blood. In osteoarthritis, these blood tests usually fall within a normal range. Doctors also can order a test of the synovial fluid in the joint, to check for an unusual level of white blood cells. Again, the fluid usually falls within normal range in cases of osteoarthritis.

OSTEOARTHRITIS VERSUS RHEUMATOID ARTHRITIS

Although osteoarthritis and rheumatoid arthritis may seem similar, they actually develop at different stages of life, have vastly differing symptoms, and affect different joints.

OSTEOARTHRITIS

Age of onset: Usually after 45. Gradual onset

Joints affected: Mostly knees, hips, back, feet, and fingers. Often affects single joints on either side of body.

Symptoms: Pain and stiffness. Inflammation, redness, tenderness only in advanced cases.

RHEUMATOID ARTHRITIS

Age of onset: Usually begins between 25 and 50. Often begins without warning.

Joints affected: Can affect almost all joints. Often appears in many joints at once, on both sides of the body.

Symptoms: Pain, stiffness, swelling, tenderness, and redness in joints. Also can cause general fatigue, and sometimes fever.

OSTEOARTHRITIS VERSUS RHEUMATOID ARTHRITIS

OA and rheumatoid arthritis are the two most common forms of arthritis. While both can result in painful joints and limited movement, rheumatoid arthritis is an autoimmune disorder and thus has different causes, diagnoses, and treatments. However, OA and rheumatoid arthritis can occur in the same joint simultaneously. This can explain overlapping symptoms.

WHAT SHOULD YOU EXPECT?

Osteoarthritis is an incurable disease. Doctors do not know how to reverse the effects of OA; at best, patients can hope for symptom relief and some improvement in range of motion in the affected joint. While a major cause of partial disability, osteoarthritis is not fatal.

Almost every patient will benefit from a combination of drug therapy, exercise, weight control, and possibly surgery. Unfortunately, the progression of osteoarthritis is extremely unpredictable. Some patients will suffer only minor pain, while others with the same radiographic features will develop far worse symptoms. One small study found that 28% of people with radiographic evidence of OA in the knee showed no worsening of their condition over a period of five years. At present, doctors are unable to determine which patients are more likely to worsen. Several factors—including obesity, the presence of Heberden's nodes in the hand, and osteoarthritis appearing in several joints—seem to place people at risk for further progression of the disease as seen on x-rays. But, again, radiographic changes do not always lead to worsening symptoms.

HOW IS IT TREATED?

Because there's no cure for osteoarthritis, doctors must focus on relieving the symptoms of the disease. Most treatment plans address the need to ease pain and increase joint mobility. While components of each plan are customized to the patient's individual needs, most include a regimen of exercise and pain medication, plus nutritional guidance with the goal of losing weight or maintaining a healthy weight. Joint-replacement surgery is sometimes an option in cases of advanced osteoarthritis.

EXERCISE

People with OA often are concerned that exercising arthritic joints will worsen their condition. But research shows that placing mild stress on weight-bearing joints does not cause cartilage breakdown. In fact, the opposite is true. Cartilage needs work to stay healthy. Walking, for example, places weight on the cartilage of the hips, knees, and feet. When the weight is released, the cartilage absorbs fluids from the surrounding joint that keep it supple and healthy.

EXERCISE FOR OA

Exercise programs should be developed with three goals in mind.

- Improving the range of motion and strength in the affected joint;
- Protecting the joint and other joints from future damage by improving their function; and
- Improving the patient's health, including weight loss, better sleep, and elevated mood.

Exercise regimens must be developed on a case-by-case basis. But almost all programs will include some kind of low-impact exercise, such as swimming or walking. Physical therapy is often indicated for patients who are suffering from loss of motion in the hands, knees, and other joints. In OA of the knee, doctors recommend strengthening the thigh muscles (quadriceps) to help stabilize the joint. When done together, regular exercise and physical therapy have been shown to lessen OA symptoms, allowing patients to walk farther and reducing the chances that a patient will need joint-replacement surgery.

WEIGHT MANAGEMENT

In addition to stimulating the joints, regular exercise can help promote weight loss or maintenance. Weight loss has not been linked with improvement of OA symptoms in all cases, but studies have shown several positive connections. For instance, obese people with OA in one knee are at greater risk of developing the condition in the other knee than are those of normal weight. Obesity even has been linked with increased incidence of osteoarthritis of the hand. In cases where obesity is believed to play a role in osteoarthritis, doctors may recommend that a patient receive nutritional counseling in addition to exercise therapy.

BASIC PAIN MEDICATION

Use of pain-killing drugs is the most common, and often the most effective, way to handle the symptoms of osteoarthritis. Doctors begin with proven medications that involve the fewest side effects, and only move to more powerful drugs when these front-line medications fail to offer sufficient pain relief.

Acetaminophen. Guidelines from the American College of Rheumatology suggest that doctors begin with simple acetaminophen, especially in osteoarthritis of the knees and hips. It is known better by the brand name Tylenol and offers generalized pain relief with a minimum of side effects. It does not reduce inflammation, which is a rare component of osteoarthritis. Although dosages may vary, the maximum dosage per day is usually about 4000 mg (4 g). This is taken in several divided dosages throughout the day (usually every four to six hours).

Acetaminophen is associated with few side effects when taken at regular dosages. It has been known to cause liver toxicity patients who are otherwise at risk for liver damage, such as heavy drinkers, and with long term, excessive use (more than the maximum daily dose). Tylenol can lead to renal failure in some patients, though this is also very rare when taken at regular dosages. Patients should consult their doctor before taking any acetaminophen.

Nonsteroidal anti-inflammatory drugs. If acetaminophen consistently fails to relieve pain sufficiently, the next choice is usually a nonsteroidal anti-inflammatory drug, or NSAID. Although there currently is no good evidence to suggest that NSAIDs are indeed more effective than acetaminophen for OA, they have consistently shown to be effective in people with osteoarthritis and recent studies suggest that patients slightly favor NSAIDs over acetaminophen for management of their OA. Acetaminophen does have fewer side effects than NSAIDs and is generally better tolerated. NSAIDs also can work to reduce inflammation in a joint affected by severe osteoarthritis. Aspirin was the first, and remains the best known, NSAID, but there are now more than a dozen NSAIDs in prescription and non-prescription strengths that can help with OA. In fact, the American College of Rheumatology considers all these NSAIDs to be equally effective against osteoarthritis, although their individual toxicities may vary.

Unfortunately, NSAIDs often are more expensive than acetaminophen, particularly the prescription-only varieties. They also carry side effects that can range from mild to serious for some people. The most common side effects with NSAIDs include stomach upset, ulcers, skin rashes, dizziness, nausea, ringing in the ears, and reduced blood-clotting capacity. More serious problems include kidney and liver failure. It's important to notify doctors of any conditions that arise because of NSAID use.

NSAID use is not recommended for everyone despite the fact that some are available without a prescription. Patients who have experienced asthma or any allergic-type reactions to aspirin or other NSAIDS should avoid all types of NSAIDs. NSAIDs can worsen certain pre-existing conditions, such as congestive heart failure, high blood pressure, and liver or kidney problems and usage should be avoided or limited in these patients. NSAIDs are associated with stomach ulcerations and bleeding and those particularly at risk include persons over 65, those on blood-thinning drugs, and those with a history of stomach ulcers and/or bleeding. Using the lowest dose possible for the shortest period possible is recommended but this may not always be feasible in more severe forms of OA.

COMMON NSAIDS

Here's a list of some common NSAIDs used in osteoarthritis:

Aspirin. Available under many brand names, including Bayer and Bufferin. Taken in divided dosages up to a maximum of 6g/day. No prescription necessary.

Ibuprofen. Motrin and Advil are commonly known brand names. Available without a prescription. Has been shown to have the fewest side effects of any NSAID when taken in low doses (1600 mg/day or less). The maximum daily dose is 3200mg. Ibuprofen is often the first option doctors consider when trying NSAIDs for people with osteoarthritis.

Indomethacin. Known by Indocin and numerous other brand names. Has a higher toxicity level than other similar NSAIDs, and is not recommended as a front-line treatment. Available by prescription only.

Diclofenac. Available in slow-release and immediate-release formulas. The drug is available in generic form by prescription only. A new drug, Arthrotec, combines diclofenac with misoprostol, which helps protect the stomach lining.

Naproxen. Aleve and Anaprox are common brand names. Available in prescription and non-prescription formulas.

Fenoprofen. Sold under the brand name Nalfon. By prescription only.

Piroxicam. Brand name is Feldene. Available by prescription only. Is longer-lasting than other NSAIDs; this means it can be taken only once or twice daily. The risk of serious side effects is higher than shorter-lived NSAIDs, however.

Diflunisal. Brand name is Dolobid. Available by prescription only. Also a long-lasting NSAID, with higher risk of side effects.

NSAIDs are sometimes combined with acetaminophen. This allows for a lower dosage of NSAIDs that patients may tolerate better. Under no circumstances should patients take more than one NSAID at a time, as this can greatly increase the risk of side effects. And patients should always consult their doctors before taking any NSAIDs.

Doctors may prescribe other drugs to counter the side effects of NSAIDs. These include antacids that help prevent heartburn and stomach ulcers or agents that protect the stomach lining from NSAID use such as misoprostol (Cytotec), and others that can help reduce the production of stomach acid and fight duodenal ulcers, such as ranitidine (Zantac) or omeprazole (Prilosec)/lansoprazole (Prevacid). It is strongly recommended that patients be tested for liver or kidney function problems before beginning NSAID therapy for osteoarthritis.

COX-2 inhibitors. All NSAIDs work by inhibiting enzymes called cyclooxygenases. These enzymes help produce prostaglandins, fatty acids that regulate a number of body functions, including pain and inflammation in osteoarthritic joints. But most NSAIDs are nonspecific; that is, they inhibit all prostaglandin production. This can have adverse affects throughout the body. The enzyme cyclooxygenase-1 (COX-1), for instance, helps produce chemicals that protect the stomach lining from gastric juices. It also helps maintain proper blood flow to the kidneys. Most side effects from NSAIDs come from blocking COX-1 production.

A new generation of NSAIDs now selectively blocks only cyclooxygenase-2 (COX-2)—the enzyme which helps produce the prostaglandins responsible for pain and swelling in OA. These drugs are called COX-2 inhibitors, and they represent a step forward in the treatment of osteoarthritis. COX-2 inhibitors are no more effective than older NSAIDs, but they seem to be much better tolerated by the body. That allows people to take medication regularly with fewer stomach and blood clotting-related side effects.

•Celecoxib. Celecoxib was the first COX-2 inhibitor approved by the U. S. Food and Drug Administration for use in osteoarthritis. It is available by prescription under the brand name Celebrex. Clinical studies with celecoxib found the drug to be effective in relieving pain and stiffness in OA, with a significant decrease in stomach ulcers and blood clotting problems, two of the more serious side effects from older NSAIDs. The studies also found celecoxib to be as effective as naproxen in relieving OA pain and inflammation. Patients using Celebrex reported having less trouble performing everyday tasks, such as bending, bathing, and climbing stairs, than those who were given placebos. The recommended dosage for Celebrex in cases of osteoarthritis is 200 mg per day, taken orally in either one dose or two divided 100 mg dosages. While it lacks many of the side effects of older NSAIDs, celecoxib still can cause heartburn, stomach pain, diarrhea, and kidney problems in some people. In patients who are allergic to sulfa or any sulfonamides, Celebrex should be avoided.

•**Rofecoxib.** Another prescription only COX-2 inhibitor, rofecoxib, reached the market shortly after celecoxib. It is sold under the brand name Vioxx, and shares many of the same properties as its cousin. Vioxx can be used in patients who have a sulfa allergy. Studies have found rofecoxib to be as effective as ibuprofen and diclofenac in relieving pain and morning stiffness from osteoarthritis, with a much lower incidence of stomach ulcers than the older comparator NSAIDs. Vioxx is typically given in total daily doses of 12.5 mg or 25 mg, and is taken orally either once or twice daily.

•**Meloxicam.** The third prescription COX-2 inhibitor for treatment if OA is meloxicam (brand name Mobic). Mobic is less of a selective COX-2 inhibitor than either Celebrex or Vioxx but more selective than traditional NSAIDs. Studies with Mobic show similar results compared to the previous two COX-2 inhibitors. Studies found meloxicam to be as effective as piroxicam, and slightly less effective than diclofenac for OA pain. The incidence of stomach-related side effects including ulcers and bleeding was much less common with meloxicam compared to diclofenac and piroxicam. Mobic is dosed from 7.5 mg to 15 mg daily. Mobic, like Vioxx, can be used in patients who are allergic to sulfa drugs.

COX-2 inhibitors offer the patient with osteoarthritis the same relief benefits of NSAIDs but with a lower risk of stomach complications or serious bleeding complications. This risk is not completely eliminated, however, with selective COX-2 inhibition. They are of particular benefit for those persons at risk of developing these specific side effects, although their safety with long-term use for more than a year is now just being established. Theoretically, their selective inhibition of the COX-2 enzyme should offer an additional advantage of protecting kidney function but this has not generally been the case. Since COX-2 inhibitors are still NSAIDs, they share similar warnings and precautions that apply to the older generation of NSAIDs. Unfortunately, the cost of these newer NSAIDs is also higher than generic older NSAIDs and about the same as the prescription NSAIDs; their cost runs anywhere from $60 to $75 per month.

TOPICAL CREAMS

Many patients get additional relief from pain flare-ups by using topical creams containing capsaicin, a substance found in hot peppers. The creams are applied up to four times a day directly on joints, typically on the hands and knees affected by OA. Research has found that the cream is effective when used four times daily in a 0.025% solution. Capsaicin cream is available over the counter, and is sold in concentrations of 0.025%, 0.075%, and 0.25%. Some patients who use the cream report local burning and stinging sensations that may be associated with some redness on the skin for the first few days of use. Doctors recommend using a glove when applying the cream, to avoid bringing it into contact with eyes and other sensitive areas.

OPIOIDS

In rare cases, even stronger pain medicines may be needed to relieve flare-ups of OA. These drugs are known as opioid analgesics. They are a powerful class of medicines used for cancer patients and others who suffer from extreme pain. Opioids are synthetic versions of opium-derived drugs like morphine and heroin. The most well known are probably codeine and hydrocodone, which are typically combined with Tylenol. Other opioids sometimes used in osteoarthritis include propoxyphene (Darvon) and oxycodone (Percodan). Opioids and opioid-like medicines should be reserved for extreme cases of osteoarthritis. They may have a place in those patients that have consistently tried and failed the other less potent, conventional drugs used to manage pain in OA. Moreover, these agents do not work to decrease inflammation, which is more prevalent in severe cases of osteoarthritis.

Most doctors avoid long-term use of these drugs for osteoarthritis because of potentially dangerous side effects and abuse potential. These may include a reduced breathing rate, drowsiness, mental confusion, nausea and vomiting, constipation, allergic-type reactions, and mild to moderate withdrawal symptoms upon ceasing use of the medication. Elderly persons and those with liver, kidney, or respiratory problems are particularly prone to developing side effects from opioids. It is recommended that patients not drink any alcohol while taking opioid medication. A recent study of 133 people with persistent OA pain, however, found that long-term oxycodone gave patients relief from pain, improved their overall mood, and helped with sleep. While these results seem encouraging, more research is needed before opioid use becomes a standard in the treatment of osteoarthritis.

Another centrally acting drug, tramadol (Ultram), has also shown promise in severe cases of osteoarthritis pain. It has properties similar to opioids, but appears to have fewer side effects.

DRUG INJECTIONS

When a patient suffers a painful flare-up of osteoarthritis in the knee or hip, doctors may suggest an injection of corticosteroids. Corticosteroids are powerful hormones that are manufactured in the adrenal glands. By injecting them directly into the cartilage, doctors can often reduce inflammation in a joint and alleviate the accompanying pain. In cases where the joint has become swollen, the doctor may first drain part of the fluid in the joint with a syringe, then inject the corticosteroids.

Corticosteroids have a proven record of reducing pain in knees and hips. But the procedure can only be repeated three or four times per year. More frequent use of corticosteroids can actually lead to cartilage and other connective tissue breakdown. Patients who require more than four injections per year in a joint are often considered candidates for surgery, including possible joint replacement. The most common corticosteroids used for injections are triamcinolone (Aristocort) and methylprednisolone (Medrol). Pain from the injection itself seems to be the most common side effect.

Researchers also are looking closely at a relatively new procedure: injecting chemicals that mimic hyaluronic acid, a basic building block of articular cartilage, into knee joints. In healthy cartilage, hyaluronic acid acts as a lubricator, keeping joint fluid viscous and allowing the cartilage to remain elastic. People with OA often have lower concentrations of hyaluronic acid in their affected joints. The treatment involves a series of injections given over a period of three to five weeks. Research has been somewhat mixed on the treatment's effectiveness, but one study has shown that the injections may be as effective at relieving knee pain than a single injection of corticosteroids. Another study found that the injections were as effective as the use of NSAIDs in relieving pain, although the injections did not improve activity levels in patients as much as NSAIDs. The two drugs approved for the injection procedure are hyaluronan (Hyalgan) and hylan G-F 20 (Synvisc). Side effects appear to be minor, but may include pain from the injections themselves and joint swelling Simultaneous therapy with corticosteroid injections is not recommended.

SURGERY

Surgery may be indicated for patients who cannot find pain relief or improved joint motion through medication, exercise therapy, or other methods.

Arthroscopic surgery. This is the least invasive method, and is typically performed on the knee. It is reserved for patients with cartilage tears, bone spurs, or other features that make the underlying osteoarthritic condition worse. During the procedure, surgeons make several punctures in the knee and operate with tiny instruments that they direct with the help of a small camera placed in one of the holes. Surgeons typically trim torn pieces of cartilage and shave its rough edges; remove any loose pieces of cartilage or other material in the joint; and remove bone spurs with a shaving tool. During the procedure, surgeons also perform *lavage* on the joint, which involves washing it out with several liters of a warm, sterile saline solution. Lavage is sometimes performed without any trimming in the joint. This can remove loose particles in the joint and may help with pain by washing away inflammatory chemicals.

While arthroscopic surgery can restore some function and relieve pain in the joint, it is not a cure for OA. The surgery has no effect on the progression of the disease. In fact, a small pilot study found that the placebo effect might account for part of the surgery's success rate. Men who received fake surgery in the study reported similar pain relief after the procedure as those who had full arthroscopic surgery.

Osteotomy. This procedure is sometimes available to patients with osteoarthritis in the hip or knee. It involves cutting and reshaping the ends of bones to improve the motion in the affected joint. This is used only when patients have a severe misalignment of bones from the progression of OA in the joint.

Joint-replacement surgery. Also known as arthroplasty, joint-replacement surgery is a very invasive, but usually effective way to restore function and relieve pain in joints ravaged by osteoarthritis. The surgery is among the most common procedures in the country; more than 137,000 hip replacements are performed each year in the United States, along with more than 245,000 knee replacements. Replacements are available for other joints, such as the ankle and shoulder, but they are not as effective and are used much less often.

Joint replacement is reserved for people who fail to receive sufficient pain relief from medications and other methods. Patients also must suffer loss of mobility so severe that they're unable to perform even daily tasks like walking short distances or climbing stairs. The procedure involves removing the cartilage and bone ends in the joints and replacing them with stainless steel pieces that are capped with a Teflon-like substance to simulate cartilage. The pieces are cemented to the existing bone with an acrylic polymer.

The surgery has been performed since the 1970s in the United States. Complications from the procedure are very rare, and results are usually excellent. More than 95% of patients receiving hip replacements report dramatic pain relief, and about half are still able to perform housework and other light chores twenty years after the procedure. The knee joint has proven more difficult to replace, though the vast majority of patients report reduced pain and increased function in the joint. Artificial joints are not perfect. While most people feel less pain and are able to function better than before the surgery, they rarely return to levels similar to that of people with no damage to their joints. Significant physical rehabilitation periods, lasting weeks or months, are needed to gain maximum benefit from the procedures.

The surgery is usually performed on older patients; about three of every four knee-replacement patients are over 65, as are two of every three people who receive hip replacements. There are two reasons for this. First, osteoarthritis usually does not progress to the point where arthroplasty is needed until a patient is older. Second, the artificial joints can loosen or wear out after a decade or so of use, so younger patients might require additional surgery to repair or replace the joint later in their lives. About 20% of artificial knees may need to be replaced after ten years. Hips tend to last longer; about 85% of people report having their original transplanted joint twenty years after the surgery. New joint replacements that allow natural bone to grow into the structure may help fix this problem.

Arthroplasty is not for everyone. People with blood-clotting disorders are not good candidates, nor are those who have underlying conditions of the heart or lungs that make any kind of surgery unwise. In addition, obese people have more problems with joint loosening, since they place much more stress on the artificial joints.

After deciding to have the surgery, it's wise to search for a facility that handles a high volume of joint replacements. A recent survey found that hospitals where more than one hundred such surgeries are performed each year have far lower rates of infection, complications, and mortality from joint replacements than those that handle six or fewer such surgeries each year.

ALTERNATIVE TREATMENTS

Glucosamine sulfate and chondroitin sulfate. The unsuccessful search for a medical cure has led many discouraged patients to try alternative treatments for osteoarthritis. The best known of these methods is the use of glucosamine sulfate and chondroitin sulfate in supplemental pill form. Both substances naturally occur in cartilage. Glucosamine is a sugar molecule responsible for helping to build collagen and proteoglycans. Chondroitin is a major component of the proteoglycan structure in joints, helping to attract fluid into the cartilage to provide shock absorption for bones and nutrient intake for the cartilage tissue.

Researchers in Europe have produced a number of studies over the past twenty years that show that taking glucosamine and chondroitin can alleviate pain in an osteoarthritic joint. Of even greater interest are studies that found these supplements might actually be able to slow, stop, or even reverse, the deterioration of articular cartilage. If this were the case, these supplements would be the first true cure for osteoarthritis. Unfortunately, a number of experts have reviewed the European studies and found them to be unsound. The studies were not conducted properly, and may have exaggerated the effect the substances had on cartilage destruction. Several studies in the United States are now looking at the effects of glucosamine hydrochloride and chondroitin sulfate; to date, none have duplicated results of the flawed European research that found the drugs might help cartilage regenerate. Preliminary research suggests that they can relieve pain with fewer potential side effects compared with NSAIDs. The pain relief is not immediate, however; the supplement must be taken for a period of days or weeks before any effect is achieved. Since the precise benefit and role of glucosamine and chondroitin in OA remains unknown at this time, anyone considering taking these supplements should consult with their doctor beforehand.

S-Adenosylmethionine. S-Adenosylmethionine, better known as SAMe ("Sammy") is another European import that has found favor with some American OA sufferers. SAMe is an amino acid compound that helps regulate a number of body functions, including the construction of cartilage. It has been used for years overseas as a treatment for diseases ranging from depression and fibromyalgia to osteoarthritis. Many European studies have found that SAMe is as effective as some NSAIDs in controlling pain in osteoarthritis, with fewer side effects (mild stomach upset). Only one small study completed in the United States found that some patients receiving SAMe supplements got better pain relief than those who took a placebo. This effect only applied to those with mild cases of OA and only after several weeks of taking SAMe; people with more severe cases did not appear to benefit. There's no proof that SAMe helps regenerate cartilage. The supplements also are very expensive, ranging from $60 to more than $200 per month. Experts believe people can get the same results more cheaply, with a less expensive alternative and equally low side effects, by taking COX-2 inhibitors although there are no studies directly comparing these agents. More studies are needed to define SAMe's place in therapy for OA and the safety of taking supplements in combination with other OA drugs such as NSAIDS. Patients should never take SAMe or other supplements without first talking to their doctor.

Acupuncture. Like SAMe and glucosamine/chondroitin, acupuncture treatments have a mixed clinical record with OA. One study found that people using acupuncture treatments along with their regular medication reported less pain, stiffness, and loss of function than those not receiving acupuncture. The effect seemed to disappear four weeks after treatment stopped. However, the researchers were not able to control for the placebo effect; patients may simply have believed the treatments were helping them whether or not they actually did. In fact, a 1994 study of forty people with knee osteoarthritis showed no difference in pain relief between people receiving acupuncture and those receiving a fake version of the treatment.

HOW IS IT PREVENTED?

The causes of osteoarthritis remain poorly understood, so experts have a difficult time outlining a plan to prevent the onset of the disease. The most important controllable risk factors appear to be obesity and occupational or recreational activities that place abnormal stress on weight-bearing joints. *The single best recommendation for prevention is to reach and maintain an ideal body weight.* People with poorly aligned knee or hip joints should avoid distance running, heavy lifting, and other high-impact exercise or activities that could hasten osteoarthritic changes in the joint. No one should exercise or work to the point of causing pain in a joint.

WHAT RESEARCH IS BEING DONE?

The search continues for an osteoarthritis cure, although researchers do not appear close to finding a way to stop or reverse progression of the disease. Most research is focused on methods that would slow or stop the effects or collagenolytic agents—chemicals that cause the body to break down collagen, the major building block of cartilage. These methods may include giving test subjects forms of tetracycline or other compounds that would inhibit metalloproteinase and/or interleukin-1. Both these substances stimulate the body to destroy cartilage.

Researchers also are experimenting with creating new chondrocytes and injecting them into damaged cartilage. Chondrocytes are responsible for building new cartilage. In theory, taking chondrocytes from a person, growing more in a laboratory, and then placing them inside an osteoarthritic joint could stimulate new cartilage growth. This has not been done successfully to date.

WHAT YOU CAN DO NOW

Patient involvement plays a key role in the treatment of osteoarthritis. Patient education, regular exercise, weight reduction and other factors are among the most vital components of any treatment plan. People with osteoarthritis can take steps on their own that may slow the progression of the disease or at least make it more manageable. These include losing weight, exercising, eating better, and learning to take medication in proper doses and at the most effective times. It's also important for patients to learn more efficient ways to handle everyday activities that osteoarthritis can complicate, such as climbing stairs or opening jars. Since depression is common among people with all types of arthritis, patients and caregivers also must take action to ensure that osteoarthritis doesn't begin to affect a person's mental well-being. While it can be difficult to live with, osteoarthritis should not deprive anyone of a largely normal, full lifestyle.

Patient education. If you or a loved one has osteoarthritis, the most important first step is learning more about the disease, including its causes and treatment options. Researchers have found that those who simply read pamphlets and other materials about OA are more likely to reduce pain and increase mobility. The positive effect becomes even stronger when patients take additional steps, such as attending self-care classes. Patients who go to these classes have been shown to get better results in pain management and overall function than those who don't. Many classes teach people with OA how to perform simple tasks, like climbing stairs, using canes, and opening jars more efficiently. Educational materials are readily available through nonprofit groups like the Arthritis Foundation. The foundation's local chapters also offer classes. Contact information can be found at the end of this chapter.

Support systems. Many patients find attending support groups helpful in learning to deal with the anxiety and everyday problems that osteoarthritis can cause. Numerous support groups are available in most areas. Doctors can play a positive role by staying in contact with their OA patients. Monthly check-up calls from trained arthritis experts have been shown to improve a patient's chances of reducing pain.

Losing weight and maintaining a healthy diet. Obesity is a major risk factor for osteoarthritis. And poor eating habits, more than anything else, are responsible for obesity. There are no magic foods that can improve osteoarthritis, but research shows that it's important to get enough of several key vitamins, including vitamin D and the antioxidant vitamins A, C, and E. If there is doubt that a person is meeting recommended daily vitamin requirements, consider taking a daily vitamin supplement. It also helps to drink skim milk and eat at least five servings of fruits and vegetables each day.

It's not entirely clear that weight loss helps control symptoms in people with OA, though some research is promising. It has been shown, however, that losing weight can help prevent developing OA in additional joints. Patients who have had trouble losing weight, can talk with their doctor, who may recommend a nutritionist to help devise an eating plan that will address the patient's dietary needs and weight loss concerns.

Exercise. Regular exercise is vital to maintaining joint function and patient mobility. It also can help aid in sleeping, losing weight, and fighting off depression and anxiety. Health care providers can recommend an exercise program that includes muscle strengthening, stretching, and low-impact aerobics.

Aerobic exercise can take many forms:

- Swimming places little stress on the knees or hips.
- Walking is a superb exercise that gives the cartilage in knees and hips a chance to perform under mild stress; this helps keep the cartilage elastic.
- Rowing and bicycle riding are also low-impact activities.
- Exercising with a partner or in a group can keep interest levels higher, as can using a variety of exercises.

There's little doubt that regular exercise can help improve joint function. An eighteen-month study of three hundred sixty-five patients age 60 or older, all with osteoarthritis of the knee, found that those who did aerobic exercise at least three times a week for one hour improved their walking capacity significantly more than those who simply took a health education course. These results have been repeated a number of times in different settings.

Patients should never begin an exercise routine without first consulting their doctor. Some exercises may not be appropriate for particular types of OA or for other health conditions the patient may have.

Use a little ice. Never exercise a joint to the point of pain. But if there is pain after working out, joints sometimes respond well to ice. Always place a thin towel between the ice pack and the joint, and limit the icing to about 20 minutes or so. This can be repeated several times per day. Sometimes, applying ice to a joint before exercise can reduce pain during the workout.

Use medicines properly. Always follow the exact instructions for any drugs to be taken. Patients should inform and consult with their doctor before using nonprescription drugs (aspirin, ibuprofen, acetaminophen, naproxen). Many NSAIDs, even those of newer variety (Celebrex, Vioxx, Mobic), can cause stomach upset, so it's usually recommended to take them with food and water. It also may help not to lie down for an hour or so after taking them, to help keep stomach acids out of the esophagus and prevent heartburn. Avoid or limit alcohol intake when using Tylenol or any of the NSAIDs. If the patient has other conditions that require medication, always inform the doctor about them. Other medications can interact with osteoarthritis drugs and supplements. Consult the pharmacist if you are concerned about potential drug-to-drug interactions. Younger women should immediately inform their doctors if they become pregnant, some medications are not recommended for use during pregnancy.

ADDITIONAL RESOURCES

WEB SITES

American College of Rheumatology

www.rheumatology.org/index.asp

Arthritis Foundation

www.arthritis.org

Centers for Disease Control and Prevention

www.cdc.gov/nccdphp/arthritis.htm

The National Institute of Arthritis and Musculoskeletal and Skin Diseases

www.nih.gov/niams

Parkinson's Disease

In recent years, Parkinson's disease, often referred to as PD, has assumed a public face with the disclosure of several celebrity cases—Attorney General Janet Reno, actor Michael J. Fox, and former boxer Muhammad Ali. Watching Reno's press conferences during the years she was in Washington, the public watched the degenerative nature of this disease, as her symptoms have progressed from slight trembling in one hand to sometimes-violent chopping motions with both arms. Less typically, Fox was diagnosed at the young age of 30.

SIGNS & SYMPTOMS

- Abnormal slowness of voluntary movement, leading to a characteristic shuffling gait
- Rigidity
- Tremors (shaking)
- Lack of stability when standing
- Difficulty initiating voluntary movement, feeling "stuck" in place, "frozen" in one position
- Drooling
- Fixed facial expression with infrequent blinking
- Decreased volume in speaking
- Illegible handwriting
- Lack of arm swing
- Depression, anxiety, sleep disturbance
- Urinary incontinence
- Cognitive impairment

WHAT IS IT?

Parkinson's disease is a chronic, progressive neurological disorder characterized by slowness of movement (bradykinesia), tremor (shaking), difficulty walking, stiffness, and problems with balance. It is a relatively common disease—the second most common degenerative neurological disease after Alzheimer's—affecting more than one million Americans. It most often strikes after the age of 50, and becomes increasingly prevalent in older people. It is named for James Parkinson, the British physician who first described it in 1817.

The symptoms of PD are a result of the degeneration of a part of the brain involved in movement control, the substantia nigra, a small area within the brainstem. Cells in the substantia nigra produce the neurotransmitter dopamine, a chemical that is part of the brain's message transmission system. Dopamine helps regulate the movement control centers of the brain and without it, the uncontrollable shaking or abnormally slow movements that are a hallmark of Parkinson's occur. Many parts of the brain are affected by the loss of dopamine. Other neurotransmitters (for example, norepinephrine) may also be depleted, and this may contribute to the depression that is seen in many PD patients. The latest investigations into what happens in the brain of a person with PD are focusing on the oxidization of dopamine and the possible role of antioxidants, the same nutritional supplements that are believed to have a role in preventing heart disease and some types of cancer. Most investigators believe that PD is caused by the effect of toxins—whose identity is as yet unknown—on a genetically susceptible individual.

Drugs that interfere with the brain's use of dopamine, such as haloperidol (Haldol) and similar drugs used to treat mental disorders, as well as the antinausea drug metoclopramide (Reglan), can cause "parkinsonism," a Parkinson's-like syndrome. The symptoms of parkinsonism typically vanish within six to twelve months after the patient is taken off these drugs.

WHO IS AT RISK?

Like many diseases, the biggest risk for developing Parkinson's disease is simply growing older. Approximately 1% of people over 65 and from 1.5 to 2.5% of people over the age of 70 have PD. More than half of all people over the age of 85 have some parkinsonian features (but not Parkinson's disease). Fifteen percent of cases are diagnosed before the age of 50.

PD is seen in people of all ethnic groups and almost equally in men and women.

There is a range of estimates of the prevalence of PD. The National Parkinson's Foundation puts the number as high as 1.5 million Americans. By the year 2040, the U.S. Department of Census predicts there will be 1.3 million to 1.7 million cases in the United States.

OTHER MOVEMENT DISORDERS

A number of other movement disorders can impair a person's functioning and some of these may appear to PD at first. These include:

Essential tremor. This is characterized by involuntary shaking of a body part, usually the hands or arms. The head and voice may also be affected. It progresses slowly and may remain mild throughout life. However, it may cause disability, affecting handwriting and performance of other fine motor tasks with the hands. This disorder is very common, affecting as many as ten million Americans—20 times more common than PD.

Progressive supranuclear palsy. This degenerative disease is one of a number of parkinsonian syndromes. It often progresses rapidly and the cause is unknown. It is fairly rare, appearing after the age of 45 and, typically, twice as frequently in men as in women. The condition is characterized by unstable posture and frequent falls; difficulty swallowing and speaking; bradykinesia; the inability to look downward; and other visual disturbances. It is often misdiagnosed initially as PD.

Dystonia. Dystonia is characterized by continuing muscle contractions, causing involuntary twisting or turning movements or abnormal postures. Dystonia is thought to result from the brain's difficulty in processing neurotransmitters. Many types of dystonia have been described, depending on the location of the impairment. Some dystonia begins in childhood. The condition is rarely responsive to low doses of levodopa (L-dopa), the dopamine-replacing medication that is used for PD

Restless legs syndrome. This chronic condition, characterized by a compulsion to move the limbs, often runs in families and has been estimated to affect as much as 10% of the population. It is common in pregnancy. The symptoms are unpleasant creeping sensations felt deep within the legs, and sometimes arms, which often affect sleep. It sometimes responds to L-dopa and other drugs.

Tourette's syndrome. This syndrome, thought to be inherited, is characterized by multiple voice or motor tics (involuntary, uncontrollable, repetitive sounds or actions). It usually begins in childhood, is more commonly seen in boys, and can range from mild to severe. Examples of tics are eye blinking, head jerking, foot stamping, body twisting, coughing, grunting, or yelping. Tourette's is treatable with several different medications. The condition is not degenerative, and the symptoms lessen with age.

Little is known about what causes PD and if there are any specific risk factors. There is evidence that genetics are involved in early-onset PD (before the age of 50). While there may be some genetic susceptibility involved with later-onset PD, environmental factors are possible triggers, and this is the direction in which most researchers are looking.

A very small minority of people with PD trace the beginnings of their disease to a head injury of some sort or another type of trauma, even an emotional trauma, but neurologists doubt there is a direct link. It is known that exposure to a chemical known as MPTP causes Parkinson's in humans and research monkeys. Used as an illicit recreational drug, MPTP is converted in the body to a neurotoxin that selectively destroys the substantia nigra. Scientists are investigating the possibility that PD is associated with environmental toxins such as herbicides and pesticides. One study that compared nearly five hundred newly diagnosed PD patients to a slightly larger control group drawn from the same population found that individuals with a history of exposure to pesticides or herbicides in the home (that is, not industrial usage) had a 70% increased risk of developing PD. Another study has linked the development of parkinsonism in laboratory rats to rotenone, a pesticide widely used for commercial and home-gardening uses. Rotenone is a natural substance made from extracts of tropical plants and has long been thought to be relatively safe. Scientists continue to investigate the possible association between PD and environmental toxins.

HOW IS IT DIAGNOSED?

Parkinson's disease is diagnosed on the basis of a number of symptoms. The four most common and significant are motor signs:

- Bradykinesia, or abnormal slowness of voluntary movement, leading to a characteristic shuffling gait
- Rigidity
- Tremor (shaking). In PD, tremor typically begins in one hand in contrast to essential tremor, which from the beginning, affects both hands
- Lack of stability when standing

Other symptoms vary from person to person and in severity, according to the state of the disease. They may include:

- Difficulty initiating voluntary movement, feeling "stuck" in place, "frozen" in one position
- Drooling
- Fixed facial expression with infrequent blinking
- Decreased volume in speaking
- Illegible handwriting (known as micrographia, for small handwriting)
- Lack of arm swing
- Decreased ability to smell (rarely)
- Dandruff or oily skin
- Depression
- Anxiety
- Sleep disturbance
- Constipation
- Sweating
- Urinary incontinence
- Impotence
- Cognitive impairment (although this is a very late complication of PD and is not an inevitable feature of all cases)

TESTS

Parkinson's is usually diagnosed based on a neurological exam. There are no tests that are specific for PD, but tests help to rule out other conditions with similar symptoms. On average in the United States, there is a lag of eighteen months between early symptoms of PD and diagnosis, because of the subtlety of the symptoms. When seeking diagnosis for Parkinson-like symptoms, it is important that a patient be examined by a board-certified neurologist experienced in movement disorders.

A relatively new type of imaging called single-photon emission computed tomography (SPECT) has been used to examine the dopamine transporters in the brain. These studies have been able to detect decreases in dopamine production before PD symptoms become noticeable. In the future, SPECT may have a role in early diagnosis of Parkinson's.

WHAT SHOULD YOU EXPECT?

The course of Parkinson's varies from one patient to another. There is no cure for Parkinson's yet, but during the early and middle stages, medication is usually very effective in controlling the symptoms. After ten years or more, it can be difficult to treat. However, PD generally does not shorten life. People with PD, especially women, are more likely to require residence in some sort of care facility. The predominance of women needing institutional care may be related to the fact that women so often are the caregivers, but may not have caregivers available for them in their homes when infirmity makes it difficult to tend to their own daily needs. Moreover, women in general live longer than men, whether they have PD or not.

Treatments available for PD now allow many people with the disease to maintain an acceptable level of functioning throughout their lives, and research continues to turn up improved therapies. Symptoms and responses to treatment vary so much from one person to another that it is hard to describe a typical course of the disease, but many people will need some assistance with activities of daily living after ten to fifteen years with PD.

The tremors of PD begin episodically, in just one hand or on one side of the body (although not everyone with PD experiences tremors). Over time, tremors are accompanied by slow movement and stiffness, particularly on the side of the body where symptoms began. Symptoms may then progress to the other side, but they usually remain more pronounced on the primary side. Persons with PD may also experience gait and balance problems, with particular difficulty walking stairs, getting through doorways, and turning corners.

Pneumonia is the most common cause of death in people who die of complications from PD. Factors that contribute to pneumonia in PD include immobility, poor cough and inability to clear secretions, and repeated episodes of aspiration. However, it is worth noting that most people with PD die of unrelated causes (for example, cancer or heart disease).

HOW IS IT TREATED?

There is no cure for Parkinson's disease, and treatment is aimed at controlling the symptoms. PD can be treated with medications or, in more severe or advanced cases, surgery. In addition, some lifestyle changes may lessen some symptoms.

MEDICATIONS

L-Dopa. Oral medications are the first-line treatment for Parkinson's disease. Orally administered dopamine cannot be absorbed directly by the brain so a chemical called levodopa, or L-dopa, which is converted to dopamine, is given. L-Dopa has become the gold standard of PD treatment. It is very effective for most patients, at least at first. However, with time it can have serious side effects and there is a diminution in potency after a period of usage.

Levodopa revolutionized the treatment of Parkinson's when it was introduced in the early 1970s. It is given with another drug, carbidopa, which increases the absorption of L-dopa into the brain and reduces nausea. L-Dopa is very effective in alleviating PD symptoms. It is generally tolerated well. The most common early side effect is mild nausea. In the later stages of PD, it can contribute to mental confusion and hallucinations and uncontrollable twitching or jerking (dyskinesia). Half of patients taking L-dopa have fluctuations in their motor functioning after five to seven years, and 84% after ten to twelve years.

Perhaps the biggest problem with this drug, however, is that for many people its effectiveness lessens over time. Most people get the best results for a few years after beginning the drug, and then will find that the doses work for progressively shorter period of time. This is called the "wearing off" phenomenon. For some people, an "on-off" effect causes symptoms to come and go unpredictably. There is scientific debate about wearing off—some think that L-dopa paradoxically damages the neurons that produce dopamine, while others believe it is related to the natural progression of the disease. Because of its limited effectiveness, doctors often do not prescribe L-dopa until PD symptoms seriously interfere with a person's normal functioning.

Dopamine agonists. Dopamine agonists stimulate the same centers of the brain that dopamine acts upon. They are used with L-dopa or instead of it, and many doctors now start their PD patients on dopamine agonists to put off

425

using L-dopa. A five-year study found that one dopamine agonist, ropinirole (Requip), was successful in controlling PD symptoms with a decreased risk of dyskinesias. A two-year study found equally good results for avoiding dyskinesias with pramipexole (Mirapex), another dopamine agonist. It was not as effective as L-dopa in alleviating symptoms, but most people who took it said they were satisfied with the results. Although the dopamine agonists are generally well tolerated, they do have potential side effects: somnolence, hallucinations, and swelling. The falling-asleep problem—labeled "sleep attacks" for their often sudden and unexpected onset—could be an issue for people with PD who drive motor vehicles.

COMT inhibitors. COMT inhibitors are used with in combination with L-dopa. They block an enzyme that breaks down L-dopa, allowing L-dopa to work more efficiently. Examples of COMT inhibitors are tolcapone (Tasmar) and entacapone (Comtan). Tolcapone can cause liver damage, and people taking it should have their liver function monitored. Some patients have low blood pressure, which can be treated with midodrine HCl (ProAmatine) or fludrocortisone acetate (Florinef). Selective serotonin re-uptake inhibitors and tricyclic antidepressants are often prescribed for depression or anxiety, although they should not be used by patients taking selegiline. Sildenafil citrate (Viagra) is used for treating sexual dysfunction in men with PD.

A number of other drugs are also used to treat PD. Selegiline (Eldepryl), a drug classified as a monoamine oxidase inhibitor, is often prescribed when L-dopa starts losing effectiveness. There is evidence to suggest it may also protect the brain when used early in the illness, thus delaying the time before L-dopa is needed. Amantadine (Symmetrel) is an antiviral medication used to treat the flu, but has also been shown to reduce some of the symptoms of PD. In PD there is an imbalance of neurotransmitters: dopamine is depleted and the brain chemical acetylcholine is relatively excessive. So anticholinergic drugs are also effective in treating tremors and rigidity in early PD because they block acetylcholine. Commonly used anticholinergics include benztropine (Cogentin) and trihexyphenidyl (Artane). However, they may cause side effect, including dry mouth, constipation, urinary retention, blurred vision, confusion, and hallucinations. There is some debate about the order in which to use the various medications. It is often helpful for the patient to get a second or even third opinion when medications are prescribed, to get a complete understanding of the risks and benefits of each.

SURGERY

Because so many medications are proving effective against PD, surgery is reserved for advanced cases of Parkinson's and for patients who have a poor or inconsistent response to medications. But surgery can play a significant role in treatment, especially for early-onset patients. Enhanced imaging and other adjuncts to surgery are making surgical therapies for PD increasingly safe and effective. In a recent informal survey, physicians specializing in treatment of PD indicated that 10 to 30% of cases are appropriate for surgery.

In the 1930s, neurosurgeons discovered that inflicting tiny wounds (lesions) in certain sections of the brain could substantially alleviate PD symptoms. This is called ablative surgery. Surgery was first done on the region of the brain called the globus pallidus, and then in the thalamus. These procedures were refined with the use of devices that accurately position and stabilize the area to be operated on. Patients are awake and alert during the procedure (under local anesthesia) and can react to electrical stimulation of a small area of the brain, which is then selected for the placement of the lesion. Lessening of tremor has been the result in up to 90% of patients who received stereotactic thalamotomy, and up to 80% of patients who receive stereotactic pallidotomy experience more "on" time (periods of improved functioning) and less dyskinesia. However, in as many as one-quarter of surgical cases, there are adverse side effects, ranging from bleeding to partial paralysis to speech impairment and mental changes. The highest risks are in older patients and those who have the procedure done on both sides of the brain.

The next refinement of surgery was to use the electrical stimulation itself as the therapeutic mechanism. This is known as deep-brain stimulation (DBS) and is one of the most fertile areas of clinical study in PD. Electrodes are implanted in an area of the brain known as the subthalamic nucleus, located near the globus pallidus, which is pathologically overactive in Parkinson's. Wires run from the electrodes to an implanted pulse generator just over the collar bone. Patients can turn the device on and off with a hand-held magnet. Studies have found improvements in motor function of patients undergoing DBS. Despite its general safety, there are potential side effects, including paresthesia (abnormal sensations such as burning, tingling, or numbness), mental slowness, memory decline, headache, and gait disorders.

The most recent surgical approach involves implantation of fetal substantia nigra (brain) cells into the brains of people with PD. This still-experimental technique has been very controversial because the tissue comes from aborted fetuses. Politics aside, however, it has been demonstrated that implanted cells can replace the degenerating substantia nigra in the Parkinson's patient and restore dopamine production. The procedure has been done on only about one hundred and fifty patients and results have been inconsistent, but many of the patients have shown improvement, and the need for much lower doses of L-dopa. In one case, the benefits of the fetal cell implantation continued for ten years. However, there have also been reports of severe dyskinesias resulting from implantation, perhaps as a result of overgrowth of the implanted tissue. Clearly, this is an area where further research is needed before this technique can be broadly applied.

LIFESTYLE CHANGES

Exercise and targeted physical therapy can be effective in lessening the symptoms of Parkinson's. Physical and occupational therapy can supply ways to compensate so that disability is reduced. Therapy programs have to be designed individually, taking into consideration the needs of patients and their caregivers. Also, patients' capabilities and responses often vary hour by hour, depending on the medication cycle, and so different movement strategies might be taught at different times.

Many physical and occupational therapy techniques can be applied to the different motor problems experienced by people with PD. For example, sometimes visual cues, such as chalk marks measuring lengths of steps, are helpful with walking. Mental rehearsal and breaking down an action into a sequence of steps can aid rolling over and getting out of bed and other complex activities. Keeping a log detailing incidents of falling can often indicate patterns or conditions (only falling in the morning, or stumbling over a particular rug, for example) that both patients and caregivers can avoid. Practicing reaching, grasping, and handwriting with large strokes can be helpful. There should be an emphasis on maintaining fitness with activities such as walking, swimming, yoga, golfing, or cycling on a track. One recent study suggested that music therapy was also effective in relieving PD symptoms.

No special nutritional guidelines are recommended for people with PD, but a healthy, well-balanced diet can help maintain general good health. Constipation is experienced by many people with PD, and this can be reduced by a diet high in fiber and fluids. Doctors recommend that patients with a poor response to L-dopa try eating most of the protein in their diet at their evening meal, because protein can make L-dopa less effective. Doctors or other health care professionals can help patients develop good dietary habits.

WHAT RESEARCH IS BEING DONE?

Many efforts are ongoing in Parkinson's research, in a number of different areas. Scientists are looking at new drugs or better ways to use existing drugs to alleviate symptoms, including lessening side effects of L-dopa and other medications. They are attempting to develop drugs that improve the underlying disease, reversing or slowing the degeneration of the nerve cells that produce dopamine. They are investigating the various surgical techniques used to treat PD, and analyzing the advantages of each. There is no cure yet for this disease, but many researchers think that science is moving in that direction.

Some of the most provocative work comes with compounds called neuroimmunophilins, which have shown the ability in animals to regenerate nerves that have been damaged by injury or disease. Neuroimmunophilins have also demonstrated that they can pass through the blood-brain barrier, the protective mechanism that limits the passage of some drugs, chemicals, and toxins in the brain; therefore, these compounds can be given by mouth. Researchers are learning more about how to use these compounds so they will not have significant side effects, and will soon move their efforts from laboratory animals to PD patients who may benefit from the treatment and point the way, with their results, to future usage. One neuroimmunophilin has reached the clinical trial stage.

In surgery, deep brain stimulation is already a treatment option, but it is in its infancy and continuing studies are determining how it can be used best. The other surgical procedure under investigation is tissue implantation. Because of the shortage of human fetal brain tissue, and the political and ethical debate surrounding its usage, scientists are looking for other sources to provide tissue that has the potential to regenerate dopamine-producing cells. Experimental work is being done with fetal pigs, which have neurons physiologically similar to humans. So far, the work has been moderately successful in humans, and immunosuppressive drugs may be needed because it is a transplant between species (xenotransplantation).

TIPS FOR CAREGIVERS AND PATIENTS

Some of the best and most knowledgeable advice for caregivers comes from the organizations that represent people with PD and their families. The following tips are from the American Parkinson Disease Association.

For the caregiver

• Appreciate that "normal" has changed and may never be the same again.

• To deal with the frustration of bradykinesia (slowness of movement), have something to do such as listening to music, reading, or knitting.

• Always allow plenty of time to get to places and don't pressure the person with PD. It only causes stress and makes things worse.

• The person with PD may need reminders, especially when the disease affects cognition.

But prioritize your reminders so that your helpfulness is not perceived as nagging.

• Be aware that PD may cause personality changes. These may be subtle or obvious. Be prepared to live with these changes, but also look beyond them for reasons that may be treatable such as depression or anxiety.

• One of your own reactions to the frustrations of PD might be anger. If the anger becomes more than occasional, seek counseling.

• Look for a support group (see following section). Be attentive to your own needs. If the burden begins to feel overwhelming or depression sets in, seek counseling.

For the person with Parkinson's

• Change clothing styles to eliminate difficult but-

Continuing research has also brought new insights into the genetics of PD, and two genes have been located that may be implicated in certain cases of PD. However, genetic factors are thought to be involved with only a small percentage of PD cases, mostly early-onset disease.

Gene therapy is another area of active medical research for many conditions, although so far it has not delivered the promise that many had hoped for in treating disease. But a recent report documented that injection of a gene promoting the production of dopamine could stimulate the brains of monkeys with chemically induced Parkinson's to produce dopamine, and it relieved symptoms. Not only did the gene treatment prevent further degeneration of the substantia nigra, but the cells regenerated, and the results were still evident eight months after the treat-

tons, belts, or zippers. Use Velcro fasteners whenever possible.

• A "fanny pack" may be easier to access than a wallet or pocketbook.

• Men with PD may want to grow a beard to avoid shaving problems.

• Short hair and easy "wash-and-wear" hairstyles can make this aspect of grooming more practical for women with PD.

• In the house, remove scatter rugs and thick pile carpet.

• Tub seats and rails, hand-held showers, and raised toilet seats can help make bathroom tasks safer and easier and preserve independence in this intimate area.

And from the National Parkinson Foundation:

• Make a conscious effort to lift your feet when you walk, to avoid shuffling, foot drag, and falls.

• Don't stand for too long with your feet close together; it increases the risk of falling.

• Turn by walking in a U, rather than trying to pivot.

• To help with balance, use a rubber-tipped cane.

• When you feel frozen to the floor, try rocking slightly from side to side to get moving again. Or step over an imaginary obstacle to continue forward.

• Swing both arms when walking to keep your balance.

• Never carry objects in both hands when walking.

• Don't try to do other things when you are walking, such as carry on a conversation. Focus on the task at hand.

ment. This work is still very preliminary, and safety will have to be assessed before it can be used in humans, but it presents an encouraging avenue for scientists to investigate.

Another intriguing area of interest in Parkinson's research is antioxidants. Oxidation of neural cells is thought to be part of the reason they degenerate, and scientists are looking at whether dietary supplementation with antioxidants (vitamins A, C, and E, and coenzyme Q-10) can be protective of the neurons that produce dopamine, and have a role in preventing PD. These effects are still not proven, however.

Sometimes scientific research turns up unexpected findings. Nicotine is not thought of as a healthful substance, but it seems to have a positive effect on

Parkinson's patients. Experiments with nicotine patches have found that the nicotine lessens both motor and cognitive symptoms in PD patients. This is another area in which research will continue, to gain further understandings of a preventive and/or therapeutic role for nicotine.

Clearly, more research is needed before the best way to use existing pharmaceuticals, alone or in combination, is best understood. New methods of drug delivery—i.e., via a skin patch or implanted pump—are also under investigation

HOW CAN IT BE PREVENTED?

At present, there is no way to prevent Parkinson's disease and other movement disorders. Many of the research efforts mentioned above are looking for methods of prevention. Interestingly, caffeine has been found to have a role similar to nicotine in some studies. A large population study of Japanese-American men found that high coffee/caffeine intake was associated with a significantly lower incidence of PD. Men who didn't drink coffee were five times more likely to develop PD than those who drank four to five cups a day. However, there is no evidence that persons with PD benefit from increasing their consumption of caffeine.

Other chemicals that may have a role in preventing PD are antioxidants and estrogen, but much more study needs to be done before these mechanisms are understood and their benefits applied.

WHAT YOU CAN DO NOW

FOR THE CAREGIVER

Parkinson's disease is an insidiously progressive condition that begins slowly and is not, in itself, life-threatening. But it takes its toll on the caregiver as well as the patient in a number of distinctive ways. Caregiving is stressful and sometimes overwhelming. It is not uncommon for caregivers to have periods of denial, depression, and overcompensation.

Understanding this disease will give insight into what the patient is experiencing, an important element of compassionate caregiving. It is also important that caregivers have an ongoing relationship with the physician and other health care providers so they stay aware of the range of treatments available and the risks and benefits of each. To safeguard their own physical and mental health and well-being, caregivers need to pay attention to their own needs, seek the help of close friends and other family members, and join a support group to learn how others handle similar challenges.

A diagnosis of Parkinson's disease can be frightening for patient and caregiver both. One of the most common reactions for a caregiver is to overcompensate, to try to do more for the patient than is necessary. This is likely to cause an overdependent relationship and increase the feeling of disability. A more constructive approach is to highlight a person's capabilities and work from there. Patience is a very important quality for caregivers. Caregivers who are feeling overwhelmed should also consider asking for help from other family members, hiring outside help, or seeking respite from an adult day care center.

ADDITIONAL RESOURCES

ORGANIZATIONS AND WEB SITES

American Parkinson Disease Association Inc.

1250 Hylan Boulevard

Suite 4B

Staten Island, NY 10305

800-223-2732

www.apdaparkinson.com

National Institute of Neurological Disorders and Stroke

www.ninds.nih.gov

National Parkinson Foundation, Inc.

1501 N.W. 9th Avenue

Miami, FL 33136-1494

800-327-4545 . In Florida: 800-433-7022

www.parkinson.org

Parkinson's Disease Foundation (PDF)

710 West 168th St.

New York, NY 10032-9982

800-457-6676

or 833 West Washington Boulevard

Chicago, IL 60607

312-733-1893

www.pdf.org

www.parkinsons-foundation.org

Parkinson's Action Network (PAN)

840 Third St.

Santa Rosa, CA 95404

800-850-4726

www.parkinsonaction.org

Young Parkinson's Information and Referral Center

Glenbrook Hospital

2100 Pfingsten Road

Glen View IL 60025

800-223-9776

Young Parkinson's Support Network

142 Perkins Row

Topsfield, MA 01983

978-887-8544

BOOKS

Argue, John. *Parkinson's Disease & the Art of Moving.* Oakland, Calif.: New Harbinger Publishers, 2000.

Goldmann, David R., and David A. Horowitz, (eds). *American College of Physicians Home Medical Guide: Parkinson's Disease.* New York: DK Publishers, 2000.

Grady-Fitchett, Joan. *Flying Lessons: On the Wings of Parkinson's Disease.* New York: Forge Publishers, 1998.

Hauser, Robert A., et al. *Parkinson's Disease - Questions and Answers,* 3rd ed. Coral Springs, Fla.: Merit Publishing International, 2000.

Hutton, J. Thomas, et al. (eds). *Caring for the Parkinson Patient: A Practical Guide.* Amherst, N.Y.:Prometheus Books, 1999.

Morgan, Eric R. *Defending Against the Enemy: Coping With Parkinson's Disease.* Fort Bragg, Calif.: Q.E.D. Press, 1997.

Waters, Cheryl H. *Diagnosis & Management of Parkinson's Disease,* 2nd ed. Los Angeles: Professional Communications, 1999.

Prostate Cancer

| **SIGNS & SYMPTOMS**

There are hardly ever any warning signs for prostate cancer. Prostate cancer begins in silence, growing very slowly, producing no symptoms for years. Regular screening for this disease is critical, so that prostate cancer may be caught and cured before it grows into a fatal tumor.

The statistics are sobering: This year, an estimated 31,900 American men—about one every sixteen minutes—will die of prostate cancer, and more than 180,400 American men will be drafted, by diagnosis, into the "reluctant brotherhood" of men with prostate cancer. Prostate cancer is the second leading cause of cancer death in men, behind only lung cancer. But the picture used to be much worse. In 1988, the number of men who died from prostate cancer was far higher—an estimated 44,000. The good news is that over the last twenty years, there has been a revolution in prostate cancer detection and treatment.

WHAT IS IT?

The prostate is a small gland—about the size and shape of a walnut—that sits at the base of the bladder, millimeters away from the rectum, in a densely packed area of anatomy. It encircles the urethra, the tube that carries urine from the bladder and out of the body. When it becomes enlarged, as it does in a harmless but annoying disorder called benign prostatic hyperplasia (BPH, also called "enlargement of the prostate"), it can cause hard-to-ignore symptoms right away, including difficulty in urination or increased urgency and frequency of urination.

But when cancer grows in the prostate, it's usually not near the urethra, and usually has little effect on urination. As a result, *there are hardly ever any warning signs for prostate cancer*—no telltale symptoms that, if picked up promptly

435

by an astute clinician, can guarantee that this often-deadly disease will be detected and treated in time. Instead, prostate cancer begins in silence, growing very slowly, producing no symptoms for years. It is during these early years in the life of a prostate tumor—when it is small and localized (restricted to the prostate, and not yet spread beyond it)—that cancer is most vulnerable, and easiest to kill. This is the crucial "window of opportunity" for treatment, and this is why regular screening for this disease is so important—so that prostate cancer may be caught and cured as quickly as possible.

WHO IS AT RISK?

In all men, prostate cancer takes years to develop. But there are three major risk factors for prostate cancer—age, family history, and race (being of African-American descent)—that can increase the odds that a cancer will form. Because men with a family history of prostate cancer and African Americans are more likely to develop the disease at a younger age, they need to begin yearly testing earlier, as well—at age 40, instead of 50. More on these risk groups in a moment.

Briefly, this is how scientists believe most prostate cancer happens: Like many cancers, it is caused by damage to DNA, the vast chain of chemical combinations that make up our genetic blueprint. Every gene is a chemical building block, with its own particular sequence of DNA codes, and every gene plays a small but important part in the production of specific proteins that control body functions. Each time a cell divides, the genetic code must accomplish a miracle—it must make a perfect copy of itself. This is a complicated business, with much potential for mistakes. As safeguards, our bodies have numerous "back-up" systems in place, protective mechanisms to prevent malfunctions in cell division—and most importantly, to keep cancers from developing. In prostate cancer, scientists believe, our own cellular metabolism—the everyday processing of nutrients and other chemicals—goes awry. Countless times a day, our metabolism creates a toxic byproduct—oxygen radicals, also called free radicals. The name sounds dangerous, and these tiny, electrically charged molecules are highly reactive and unstable. Free radicals can do great harm —called oxidative damage—to tissue. Normally, cells have specialized "bodyguards," called scavenger enzymes, that work hard to convert these free radicals into harmless, water-soluble products. But in prostate cancer, the most common of these protective, free radical-fighting enzymes is knocked out—even in early disease. Because prostate cancer cells lack this key enzyme (called glutathione-S-transferase), the normal oxidative damage has a much greater effect. Scientists believe that most of the risk factors linked to prostate cancer somehow result in increased oxidative damage. Mutations or changes in the DNA code occur gradually, over time, as oxidative damage takes its toll. Which brings us to the most important risk factors in prostate cancer:

Age. The incidence of prostate cancer rises dramatically with age—more so than any other cancer. An American man in his mid- to late-70s is much more likely to develop prostate cancer than a man in his mid- to late-40s. For men in their forties and fifties, the risk of developing prostate cancer is one in 53. But once men reach their 60s and 70s, the risk is much greater—down to one in seven.

Scientists estimate that it takes roughly eleven or twelve years (about a year less in African- American men) from the beginning of prostate cancer—when those first few cells go bad—to its clinical presentation, when it causes a significant change in prostate-specific antigen (PSA)—a prostate cancer screening test, or when it's big enough for a doctor to feel during a rectal exam.

Race. African Americans have the highest risk of prostate cancer of any ethnic group in the world. Worse, black men seem to get more severe forms of prostate cancer, are more likely to have cancer recur after treatment, and are more likely to die from the disease than white men of comparable age—which, again, is why these men need to start regular screening at age 40, and to continue it vigilantly. Exactly why black men are hit so hard by this disease remains uncertain, although it is a major focus of genetic research in prostate cancer.

Family history. Some forms of prostate cancer are hereditary. As characterized by scientists at Johns Hopkins, the risks of hereditary prostate cancer break down like this: If your father or brother has had prostate cancer, your risk of developing the disease is twofold greater. If three family members (such as a father and two brothers) have developed prostate cancer, or if the disease occurs in three generations in your family (grandfather, father, son), or if two of your relatives have developed the disease at an early age (younger than 55), then you may have a hereditary form of prostate cancer. Scientists at Johns Hopkins, the National Human Genome Research Institute, and elsewhere are closing in on the genes responsible for hereditary prostate cancer. When they are found, genetic testing will be available.

Environment. Environment—mainly meaning diet—also plays a role, although exactly how big it is and how it works are still being determined. Scientists began considering environment part of the equation of prostate cancer when they noticed a remarkable phenomenon. Autopsy studies from around the world have found that about half of all men—no matter where they live, or what color their skin is—develop small, "incidental" clusters of prostate cancer by the time they are 80 years old. This cancer seems to be harmless; it seems quite content in the prostate, rarely grows, and hardly ever spreads. Even Asian men get this "incidental" cancer—a fact remarkable in itself, because these men almost never develop the kind of prostate cancer that needs to be treated. In Asian men, the risk of developing significant prostate cancer is very low until these men migrate to Western countries. Then their risk of developing prostate cancer increases over time. Thus, scientists believe that the steps that spark cancer—even if it's just the "incidental" kind—are universal. But in some men, this spark simply smolders; in others, it becomes a wildfire. The big difference must be environmental. Is it the fault of the Western diet—too few vegetables and fruits, too much red meat and fried food—or is it one or more beneficial components of the Asian diet, such as soy or green tea? Or is it some other factor—something in the soil where we grow our vegetables, or even a difference in how much sunlight we get? The answers to these questions may enable scientists to prevent prostate cancer someday, or at least delay its onset for many years.

HOW IS IT DIAGNOSED?

It used to be that prostate cancer was diagnosed mainly when it produced symptoms, such as back pain or urinary obstruction or when it had grown big enough to feel, during a digital rectal examination (when a doctor's gloved, lubricated finger, inserted in the rectum, palpates the prostate, feeling for hard or abnormal places).

SCREENING AND THE PSA TEST

Then came the PSA test, which measures levels of an enzyme called prostate-specific antigen in the blood. In the late 1980s, the PSA test began to be used, along with the digital rectal exam, as a means of screening men yearly for prostate cancer. This diagnostic combination has proven highly effective: Now doctors can detect cancers at an earlier, more treatable stage than ever before—about five to seven years sooner than in the decades before PSA. The average age of diagnosis has dropped from 72 to 69. And most importantly, the rising tide of prostate cancer deaths seems to have turned: Before 1991, deaths from prostate cancer in the United States were increasing by 1 to 2% a year. But since 1991, this number has been falling, on average, by about 1.5% a year. Men who are at higher risk—African-American men, or those who have a family history of prostate cancer (as described above)—should start yearly screening, with a PSA blood test and a digital rectal examination, at age 40.

What about men at normal risk? Conventional wisdom has been that most men should start yearly screening at age 50. But recently, using a highly sophisticated computer model, which mathematically simulated progression of prostate cancer in a hypothetical group of men, Johns Hopkins scientists found that men at normal risk should have their first digital rectal exam and PSA test at age 40, then again at age 45, and then beginning at age 50, be tested every other year, until old age or ill health suggest that a man's life expectancy is less than ten or fifteen years.

Screening for prostate cancer with a yearly PSA test, in addition to the rectal exam, is itself somewhat controversial. For much of the 1990s, some doctors opposed this, basing their argument on the fact that millions of American men have prostate cancer that will never bother them during their lifetime. (This is the "incidental" prostate cancer, discussed above, which rarely becomes aggressive and rarely needs to be treated.) These doctors argue that regular screening will subject many men without cancer to unnecessary worry and diagnostic procedures. Furthermore, they say, even if cancer is diagnosed, there's no way to know whether the current testing and treatments—all of which have side effects—will change the outcome or improve the health of the patient. The arguments against PSA testing are not nearly as compelling as they were a decade ago, mainly because of the decrease in deaths from prostate cancer since its widespread use began in the late 1980s.

As valuable as PSA testing is, many scientists studying prostate cancer have spent the last decade figuring out how to understand its many subtleties, and make PSA testing even better. PSA testing is not a foolproof crystal ball: For example, a man can have prostate cancer even if his PSA is low. This is true of about 25% of men who are diagnosed with prostate cancer every year—and this is why the digital rectal examination is the other half of the diagnostic coin. The tests complement each other; either test can pick up cancers the other may miss.

And, just as having a low PSA doesn't mean a man doesn't have cancer, having a high PSA doesn't necessarily mean that he does; other prostate problems—such as enlargement, infection, inflammation, or trauma (from biopsy of the prostate, or even a vigorous rectal exam) can elevate PSA. Normally, a man doesn't have much PSA in his blood. The prostate makes part of the seminal fluid, and PSA's role seems to be as a kind of anticoagulant (anticlotting agent) to ensure the consistency of semen. PSA is secreted in high concentration into the semen, via the prostate's network of drainage ducts. However, when a man has cancer in his prostate, these ducts don't work very well. As a result, instead of draining into the urethra, PSA seeps out of the prostate and into the bloodstream. Having an elevated PSA doesn't automatically mean cancer; but it suggests that something is happening in the prostate that needs to be investigated.

More "cancer-specific" approaches to PSA. Scientists are taking many innovative approaches to PSA, looking for ways to make it a more cancer-specific test. One of the most promising of these is the discovery and measurement of "bound" and "free" PSA—the two forms of PSA that can be present in the bloodstream. In one form, PSA is tied, or chemically "bound," to other proteins; in the other form, PSA floats around in the bloodstream by itself—it's "free." (Note: The routine PSA blood test only measures "total" PSA. Having the PSA broken down into its free and bound forms requires a separate blood test.) We know that when a man has an elevated PSA because of BPH, he's got more PSA in the free form. *But men with prostate cancer are more likely to have low levels of free PSA* (also known as "percent-free" PSA). Thus, if a man has an elevated PSA and most of it is bound, then the PSA elevation is probably coming from cancer. *If a man's free PSA is less than 20 to 25% of the total PSA, this strongly increases the likelihood that he has cancer. If his free PSA is greater than 25%, the high PSA is probably due to BPH.*

PSA density. This is determined by the volume of the prostate, which is measured with transrectal ultrasound. (The next step in diagnosis, if cancer is suspected, is for a man to undergo a biopsy of the prostate, which is done using transrectal ultrasound, discussed below.) The idea here is that most men in the age group for prostate cancer are old enough to have at least some BPH, which can elevate PSA, too. PSA density is the PSA score divided by the volume of the prostate. Basically, if a man has benign disease, his PSA should be approximately 10%, and no higher than 15%, of the weight of his prostate (which translates to a PSA density of 0.1 to 0.15). For example, if a man has a PSA of 9 and his prostate weighs 90 grams, most of the PSA is probably coming from BPH. But if his prostate weighs only 30 or 40 grams, his PSA level is too high to be explained by BPH alone.

PSA velocity or PSA's rate of change from year to year. PSA usually rises much more quickly in a man with prostate cancer than it does in a man with BPH. To get a good idea of PSA activity—whether it's going up or changing, and how quickly—requires more than several tests over time, at least three PSA measurements that span more than eighteen to twenty-four months. In men without cancer, PSA should not increase more than 0.75 per year. There is, however, a natural fluctuation—as much as 15 to 30%—in PSA readings. Thus, having two PSA tests in a short span of time—two or three months apart—is not terribly helpful, and any change may be meaningless. Say a PSA test result is 3.5; two months later, the next PSA test is 3.9. This could be a normal variation, yet it could cause needless anxiety.

PSA and age. It's a fact of life: Your prostate gets bigger as you get older. Thus, it doesn't make sense that the PSA cutoff point should be the same for a 40-year-old man as for an 80-year-old man, who probably has at least some BPH. The younger man almost certainly has a much smaller prostate. Because of this, instead of a "one-size-fits-all" PSA standard (which means, basically, that anything under 4 nanograms per milliliter is okay), many urologists now recommend a cutoff of 2.5 ng/mL for men in their 40s, and a cutoff of 3.5 to 4.0 ng/mL for men age 50 to 70 years. Note: Before a man has his PSA blood test, he should make sure his doctor draws his blood before he undergoes the digital rectal examination. Otherwise, the rectal exam can ruin the PSA reading, artificially raising it and creating needless worry. Also, because sexual activity can raise PSA, men should not ejaculate for at least two days before having this blood test. In contrast, the drug finasteride can artificially lower PSA. Men taking this medication (in the form of Proscar, for BPH, or Propecia, used to fight hair loss) should be sure to inform their physicians, so the PSA reading can be readjusted to compensate for this drug effect.

BIOPSY

If prostate cancer is suspected, the next step is a needle biopsy, an outpatient procedure. This is done by an urologist, with the help of ultrasound, a painless type of imaging that uses sound waves. The ultrasound is focused through a probe (inserted in the rectum), which clearly outlines the edges of the prostate, allowing the urologist to capture tissue samples in a systematic way. The biopsy needle is hollow in the center, designed to capture tiny cores of tissue—each about a millimeter thick—that pathologists will then analyze under the microscope. The ultrasound technology is used only to direct the biopsy needle, and to gauge the weight of the prostate. (By itself, ultrasound is not accurate enough to determine if a man has prostate cancer.) Because there is usually more than one spot of cancer in the prostate, many urologists take twelve biopsy samples (sometimes more, if the prostate is very large). Prostate biopsy is not a perfect method for detecting prostate cancers since some important cancers are missed with biopsies, and some cancers that would not have caused harm may be detected. Note: Men taking any blood-thinning medication like warfarin or coumadin and others, including a daily aspirin, should stop taking it at least a week before the biopsy. (However, they should consult with their doctor first since some patients will need to continue with an anticoagulant such as heparin.) Antibiotics will probably be prescribed to be taken before and after the procedure, to minimize the risk of infection. Most men have minimal complications with prostate biopsies, which can include blood in the semen, urine, or with a bowel movement. If fever, chills, or unusual bleeding develop, the doctor should be notified right away.

THE GRADE OF CANCER

The needle biopsy can be negative, suspicious, or positive. One of the difficulties in interpreting the results of a biopsy is that prostate cancer cells are heterogeneous. This means that, to the pathologist trying to make sense of them, they're a mixed-up conglomeration of many kinds of cells that range all the way from the almost normal-looking, to cells that are so poorly differentiated and obviously diseased that they could never be considered normal. Well-differentiated cancer cells have distinct borders and clear centers, and their growth is relatively slow. Poorly differentiated cancer cells, on the other hand, are more blurry-looking, less well defined, and behave more aggressively. Under the microscope, the samples of tissue from a needle biopsy taken from one part of the prostate may look one way, and those from another part may look completely different.

"Suspicious" biopsies may include two diagnoses: atypical and PIN (prostatic intraepithelial neoplasia). "Atypical" means that the cells can't definitely be called cancerous, but then again, they aren't normal, either, and a second opinion from another pathologist would be wise. If a second pathologist agrees that it is atypical, a repeat biopsy should be done. Similarly, PIN cells aren't cancerous, exactly, but they are good indicators that cancer is either nearby or that it may develop soon. If PIN is found, especially if it is high-grade (grade 2 or 3), then the man is at an increased risk of harboring a cancer, and should have a repeat biopsy.

The Gleason score

If the diagnosis is cancer, the pathologist will assign what's called a Gleason grade somewhere from 1 through 5. The Gleason grade is based on specific patterns of cancer cells; the least aggressive and most well differentiated have the lowest grade. The pathologist adds the number corresponding to the most common pattern to the number corresponding to the second-most common pattern, to arrive at a Gleason score from 2 to 10. The most common Gleason score is 3 + 3 = 6. The lowest possible score (and rarest) is Gleason 1 + 1 = 2. Cancers with a Gleason score of 2 to 4 are the most well differentiated, slowest growing, and easiest to cure. Those with Gleason scores of 5 and 6 are tumors that are moderately well differentiated, relatively slow growing, and usually curable. Gleason 7 cancers are moderately aggressive tumors that need aggressive treatment if they are diagnosed at a curable stage. Gleason scores of 8 to 10 are the most aggressive, fastest-growing tumors; many of these cancers have spread to distant sites by the time a diagnosis is made.

THE STAGE OF CANCER

The stage means the extent of cancer. Is it contained within the prostate, or has it spread outside? If so, has it spread by just a few millimeters, or has it metastasized, or traveled through the blood or lymph system to distant outposts? Staging prostate cancer—predicting the extent of it—is the first step to determining the best form of treatment. This assessment is called the clinical stage. The actual stage can't be determined unless a man has surgery to remove the prostate; then, the entire gland can be studied by a pathologist, who can see if the surgery removed all the cancer—if the edges, or margins, of the removed prostate are cancer-free, or "negative," or if there is cancer present at the margins. This is called the "pathological stage."

The standard staging system for prostate cancer is known as the TNM Classification. T represents the local extent of the tumor; N indicates the presence or absence of metastases (or "spread") to the lymph nodes, and M stands for distant metastases. Many urologists use the 1992 TNM classification, which has three subcategories for early cancers that can't be felt during a rectal exam: T1a, T1b,

---

THE TNM STAGING SYSTEM

The 1992 and 1997 systems are almost the same, except that stages T2a and T2b of the 1992 system were merged into one category in the 1997 system.

1992 Stage	1997 Stage	Description
T1a	Same	Not palpable in a rectal exam; found incidentally, when benign tissue is removed by a TURP; 5% or less of the removed tissue is cancerous.
T1b	Same	Not palpable; found incidentally, but greater than 5% of the tissue removed by the TURP is cancerous.
T1c	Same	Not palpable; identified by needle biopsy because of elevated PSA.
T2a	Same	Palpable; involves less than half of one lobe of the prostate.
T2b	T2a	Palpable; involves more than half of one lobe, but not both lobes.
T2c	T2b	Palpable; involves both lobes.
T3, T4	Same	Palpable; penetrates the wall of the prostate and/or involves the seminal vesicles
N+	Same	Has spread to the lymph nodes.
M+	Same	Has spread to bone.

---

and T1c. Palpable tumors (tumors that can be felt during a rectal exam) are ranked into three categories: T2a (cancer in less than half of one lobe of the prostate), T2b (cancer involving more than half, but only one lobe of the prostate) and T2c (cancer in both lobes of the prostate). For all the stages, see "The TNM Staging System," on p. 444.

The Partin Tables

When the PSA, Gleason score, and clinical stage are known, the Partin tables, developed by urologists Alan Partin and Patrick Walsh at Johns Hopkins, can be used to make an educated estimate of the likelihood that the cancer has been diagnosed at a curable stage. These tables are the next best thing to "virtual surgery"—they help predict what would be found (the pathological stage) if the prostate were removed surgically and examined by a pathologist. Cancers that are "clinically localized" (confined to the prostate) are most likely to be curable, followed by "locally advanced" (which have penetrated the capsule, or wall, of the prostate) cancers, which are still confined to the area around the prostate (and may be curable with radiation). Today, with the help of the PSA test, most men diagnosed with prostate cancer have evidence of clinically localized disease.

These tables are designed to help a man and his doctor predict his cancer's pathologic stage, and determine the best course of treatment. For example, if have stage T1c disease, with a Gleason score of 5 and a PSA of 4.5, means there is a 71% likelihood that the cancer is confined to the prostate.

More information on the Partin Tables may be found at the Brady Urological Institute website (www.urology.jhu.edu), which has a special section on Partin Tables.

HOW IS IT TREATED?

The breakthrough in early diagnosis is only part of the story. The other part is that treatment has improved dramatically, too. Thanks to more aggressive, effective therapy—better surgery, and more precise techniques for administering radiation—doctors are not only able to diagnose most prostate cancer early, they're better able to cure it. There has been an explosion of research targeted at every aspect of prostate cancer—at pinpointing its causes, at preventing it from developing, and at treating advanced disease. For the first time, there is new hope for extending and improving the lives of men with advanced cancer (which has spread beyond the prostate, to the lymph nodes, nearby seminal vesicles, or bone). Groundbreaking research and innovative methods are starting to pay off, with promising new drugs now being tested in patients. Even though in some men it may not be possible to cure, it may soon be possible to stop prostate cancer from growing further.

What's the best treatment for prostate cancer? Because prostate cancer isn't a "one-size-fits-all" disease, the answer is: The best treatment is different for every man. There are many factors—not only the clinical stage of your cancer, but your own age and general health—to be considered. For localized disease, there are three main choices: Watchful waiting, surgery, or radiation therapy.

WATCHFUL WAITING

When cancer is well- to moderately well differentiated (Gleason score 2 through 6) and localized (confined within the prostate) it can take more than ten years to spread and cause harm. Thus, men with this kind of cancer must look at the long haul, and make a frank assessment of their probable life expectancy. It's a hard question to ask, but how long is the person with this cancer probably going to live? If the man is younger than 75 and in reasonably good health, he may live long enough to need treatment. Watchful waiting, or "expectant management," may be the best option for men who are older, or who have serious health problems. These men are not likely to die of prostate cancer, and if the cancer does progress, the symptoms can be managed with hormonal therapy.

Watchful waiting also may be a safe gamble (although a gamble nonetheless) for men with very small, low-volume cancers (smaller than 0.5 cc), that are not poorly differentiated (Gleason score 6 or below), and might be the "good" kind of cancer— the kind that probably doesn't need treatment. For younger men (in their 50s and early 60s), the immediate advantages are obvious—no unpleasant treatment, no side effects. But many urologists do not encourage healthy men under age 65 to choose watchful waiting, because of their longer life expectancy. There is no guarantee that over the next fifteen or twenty years the cancer won't change.

Many men with stage T1a disease, and some men with low-volume stage T1c disease have these "good" cancers. Researchers have determined that for these men, the safest guideline may be age: If the man is younger than 65 and in good health, he should strongly consider curative therapy. The major concern here is that from one checkup to the next, the tumor will slip past the prostate, to the point where curing the cancer is very difficult. Studies indicate that at this point, we can say that even if a man has small-volume cancer today, there is a 30% chance that on his follow-up biopsy, he will be found to have more extensive cancer—and if this happens, there is a 10% chance that the cancer will have spread beyond the ability of surgery to remove it all.

Finally, the greatest risk of all is in accepting the initial biopsy itself as gospel. Most prostate cancers tend to be underrepresented on biopsy. Think about sticking a tiny needle in a walnut, and trying to strike gold, when the "gold" in this case is one or more tiny spots of cancer. So the course of watchful waiting is one of uncertainty—in making an accurate prediction to start with, and in gambling that this cancer will remain unchanged for the rest of the individual's life.

If a man decides to take the watchful waiting path, then to make sure the cancer is as small as the doctor thinks it is, a repeat prostate biopsy should be done (with at least 12 samples taken throughout the prostate). That should be followed by a PSA and digital rectal examination every six months, and a prostate biopsy every year. This is because PSA does not always change to reflect a progression of cancer, and can't be depended on to sound the alarm if treatment becomes necessary.

CAN DIETARY CHANGES HELP?

There is intense interest in attempting to prevent progression of prostate cancer through dietary changes and supplements—antioxidants, herbal compounds, and "nontraditional" forms of healing, such as meditation and acupuncture. One day, scientists may well prove that diet can help prevent cancer from developing. But the idea that starting a diet after cancer develops can make the disease go away may be more like shutting the barn door after the horse has galloped away. The development of cancer happens through a complicated process of DNA damage, which usually takes many years. But once DNA has been damaged enough to cause cancer, there is no evidence that a man can turn back the clock.

CURATIVE TREATMENT: SURGERY AND RADIATION

For tumors that are confined to the prostate—stages T1 and T2—there are two main options: Surgery, in the form of radical prostatectomy, and radiation therapy. Radiation also is used when cancer has spread just outside the gland, to kill cancer cells and shrink the prostate. High-energy x-ray beams are aimed at the prostate and sometimes at nearby lymph nodes; sometimes this is combined with implanted "radiation seeds."

Radical prostatectomy

The gold standard of prostate cancer treatment is the radical prostatectomy. There is no better way to eradicate cancer that is confined to the prostate. But the operation is hard on two fronts.

First, to put it bluntly, it is one of the most difficult operations a surgeon can perform, and skill levels can vary greatly among surgeons. The prostate is located deep in the pelvis, surrounded by structures that are fragile and vulnerable to injury—the rectum, the bladder, the sphincter responsible for urinary control, some large blood vessels, and the bundles of nerves that are responsible for erection. This procedure is, as doctors say, "operator-dependent." The rates of cancer control and complications vary dramatically, depending on the skill and experience of the surgeon—which means that if you are considering radical prostatectomy, you owe it to yourself to find the best, most experienced surgeon available, and to have the operation at a "large-volume" hospital used to taking care of radical prostatectomy patients.

Second, even when the operation is performed perfectly, there are side effects—namely, the risks of impotence and incontinence. In men under 65 who undergo treatment by a surgeon who is an expert, the side effects of surgery and radiation therapy are similar. In men over 70, incontinence and impotence are more common.

Today at Johns Hopkins (the hospital is noted here because results vary worldwide, depending on a range of factors including the surgeons' skill and the selection criteria for patients), 86% of men who undergo surgery to remove the prostate—radical prostatectomy—regain sexual potency within one to two years, while only 2% wear a pad for urinary incontinence that they change more than once a day. Overall, in men treated since 1989, at ten years or more after surgery, 2% have local recurrence of cancer and 8% develop distant metastases, and 80% have an undetectable level of PSA. Important factors for the return of sexual function include age, the extent to which the cancer extends outside the prostate, and the extent of nerve loss—whether one or both of the bundles of nerves that control erection had to be removed during surgery. After radical prostatectomy, men have normal sensation and a normal sex drive, and can achieve an orgasm. They often have difficulty achieving an erection, particularly in the first months after surgery. This often improves with time, but a man doesn't have to wait until he has the "perfect erection" to resume sexual activity. There are many good treatments for erectile dysfunction.

Note: Before surgery, men should alert their doctor if they have had any unusual problems with bleeding in the past (from dental work, for example). Aspirin and drugs such as ibuprofen can cause excessive bleeding; men who are taking regular aspirin or a similar blood thinner or an anticoagulant drug such as warfarin or coumadin, should stop at least ten days before the operation, but be sure check with their doctor first since some patients will need to continue with an anticoagulant such as heparin. Certain vitamins—particularly, vitamin E— herbal compounds, and other dietary supplements can affect blood-clotting mechanisms, too. Men who have ever had a blood clot should make sure their doctor knows about it. This could influence the way anesthesia is administered. Men considered at higher risk of developing a blood clot may have a stronger blood-thinning medication intravenously administered throughout their stay in the hospital.

The best results with radical prostatectomy are achieved with the retropubic procedure (the most common operation), described above, which is made with an abdominal incision. There is another approach, called the radical perineal prostatectomy, in which the prostate is removed through a small incision in the perineum, the space between the scrotum and rectum. A laparoscopic procedure, popularized in Europe, has become more common. This minimally invasive form of surgery uses a small incision through which the surgeon inserts a long flexible tube (laparoscope), equipped with a video camera for viewing as well as small cutting instruments used to remove the prostate. But there are as yet no long-term study results on this procedure.

Radiation therapy

Radiation therapy is a good option for men over 70, men in poor health who aren't considered strong enough for surgery, or men who have disease that has extended beyond the prostate to the point where it can't be removed surgically (stage T3 or T4). Many urologists do not recommend radiation for younger men, because its ability to control the cancer may not last forever. Radiation does not eliminate the entire prostate; it only kills a percentage of cells. There is always some uncertainty, especially for younger men, as to whether radiation's effect will last a lifetime. There are two standard approaches: sending radiation into the tumor from the outside, with external-beam therapy, and implanting radioactive seeds directly into the tumor (called interstitial brachytherapy). Many radiation therapists have reported that they have achieved better cancer control by adding two or three months of hormonal therapy. (Long-term hormonal therapy, for advanced prostate cancer, is discussed below.)

One difficulty in evaluating the success of radiation therapy is in the way "success" is defined. After radical prostatectomy, the definition of success is simple: A PSA level of 0.1 ng/mL or lower is considered "undetectable." A PSA of 0.2 or higher is considered to signal a recurrence of cancer. But with radiation, there is no standardized, definitive PSA cutoff point between success and failure. Some physicians commit themselves to a specific yardstick—a PSA number, such as 1.0 ng/mL. Others assume all is well if a man's PSA after radiation is in the "normal" range—lower than 4.0. In most radiation studies, however, the yardstick is PSA nadir—the lowest point PSA reaches after treatment. Because radiation's effect is gradual, it generally takes two to three years for PSA to "bottom out." The definition of relapse, or "biochemical failure" (this means that PSA levels start creeping back up) after radiation therapy is unique, as well. The American Society for Therapeutic Radiology and Oncology defines biochemical failure as three consecutive rises in PSA after it reaches its nadir. The problem with this is that if a man has a blood test every year—and it takes two years after treatment for PSA to fall as much as it's going to fall—and then three more consecutive blood tests are needed to determine a biochemical failure, short-term results, especially five years or less after treatment, under this definition are not helpful.

Also, both external-beam radiation therapy and radiation seed therapy have been improved in recent years. Although this is good news, it does mean that long-term studies of patient outcomes following radiation therapy—which were based on tracking patients who underwent the old form of treatment—are essentially meaningless. The follow-up must start anew, and it takes at least 10 years to have a good sense of any treatment's long-term effectiveness. With that caveat, here are the two forms of radiation therapy:

External-beam radiation therapy. With external-beam therapy, the radiation doses are spread out over weeks, usually five days a week, for about eight weeks. Each treatment lasts just a few minutes at a time. In recent years, scientists have learned that the dose of radiation received has a lot to do with the success of treatment; men who receive higher doses of radiation have lower relapse rates than men who receive less radiation. But higher doses of radiation are associated with more side effects, and the challenge for radiation therapists has been to balance killing cancer cells with preserving healthy tissue just millimeters away.

But a new technique called three-dimensional conformal therapy allows for greater precision—allowing doctors to maximize the dose of radiation to the prostate tumor and thus sharpen the treatment's cancer-fighting ability, while reducing the damage to nearby tissue. It involves sophisticated software and imaging systems that allow three-dimensional treatment planning, and the radiation is delivered with computer-controlled programming that allows doctors to adjust the radiation dose per millimeter (or even smaller) of tissue. Refined radiation machines now deliver intense, precise levels of radiation to the prostate, but do as little harm as possible to the surrounding tissue—the rectum, bowel, bladder, bone and bone marrow, and skin.

The most common complications after radiation therapy are bowel problems (diarrhea, rectal discomfort or cramping, urgency to have a bowel movement) and urinary trouble (feelings of urgency, the need to urinate frequently, painful or difficult urination, and stress incontinence). For one third to one half of men, these symptoms become bad enough to require medication. Erectile dysfunction is another common complication, although it may take months or years to develop. This is probably due to radiation's effect on the blood vessels, resulting in an eventual decrease in blood flow to the penis. But this doesn't mean a man who undergoes radiation therapy can't still have a normal sex life. The drug Viagra can improve sexual function in men after radiation therapy, particularly in men who can achieve partial erections.

Interstitial brachytherapy (radiation seeds). In this form of radiation therapy, tiny pellets—2.5 mm long, the size of a poppy seed—are implanted directly in the prostate. As with conformal therapy, this form of treatment has benefited from sophisticated computer and imaging technology, allowing doctors to make a customized map of each man's prostate.

Brachytherapy alone (the use of seeds without something else, such as external-beam radiation therapy) is not ideally suited for men with a large, bulky tumor, a high-grade (Gleason score 7 or above) tumor, or lymph node metastases. Most radiation seed treatments don't include the seminal vesicles or tissue outside the prostate. So, if there is a risk that cancer has spread beyond the prostate, men are also treated with supplemental external-beam radiation therapy. The choice of radioactive isotopes (seed material) also varies; some doctors prefer iodine, others palladium. One problem with this still-evolving technology is that nobody has yet figured out the precise radiation dose needed to eradicate prostate cancer. There are no long-term results to show how effective these seeds are, and to determine the long-term side effects and quality of life.

ADVANCED CANCER

Data from the National Cancer Institute suggest that about 75% of men today are diagnosed with localized prostate cancer that is potentially curable with surgery or radiation therapy. That leaves 25% of men in another situation—they are diagnosed with prostate cancer that is more advanced. Further, scientists estimate that about 30% of men who undergo surgery or radiation to treat what appears to be localized prostate cancer will have a recurrence of cancer after treatment. These statistics tell a story that urologists and oncologists know well: There is a great need for better treatment for advanced disease.

When cancer advances beyond the prostate, and localized treatment no longer cures the cancer, there are several options. One is watchful waiting—following the patient closely, and eventually starting hormonal therapy—shutting down the male hormones (also called androgens) that feed the prostate and help sustain the cancer, reducing levels of testosterone to almost zero. At first, hormonal therapy—particularly when a man is suffering from pain, if cancer has invaded the bone—can cause a dramatic improvement. The prostate tumor shrinks, PSA levels drop, and, most importantly, the man feels better. But hormonal therapy (also called androgen ablation therapy) has significant side effects: it stops the sex drive in most men; can lead to osteoporosis; and may cause hot flashes, personality changes, and painful swelling of the breasts. Strategies to treat the side effects of hormonal therapy have not been shown to be very effective. More than this, although it delays progression of cancer—sometimes for many years—hormonal therapy does not stop it forever. This is because some prostate cancer cells are able to thrive even without androgens. In the late 1980s, some investigators believed that a different approach to hormonal therapy, called complete androgen blockade (blocking hormones made by the testicles and adrenal glands) would improve the survival of men with advanced prostate cancer. Unfortunately, complete androgen blockade has been shown to offer no improvement in survival over androgen ablation that removes the testosterone produced by the testicles. The quest now is to find new strategies to conquer advanced disease.

THE TREATMENT OF PAIN

Sometimes, the pain of advanced prostate cancer can be severe. No man should have to experience debilitating pain. If the pain is not being treated aggressively, a man has a right to and should find another doctor—ideally, one attuned to the particularly intense pain of cancer. Men who are able to get pain under control eat better, feel stronger, and are better able to fight the cancer than men whose energy is consumed by pain.

Drugs for milder pain include nonsteroidal antiinflammatory agents—aspirin, acetaminophen (Tylenol), naproxen sodium (Aleve), and ibuprofen (Advil, Motrin), available over-the-counter. Prescription drugs (and there are many) include sulindac (Clinoril), ketorolac (Toradol), diflunisal (Dolobid), and salsalate (Disalcid), to name a few. Drugs for moderate to severe pain include fentanyl (Duragesic), propoxyphene (Darvon, Darvocet), codeine (Tylenol with codeine), oxycodone (Tylox, Percocet, Percodan), meperidine (Demerol), methadone (Dolophine), hydromorphone (Dilaudid), hydrocodone with acetaminophen (Vicodin or Lortab), and morphine (Roxanol).

"Spot" radiation, localized external-beam radiation, generally helps ease pain in specific sites (when cancer invades bone), often for several months at a time. So does a radioactive compound called strontium-89, an isotope that is injected into the body, and absorbed by bone, where it tends to zero in on cancer. An average shot of strontium-89 lasts about six months, and a bonus here is that it acts on new areas of pain that crop up (unlike spot radiation, which treats only the target area).

Another approach to bone pain is an endothelin-blocking agent, now being tested in patients. Endothelin is a substance made by endothelial cells, which line blood vessels. It is believed to be a major component of the severe pain that can occur when cancer attacks bone; it's also linked to the particular bone damage that sometimes accompanies prostate cancer, in which the bone becomes rock-hard, almost like concrete. Endothelin is a nasty substance, linked chemically to the venom in a bee sting. Blocking it, in early studies, seems to relieve pain and improve quality of life. There is some evidence to suggest that blocking endothelin may even help fight prostate cancer itself, in addition to the terrible pain it can cause.

WHAT RESEARCH IS BEING DONE?

As noted before, prostate cancer is an exploding area of research. New drugs and treatments are in varying stages of being ready for use in humans. Research trials are being conducted at many major medical centers.

NEW CHEMOTHERAPEUTIC DRUGS

Not only are researchers developing whole new classes of cancer-fighting drugs, they're rethinking their strategies for giving them. In the past, oncologists used to wait for men to develop "hormone-refractory" cancer (cancer that does not respond to hormonal therapy), and gave chemotherapy as a "last-ditch" approach. The problem is that when cancer has defied other treatments, it often becomes even more aggressive (this is somewhat akin to bacteria becoming resistant to antibiotics). So by going after it earlier—when cancer is still relatively young and vulnerable—oncologists are hoping to change the course of the disease. Many of these drugs are aimed at containing prostate cancer, rather than eradicating it. They also have fewer side effects than traditional chemotherapy. Because these new drugs help slow down growth, the idea is that using them in men with minimal disease—men whose cancer has just begun to return after surgery or radiation, for instance—may delay further progression of cancer. One such drug currently being tested is exisulind, which is similar to a drug currently used to treat colon polyps.

Another promising medication, in a new category called "anti-metastatic" drugs, inhibits a process called angiogenesis—the development of new blood vessels to supply the cancer—and slows cell growth. Again, instead of curing the cancer, the idea is to stop it from growing, and keep it confined. Angiogenesis inhibitors such as thalidomide are being tested in other forms of cancer, as well. Another approach currently being tested in patients uses the adenovirus, a common cold virus—reengineered so that it targets only cells that make PSA. Yet another targets a pathway important to hormone-resistant cancer cells—the release of growth factors by cancer cells. Blocking steps along this pathway (which help cancer cells divide) may help starve resistant cells.

GENE THERAPY

Gene therapy trials are currently under way to determine if genetically engineered cancer vaccines can unleash the body's own immune system, and help it attack and kill cancer cells. In laboratory studies, the strengthened immune system seems able to attack not only the tumor cells, but also the blood vessels around them (another antiangiogenesis effect).

One of the most exciting approaches is the use of an antibody—a protein made by white blood cells—as a "letter bomb" that can deliver cancer-killing drugs directly to cancer cells. The beauty of antibodies is that they are exquisitely precise, and highly effective at killing foreign invaders. Our bodies dispatch antibodies all the time, to protect us from anything perceived as a threat—infection, viruses, and other invaders. Monoclonal antibodies are genetically engineered to target even specific proteins on the surface of cells. One of these proteins is called prostate-specific membrane antigen, present in nearly all prostate cancer, which increases as cancer becomes more aggressive and which is made most of all by hormone-resistant prostate cancer cells. Monoclonal antibodies may be used in the future to deliver radiation or high-powered chemotherapy drugs directly to the cancer cells.

HOW CAN IT BE PREVENTED?

Many men are interested in preventing prostate cancer, and it seems clear that, over the long term, a man's dietary choices could either protect him against cancer or make him more vulnerable to it. There is clearly an association between the intake of animal fat and the incidence of prostate cancer, although the association may be due to the fact that diets high in fat lack other foods like fruits and vegetables thought to lower the risk of cancer. It is also known that eating many fruits and vegetables—at least the "five a day" recommended by the American Cancer Society—can reduce the risk of many cancers. Changing to a healthier diet—namely, limiting animal fat (including dairy products), reducing overall calorie intake (cutting out gratuitous calories in soda, for instance), and eating mostly fruits and vegetables certainly won't hurt, and may help prevent heart disease as well as cancer. Beyond this, there is preliminary evidence that vitamin E and a nutrient called selenium, found in root vegetables, may have a protective effect against cancer. Eating more lycopenes, found in tomato products, also may help.

ADDITIONAL RESOURCES

ORGANIZATIONS AND WEB SITES

American Cancer Society

Prostate Cancer Resource Center

www3.cancer.org/cancerinfo

National Cancer Institute CancerNet–

Prostate Cancer

www.cancernet.nci.nih.gov

National Cancer Institute Cancer

Information Services

Public Inquiries, Office of Cancer Communication

National Cancer Institute

9000 Rockville Pike

Bethesda, MD, 20892

800-4-CANCER

Prostate Cancer Support Network

300 W. Pratt St., Suite 401

Baltimore, MD 21201

800-242-2383

Provides services for several support groups, self-help organizations, and their members, including "Us Too."

Prostate Health Council and the Sexual Function

Health Council

American Foundation for Urologic Diseases

300 W. Pratt St., Suite 401

Baltimore, MD 21201

800-242-2383

BOOKS

Walsh, Patrick C., and Janet Farrar Worthington. *The Prostate: A Guide for Men and the Women Who Love Them.* New York: Warner Books, 1997.

Stroke and Stroke Rehabilitation

Stroke is the third leading cause of death in this country, accounting for 150,000 deaths each year (after heart disease and all forms of cancer combined). But many more people survive stroke than die from it, and stroke is the most common cause of disability requiring rehabilitation. There are currently more than four million Americans living with some neurological deficit due to stroke. The brain damage from stroke can (and often does) cause physical, cognitive, and psychological impairment. The need for caregivers for this population is clear and compelling. And stroke survivors often require very specialized care.

WHAT IS IT?

A stroke is the interruption of blood flow to the brain, causing damage to brain cells. It is sometimes referred to as a "brain attack" or cerebrovascular accident (CVA) and can occur when blood is blocked from getting to the brain or when a blood vessel in the brain bursts. Estimates of the number of strokes each year in the United States range from 550,000 to 750,000 and strokes may sometimes go unreported or be misdiagnosed. Whatever the exact number, stroke is a major health problem and one that is increasing as the population ages. According to one projection, the number of strokes will more than double in the next fifty years.

Strokes are classified into several different categories, according to the cause of the interrupted blood flow. A blockage impeding blood flow to the brain is called ischemia or an ischemic stroke. Stroke that results from bleeding or hemorrhage in the brain is called a hemorrhagic stroke.

ISCHEMIC STROKE

Ischemic stroke is by far the most common type, responsible for 70 to 80% of all strokes. There are two main types of ischemic strokes, and another milder version that is often called a "mini-stroke."

Transient ischemic attack (TIA). This is the so-called mini-stroke, which exhibits many of the same symptoms as a stroke (see below), but resolves within an hour or less with no residual deficits. It usually lasts just a few minutes and is caused by a temporary reduction of blood flow to the brain. However, TIA is often a warning that more serious stroke is imminent, and one third of the 50,000 Americans who have TIAs each year will have an acute stroke sometime in the future.

Cerebral thrombosis. This is the most common type of stroke, occurring when a blood clot (thrombus) forms within an artery supplying blood to the brain. Usually this happens in an artery that has already been narrowed by atherosclerosis, the buildup of fatty deposits (plaque) on the interior walls of the arteries. Cerebral thrombotic strokes often happen at night or first thing in the morning.

Cerebral embolism. In an embolic stroke, a clot of blood or other particles forms somewhere else in the body and makes its way to the cerebral arteries, lodging there. Usually the floating clot travels from the heart. A frequent cause of these emboli is a cardiac disorder called atrial fibrillation, in which the atria, the two upper chambers of the heart, do not beat effectively enough to move blood along, it pools and clots, and the clots get into the bloodstream. They also can occur from clots forming in heart valves or on the inner surface of the heart following a heart attack.

Ischemic strokes can also be caused by stenosis, a narrowing of the cerebral arteries. This is usually due to atherosclerosis. Stenosis is differentiated by whether it forms in large or small arteries. A stroke in the smallest arteries, referred to as small vessel disease, creates a small area of dead brain cells, known as an infarct. This type of stenosis is most commonly caused by hypertension (high blood pressure). Stroke from small vessel disease is sometime called lacunar infarction, from the French word lacune, which means gap or cavity.

HEMORRHAGIC STROKE

The other main type of stroke is a hemorrhagic stroke. A hemorrhage, or bleeding, in the brain can be caused by a number of factors.

- An aneurysm is a weak spot on an artery wall that may stretch and eventually rupture.
- Arterial walls can break open when they are plaque-encrusted and lose their elasticity, becoming brittle, thin, and liable to crack. These changes are usually caused by hypertension.
- An arteriovenous malformation (AVM) is a tangle of defective blood vessels with thin walls that can rupture.
- Head injury can also cause hemorrhage in the brain.

Hemorrhagic strokes are further classified by where in the head the bleeding occurs. If the bleeding is actually within the brain, this is known as a cerebral (or intracerebral) hemorrhage. If the bleeding is in the space between the brain and the skull—known as the subarachnoid space—it is a subarachnoid hemorrhage. This space is where the cerebrospinal fluid (the liquid that bathes the brain and spinal cord, gives the brain buoyancy, and removes waste products from the nervous system) is contained, and the fluid is quickly contaminated with blood when a subarachnoid hemorrhage occurs. A subarachnoid hemorrhage is likely to be caused by a blood vessel abnormality, such as an AVM or aneurysm. Of all types of stroke, the subarachnoid hemorrhage is the most lethal.

WHO IS AT RISK?

Anyone can have a stroke—they happen to men and women of all ages, all races. Strokes are rare in children, but they do happen. There are conditions under which strokes are more likely to occur. Some conditions are beyond our control; these are nonmodifiable risk factors. People can't do much to change their age, gender, or ethnicity, but there are a number of other risk factors for stroke that can be changed. These are known as modifiable risk factors. When more than one of these factors is present, they compound each other and increase the risk to a greater extent than just the combination itself would imply.

NONMODIFIABLE RISK FACTORS

Age. However, like many medical conditions, age is a significant risk factor—the older you get, the greater your risk. Someone older than 65 years of age is seven times more likely to have a stroke than the general population. Two thirds of strokes are in people older than 65, and after the age of 55, the risk for stroke doubles each decade. The incidence of stroke in this country has remained relatively stable since the mid-1980s, and mortality rates declined 30% from 1960 to 1990. However, the aging population—with baby boomers creeping into old age—will certainly account for an increase in the absolute number of strokes in decades to come.

Sex and race. Men have a slightly higher chance of having a stroke than women, but women are more likely to die of stroke. This may be because women live longer than men, in general, so their strokes are likely to occur at a later age. Ethnicity also affects risk—African Americans have double the incidence of stroke of white Americans. Asian-Pacific Islanders and Hispanics also have greater risk of stroke than whites. African Americans who have a stroke between the ages of 45 and 55 are up to five times more likely to die of their stroke than whites in that age group.

Genetics. Some genetic factors may also be involved. Strokes are known to run in some families, and some of the conditions that predispose a person to strokes—for example, diabetes and hypertension—sometimes have genetic causes. Some vascular malformations also have a genetic cause. Another genetic condition, sickle cell disease, which primarily strikes blacks and Hispanics, increases the risk of stroke because the "sickled" red blood cells are less able to carry oxygen than healthy cells and may stick to blood vessel walls.

Illness and injury. Head and neck injuries may occasionally cause damage to the brain's vascular system and rarely cause stroke, as can certain infections.

Geographics. Curiously, increased risk for stroke in the United States has been tied to certain geographic areas. The southeastern United States has been called the "stroke belt" because of the higher than average incidence and mortality rate from stroke. Three states in particular, North Carolina, South Carolina, and Georgia, have a stroke mortality rate twice the national rate. Researchers have investigated this phenomenon but so far haven't been able to pin down a reason for it. Some of the working theories involve environmental factors or lifestyle factors such as diet and smoking.

> ## MODIFIABLE RISK FACTORS FOR STROKE
> - Hypertension
> - Heart disease
> - Diabetes
> - High blood cholesterol
> - Cigarette smoking

MODIFIABLE RISK FACTORS

The primary modifiable risk factors for stroke are:

Hypertension. High blood pressure is the strongest of any contributor to stroke. The risk for stroke increases by 400 to 600% in people with high blood pressure. This is a fairly ominous statistic given the fact that one-third of adult Americans— about 50 million people—have high blood pressure. Hypertension plays a larger role in strokes in younger people, compared to the elderly. A number of different drugs are used to treat high blood pressure (i.e., beta-blockers, ACE inhibitors, calcium channel blockers, diuretics, vasodilators) and studies have shown that these can decrease the risk of stroke by more than one third.

Heart disease. A history of heart disease, especially atrial fibrillation, also increases the risk for stroke. Atrial fibrillation has a greater impact as people age, and is the cause of 25% of strokes in people over the age of 80. Malformations in the heart valves and muscle can also increase the risk of stroke, as does having surgery to correct heart malformations or treat cardiovascular disease. The reason for this is that surgery can dislodge plaque in the aorta or carotid arteries, and send it traveling through the bloodstream to the arteries that feed the brain. Occasionally, blood clots may also form on artificial heart valves, later becoming dislodged and blocking a blood vessel in the brain

Diabetes. Diabetes triples the risk for stroke. Diabetics also have a higher incidence than average of hypertension, amplifying the risk. As with all potential complications of diabetes, control of blood glucose lowers the increased stroke risk.

461

High blood cholesterol. High cholesterol also increases stroke risk. The dangerous type of cholesterol is not that naturally produced by the liver, but dietary cholesterol which we ingest when we eat foods high in saturated fat and cholesterol. However, high levels of high-density lipoprotein (HDL), the so-called "good" cholesterol, are beneficial and help protect against stroke. Total cholesterol can be lowered with a healthy diet and regular exercise; if this is not sufficient, drugs are effective. Statins, one type of cholesterol-lowering drug, have been shown to decrease the risk of stroke.

Cigarette smoking. Smoking almost doubles the risk for ischemic stroke and also increases the risk of subarachnoid hemorrhage. The more a person smokes the greater the risk. Smoking is a potent risk factor because it promotes atherosclerosis, increases levels of blood-clotting agents, and weakens the walls of blood vessels.

Heavy drinking and illicit drug use. Alcohol and drugs, particularly cocaine, are also risk factors. Cocaine has been shown to decrease blood flow to the brain by as much as 30%. Other drugs, including amphetamines, heroin, and anabolic steroids, cause blood vessels to constrict and blood pressure to rise and have been linked to increased risk of stroke.

History of stroke. A history of transient ischemic attacks also increases a person's risk for stroke, as does a history of previous stroke. Up to half of all strokes are in people who have previously had a stroke or TIA.

Lifestyle. Lifestyle factors such as obesity and physical inactivity increase the risk for stroke. Some studies have linked increased stroke risk to lower income and educational levels.

Oral contraceptives. Almost since they were introduced in 1960, oral contraceptives (OCs) have been associated with increased risk of ischemic stroke. Since women of childbearing age are usually not at particularly high risk for stroke, this association has been examined by numerous studies during the forty years in which OCs have been available. A recent analysis of the studies confirmed that women taking OCs are at increased risk for stroke, even with the lower doses of estrogen currently prescribed. However, researchers concluded that the increased stroke risk translated to a small number of cases in this population and was outweighed by the benefits of birth control pills in providing effective and safe contraception. The risk is higher in women who are over 35 years old and who also smoke.

HOW IS IT DIAGNOSED?

Knowing the symptoms of stroke is particularly important for caregivers of stroke survivors, since these patients are at increased risk for another stroke. Most strokes come on suddenly; a more gradual onset is unusual but not impossible, particularly in the case of an ischemic stroke. Symptoms can appear at the moment of the actual stroke, or minutes or even hours later. Since each side of the brain controls the opposite side of the body, if the stroke is in the left side of the brain, the right side of the body will be affected, and vice versa.

SYMPTOMS OF STROKE

Like most aspects of stroke, the symptoms are individualized, depending on the location and severity of the stroke. However, some generalizations can be made. The following list of symptoms of stroke is from the National Institute of Neurological Disorders and Stroke (NINDS).

- Sudden numbness or weakness in the face, arm, or leg, particularly on one side of the body
- Sudden confusion or trouble speaking (slurred or incomprehensible speech) or trouble understanding speech
- Sudden vision loss or trouble seeing from one or both eyes
- Sudden trouble walking, or dizziness, loss of balance, or loss of coordination
- Sudden severe headache for no apparent reason

Other symptoms may include trouble swallowing, vomiting, irregular breathing, sudden deviation of the eyes in one direction, double vision, or loss of consciousness. Children having strokes may experience symptoms somewhat different from adults. These can include seizures, convulsions, sudden speech loss or other speech impairment, paralysis or weakness on one side of the body, fever or headache, or loss of expressive language such as body language and gestures.

It is critically important to get medical care immediately for anyone experiencing any of these symptoms. Studies have shown that many people initially ignore the symptoms of stroke and delay seeking medical help. The speed with which stroke is treated has a direct impact on recovery and severity of resulting disabilities.

DIAGNOSTIC TESTS

Health care providers and medical centers have a number of different imaging tools they can use to diagnose the location and magnitude of the stroke. The specific type of test used depends on many factors, including the symptoms the person had and the results of a medical examination. Diagnostic tests include:

Computerized axial tomographic scan (CAT or CT scan). This specialized x-ray, which generates a series of cross-sectional images, can help determine whether a stroke has occurred and if it was ischemic or hemorrhagic.

Magnetic resonance imaging (MRI). The MRI uses energy from a magnetic field to generate images of the brain. MRIs show soft tissue and are useful to determine the location and size of ischemic strokes. They can also identify many aneurysms and AVMs (arteriovenous malformations). Variations of MRI are magnetic resonance angiography (MRA) and functional MRI. MRA maps blood flow in the brain to determine narrowing in the arteries. Functional MRI shows brain activity by picking up signals from oxygenated blood.

Radionuclide angiography. This technique provides an image by injecting radioactive materials into a vein in the arm. They are carried to the brain where they show up clearly on an x-ray, delineating areas of the brain that have been deprived of blood flow.

Other tests highlight blood flow patterns. These include Doppler ultrasound waves near the carotid artery in the neck; carotid phonoangiography, in which a sensitive microphone on the neck records the sound of blood flow and can detect abnormalities; transcranial Doppler, which evaluates blood flow in arteries within the brain; and cerebral angiography, which visualizes the brain's blood vessels using a contrast dye, which is injected through a catheter in the leg and x-rayed as it moves through the brain.

DIFFERENTIAL DIAGNOSIS

Stroke can be mistaken for other disorders, and differential diagnosis is the process by which doctors rule out other disease possibilities by considering symptoms that are and are not present. Other conditions that are sometimes mistaken for a stroke include seizures, brain tumor, subdural hematoma, peripheral neuropathy, multiple sclerosis, hypoglycemia, encephalitis, and migraine.

WHAT SHOULD YOU EXPECT?

Mortality rates for stroke in the United States are among the lowest in the world. About 85% of people who have strokes in this country survive them. Many people completely recover from stroke, sometimes spontaneously without rehabilitation. About 20% are capable of taking care of themselves by two weeks after the stroke, with no rehabilitation necessary. More than a million survivors live today with little or no long-term impairment from their stroke. The potential for recovery is good because neurons in the brain are often damaged but not destroyed by stroke, and the damage may be reversible. An important key to recovery is prompt treatment.

However, stroke survivors frequently are left with severe physical and mental disabilities. The damage that stroke causes in the brain can affect the whole body. Twenty percent of stroke survivors will have such serious resulting disability that they will never walk again and will require assistance with activities of daily living for the rest of their lives, regardless of rehabilitation efforts. About two million survivors live with crippling paralysis, speech loss, and/or memory problems. In nearly three quarters of cases, stroke will have a significant impact on how a survivor lives his or her life. Studies have found that after stroke:

- 71% of survivors will be impaired in continuing in their jobs;
- 31% need assistance in self-care;
- 32% are clinically depressed;
- 20% need assistance in ambulation (walking or otherwise getting around);
- 16% remain institutionalized;
- 14% will experience a second stroke in the first year following a stroke.

Strokes cause a range of effects, depending on the part of the brain that was deprived of blood, and how long the deprivation continued. Effects may involve motor abilities, sensory perceptions, vision, language ability, cognition, and affect. The most common effects, according to the NINDS, are:

- Weakness or paralysis on one side of the body (perhaps whole side, or just the arm or leg)

- Muscle stiffness or spasticity or painful muscle spasms
- Balance and/or coordination problems
- Language problems, including aphasia (difficulty with spoken or written communication; difficulty remembering or understanding words) or dysarthria (slurred speech)
- Unawareness of sensations on one side of the body
- Pain, numbness, or odd sensations
- Difficulty swallowing (dysphagia)
- Problems with memory, thinking, learning, or attention
- Unawareness of the effects of the stroke
- Bowel or bladder control problems
- Fatigue
- Difficulty controlling emotions and sudden mood swings (emotional lability)
- Depression
- Difficulty with the activities of daily living
- Sexual dysfunction

CONTINUING ISSUES

In addition to the need for extended rehabilitation for some stroke patients, a number of other issues are of continuing concern for many who survive a stroke and their caregivers. Among them are the following:

Depression. It is estimated that as many as two thirds of stroke survivors experience depression at some stage after their stroke, and 10 to 27% have a major depression. In some studies, rates of depression continue to rise during the eighteen months following a stroke. Many stroke survivors feel that their quality of life has deteriorated, that they will never be the person they were before the stroke, and these despondent feelings can fuel depression. Often they find themselves unable to control their emotions. Depression may also be related to physical damage the stroke has caused in the brain. To further complicate the problem, patients who are depressed have a more difficult time regaining their cognitive function, an interaction that has been referred to as a "dementia of depression." Caregivers and family members should be alert for signs of depression in stroke survivors. Both "talk" therapy and antidepressant medications can be effective and valuable tools to help deal with depression. Another tool is counseling for caregivers—such counseling has been found to reduce rates of depression in stroke patients themselves

Problems with bowel and/or bladder control. Incontinence is one of the primary issues that concerns caregivers. It determines when a patient is ready to be discharged from a hospital or rehabilitation unit. However, many patients return home with continued continence issues, sometimes because they are embarrassed to speak of them. This issue needs to be addressed because there are solutions. Incontinence can usually be treated and sometimes cured; in other cases, it can be managed in a way that allows patients maximum independence. Medications, behavioral therapy, and surgery are all used successfully to treat incontinence. And when these fail, special absorbent underclothing is available that is no more bulky than regular underwear.

Sexual dysfunction. This is another common problem that can be associated with stroke, but is often neglected because of reluctance of patients and spouses, caregivers, and healthcare providers to discuss it. Sexual dysfunction (particularly erectile dysfunction in men) can be due to physiological, psychological, or emotional causes, or a combination of the three. Other medical problems (for example, diabetes, prostate conditions, or arthritis) or the simple reality of aging may be factors. In both men and women, studies have found that sexual activity does decrease after stroke. However, many stroke survivors have active and satisfying sex lives. Couples may need to work on finding new positions that overcome their physical disabilities. They often need to rework their relationships, taking into consideration role shifts that result from dependence caused by a stroke. People are often fearful that sexual activity will cause another stroke, although this is an extremely small risk. Patients should evaluate medications they are taking with their health care providers, to determine if the drugs contribute to sexual dysfunction. There are a number of treatments for sexual dysfunction, both mechanical and pharmaceutical. Viagra may be helpful for men who have had strokes, although it has not been specifically tested in this population. Viagra should not be used by people who take nitrates or have unstable angina. Because of the rare, but occasionally serious, complications associated with Viagra, its use should be discussed with a doctor before taking it.

Nutrition. Stroke survivors often have trouble swallowing, which can complicate the problem of providing adequate nutrition. Caregivers should consult with a qualified nutritionist to design meals that will provide the necessary nutrients and be appealing and palatable to the patient.

HOW IS IT TREATED?

Treatment of stroke is divided into two categories: Acute treatment is the immediate medical attention used to save the life of the stroke patient and stabilize the patient medically. Post-stroke rehabilitative therapy is more long-term and addresses the deficits caused by the stroke in an attempt to repair damage and prevent further deterioration

ACUTE TREATMENT

Stroke has been described in medical literature for centuries, but until the past few years, medical science had little to offer for the immediate treatment of CVAs.

Tissue plasminogen activator. In 1996, the Food and Drug Administration approved the use of tissue-type plasminogen activator (t-PA) to treat ischemic strokes within three hours of onset. This drug, known as a thrombolytic agent, interrupts a stroke by dissolving the blood clot that is blocking blood flow to the brain. t-PA has been used for years to treat heart attacks, but health care providers have been cautious in applying it to stroke because it can occasionally cause bleeding in the brain, intensifying the damage of the stroke. t-PA was approved to treat strokes after an NINDS study found that when given within three hours of the beginning of a stroke, it reduced disability by at least 30%. There is still some debate about whether enough research has been done to establish the safety of t-PA for stroke patients, but both the American Academy of Neurology and the American Heart Association now recommend that it be used within the established guidelines.

The guidelines for t-PA use for stroke require not only that the drug be given within three hours of stroke onset, but also that there is a clear diagnosis of ischemic stroke and a CAT scan has ruled out any evidence of bleeding in the brain. In addition, there should be no clinical symptoms that suggest bleeding and no seizure associated with the stroke. Also, if the patient is showing rapid spontaneous improvement, t-PA is not indicated.

These guidelines considerably narrow the number of patients who are eligible for this treatment, but even within these limitations, t-PA is not given as often as it could be. A recent NINDS statement concluded, "The vast majority of patients who might benefit from [t-PA] do not receive it." Part of the reason for underuse of the drug is lack of knowledge in both the lay and medical communities. The general public needs a greater awareness of stroke symptoms and the critical importance of getting immediate care. Health care providers need to know the proven value of t-PA. However, there is also need for caution because some studies of use of t-PA in the community did not turn up the positive results of the NINDS study. A study in Cleveland, for example, found a three times higher death rate for stroke patients given t-PA, compared to those who were not. Clearly, more research is necessary to determine the best use for this and other drugs and how they can best be delivered.

Neuroprotectant drugs. Much of the damage from stroke occurs as neurons (nerve cells) in the brain are starved for blood and the oxygen it carries. The neurons become damaged or die. A number of different drugs called neuroprotectants may protect the brain from this damage and help the cells live longer. Some of these drugs are showing promise and are under investigation but nothing has yet been approved specifically for this purpose.

Anticoagulant drugs and aspirin. Aspirin is often prescribed after ischemic stroke; it is an antiplatelet drug that decreases the activity of platelets, the clotting cells in the blood, thus reducing the risk of blood clots forming. Several other antiplatelet drugs are also available, including clopidogrel (Plavix) and a dipyridamole and aspirin combination (Aggrenox). Anticoagulants such as warfarin (Coumadin) and heparin are also used for this purpose in some stroke patients.

Surgery. In cases of hemorrhagic stroke, surgery is sometimes needed to stop bleeding or remove large blood clots. Another type of surgery, carotid endarterectomy, is used for some ischemic stroke patients whose carotid artery is partially blocked. (Totally blocked arteries usually cannot be reopened.) In this operation, the interior of the carotid artery is scraped clean and smooth. In a relatively recent variation of the procedure, a stent, a tiny cylindrical tube, is inserted to keep the walls of the artery open. The stent remains in place, and the tissue of the blood vessel soon knits around it. All these procedures have some risk and can only be used in certain people with stroke.

Dedicated stroke teams. Best outcomes for stroke treatment, both acute and long-term, come from specialized stroke centers with 24-hour coverage from dedicated teams, 24-hour CAT scan availability, and other services focused specifically on the stroke patient. Many studies have confirmed that treatment in specialized units translates to reductions in death rates, dependency, and institutionalization. In a recent statement, the Brain Attack Coalition, a consortium of health care professionals from a number of medical centers, noted that many hospitals do not have the necessary protocols in place to treat stroke patients efficiently and quickly, and they urged the establishment of acute stroke teams and primary stroke units in hospitals.

REHABILITATIVE TREATMENT

Stroke rehabilitation is still an "infant science," and guidelines for optimum care are still being established. However, an increasing number of specialists devoted to stroke rehabilitation care and a rapidly growing number of studies are shedding light on techniques that work—and those that don't—and methods to confront the challenges of stroke rehabilitation.

Stroke survivors often must deal with many losses—loss of mobility and dexterity, loss of independence, loss of connection with others, and occasionally loss of competence. Rehabilitation addresses these losses. It is estimated that 60% of stroke survivors can benefit from some form of rehabilitation. Of the other 40%, half will recover completely without rehabilitation and the other half are too severely impaired to benefit. However, the delineations between these groups are not always clear, and determining who should receive services is the first step of stroke rehabilitation. Medical professionals have a number of assessment tools they use to decide which services a patient should be offered.

For maximum effectiveness, rehabilitation should begin early in the acute stage of care—as soon as the diagnosis of stroke is known and the patient is medically stable. While most recovery occurs in the three months immediately following the stroke, improvement can continue beyond this period, especially in patients with severe disabilities. The earlier rehabilitation begins, however, the better the chance of recovering lost skills. Prolonged bed rest is not helpful and can cause additional medical complications such as bedsores, blood clots, pneumonia, and stiff joints. Patients who are reasonably alert, with stable vital signs, should be sitting in a chair (with assistance) by forty-eight hours after the stroke. Early rehabilitation efforts will include range-of-motion exercises to prevent limbs from contracting and to promote proper positioning.

The American Heart Association lists six areas of focus as the goals of rehabilitative care:

- Preventing, diagnosing, and treating other medical problems and complications that exist along with the stroke.
- Training to allow the patient maximum independence.
- Helping the patient and family cope socially and psychologically.
- Helping the patient reintegrate into the family and community, resuming home, recreational, and vocational activities.
- Learning to cope with any disability and maximizing quality of life despite the disability.
- Preventing another stroke, or heart attack, for which the stroke survivor is also at increased risk.

After the acute stage of stroke, further rehabilitation varies in intensity from one patient to another, needing an individualized approach tailored to the patient's capacity. To benefit from rehabilitation, the stroke survivor must be medically stable with enough endurance for at least minimal level rehabilitation activities, and able to learn. In people whose stroke has caused severe cognitive disability, the ability to learn new strategies may be severely impaired and they are not likely to benefit from rehabilitative treatment. The amount of damage to the brain, the attitude of the patient, the cooperation of family and friends and involvement of the caregiver, and the timing of rehabilitation all influence the success of rehabilitation. It is important that caregivers and family members be educated about what to expect in the way of recovery and what they can do to help.

Sometimes rehabilitation is indicated even if the person doesn't appear to want it. Because of their cognitive impairment, some patients may insist that they don't need rehabilitation, while others may be too depressed to participate or too frustrated by their communication disabilities. As caregiver, you have a critical role in motivating the stroke survivor towards rehabilitation, and to prevent patients in denial about their impairment from driving, using hazardous machinery such as power tools, or engaging in other potentially dangerous activities.

THE TREATMENT TEAM

Good stroke rehabilitation requires several different types of therapy, thus a team approach. The most important members of the team are the patient and family and caregiver. It is crucial that patients' wishes be known; sometimes, in patients with communication disabilities, it is up to you as caregiver to interpret these wishes. Make sure that team members appreciate the desire of the patient to be part of caregiving decisions and help state the patient's questions and opinions.

Among the professional members of most teams, you will usually find the following:

Physician. A physician usually coordinates the rehabilitation team. The physician may be a neurologist, physiatrist (specialist in physical medicine and rehab), family doctor or internist, or geriatrician (specialist in treating elderly patients).

Rehabilitation nurse. The rehabilitation nurse is an important part of the team, providing and overseeing the nursing care that is critical for stroke patients. The nurse is also often the contact person for the family, and helps educate family members and caregivers about their role in rehab. Nurses are often the first to notice any deterioration in condition. They monitor patient bowel and bladder function and address concerns related to skin (bedsores), medication, comfort, safety, emotional, and sexuality issues.

Physical therapist. The physical therapist uses exercises, training, and manipulation to help the patient relearn movement, balance, and coordination, leading to sitting, standing, walking, lying down, and switching from one movement to another.

Occupational therapist. Occupational therapy teaches stroke survivors to handle the activities of daily living, such as eating and drinking, dressing, bathing, cooking, reading and writing, and toileting, with the goal of independent living. Often new approaches to these standard tasks must be learned to overcome deficits caused by stroke.

Specific goals of rehabilitation will vary, depending on personal circumstances. Goals must be realistic or patients, therapists, and caregivers may become discouraged and lose motivation. About 75% of stroke survivors will eventually be ambulatory, although walking might involve a cane or walker. Caregivers should be aware of the risk of falling during this time. Other goals might include independently accomplishing some of the tasks of daily living, such as eating, toileting, bathing, and dressing; driving a car; and working at a job or volunteer activity.

Speech therapist. Also called speech or language pathologist, this member of the team helps patients relearn language and speaking skills, or alternative means of communication when necessary. Communication can be a very frustrating process for stroke survivors, making them feel helpless and isolated, and the speech therapist helps patients develop coping skills to deal with their language deficits. Also, speech therapists evaluate patients for any swallowing problems and make appropriate recommendations for safe swallowing.

Psychologist/psychiatrist. Among the most common post-stroke disabilities are psychological problems such as depression, anxiety, anger, and frustration. One third to one half of stroke survivors are estimated to suffer from depression, and it is also a common problem among caregivers.

Social worker. Many families will benefit from social services. Social workers help evaluate the patient's coping skills and social supports and help with transition back to the community. They also help to make arrangements for care or therapy after discharge, and help get any equipment recommended by the team.

Nutritionist. Stroke survivors often have eating, drinking, and swallowing problems, leading to nutritional issues. A nutritionist can help design meal plans that are practical for the patient and provide the necessary nutrients. As caregiver, you will often be involved with meal planning and eating, and will consult with the nutritionist.

Recreational therapist. These therapists augment the work of physical therapists in helping patients resume recreational and athletic activities they enjoyed before their stroke. Techniques they use may include music, art, and games.

Setting for stroke rehabilitation

Rehabilitation therapy is expensive. In today's climate of managed care and increasing scrutiny of the bottom line in medical treatment, the setting for stroke rehabilitation has become an issue of some debate. Generally, rehabilitation programs fall into one of four categories: hospital programs, in either acute or rehabilitative facilities; long-term care facilities with specialized nursing and therapy; outpatient programs; and home-based programs.

Although most evidence points to best recovery from concentrated care in a specialized stroke center, there have been some studies that have found that home-based rehabilitation can also be effective, at least for some patients at some point in their care. However, one study did identify a potential risk of at-home care—the mental health of the caregiver. Caregivers for people who received their rehabilitation therapy at home rather than a hospital scored significantly lower in mental health evaluations. Care for a stroke patient can be very consuming—as a caregiver, it is important that you take time to attend to your own personal needs. These factors must be considered in deciding how long institutional care can be delivered and when the primary site of rehabilitation can be switched to the home. Of course, one of the major factors in this decision will be the reimbursement policy of the health insurer.

Almost all patients receiving rehabilitation will transfer from one facility to another, or from a facility to home, during the course of treatment. Continuity of care is important, and close communication between the treatment team and the patient, family, and caregiver are necessary to avoid gaps in care.

Types of therapy

There are a number of different schools of therapy, particularly physical therapy, and no single method stands out as best for stroke rehabilitation. Muscles in a stroke-affected area may be flaccid (limp and weak, of decreased tone) or spastic (stiff, of increased tone), producing different types and degrees of paralysis or contracture. Preventing contracture is one of the first goals of physical therapy, and involves range-of-motion exercises and proper positioning. Range-of-motion exercises should begin on the day of the stroke, with the patient learning how to use an unaffected limb to move a paralyzed one. Positioning can be accomplished with braces or other devices—for example, an ankle brace to prevent shortening of the Achilles tendon.

Some types of physical therapy emphasize flexing of limbs, others inhibit movement to prevent spasticity. Electrical stimulation can also increase strength and prevent muscle wasting and promote use of a function. Electromyographic biofeedback, in which a patient can see his or her responses to electric shocks to the muscle, is another technique that is useful for some patients. It is necessary for a patient to be fairly mentally aware for biofeedback to be effective.

Medications may also play a role in stroke rehab. An injection of Botox, a botulism toxin (thought of by most people as a poison, but safe when used in controlled medical situations) can reduce spasticity and help muscles relax. Tizanidine (Zanaflex) is an oral medication that reduces muscle spasticity without weakening the muscles. In another relatively recent therapy option, an implanted pump delivers baclofen, an antispasticity medicine, directly to the spinal fluid that bathes the nerves extending from the spine to the muscles. Medications are also used to address cognitive issues. Methylphenidate (Ritalin), the drug commonly used to treat children with attention deficit disorder, and other stimulants may be helpful in aiding some stroke survivors to focus on a task.

As many as 70% of stroke survivors need some sort of treatment for shoulder pain. Shoulder pain after a stroke can be a result of inadvertent injury during transfers (for example, from bed to chair), poor positioning in the bed or chair, or rotator cuff weakness. Shoulder-hand syndrome—in which there is pain, swelling, and other changes in the hand as well as shoulder—is also common, sometimes developing a month or two after the stroke. Range-of-motion exercises are usually effective to alleviate these pains; sometimes pain-relieving medications or steroid injections to the joint are prescribed. In the most serious and stubborn cases, a nerve block can be injected to block the pain.

Retraining the brain

In recent years, a relatively new approach to treatment called constraint-induced movement therapy has gained approval in stroke rehab. This therapy opposes the natural instinct of an intact limb to take over the functions of an impaired limb. The basic premise is that if the impaired limb is forced to perform, it will. This is achieved by restraining the other limb; for example, keeping the good arm in a splint for 90% of waking hours. When this is done for a period of about two weeks, many patients demonstrate considerable improvement in motor ability. The therapy is also applied to lower limbs for walking, climbing, and balance and support exercises, by supporting the body in a harness to take the weight off the weak leg.

Imaging of the brain has shown that one of the mechanisms responsible for the success of constraint-induced therapy is a reorganization in the cortex of the brain—the outermost layers of cells that play a large role in movement, sensation, language, thinking, and emotions. A certain amount of reorganization occurs automatically when body parts are affected by the stroke and the brain begins to compensate to take over their function. The constraint-induced movement seems to help healthy areas of the brain learn the functions of injured areas. Studies have shown that just a brief period of treatment (two weeks or less) can cause long-term improvement.

The approach is new and needs to be studied over longer periods to know if the improvement will be permanent. It definitely does not work for everyone with stroke, especially people with total paralysis. But many health care providers are very encouraged by the results of this approach to therapy, especially since it does not involve the risks of medications or adverse side effects.

Progressing in therapy

Individual goals in therapy should be set early in the process. A logical progression of tasks follows for most patients. First, they will roll in the bed independently, then roll to a sitting position on the side of the bed. Often it is helpful for a person to use an unimpaired limb to move an impaired one, either lifting one arm with the other, or hooking the normal ankle around the weak leg and pulling the weak leg where it should go. Sitting may initially result in dizziness, especially in someone who has been lying down for a few days. Therefore, even this early step should not be done without supervision.

From sitting on the side of the bed, the next step is standing and either taking a few steps or transferring directly to a chair. Transfers to a chair and to the toilet should be carefully supervised; in the first days after a stroke, this will usually be done in the hospital with care from nurses and therapists, but the caregiver needs to learn how these procedures work and how much assistance the patient will need. Caregivers should be very aware of the potential for falls. Falls are a significant cause of injury for stroke patients.

About three quarters of stroke survivors will eventually walk, although they may need some time in a wheelchair before they are on their feet, and they may need some sort of support when they are walking. A number of devices are available to make walking and other activities easier for people who have had strokes, or other brain or spinal cord injuries.

Assistive devices

Several different types of equipment are useful in helping stroke survivors regain function or compensate for lost function. These are known as assistive devices.

They range from canes, walkers, and wheelchairs to special eating and grooming utensils.

Wheelchairs. Wheelchair adaptations are often necessary to address the needs of stroke patients. Usually the seat of the wheelchair used by a person who has had a stroke will be about two inches lower than the seat of a standard wheelchair. This is to enable the person to help propel the chair by making firm contact with the floor with his or her unaffected foot. Wheelchair users can also use the stronger hand and arm to turn the wheel and steer. Brake extenders can help the patient reach across with the strong arm to lock the wheel. If the person has one partially paralyzed arm, a lap board provides a good place to support it and keep the arm from falling over the side of the chair, where it can get caught in the wheel. A clear board is recommended so the patient can see his feet and the ground beneath the chair.

Canes and walkers. Canes or walkers support weight that the weak leg can't handle and help with balance when walking. Many stroke patients have trouble with a walker because they cannot supply the strong two-handed grip it requires. At least three different types of canes are used: the standard J-neck cane; a four-pronged quad cane, which provides improved balance with its four-footed stand but may be difficult to use in stairs or crowds; and the walker cane, also called a hemiwalker, which has four widely separated legs (similar to a walker) that meet in a crossbar that is gripped by the user. Canes should always have rubber tips to avoid slipping. They should be carried in the unaffected hand, and patients and caregivers should be alert for early signs of compression nerve damage in that hand. Some training is usually necessary to establish a comfortable gait that takes best advantage of a device and for specialized tasks such as stair-climbing.

Braces. Orthotics are braces, usually for the lower extremities, and they are useful for stroke patients in a couple of ways. Walking is a complex operation involving several different muscle and bone movements—second nature to the able-bodied, but difficult or painful for many stroke survivors. When there is ankle weakness, an ankle-foot orthosis (AFO), sometimes with a hinged ankle joint, can help with gait. Braces are also useful in the case of knee weakness to keep the knee from buckling. Wrist-hand orthoses prevent wrist and finger contracture and may help with relearning fine motor activities. Orthotics must be carefully monitored by caregivers—they can cause pressure areas if not appropriately designed and fitted, and they may impair some movements while improving others. Consult with your doctor and physical therapist to find an experienced

ASSISTIVE DEVICES

As caregiver, it is important to understand the sense of independence that a patient feels with self-sufficiency in dressing, going to the bathroom, eating, and other daily activities. Many assistive devices are available to help with the activities of daily living. In addition, it may be necessary to adapt the home to the needs of the stroke survivor with wheelchair ramps, widened doorways, and rearranged furniture. Ask your occupational therapist about specific devices including:

- special eating utensils with easy-to-grip handles
- bedside commodes
- Velcro closings on clothing
- elastic shoelaces
- dressing sticks and reaching sticks
- grab bars, special chairs, hand-held shower nozzles, or other adaptations for the tub and shower

orthotist (person who fits braces) who works with stroke patients.

Discharge—going home

The average length of stay in an inpatient rehabilitation unit or rehabilitation hospital is about two to three weeks for the stroke patient. Going home is the goal, and planning for discharge should begin with the first signs of recovery. Often discharge planning is done with a social worker. Sometimes a therapist may want to visit the home to determine any physical modifications that would make life easier for the stroke survivor. This can include things as simple as moving scatter rugs from a hallway or putting a chair in the shower. A therapist, social worker, or home care coordinator can also help with assessing equipment needs, getting a handicapped parking permit, connecting with community services, and other tasks. Continuing services from members of the treatment team will be necessary for many people, and continuing communication among team members is important during outpatient follow-up.

One of the most important parts of discharge planning is educating caregivers to anticipate and know how to deal with the many responsibilities that are associated with caring for a stroke survivor. Hands-on training sessions for caregivers by therapists and nurses are very helpful. Counseling may also be helpful for caregivers. Often family members are so consumed with the needs of the patient that they may overlook their own needs. A home health aide for several days a week after discharge can assist with bathing and other personal care activities and provide needed relief and support for caregivers and family members.

As recovery progresses, the professional therapists will project further goals and determine the necessity for continued therapy. Sometimes it is hard for a patient and family to face the conclusion of therapy—they may interpret this as the end of recovery, a hopeless situation. In fact, recovery may continue for many people, although it will slow down considerably. Home exercise programs may be recommended to maintain gains or to promote new improvements. Again, there is an important supportive role for the caregiver to address patient morale and motivation.

WHAT RESEARCH IS BEING DONE?

Both laboratory and clinical researchers are investigating methods to improve rehabilitation for stroke survivors. They are trying to learn the mechanisms of recovery and how skills are relearned after damage to the cells of the central nervous system. One of the most active areas of study is cortical reorganization—sometimes called rewiring, how brain cells reorganize themselves after they have been damaged so that healthy cells take over the function of injured or destroyed cells. New advances in brain imaging are providing new insight in this area.

The American Heart Association recommends that stroke research:

- Expand knowledge about brain physiology and mechanisms associated with stroke recovery.
- Develop instruments to measure improvement after stroke.
- Determine the type of treatment unit that contributes most to success in rehabilitation, and the different types of treatments and regimens that are most effective.
- Determine the outcomes produced by different types of strokes.
- Investigate the use of medications on recovery of motor, language, and cognitive functions.

Much remains to be learned about how specific interventions can help stroke survivors walk and perform other physical activities; talk, understand, and regain communication abilities; and reacquire their prestroke cognitive aptitude. Researchers are adding to knowledge about the roles of different parts of the brain by studying what the implications are for the injuries suffered by various regions

479

of the brain during stroke. They are seeking answers to questions about the first and second wave of damage to brain cells when blood is cut off and the role of chemical messengers between brain cells.

The U.S. government's post-stroke rehabilitation clinical practice guidelines suggest several areas for prioritization in advancing stroke rehab:

- Identification of patients most likely to benefit from stroke rehab
- Determination of which program will work best for each patient
- Determination of effectiveness of specific treatments and combinations of treatments
- Identification of best timing, duration, and intensity of rehabilitation therapy
- Standardized measurement of outcomes of post-stroke rehab

In other more general stroke-related research, scientists are looking at vasodilators, drugs that expand blood vessels, and the role they can play in preventing or treating strokes. Another area of investigation is gene therapy and how it can be applied to protect brain cells, prevent inflammation, and repair cells.

The processes at work in animal hibernation have long piqued the interest of brain researchers. In hibernating animals, there is a dramatic decrease of blood flow to the brain along with generally slowed-down metabolism, yet animals awaken from hibernation with no brain damage. Unlocking the secrets of hibernation may have human applications in the treatment of strokes and other brain dysfunction.

Currently, there are more than 100 clinical trials under way in the United States to investigate various aspects of stroke. Specific ongoing studies are looking at:

- Effectiveness of aspirin compared to warfarin, an anticoagulant, and other drugs in preventing second strokes
- Role of certain proteins (antiphospholipid antibodies), which are often elevated in people who have strokes
- Value of stenting to treat carotid atherosclerosis
- Genes found in persons who are at high risk for stroke
- Relation of patent foramen ovale, a heart defect, to stroke
- Use of vitamins (B6 and B12) to prevent stroke
- Effect of estrogen therapy to prevent stroke in postmenopausal women

HOW CAN IT BE PREVENTED?

In many cases, stroke is a preventable condition. NINDS scientists predict that with current technologies and developments on the horizon, 80% of strokes will be preventable ten years from now. The information about modifiable risk factors can be directly translated to ways of preventing stroke. If you reduce the influence of these factors in your life, you can reduce your risk of stroke and maybe prevent it altogether. This means:

• Keep your blood pressure down. High blood pressure (hypertension) is one of the chief contributing factors to stroke. Have your blood pressure checked regularly, follow your doctor's advice about lowering it, and take any blood pressure medications as advised. Treating high blood pressure lowers the risk of both ischemic and hemorrhagic stroke.

• If you smoke, stop. Quitting smoking decreases the risk of stroke.

• Have your blood cholesterol monitored, beginning in your 30s. If it is high, try to lower it through exercise, dietary changes, and medication if necessary.

• Once you reach the age of 50, have your health care provider listen carefully to your heart for sounds of murmurs and also to your carotid arteries for the telltale signs that they are narrowing.

• If you have diabetes, do what you can to keep your blood glucose within the target range. This means taking medications regularly, adhering to your diet, and frequent monitoring of blood glucose.

• If you are obese, lose weight through common-sense dieting and exercise. If your lifestyle is sedentary, perk it up. Consult your health care provider about how to best accomplish weight loss and begin an exercise program.

• Also consult with your doctor about taking aspirin daily as a preventive measure against stroke and heart disease.

Once a person has had one stroke, he or she is at increased risk for a second, and a number of measures can be taken to prevent that. First, obviously, follow the recommendations listed above. Then, if tests show that there is more than a 70% blockage of either of the carotid arteries, consider surgery to open the blockage. This procedure, called carotid endarterectomy, has been found to reduce the risk of stroke by more than 15%.

Some drugs also are proving to have a role in preventing first and recurring strokes. While use of aspirin has become a mainstay, other drugs with antiplatelet activity are also effective. Drugs that are being used include clopidogrel (Plavix), dipyridamole (Persantine), and Aggrenox (a combination of aspirin and dipyridamole). Statins, which lower cholesterol, also seem to reduce risk of stroke. Warfarin, an anticoagulant, reduces the stroke risk for some patients, especially those with atrial fibrillation and other types of heart conditions causing stroke. Studies are underway of all of these drugs—including aspirin—to determine the most effective and safest doses to be taken.

WHAT YOU CAN DO NOW

As caregiver, you will need to learn a great deal to look after a stroke survivor—nursing tasks; the basics of therapy, what it aims to accomplish, and how; nutrition; dealing with incontinence; dealing with depression—the list goes on. The special skills you will require depend on the specific needs of your patient. Training is necessary. Unless you are a nurse or similar health care professional, you will need formalized instruction for the tasks that await you. You can arrange for training while the patient is still in the acute phase of treatment. If you have questions, speak to a nurse, doctor, therapist, or social worker about how this can be accomplished.

Taking care of a stroke patient can be a demanding, exhausting, and isolating job. Caregivers often forget to take care of themselves and may end up with their own depression or other illness, or become too fatigued to function. One of the most beneficial things you can do for yourself as a caregiver is to find others facing similar challenges and share your experiences. Support groups for both caregivers and stroke survivors can be found around the country. You can find support groups in your area through the American Stroke Association (see following section) and the American Red Cross.

The NINDS recommends a number of tips to reduce stress for both caregivers and stroke patients, in the difficult period as the transition is made from hospital to home care. Your health care providers, therapists, and social worker may be able to help with some of these suggestions.

• Remain hopeful, don't give up. One of the most important things a caregiver can do is keep hope alive. Today may have been difficult but tomorrow can be better. Take one day at a time.

• Progress is likely to be slow and incremental. Appreciate small gains. Learn from your mistakes to come up with better ways to do things.

• Appreciate that caregiving skills are learned through experience and you will get better as you go along. Experiment to find the techniques that work best for you and the person you're caring for.

• Plan breaks so you can get some time for yourself as family members and friends take over for a few hours, or a day.

• Plan activities to get out of the house, for both you and the stroke survivor.

• Avoid comparing life now to life before the stroke.

• Research the field of stroke rehabilitation, and read as much as you can find about people in similar situations. There are many books written by stroke survivors and their family members (see below).

• Find a support group where you can share your feelings and frustrations. Talk to people who have been in the same situation. If you live in a remote area, you may find support on the Internet.

• Don't blame your charge for your frustrations. Appreciate that this relationship is also difficult for the other person in the relationship, the stroke survivor. Treat each other with kindness. If you have trouble with this very important part of care, you may need counseling to continue working effectively.

ADDITIONAL RESOURCES

ORGANIZATIONS

Agency for Healthcare Research and Quality

AHRQ Publications Clearinghouse
P.O. Box 8547
Silver Spring, MD 20907
800-358-9295
www.ahcpr.gov

American Stroke Association (division of American Heart Association)

7272 Greenville Avenue
Dallas, TX 75231-4596
800-AHA-USA1 (800-242-8721)
Fax 214-987-4334
www.americanheart.org

Brain Aneurysm Foundation

295 Cambridge Street

Boston, MA 02114

617-723-3870

Fax 617-723-8672

National Aphasia Association

156 Fifth Avenue, Suite 707

New York, NY 10010

800-922-4622

www.aphasia.org

National Family Caregivers Association

10400 Connecticut Avenue, Suite 500

Kensington, MD 20895-3944

800-896-3650

www.nfcacares.org

National Stroke Association

9707 East Easter Lane

Englewood, CO 80112-3747

800-STROKES (800-787-6537)

or 303-649-9299

Fax 303-649-1328

info@stroke.org

www.stroke.org

NIH Neurological Institute

P. O. Box 5801

Bethesda, MD 20824

800-352-9424 or 301-496-5751

Stroke Clubs International

805 12th Street

Galveston, Texas 77550

409-762-1022

strokeclub@aol.com

BOOKS

Caplan, Louis R, J. Donald Easton, and Mark L. Dyken. *American Heart Association Family Guide to Stroke Treatment, Recovery, and Prevention.* New York: Times Books, 1994.

Burkman, Kip. *The Stroke Recovery Book: A Guide for Patients and Families.* LPC Publishers, 1998.

Burton, Carol, and Geoffrey A. Donnan . *After a Stroke: A Support Book for Patients, Caregivers, Families and Friends.* (The Family Health Series). Berkeley, Calif.: North Atlantic Books, 1992.

Hay, Jennifer. *Stroke. Questions You Have ... Answers You Need.* Allentown, Pa.: Peoples Medical Society, 1995.

Hinds, David M., and Peter Morris. *After Stroke.* Wellingborough, U. K.: Thorsons Publishers, 2000.

Klein, Bonnie Sherr. *Slow Dance: A Story of Stroke, Love, and Disability.* Berkeley, Calif.: Pagemill Press, 1998.

Larkin, Marilynn, and Lynn Sonberg. *When Someone You Love Has a Stroke.* New York: Dell Publishing Company, 1995.

McCrum, Robert. *My Year Off: Recovering Life After a Stroke.* New York: W. W. Norton & Company, 1998.

Rocket, Howard, and Rachel Sklar. *Stroke of Luck: Life, Crisis and Rebirth of a Stroke Survivor.* Toronto: Hushion House, 1999.

Senelick, Richard C. , et al. *Living With Stroke: A Guide for Families, Help and New Hope for All Those Touched by Stroke.* Chicago: Contemporary Books, 1999.

Sife, Wallace (ed.). *After Stroke: Enhancing Quality of Life.* Binghampton, N.Y.: Haworth Press, 1998.

Weiner, Florence, et al. *Recovering at Home After a Stroke: A Practical Guide for You and Your Family.* Body Press, 1994.

Substance Abuse and the Elderly

S ubstance abuse is most often perceived as a problem of young people. In fact, it is a broad problem that encompasses many different substances and a variety of types of abuse, and some aspects of abuse are very common in older adults. Most notably, those who care for the elderly are likely to encounter the following patterns:

- alcohol use and abuse
- misuse of prescription and over-the-counter drugs
- cigarette smoking

Elderly alcohol users and abusers fall into two categories: those who have lifelong patterns of alcohol use and those who began drinking late in life. The elderly substance abuser who takes illegal drugs is probably someone with a long-standing addiction and perhaps a lifelong pattern of multiple drug use. This last, however, is a very small category. Many illegal drug users simply do not make it to old age because of the health risks of their behavior and the lifestyle associated with it.

The categories of legal drug use listed above, however, can be applied to millions of older adults in this country. A recent publication by the government's

SIGNS & SYMPTOMS

- Forgetfulness, cognitive impairment, or dementia
- Anxiety, confusion, or delirium
- Self-neglect, resulting in poor grooming, cleanliness, nutrition, etc.
- Sleep disorders
- Depression or mood changes
- Malnutrition
- Gait disorders or falls
- Muscle weakness
- Flushed face or other skin problems
- Bladder or bowel incontinence
- Persistent family discord
- Pattern of doing well when hospitalized but poorly at home
- Change in usual social patterns, such as churchgoing or attending regular social functions

NOTE: The above *may* be symptoms of substance abuse, but since many symptoms mimic those of other conditions—other disease symptoms, side effects of medications, or even just signs of aging—they may indicate something else, so consult your health care provider if these are observed.

Center for Substance Abuse Treatment (CSAT) labeled abuse of alcohol and legal drugs as an "invisible epidemic" that affects nearly one fifth of Americans over the age of 60. Because it cannot be seen, it is a difficult problem to quantify. According to one study, 2.5 million older adults and 21% of all hospitalized patients over the age of 65 have alcohol-related problems. Another estimated that 15% of people over the age of 60 consume the equivalent of four or more drinks daily. Other studies have found that more than 40% of elderly hospital patients have alcohol-related problems. In one survey, more elderly people were hospitalized for alcohol-related health problems than for heart attacks. And misuse of prescription drugs, even more difficult to tally, has been found to be a problem among a significant percentage of the senior population.

Caregivers and health care providers are likely to overlook substance abuse issues in older adults for a number of reasons. The elderly substance abuser usually does not fit the stereotype of a "typical" alcoholic or drug user. Often the symptoms overlap symptoms of other conditions common in the elderly, such as dementia and depression. Also, for many people, alcohol abuse and/or drug misuse is cloaked in shame and denial—in particular, adult children of people with problems related to alcohol or drug misuse are often ashamed of their parents' behaviors. The elderly and their caregivers are not likely to seek help for a problem they don't want to acknowledge. Consequently, thousands of senior citizens could benefit from treatment for substance abuse problems but don't receive it. This can have negative effects on all aspects of their lives—physical health, mental health, cognitive functioning, and social functioning.

Alcohol is even more of a threat to the physical health of senior citizens than it is to younger drinkers. Because the liver loses some efficiency as a person ages, alcohol metabolizes more slowly, and it takes less to have an effect as a person gets older. A 40-year-old may barely feel the effects of two or three drinks that will make a 70-year-old feel intoxicated. The elderly are also more fragile and at greater risks for falling, household accidents, and auto or pedestrian accidents—risks that are exacerbated by the use of alcohol. Other complications of age and drinking are the medications that many older people take. They can interact negatively with alcohol. Or drinkers may forget to take medications, or forget that they have taken them and take them twice.

WHAT IS IT?

There are a number of different definitions of alcoholism and substance abuse, and health care providers use these for diagnostic purposes. However, this isn't a problem that can be easily pinned down by lab tests or clinical observations, and definitions have only recently been reviewed and revised so that they are beginning to address the specifics of elderly substance abuse. CSAT and the National Institute on Alcohol Abuse and Alcoholism (NIAAA) both recommend that older drinkers consume no more than one drink a day. Elderly alcohol abusers are divided into two groups: most are estimated to have a pattern of alcohol use that dates back to earlier in their lives, while the second group did not begin drinking until they were more advanced in years. The first group can often be identified by previous dysfunctional behavior and problems caused by alcohol use such as legal troubles, family problems, and difficulties with employment. The drinking problems of the late-onset group are often more subtle and often are related to life situations such as retirement, death of loved ones, loneliness, illness, or a combination of these factors. Among the group that appear to be late-onset drinkers, there may well be some persons who had well-hidden problems with alcohol early in life.

WHO IS AT RISK?

The biggest single risk factor for substance abuse problems for the elderly is a history of substance abuse in their younger years. Family history and genetics also play a role, as they do for many diseases at any age. Beyond that, however, the risks for developing chemical dependency and other substance abuse problems are somewhat different for the elderly than they are for younger people. Critical factors that influence youthful substance abuse such as poverty, low self-esteem, history of child abuse, and low educational attainment are often not in play with older people. Rather, substance abuse among the elderly is related to the losses and other similar life-changing events that they face.

Alcohol use is more common among elderly men than women, although since women outlive men, there is a preponderance of women in the oldest age brack-

LIFE EVENTS AND SUBSTANCE ABUSE

There is some dispute about the significance of life events, a difficult and subjective topic to study. However, many clinicians and researchers observe the following as precipitators of alcohol or drug abuse or misuse later in life:

- Illness and disability, especially chronic illness associated with pain
- History of depression or other psychiatric disorders
- Becoming a widow or widower. Men who lose a spouse are more likely than women to seek solace in drinking
- Loss of friends and other relatives
- Retirement
- Loss of meaningful role or function in life, feeling of uselessness
- Loneliness
- Having a spouse or partner who is a substance abuser

ets and thus more female problem drinkers in raw numbers. A large study of the drinking habits of the elderly found that 3% of men and 0.5% of women were alcohol abusers or dependents, and another 3 to 4% of all elderly had problems with alcohol use, but not severe enough for them to be classified as alcoholics.

Unlike alcohol, prescription drugs are more likely to be misused by women than men. The drugs most likely to cause trouble are sedatives or hypnotics (sleeping medications) and anxiolytics (antianxiety drugs). These include benzodiazepines like Valium, which are very widely prescribed. One study found that nearly one quarter of people over 65 had been prescribed some sort of psychoactive drug in the previous year. Generally it is recommended that these drugs be used for four months or less. However, studies have determined that elderly people are more likely than younger ones to take these drugs beyond the recommended period.

Tobacco is a different issue, with different risk factors, although using alcohol or other drugs increases the likelihood that a person will also be a smoker. The good news is that growing older is associated with increased success in quitting smoking. An estimated 60% of elderly women and 70% of elderly men who were smokers earlier in their lives have already quit, according to the Department of Health and Human Services. This is due to a combination of more effective cessation methods and the fact that smokers who did not quit tended to die earlier. But among the elderly who do smoke, 10% per year quit.

As today's middle-aged baby boomers move toward old age, some predict that the problem of substance abuse among the elderly may increase in the future for two reasons. First, there will be more senior citizens than ever before; and second, this group has always had liberal attitudes about drug use. In one study of women drinkers, researchers estimated that by the year 2020, there will be as many as 300,000 women over the age of 65 with symptoms of alcohol dependence. And more marijuana and other drug use among senior citizens is likely to be seen in coming decades.

HOW IS IT DIAGNOSED?

There are many tools used to diagnose alcohol and drug use, and many of them have excellent track records, but few have been evaluated for use in an elderly population. Substance abuse in the elderly can be a very difficult problem to diagnose. Drinking and drug use by senior citizens is often done in secret. When questioned by caregivers, family members, or health care providers, many older people have a tendency to minimize the amount consumed. Family members may enable the secret usage. Denial can be major factor impeding diagnosis.

Nearly 90% of elderly people see a doctor regularly. But doctors often fail to detect substance abuse in the elderly more often than in younger patients. The symptoms of substance abuse are often overlooked or misinterpreted. In retired people who live alone, don't drive, and don't have regular social contacts, they can go undetected for months or even years. Symptoms of substance abuse may be similar to other disease symptoms, or side effects of medications, or even just signs of aging. They can be intellectual or behavioral or physical. The following may be symptoms of substance abuse—but they may indicate something else, so further diagnostic efforts are necessary if these are observed:

- Forgetfulness, cognitive impairment, or dementia
- Anxiety, confusion, or delirium
- Self-neglect, resulting in poor grooming, cleanliness, nutrition, etc.
- Sleep disorders
- Depression or mood changes
- Malnutrition
- Gait disorders or falls
- Muscle weakness

- Flushed face or other skin problems
- Bladder or bowel incontinence
- Persistent family discord
- Pattern of doing well when hospitalized but poorly at home
- Change in usual social patterns, such as churchgoing or attending regular social functions

Many medical diseases are commonly found among older problem drinkers. Some, like hypertension, diabetes, and gout, may be pre-existing conditions made worse or unstable by alcohol. For others, like cardiac disease, including heart failure and atrial fibrillation, alcohol may play a contributing role as a cause. For still others, the disease may appear different in older patients from what is typical for younger drinkers. For example, alcoholic liver disease is more likely to be first noticed at the late stage of scarring (cirrhosis) than at the earlier stages of inflammation (hepatitis). Effects on the pancreas are more likely to be noticed first as late-stage chronic pancreatitis with diarrhea and weight loss, than as an earlier stage of acute pancreatitis with abdominal pain and vomiting. In older patients, syndromes similar to these are more commonly caused by other diseases, necessitating a careful workup for conditions such as malignancy or gallstones before drinking can be assumed to be the cause.

A laboratory finding of abnormal blood counts (for example, enlarged red blood cells, mild anemia, or diminished platelets or white blood cells) can be an indicator of a drinking problem. When drinking is combined with poor diet, alcohol can create or contribute to vitamin deficiency, particularly thiamine (vitamin B1) and folic acid (known as folate). The combination of alcohol use and low dietary folic acid can be particularly damaging to blood counts. The elderly face many causes of abnormal blood counts that are unrelated to alcohol, so abnormal blood counts require careful review by a doctor.

Difficulty in diagnosis is also compounded by the fact that the amount of alcohol or other drug consumed may be smaller than an amount that would suggest a problem in younger people, because of lowered tolerance and increased sensitivity in the elderly. In older people, small amounts may cause major problems.

A CSAT study of the problem recommends that a variety of caregivers be involved with the process of screening for substance abuse problems: friends and family, senior center staff members, drivers and volunteers who see the person on a regular basis, social workers, and health care professionals. Primary care physicians are in a good position to detect clues, although they are not always attuned to substance abuse. The CSAT report advises that everyone over age 60 be screened for substance abuse or misuse as part of their regular physical exam.

Meetings of senior's clubs and get-togethers at senior centers and retirement centers can provide opportunities for self-scored mass screening. Caregivers can also slip simple screening questions into conversations, if they suspect a problem. But it is important not to use pejorative or stigmatizing language as these subjects are introduced.

Health care professionals use a standard screening test called CAGE to detect alcohol problems. In many cases, "substance use" can be substituted for "drinking" to broaden the scope of the test, and the CAGE questions can also be modified for smoking. It consists of four simple questions (the name is an acronym for a key word in each question).

1. *Have you ever felt you should Cut down on your drinking?*
2. *Have people Annoyed you by criticizing your drinking?*
3. *Have you ever felt bad or Guilty about your drinking?*
4. *Have you ever had an Eye-opener, a drink first thing in the morning to steady your nerves or treat a hangover?*

One or more positive answers to CAGE questions may indicate a problem that should get further attention. However, binge drinkers and other more specialized types of substance abusers may "pass" the CAGE and have their substance abuse go undetected. Some people feel that the CAGE questions may be less sensitive for older adults with drinking problems than for younger adults.

Another commonly used questionnaire, the Michigan Alcoholism Screening Test, has a special geriatric version (MAST-G). It includes 26 questions, asks about a variety of habits, and is much more specific than the CAGE. Examples of the more age-specific questions are: *Does alcohol make you sleepy so that you often fall asleep in your chair? Did you find your drinking increased after someone close to you died? Are you drinking more now than in the past?* Five or more positive responses in the MAST-G indicate a possible alcohol problem. The Alcohol Use Disorders Identification Test (AUDIT) is another questionnaire that asks about how much and how often a person drinks and the effects of one's drinking. Many doctors will ask elderly patients how much they drink on an average day, how much they drink in an average week, and how many drinks they have at any one time. Answers of more than seven drinks per week, or more than three drinks at a time, may indicate a problem.

Breath, urine, and blood tests can be used to confirm alcohol or substance use. Lab studies might include blood alcohol concentration, tests of liver function, drug screens, and other biochemical markers. Brain imaging (i.e., CAT scan or MRI) can rule out neurologic causes of symptoms.

WHAT SHOULD YOU EXPECT?

Drug use takes its toll. There are many possible consequences of alcohol and other substance abuse in the elderly. That is obvious. What might not be so apparent is the more positive fact that treatment works, and older people have even better success in overcoming their addictions than their younger counterparts.

It can be difficult to sort out whether a change in a person is because of alcohol or aging. Alcohol abuse accelerates the process of aging and promotes physiologic decline. It increases the elderly's risk for accidents, injuries, and illness. Broken bones are a common problem in elderly people who drink too much. So is depression, but it is often unclear whether alcohol use caused depression, or vice versa. But alcohol abuse is definitely associated with an increased risk of suicide in older people. It contributes directly to more than twenty different diseases. If liver disease develops and drinking continues, the prognosis is very poor. Alcohol misuse also contributes to arrhythmias, heart failure, some cancers (liver; head and neck), gastrointestinal bleeding, pancreatitis, and susceptibility to infection. Some degree of cognitive impairment is seen in many people with drinking problems, particularly if there is a history of vitamin deficiencies (especially thiamine), or falls and head trauma. Various studies indicate that elderly alcoholics can have full or irreversible dementia that ranges from 25 to 60%.

The worst of these outcomes are seen in alcoholics, the heaviest of drinkers. But again, what might be considered moderate drinking in younger people can contribute to many adverse health effects in the elderly because of the slowed metabolism and increased sensitivity that aging causes. Older people often take medications that can negatively interact with alcohol. Warfarin (Coumadin) is a commonly prescribed drug that interacts directly with alcohol, and so can cause gastrointestinal or other internal bleeding.

Alcohol abuse is also thought to cause a number of neurologic syndromes, as a result of deficiencies of vitamins such as thiamine, niacin, and possibly others. Some of the neurologic syndromes may relate more to the direct toxic effects of alcohol on the nervous system. These neurologic signs and symptoms may include:

- memory impairment
- gait disorders
- problems with balance and coordination
- hallucinations, seizures, and other syndromes of alcohol withdrawal

An elderly person who has hallucinations, seizures, and other signs of withdrawal may require urgent hospitalization.

Overuse of prescription drugs such as benzodiazepines, sedatives, and hypnotics can cause impaired cognition, daytime sedation, and attention and memory problems. Misuse causes physical dependence or addiction. Older people have less tolerance for these drugs than younger people. Using sleeping pills often causes a daytime "hangover" effect in the elderly, impairing their ability to perform daytime tasks. Falls and fractures are also seen more often in those who misuse medications. Imaging of the brains of long-term benzodiazepine users has found brain atrophy, suggesting that the damage may be permanent. Chemical dependence may also cause problems in managing medications, keeping appointments, and handling other aspects of illness and disease.

The effects of tobacco and cigarette smoking are well known. Smoking is linked to lung conditions such as lung cancer, chronic obstructive pulmonary disease, and emphysema. It contributes to heart disease and stroke. It is associated with lung, head and neck, and bladder cancers. Smokers have increased rates of osteoporosis. They also are more likely than nonsmokers to suffer vision loss due to age-related macular degeneration.

HOW IS IT TREATED?

Concern of friends and family is the most common reason for seeking treatment. For many older substance abusers, a little bit of supportive care can go a long way. Caregivers can play an important role in detecting alcohol or drug problems and preventing them from progressing. Caregivers can also help in breaking down denial and readying a person for treatment. Treatment readiness is critical in substance abuse therapy. No treatment will work if a patient is too much in denial to be a partner in the process. The first line of treatment options is simply interventions, which can range from unstructured counseling and feedback to more formal therapy:

Brief intervention. This may consist of one or more counseling sessions, which broach the problem, discuss the need for change, and set goals. It is a four-step process from the therapist's point of view: ask, assess, advise, and monitor. It is often helpful to discuss categories of drinkers (or prescription drug abusers), how the patient's behavior fits him into a specific category, and the reasons for and consequences of alcohol or drug use. Reasons to cut down or stop drinking or drug use can be reviewed, as well as strategies for accomplishing this. Many counselors use a "prescription" approach to put in writing the agreed-upon limits.

Formal intervention. A more formal intervention involves a professional counselor and other significant people in the patient's life. For the elderly, it is usually advisable to have only one or two close relatives or friends involved. The participants will discuss their personal experiences with the patient's substance use.

Motivational counseling. This approach has been successful with elderly people. The patient begins by presenting his view of the problem to an understanding and supportive counselor. From there, they can identify the consequences of the substance abuse and empower the patient to take responsibility for solving the problems.

For some people, these interventions will suffice and no further treatment will be necessary. For many others, though, these are pretreatment efforts that will pave the way for treatment.

ABSTINENCE

Clearly, for younger persons and for those with lifelong problems, the goal should almost always be total abstinence. If potentially lethal problems such as emphysema and heart disease, cirrhosis, a history of drunk driving, or attempts at suicide are issues, total abstinence in the habits contributing to them (whether smoking, drinking, or prescription drug misuse) must be the goal. In particular, if someone has tried and failed in the past to control their drinking, many doctors consider that a red flag meaning that abstinence from alcohol is required.

TAPERING

There is continuing debate in the medical community about what the goal should be in treating elderly substance abusers. Abstinence is always a goal, but in some cases, particularly in an elderly population, an outcome short of total abstinence can achieve desirable medical, psychological, cognitive, and behavioral goals. For substance abuse, as for many chronic diseases, "cure" and "relapse" for elderly patients may be defined in less than absolute terms. Most health care providers will consider the degree of addiction or abuse, the age of the person, the substance abuse history, and other medical factors in determining a successful outcome. Each case must be considered individually.

However, many practitioners believe that many elderly people can be helped enormously with an approach that helps them reduce their consumption: tapering down the use of the substance. For example, an older woman could cut back from her daylong rum sipping and bottle of wine in the evening, to a single glass of wine with dinner, she might still feel she had something to look forward to but not be posing real risks to her health. The plausibility of this goal may depend on many individual circumstances, such as whether the woman lives alone, the extent and quality of her social support, how long she has been drinking too much, and whether she has any complicating medical conditions. For others, smoking a cigarette or two a day would pose much less of a health risk than smoking a pack or two a day, and for some that might be a more realistic goal than quitting smoking completely. With prescribed medications, occasional and nonescalating use of psychotropic drugs can be appropriate. Used judiciously, these drugs can be very effective in treating anxiety, insomnia, depression, and other problems of the elderly.

STRUCTURED TREATMENT PROGRAMS

Increasingly, treatment programs tailored specifically to the elderly are becoming available. In one study, patients finishing age-specific programs had more than twice the chance of being abstinent a year after treatment as those in mixed-age groups. Treatment should be in an age-specific setting whenever possible, flexible, and holistic, addressing psychological, social, and physical problems of the patient.

A number of different approaches are used successfully: cognitive behavioral therapy, which teaches skills for overcoming grief, loneliness, and depression; educational sessions; individual counseling; group therapy; family therapy; individual psychotherapy; and community support programs such as Alcoholics Anonymous. Groups can be very important in helping a person to realize he/she is not unique or alone, and many others have comparable behaviors When groups are used, it is important that they accommodate a person's sensory deficits, using enlarged print for educational materials, for example, and microphones or other audio enhancers as necessary. When looking for an AA group, try to find one with a geriatric orientation—an estimated one third of all AA members are over 50 and many groups have primarily older participants.

Treatment is also classified by the duration and setting:

- Self-help groups like AA, where the commitment might be lifelong
- Outpatient, lasting six months to a year and longer
- Inpatient residential care, typically lasting two to four weeks
- Detox, usually up to a week in an acute hospital unit

In general, treatment should be attempted from least intensive to most intensive options. Ideally, treatment should come from qualified substance abuse treatment professionals, although studies show that brief counseling by a primary care physician can significantly reduce a person's alcohol consumption.

For more serious addiction problems, detoxification may be necessary. For most elderly people, particularly if there are complicating medical problems, detox is done in an inpatient hospital setting. Decisions about inpatient or outpatient setting will depend on the severity of the symptoms. Hospitalization is usually necessary if serious withdrawal symptoms are likely, if the patient has expressed suicide threats, if psychological problems are present, if there is an unstable medical condition, if there is more than one addiction (for example, alcohol and Valium), or if there is a lack of social supports in the patient's home. If drugs are used for withdrawal, they should be begun at lower than usual adult doses and tapered upward as they are tolerated. Supplying adequate nutrition and hydration is also an important part of the detox process. Older patients do well in detox programs, but their recovery time may be longer than a younger person's.

It is often helpful, when prescription drugs are concerned, for caregivers to consult with physicians about an "unprescribing" plan to taper dosages and gradually eliminate some of the drugs that a person takes. It is important that the health care provider have an overview of all the medical problems that are involved, all the drugs that are used, and how symptoms respond to cutting back on drugs. The concept of drug "holidays" can also be useful—discontinuing certain drugs for a period of time and observing how this affects symptoms and behavior. But this is not something a caregiver should ever do alone—it is essential that a physician supervise drug tapering and holidays.

LIFESTYLE CHANGES AND BEHAVIOR MODIFICATION

There are many behavioral alternatives to pharmaceuticals, but these therapies can be time consuming, expensive, or difficult to implement. For example, to reduce use of sleeping pills in an insomniac, a "sleep hygiene" program that eliminates caffeine from the diet, emphasizes daily exercise, and structures bedtime habits can be very effective. Likewise, using massage or heat can sometimes help with pain as much as pills. These approaches require some effort, and a conscientious caregiver can play a critical role. Strategies should be supportive and nonconfrontational.

TREATMENT FOR ALCOHOLISM

Symptoms of alcohol withdrawal can begin within several hours after the last drink or frequently, the next morning. Nervousness, irritability, nausea, and vomiting are common. Peak symptoms may occur one or two days after the last drink and subside in five to seven days, although mild symptoms including insomnia may last for ten days. In the most serious cases of withdrawal following extended periods of abuse, seizures, delirium, or hallucinations may occur. Depending on the seriousness of the alcohol abuse, and any associated medical conditions, you should talk to a doctor about possible hospitalization in view of the risks of cardiovascular instability (changes in heartbeat and blood pressure) and even death.

Chlordiazepoxide (Librium) or oxazepam (Serax) are commonly prescribed to treat the symptoms of alcohol withdrawal. Thiamine is often given to prevent neurological complications such as Wernicke's syndrome. Other drugs such as anticonvulsants, short-acting benzodiazepines, and beta blockers are sometimes used to ease the symptoms of alcohol withdrawal and prevent relapse. Disulfiram

497

(Antabuse) is often used with younger patients to prevent relapse, but not usually recommended for the elderly because it can have dangerous side effects and adverse interactions with other medications. Naltrexone (ReVia) may be a safer pharmaceutical option. These are drugs for remission maintenance and not for the period of withdrawal.

Alcoholism is a chronic illness, and a true "cure" can be elusive. Treatment is likely to be an ongoing process. However, if treatment is viewed in terms of maximizing function, minimizing suffering, and halting the progression of related disease, quality of life can be considerably improved and results can be very satisfying. Some practitioners have observed that during the first six months of recovery, elderly people are likely to feel angry, feel that the fun is gone from their lives, and grieve the loss of alcohol or drugs. Then they are likely to show improvement, getting on with their lives and getting over their addictions.

TREATMENT FOR PRESCRIPTION DRUG ABUSE

There has not been much systematic study of treating prescription drug abuse problems in the elderly, but if a person has a serious problem, hospitalization is advised. Usually doses are gradually tapered, until the drug is stopped completely. It may take months to become drug-free. There is evidence that tapered withdrawal is effective and well tolerated by the elderly, and they can move on from an addiction.

For complete recovery, the patient must understand the underlying causes of the addiction, which can be accomplished through individual, group, or family therapy, according to individual circumstances. It is important that the primary care physician and any other doctors who write prescriptions for this individual be aware of the problem that has developed and be part of the treatment team. In the cases of elderly substance abusers with underlying depression, antidepressive medication can be an important adjunct to treating the addiction problem. In some cases, doctors try to substitute safer, less addictive drugs for the patient; for example, clonazepam (Klonopin) for diazepam (Valium) or alprazolam (Xanax).

TREATMENT FOR TOBACCO ADDICTION

Ninety percent of smokers who quit, quit on their own, without the help of a program or counseling or even a nicotine patch. Nevertheless, there are many different approaches to help people stop smoking, ranging from hypnosis to acupuncture to aversive therapy to cognitive therapy. Often a health crisis, like a heart attack or hospitalization for pneumonia, will be the stimulus for a person to finally try to break a decades-old habit. Elderly smokers may argue that it's too late for them to quit—that the damage has already been done and can't be repaired. In fact, this is untrue. No matter how long they have been smoking, most smokers will feel immediate relief of some symptoms when they quit—the ability to breathe deeper, the absence or lessening of a previously persistent cough. And while it's true that permanent damage has been done to a longtime smoker's lungs and cardiovascular system, it is not totally irreversible and the body will work to repair itself after smoking cessation. The health benefits of stopping smoking are significant at any age.

(For more information on treatment options for smokers who want to quit, see "Smoking cessation" in the Chronic Obstructive Pulmonary Disease chapter on p. 86, especially the sections entitled "Nicotine replacement therapy" and "Drug therapy.")

WHAT RESEARCH IS BEING DONE?

This nation's "war on drugs" includes a substantial research agenda, and several well-funded government and private agencies are devoted to various aspects of substance abuse (i.e., the Center for Substance Abuse Treatment, the Center for Substance Abuse Prevention, the National Institute on Drug Abuse, and the National Institute of Alcohol Abuse and Alcoholism). However, only a relatively small number of researchers are looking specifically at substance abuse in the elderly and the amount of literature on the subject is sketchy. As more and more baby boomers become senior citizens, it is likely that there will be increasing interest in geriatric substance abuse problems.

Some of the ongoing studies about geriatric substance abuse are investigating treatment for people suffering from both alcoholism and depression, and the effects of various treatment interventions. In general, substance abuse researchers are investigating the genetics of addiction, the way brain chemicals behave when people drink or use drugs or become addicted, and how substance abuse can be prevented. Discovery of details about brain chemistry and substance abuse has the potential to lead to more effective pharmaceutical treatments.

HOW CAN IT BE PREVENTED?

A substantial public health effort is devoted to preventing substance abuse, but it is primarily targeted at youthful potential drug users, down to elementary school age. The elderly are a considerable afterthought in the realm of prevention. However, a number of techniques and philosophies have been discussed and applied in both primary and secondary prevention.

The best way to prevent late-onset substance abuse in the elderly is to reduce risk factors. Of course, the losses and life changes that are inevitable with aging cannot be eliminated. Learning how to cope with late-life stresses and education about potential pitfalls of substance abuse can be an effective deterrent to problems ever arising for many seniors. For example, grief work, or bereavement counseling, such as that provided by many hospice organizations, may be crucial in helping an older person recover from the death of a spouse.

Secondary prevention keeps a problem from getting worse, and caregivers can play a significant role here. Recognizing early warning signs and bringing them to the attention of an individual is an important step and may be sufficient to keep a problem from getting worse. The importance of education cannot be overemphasized, and people can be educated in various ways according to their own preference and aptitudes—through printed materials, videos, one-on-one discussions, group sessions, or other methods. Remember, one size does not fit all for older adults. They have a tremendous range of learning styles, life experiences, and interests, based in part on varying life experiences and different degrees of health and fitness.

Trouble with prescription medications sometimes begins with confusion over how much of which pill to take, and how often. As caregiver, you can work with health care providers to come up with an easy-to-follow schedule of medications with written directions. Many elderly people take many pills a day and compartmentalized daily or weekly medication supply boxes can be helpful. For the person with impaired vision or reading limitations, color-coding or another easily discernible classification system can prevent mistakes. Some caregivers may wish to monitor pill taking, which should be done in a cooperative and not overbearing or critical way.

Health care professionals can play a preventive role by screening their patients for substance abuse issues, advising and educating patients who seem to have a present or potential problem, and detailing the medical consequences of substance abuse. Also, it is ultimately up to the doctor, or doctors, to know what drugs are being prescribed and how they might interact. As much as possible, you or your loved one should use one pharmacy. The condition of polypharmacy—or the prescription of many drugs for the same patient, often with no single health professional being aware of the full extent—can be the result of multiple doctors, or multiple pharmacists.

WHAT YOU CAN DO NOW

If you are a caregiver or otherwise closely involved with an elderly person whom you suspect is having a problem with alcohol or other drugs or tobacco, it is important to confront the situation directly. This is not usually a problem that solves itself—more likely, it will worsen without attention. Denial is so often a prominent feature—"Sure, I enjoy a couple of drinks, but I certainly don't have a problem," or "I don't cough that much"—that you might feel the subject is unbroachable. You might fear that continual harping on the theme will poison your relationship, but a progressive substance abuse problem in someone's life can poison everything.

The goal of working through denial is usually acquiescence to some form of treatment, but there might also be other goals that are closer to home. Rearranging a schedule, changing a routine, helping someone fill empty hours with activities and recreation, providing companionship, reintegrating a person into their community—these are approaches that deal with the substance abuse problem indirectly but get to some of the underlying causes and can be helpful if a problem is not too serious.

When trying to break through denial, it is important to remember that this can be a lengthy and ongoing process. Even if a person accepts the notion that there is a problem, he or she may continue to deny its magnitude, or resist the steps necessary to address it.

Acknowledging a problem with drinking or prescriptions or smoking requires confronting some difficult realities as basic as a person's self-concept, the real danger of continuing current behaviors, and the re-examination of relationships and

501

time spent. It is not uncommon for there to be other substance abusers in the family, which can enable the elderly person. Sometimes it is helpful to engage in a preliminary contract of abstinence or cutting back, even if a person doesn't admit a problem, so that behaviors in the abstinent period can be compared to previous behaviors.

Caregivers also fill an essential role in helping with the logistics of arranging and then receiving treatment. Many elderly people with substance use problems are frail and need transportation, assistance with meals, and help with other household tasks.

Like youth, older people with substance abuse disorders often have low self-esteem or despair about their lives. They may have tried cutting back or quitting drinking or substance use in the past, and been unsuccessful. It is very important for the caregiver to

- remain optimistic about the future,
- be supportive and positive,
- be certain that treatment can help the problem, and
- avoid assigning blame or imparting guilt.

Enlist the doctor or other health care providers, both to support your role as caregiver and to authenticate the message you are delivering. If the doctor does not have knowledge of treatment referral possibilities, work with him or her to find resources. Caregivers can also gain understanding of substance abuse or misuse through participation in groups such as Al-Anon, Nar-Anon, and the National Association of Adult Children of Alcoholics (NACoA).

ADDITIONAL RESOURCES

ORGANIZATIONS AND WEB SITES

Agency for Healthcare Research and Quality
"Help for Smokers: Ideas to Help You Quit"
http://www.ahrq.gov/consumer/helpsmok.htm

Al-Anon
World Service Office
Virginia Beach, Virginia
888-4AL-ANON
www.al-anon.alateen.org

Alcoholics Anonymous

475 Riverside Drive

11th floor

New York, NY 10115

212-870-3400

www.alcoholics-anonymous.org

Concerned About Your Drinking? Alcohol Screening Self Assessment

Harvard University Faculty and Staff Assistance Program

http://fsap.harvard.edu/alcoholtest.html

Hazelden Foundation

P.O. Box 11

CO 3

Center City, MN 55012-0011

800-257-7810

www.hazelden.org

Join Together

www.jointogether.org

Just the Facts: Chemical Dependency and the Elderly

National Clearinghouse for Alcohol and Drug Information

www.health.org

National Association for Children of Alcoholics (NACoA)

11426 Rockville Pike

Suite 100

Rockville, MD 20852

888-5541-2627

www.nacoa.org

National Clearinghouse for Alcohol and Drug Information (NCADI)

P.O. Box 2345

Rockville, MD 20847-2345

800-729-6686

www.health.org

National Drug and Treatment Referral Routing Service (a SAMHSA service)

1-800-662-HELP (24-hour treatment referral service)

National Institute on Drug Abuse (NIDA)

6001 Executive Boulevard

Bethesda, MD 20892-9561.

301-443-1124

www.nida.nih.gov

National Institute on Alcohol Abuse and Alcoholism (NIAAA)

6000 Executive Boulevard, Willco Building

Bethesda, MD 20892-7003

301-496-1993

www.niaaa.nih.gov

Substance Abuse & Mental Health Services Administration

U.S. Department of Health & Human Services

Room 12-105 Parklawn Building

5600 Fishers Lane

Rockville, MD 20857

301-443-4795

www.samhsa.gov

BOOKS

Colvin, Rod. *Prescription Drug Abuse: The Hidden Epidemic: A Guide to Coping and Understanding.* Omaha, Neb.: Addicus Books, 1995.

Drummond, Edward H. *Benzo Blues: Overcoming Anxiety Without Tranquilizers.* New York: Plume, 1998.

Eisenberg, Arlene, Howard Eisenberg, and Al J. Mooney. *The Recovery Book.* New York: Workman Publishing Company, 1992.

Fanning, Patrick, and John O'Neill. *The Addiction Workbook: A Step-By-Step Guide to Quitting Alcohol and Drugs.* Oakland, Calif.: New Harbinger Publications, 1996.

Fields, Richard. *Drugs in Perspective: A Personalized Look at Substance Use and Abuse.* New York: WCB/McGraw-Hill, 2000.

Rogers, Ronald L., and Chandler Scott McMillin. *Freeing Someone You Love from Alcohol and Other Drugs: A Step-By-Step Plan Starting Today!* New York: Perigee, 1992.

Volpicelli, Joseph and Maia Szalavitz. *Recovery Options: The Complete Guide.* New York: John Wiley & Sons, 2000.

Washton, Arnold, and Donna Boundy. *Willpower's Not Enough: Understanding and Recovering from Addictions of Every Kind.* New York: HarperCollins, 1990.

West, James W. and Betty Ford. *The Betty Ford Center Book of Answers: Help for Those Struggling With Substance Abuse and for the People Who Love Them.* New York: Pocket Books, 1997.

Eric Hardt, M.D., is Clinical Director of Geriatrics and Associate Professor of Medicine at Boston University School of Medicine in Boston, Massachusetts.

Urinary Incontinence

Urinary incontinence, the involuntary leakage of urine, is not a normal part of aging. It is very common, affecting about one out of every ten people age 65 and older, an estimated 13 million adults in America alone, but it is not inevitable, and most people who suffer from it can be helped. Unfortunately, urinary incontinence is often a silent problem, hidden from family, friends, and even the family doctor, sometimes for years. In fact, the average length of time before a woman seeks medical help for urinary incontinence is about eight years.

This is a great shame because urinary incontinence is often a profound source of embarrassment, anger, depression, and isolation. For families or caregivers, it can be a serious burden, and because many caregivers may not realize that most incontinence can be controlled, if not cured, it is often the major deciding factor in nursing home admission. Worse, even though incontinence itself is not a life-or-death disorder, it is a major health problem (and a $24 billion-a-year industry in the United States) whose complications and indirect consequences sometimes can be lethal. For example, losing independence and dignity—and needing the help of someone else to manage one of the most personal bodily functions—or experiencing social isolation, and not going out for fear of "having an accident" can lead to depression and may decrease life expectancy. Ongoing skin irritation and breakdown can lead to infection. The chronic use of a catheter may lead to scarring, kidney damage, stones in the urinary tract, and even serious, life-threatening infection.

And yet, for most people with urinary incontinence, the greatest obstacles to treatment are usually the first few steps: getting past the stigma of losing urinary control, admitting the problem, and seeking medical help. No matter what anyone may have told you—even if urinary incontinence has made life miserable for you or someone you love, there is much hope, and this is a highly treatable problem.

WHAT IS IT?

The involuntary leakage of urine is called urinary incontinence. Normally, our kidneys manage more than 30 gallons of water a day, constantly refining and processing, over and over again, all of the liquid we consume. The waste—the fluid that can't be reabsorbed by the body—filters in concentrated form to the ureters, long tubes that "milk" urine onward to the bladder.

Perched atop the pelvic floor, the muscular "hammock" that runs between the pubic bone and the base of the spine, the bladder is a complicated reservoir that holds between two and three cups of fluid. It is laced with stretchy connective tissue, which allows the bladder to expand like a balloon when it fills, and shrink when it's emptied. Nerves in the bladder keep the brain and spinal cord up-to-date on the bladder's status. The brain, in turn, sends chemical signals (called neurotransmitters) to all the muscles in the urinary tract, using biochemical nerve highways called the cholinergic and adrenergic systems. (This is important, because one way to control certain types of incontinence is with drugs that work along these same pathways.) The brain tells the bladder to relax and expand, and as the bladder swells, our response is voluntary. We signal muscles in the pelvis to contract, to stop or delay urination until a convenient time. Normally, when we choose to urinate, nerves in the spinal cord activate chemical switches to prompt the voiding reflex in which the detrusor, the powerful muscle that surrounds the bladder, contracts and the internal sphincter, a muscular valve in the bladder neck, relaxes automatically.

The bladder neck, rather like large faucet, allows urine to flow into yet another muscular tube, called the urethra, which takes it from here, passing urine out of the body. In men, the urethra tunnels through the prostate on its way to the penis; in women, the urethra is much shorter (about two inches, compared to about ten inches in men). At the end of the urethra is a final door—one normally under our control—called the external sphincter, a voluntary muscle. When we urinate, we tell this sphincter to relax, and muscles in the bladder and pelvic floor to contract.

After urination, this outside door closes; the sphincter contracts again.

What can go wrong? It's important to note that incontinence itself is not a disease. Rather, it's a symptom, a signal that at least one aspect (and often, more than one) of the urinary process has gone awry. Many conditions can result in temporary incontinence, which goes away after treatment. These most commonly include infection or irritation of the urinary tract or vagina. Consuming alcohol can worsen temporary incontinence, as can certain medications. Some foods also may make the problem worse, as can, quite simply, fluid overload (drinking more than the body can handle at one time). For more foods and medications that can make incontinence worse, see "What You Can Do Now," below.

Chronic incontinence is a different problem, one that almost never goes away on its own. It happens when one or more of the body's mechanisms for holding back urine can no longer do its job. Chronic urinary incontinence can be caused by many factors, including:

- weakened muscles in the urethral sphincter
- weakened pelvic muscles (which support the bladder)
- weakened muscles in the bladder, or the opposite
- overactive muscles in the bladder
- restriction of the urethra (often caused by an enlarged prostate)
- neurologic disorders
- imbalance of hormones in women
- physical limitations (such as needing help to get to the bathroom)

Incontinence is a complicated problem, and it may manifest itself in one or more of several forms. These include:

STRESS INCONTINENCE

This form of incontinence is mechanical—muscles, valves, or the nerves that control them don't function properly, and as a result, urine leaks at the proverbial "drop of a hat." Pressure on the bladder, such as a cough, sneeze, or laugh, can be enough to trigger a spurt of urine. Almost any form of exercise—swinging a golf club, lifting a grandchild or a bag of groceries, or simply standing up after sitting for a while—can cause leakage. The key here is activity. Incontinence only happens when some movement puts pressure on the bladder.

In men, stress incontinence is almost always the result of damage to the internal sphincter, caused by treatment for prostate cancer or benign prostate enlargement. In women, several factors may be at work. When the pelvic floor muscles become weakened, damaged, or stretched (most often from childbirth), the pelvic floor starts to sag. The bladder, in turn, droops. This prolonged muscular slouch (and the extra pressure this puts on the bladder neck) can even shift the angle at which the bladder connects to the urethra, sometimes preventing the internal sphincter from forming its usual tight seal, and obliging the urethra to stay open (a condition called urethral hypermobility). Women, too, may suffer damage to the sphincter, urinary tract nerves (which control the muscles), or pelvic floor muscles from surgery (mainly hysterectomy). Significant weakening or damage to the sphincter muscles (called ISD, intrinsic sphincteric deficiency) also can cause the bladder neck and urethra to slacken. Although some women are born with ISD, it can be a complication of injury, surgery, or radiation. Another mechanical problem that can occur in postmenopausal women is caused by the loss of estrogen. The urethra thins, and the effect is like an inadequate washer on a faucet—a faulty seal, which can't close tightly enough to do the job.

URGE INCONTINENCE

The element of surprise is not a major part of urge incontinence, as it so often is with stress incontinence. People with urge incontinence know all too well that they need to go to the bathroom. The problem is that the interval between "early warning" and the time urine can no longer be controlled is often very short—at most, a matter of minutes. If stress incontinence is a structural problem, urge incontinence is more the result of bad wiring—inappropriate or missing communication between the bladder and the brain. Many doctors describe urge incontinence as an overactive, or "irritable" bladder (similar to irritable bowel; in fact, some of the same medications that are effective in treating irritable bowel can help calm irritable bladder). Nerves in the bladder signal the muscles to contract too often, many times more than necessary, and the bladder becomes, in effect, overenthusiastic. When the bladder sends the message to the brain that it's full, the response is immediate: an urgent need to urinate that overrides the brain's message of "Not now—wait until you get to the bathroom!" Instead, urination often begins on the way to the bathroom. Urge incontinence means using the bathroom very often—

more than every two hours while awake, and awakening more than once during sleep because of an urge to urinate. More than that, it means that your life starts to revolve around proximity to the toilet—not going to the movies, theater, church, or a sports event, for example, because it's too embarrassing to keep getting up to use the bathroom. Sometimes, the need to urinate can be triggered by suggestion—just hearing the sound of running water, for instance, or washing your hands, or by drinking a few sips of any beverage.

Many men with benign prostate enlargement suffer a series of events that leads to "detrusor instability." The bladder becomes overmuscled from years of distension, because of poor urine flow through the urethra, which in turn is being squashed by the growing prostate. But the nerves involved in urination can be damaged or hampered by many conditions and simply as a result of aging itself. Some of these include neurologic ailments, such as Parkinson's disease, multiple sclerosis, stroke, or spinal cord injury. Anxiety (a factor in irritable bowel as well), depression, and infection also may interfere with bladder-brain communication. It may be that coronary artery disease—which affects the blood vessels—somehow damages the small blood vessels that supply the tissue in the bladder. Diabetes, whose ravages can be felt throughout the body, also may play a role.

OVERFLOW INCONTINENCE

Here, the problem is in the bladder. For some reason—usually either a blockage that impedes the normal outflow of urine, or a weakness of the bladder muscle itself—the bladder cannot empty itself completely. It's always at least partly full, and the stress of continuous distension on the muscle eventually takes a toll on the internal sphincter, as well. Imagine the neck of a water balloon, overstretched and leaky.

FUNCTIONAL INCONTINENCE

This is often the most difficult type of incontinence to treat. Here, the machinery below the waist may work perfectly well, but for some reason—mental illness, including severe depression, neurologic illnesses such as Parkinson's disease, Alzheimer's disease, or other forms of dementia—the signal that says "It's time to go to the bathroom" either is not received or understood. Functional incontinence also affects people who are severely disabled, who have great difficulty reaching the bathroom on their own.

WHO IS AT RISK?

The biggest risk factor for urinary incontinence is age. Several things happen to the aging body that can make incontinence more likely. Among them is that the ability to postpone urination lessens, as does the holding capacity of the bladder. Older people are more susceptible to spontaneous bladder contractions, or an overactive bladder; also, mobilization of fluid trapped in the lower extremities when lying down makes night-time urination more common. As we age, the tone of the muscles in the pelvic floor, bladder, and urethral sphincter slackens.

In men over 50, the prostate often enlarges and tightens around the urethra, impeding urine's journey from the body, and sometimes making it impossible for the bladder to empty completely (so it's always at least partly full). Many men who have been treated with surgery or radiation for prostate cancer experience incontinence, as well.

But women are much more likely to develop urinary incontinence than men. In fact, women make up six out of every seven cases of incontinence in adults, mainly because of the burden of pregnancy, labor, and delivery on the muscles in the pelvic floor, uterus, and urethra. The odds of incontinence are higher for women who have had more children, but the damage can be sustained during the first pregnancy. Women who have their first baby later (over age 30) are at slightly higher risk of developing incontinence, as are women who have difficult, or "assisted" labors (with contraction-inducing drugs such as oxytocin [Pitocin], or with forceps, vacuums, or other potentially damaging devices).

Another risk factor is high-impact exercise, which seems to take a greater toll on the pelvic muscles and nerves in women than men; particularly those who perform gymnastics, or who play volleyball, softball, or basketball. Women athletes with a low or flat foot arch—which provides less of a "shock absorber" to the pelvic area during running and other exercise—are even more likely to develop incontinence.

Being overweight—and thus subjecting the pelvic muscles to greater long-term strain—is a risk factor. (People with the "apple" shape, with weight concentrated around the midsection, are at slightly higher risk than people with a "pear" shape, with the greater weight below the waist.) And smoking has been shown to raise the risk of incontinence, perhaps because of long-term damage to connective tissue (such as that which helps hold the bladder in place).

HOW IS IT DIAGNOSED?

Unfortunately, incontinence is seldom diagnosed if the patient doesn't speak up and ask the doctor for help. Many doctors—two thirds, by some estimates—don't even ask their patients if they're having trouble with involuntary leakage of urine, possibly because they don't realize how treatable incontinence is today. There is room for improvement on both sides, however. Fewer than half of the people who suffer from incontinence receive medical help, because they're too embarrassed or ashamed to ask for it.

Whenever incontinence begins to bother a person, disrupts their life, or diminishes their quality of life, it's time to see a doctor. Some people take years to reach this point; others seek help after only a few episodes. Doctors can learn a great deal from a detailed medical history and physical exam, so it's very helpful to keep a journal for at least 48 hours, noting the amount of fluid drunk each day, and writing down whenever urination occurs—planned or otherwise. Patients should come prepared to list any other medical conditions, previous surgical procedures (and their dates), and any pregnancies and deliveries.

PHYSICAL EXAMINATION

The doctor will examine the abdomen, vaginal or genital area, and rectum, looking for weakness in the pelvic floor, assessing muscle tone, feeling whether the bladder moves or shifts when the patient bears down on the doctor's gloved finger or a speculum, and checking the angle of the urethra to see if the bladder is lower than it should be. Because the bladder is, in effect, a "window" to the nervous system, if the doctor suspects that a neurologic disorder is involved, he may also look for abnormalities in the patient's movement and walking, for numbness or tingling, loss of balance, or double vision.

DIAGNOSTIC TESTS

Depending on the results of the history and physical, further diagnostic tests may be needed, several of which fall under the category of "urodynamic testing." Among other things, these tests can monitor the muscle pressure in the abdomen, rectum, pelvis, and bladder; and dissect complex problems—whether more than one form of incontinence is involved, for instance. They can determine whether the bladder is "distensible"—if it can relax and contract—or whether it's hyper-

WHAT YOUR DOCTOR MIGHT ASK

Doctors can learn a great deal from a detailed medical history and physical exam. Here are some questions the doctor might ask.

When did this problem begin? What prompts urine loss—any particular activity, such as a sneeze, or laughing?

How often have you been having this urine leakage?

About how many times a day do you urinate?

Do you ever have to get up at night to urinate? If so, how many times?

Do you experience a strong urge to urinate?

About how much urine do you estimate is lost each time?

About how much fluid do you drink each day? Do you drink caffeine or alcohol—and if so, how much?

When you urinate, does your bladder feel empty afterward, or do you have the urge to keep pushing?

Have you noticed anything unusual in the urine—blood, discharge, or any odor?

Would you describe your urinary stream as forceful, or halting? Do you have problems with the urinary stream starting and stopping? Is there dribbling?

Have you felt any pain or burning when you urinate?

Are you taking any medications, or nutritional supplements?

Do you wear pads to contain urine loss? If so, how many pads per day?

reactive (whether it reacts before it's time to urinate). Does the sphincter relax in response to urination, or does it contract? Does the bladder empty completely, as it should, or is there always urine left behind? These tests can pinpoint the problem and guide subsequent treatment; best of all, the results are usually immediate (unlike some imaging studies, which may take days for a specialist to interpret).

For many people, it takes courage simply to overcome modesty and embarrassment and ask for medical help. It's no exaggeration to say that for some patients, the thought of having to "perform," or "urinate on demand," is dreadful. This is a common reaction and patients should feel free to discuss their concern with their doctor, nurse practitioner, or incontinence nurse specialist. It may help to know that—although nobody would describe this process of diagnosis as fun—these tests offer the best chance of finding the right treatment. Many people are helped by talking to others who are struggling with incontinence. Some communities have urinary incontinence support group meets in your community, often sponsored by a hospital or clinic.

HOW IS IT TREATED?

Treatments for urinary incontinence range from the very simple (muscle-strengthening exercises) to the highly sophisticated (electrically stimulating muscles in the pelvis or lower back). Many forms of treatment are available—dozens of surgical procedures, devices, pads of every size (see "What You Can Do Now"), and an arsenal of medications. Which approach will be best for any given patient depends on the type and degree of incontinence, on the patient's physical abilities, and also on their motivation—whether they are committed to muscle-strengthening exercises, for example, or prefer a quicker surgical solution.

BEHAVIOR TECHNIQUES AND EXERCISES

Kegel exercises. Exercises to strengthen the muscles in the pelvic floor, also called Kegel exercises, are effective in helping people with mild to moderate stress incontinence. They can also help people with urge and mixed incontinence (but may need to be combined with other treatment if there is significant nerve damage). As many as 75% of people who try these exercises report a significant improvement in urinary control, even elderly people, who have lived with this problem for many years.

In doing Kegel exercises, the patient learns to identify, isolate, contract and relax the pelvic muscles—and ultimately, learn to use these muscles to their greatest potential, to prevent urinary incontinence. Patients can learn to achieve a tight "seal" by learning to tighten the pelvic floor muscles, which help to support the bladder and open and close the urethral sphincters. Most people have trouble finding these muscles and require biofeedback to help with muscle identification and isolation. Periodically interrupting (stopping) the urine stream while urinating may help patients identify the pelvic muscles involved. This technique is meant to help identify the pelvic muscles; it is not an exercise, and stopping the flow too often can lead to incomplete urination.

TESTS FOR URINARY INCONTINENCE

Urodynamics. This test measures the bladder's function—checking pressures, and measuring how much fluid it can retain—using a catheter (a narrow tube inserted into the urethra, and threaded into the bladder). The doctor or nurse injects a steady stream of sterile fluid into the bladder, until the patient feels the urge to urinate, until the bladder begins to contract, or until spontaneous urination occurs. In cases of urge incontinence, it probably won't take much fluid (less than 200 mL, approximately 7 ounces or 1 cup) to prompt a bladder reaction, or generate the need to urinate. A tiny tube may be inserted in the rectum to measure abdominal pressures, and sensors are placed in the perineal area, to detect pelvic floor muscle activity. X-rays may be taken, as well.

Tests for stress incontinence. These tests are performed on women with a full bladder (in fact, they may be performed after cystometry, while the bladder is still full). Patients lie are their back and are asked to give a strong cough. Women who have stress incontinence often experience leakage from this. Remember the tilted urethra associated with stress incontinence, discussed above? The test is repeated, but with the urethra tilted up at a more normal angle. If a patient has stress incontinence, they probably won't experience leakage this time. Sometimes patients are asked to cough a third time, from a standing position. Sometimes a cotton swab is inserted into the urethra to note its tilt during straining, indicating a descent of the bladder.

Urinary flow rate (uroflowmetry). As it's name implies, this test measures speed and flow of urine: how much urine is coming out, and how long it takes the patient to void, or urinate, a certain amount of fluid? Several hours (usually two to four) before taking this test, the patient is asked to drink four cups of fluid. Then, he or she will be asked to urinate into a funnel hooked up to a "flow meter." A narrow catheter may be inserted through the urethra and into the bladder, so that pressures there can also be measured. (This does not interfere with the patient's ability to urinate.) If the flow is lower than it should be, this could signal a problem with urinary obstruction (especially in men with

Biofeedback may help patients get the hang of the Kegel exercises. (Note: Many doctors use the terms "biofeedback" and "pelvic floor strengthening" interchangeably.) This approach involves a probe, inserted in the vagina or rectum, that quantifies the contractions, telling the patient how strongly their muscles are tight-

benign prostate enlargement), or it may indicate another problem, such as bladder stones or nerve damage within the bladder.

Cystoscopy. The cystoscope—like the endoscope, colonoscope, or other "scopes" used in medicine—offers an "inside view" that's much more detailed than an x-ray or ultrasound. It is a small, lighted tube with a miniature video camera, which is connected to a television screen. Threaded through the urethra, it reaches to the bladder, and allows the doctor to check for inflammation, structural problems, or tissue abnormalities. The bladder is filled with water to inspect the lining.

Measuring postvoid residual urine. Is the bladder emptying completely? This test measures what's left behind after urination. There should not be more than about an ounce of urine; the continuous presence of leftover urine can make infection more likely, may stimulate excessive bladder contractions, and may lead to overflow incontinence. The "postvoid residual" can be measured with a catheter, or through ultrasound.

Intravenous pyelogram (IVP). An IVP—much like a similar test, a barium enema—involves a special dye that appears on an x-ray, making the urinary tract visible. This allows doctors to trace urine's path from the kidneys out of the body, and highlights any blockages. Some people may be allergic to this day. If a person has ever had an allergic reaction to iodine, shellfish, or Betadine, the doctor or imaging technician should be alerted to this before any testing begins.

Electromyography (EMG). This test is like an electrocardiogram; it uses electrodes to monitor the electrical activity in muscles in the sphincter, bladder, and pelvic floor.

Urinalysis. A urine specimen is tested for blood infection, sugar, or proteins.

Urine cytology. Rarely, a urine specimen is sent to the lab to look for cancer cells.

Creatinine. A blood test that is sometimes used to determine the effectiveness of the kidney's filtration ability, if an obstructed bladder or abnormal x-ray image is found.

ening, and whether they're using the right muscles. Some hospitals rent out monitors, so patients can practice in the privacy of their home.

Vaginal cones and weights. For women, small cones or weights, in graduated sizes (ranging from less than an ounce to more than two ounces), are used to help strengthen the pelvic floor muscles. The weights are inserted in the vagina, and women must identify and use their pelvic muscles to hold the weights within the vagina. More than 70% of women (with stress and urge incontinence) who practice with these cones for several months are not only able to hold in the lightest one, but to "build up" their muscles and work up to the heaviest weight and thus significantly improve their urinary control.

MEDICATIONS

Numerous medications can help the bladder relax (so it can hold more), inhibit bladder contractions, and/or strengthen the internal sphincter. Although these drugs are often prescribed as a "medical fix" for all forms of incontinence, they are of greatest benefit in treating urge incontinence. Here are the basic medications used to treat urinary incontinence.

Anticholinergic drugs. Anticholinergic drugs are the major weapon in the arsenal against urge incontinence. They can have an antispasmodic effect; in other words, they can relax the bladder muscle and discourage bladder contractions and can also enable the bladder to hold more urine. Oxybutynin (Ditropan XL) and tolterodine (Detrol) are the current treatments of choice for overactive bladder. Other anticholinergic medications include hyoscyamine (Cystospaz, Levbid, Levsin) and propantheline (Pro-Banthine). These drugs are not without side effects, however. They can cause dryness of the mouth and eyes, constipation, and headache, and may increase the heart rate. Other common side effects can include blurred vision, drowsiness, decreased sweating and decreased heat dissipation (creating risk of heat stroke in the elderly), and confusion in the elderly. Rarely, they can exacerbate some cases of glaucoma, so doctors must prescribe their use with caution. Tolterodine, a newer drug, mainly targets the bladder, and may have fewer or milder complications than other drugs with more sweeping effects.

Estrogen replacement therapy. Postmenopausal women often experience both stress and urge incontinence. One result of menopause is a mechanical problem, a thinning of the cells lining the urethra that creates an inadequate seal (the "faulty washer" described earlier in this chapter). Another consequence of the loss of estrogen is that it can make the bladder more reactive and less stable. Replacing the hormones, preferably with topical vaginal estrogen cream, can thicken this lining and bulk up the seal, and can calm the bladder. Because estrogen replacement therapy has its own complications (a slight increase in the risk of stroke, heart attack, blood clot, and endometrial cancer), women should discuss this with their doctor before starting any course of treatment, particularly if they have a history of heart disease or breast cancer. Women being treated with estrogen must have annual mammograms and Pap tests.

Tricyclic antidepressants. Although depression itself is not a major cause of incontinence, the same chemical pathways involved in depression can be linked to urge incontinence. Antidepressant medications, which can relax the bladder and improve muscle tone in the internal sphincter, often help people with urge as well as stress incontinence. Some of these include imipramine (Tofranil) and amitriptyline (Elavil). Again, there are many side effects—including dryness of the mouth, drowsiness, constipation, blurred vision, heart arrhythmias, and a decrease in blood pressure.

SURGICAL PROCEDURES

The list of surgical procedures to treat incontinence is huge—nearly two hundred procedures, many named after the surgeons who refined them. The goals of surgery for stress incontinence are to return the bladder (and anything else in the pelvis that may have slipped lower than it's supposed to be) and angle of the urethra to normal. Many procedures involve open surgery, making an incision in the abdomen, and sewing the bladder neck and urethra into a more correct position, anchoring them to the pelvic bone or other nearby supports. In all of these procedures, there is a slight risk of overkill—obstructing the bladder, leading to residual urine, or restricting the bladder neck or urethra. As with any surgery, your best hope of success is to find the best surgeon, one who specializes in this procedure, and whose success rates are high.

Open surgery. In the Marshall-Marchetti-Krantz procedure, the bladder neck and urethra are sewn (sutured) to surrounding cartilage. The Burch procedure takes this a step further, fastening the bladder neck and urethra to muscle tissue adjacent to the pubic bones. (For years, many gynecologists have performed this procedure at the time of hysterectomy.) Both of these procedures have very good success rates (as high as 80%) and are a good choice if an abdominal procedure is already planned.

A variation of this procedure, done either through the vagina alone, or through the vagina and with a smaller abdominal incision, is called transvaginal needle suspension. Here, the surgeon stitches through the vaginal wall to tissue near the bladder neck and urethra, and then (switching positions and working through the abdominal incision) fastens these stitches to the walls of the abdomen or pelvis. Because the walls of the abdomen or pelvis must be tough enough to hold these stitches, this operation may not be as successful in an elderly woman. Most recently, laparoscopic procedures (done through a small tube, leaving a much smaller incision) have been attempted. Although there are no long-term results yet, early results suggest the laparoscopic procedure may not be as durable, and that the failure rate is high—from 65 to 83% after about five years.

The Sling procedure. In recent years, the Sling has become the procedure of choice for many surgeons treating stress incontinence, because it improves a weakened sphincter as well as a fallen bladder. Performed through the vagina and often requiring a superficial abdominal incision, it has even been shown to help some women with urge incontinence. In this procedure, the concept of "sling" is taken literally. Using tough connective tissue overlying the woman's abdominal or leg muscles, the surgeon creates a sling to replace a slack pelvic floor—a new, sturdy hammock to support the urethra and bladder neck. Then, the entire sling is sewn to the pelvic bone and abdominal wall.

There are variations on this procedure, too. One of them involves no sutures, but uses a gauze adhesive called "tension-free tape" to stick the bladder neck and urethra in their proper places. However, a risk here is that holes can be poked in the bladder as the surgeon blindly feels for the right places to attach the tape. Again, because it's new, there are no long-term results, but early studies suggest that the tape is not nearly as durable as the hammock created in the Sling procedure. Another new variation, which seems to be helpful for men with incontinence after a radical prostatectomy for prostate cancer, is the bulbourethral sling. This procedure seems less likely to be helpful in men who have radiation therapy for prostate cancer.

Artificial sphincter. An artificial sphincter, used only for severe incontinence, is somewhat more complicated than a real one—you have to open it when you want to urinate, by releasing a valve. This, in turn, deflates the rubbery, silicone ring that encircles the urethra. As with any biomechanical device, there are two main considerations. One is the risk of infection, which can harm the tissue of the nearby urethra or bladder neck, making the incontinence even worse. Infection also may necessitate removing the sphincter, which can't always be replaced. The other consideration is that the device itself may fail, although with new generations of sphincter design and refined surgical techniques, this is becoming less of a worry.

Collagen injections. Collagen, a natural protein found in muscles, bones, and connective tissue, is a "bulking" agent. It adds heft to flimsy tissue, and inserting it into the urethra (or the nearby skin) can tighten the urethra's seal, helping women with stress incontinence (but not those with vaginal prolapse, or poor pelvic muscle support), and men with mild incontinence after surgical treatment for prostate cancer. (Note: Collagen injections are not terribly helpful for men with severe incontinence after prostate surgery, nor for men who have been treated with radiation for prostate cancer.) As procedures go, this one is easy—less than half an hour in the doctor's office. Rarely, self-catheterization is needed for the first few days (to give the collagen time to settle). Some people see an immediate improvement in symptoms; for most people, however, it takes months for symptoms to improve noticeably. As with collagen injections elsewhere in the body (the lips for instance, in cosmetic surgery), there is a risk that the collagen inserts may shift, or that they may lead to infection. Also, the collagen becomes re-absorbed over time, and more than one treatment is often necessary (patients may need replacement collagen as often as every year). Newer materials now available for injection, such as carbon spheres (Durasphere) or silicone spheres, may be more durable than collagen.

Electrical stimulation. Electrical stimulation can be delivered to the nerves that regulate bladder function in a number of ways. Noninvasive ways to deliver electrical stimulation include patches placed on the skin (transcutaneous stimulation) or a probe placed in the vagina or rectum. When treating urinary incontinence, a vaginal or rectal probe that remains in place for ten to fifteen minutes a day is best. The type of electrical current is determined by the type of incontinence: low-frequency currents are best for urge or mixed incontinence and higher-frequency currents are best for stress incontinence. Patients themselves determine how much voltage is applied; they must apply enough current through the probe to feel the stimulation, but never enough voltage to cause pain. For women, transvaginal electrical stimulation has proved effective for treating urge or mixed incontinence, and it has shown mixed results in the treatment of stress incontinence.

A variation of this therapy is the use of a magnetic field to stimulate the pelvic floor muscles and treat stress, urge, or mixed urinary incontinence. One device involves sitting in an electromagnetic chair (Neotonus). However, this approach is still too new for long-term results to be known.

A surgical implant is used in some people who fail to respond to other treatments for urge incontinence. After an elaborate screening process, in which the sacral nerves that run in the lower back are identified and tested, electrodes are implanted to block or intercept messages from the bladder to the spine. The electrodes are powered by a small generator, implanted in the abdomen. In one study, nearly half of patients were completely dry at six months, and about 75% of patients with severe incontinence experienced significant improvement. The long-term results are not so promising, however; in some people, symptoms become worse, or the electrodes are so uncomfortable (at the site of the implants, and throughout the lower back) that they are removed. Also, some studies have shown significant side effects in people who receive the electrical muscle stimulation from implants, including diarrhea, abdominal cramps, infection, and bleeding.

Catheterization. The last resort for treating incontinence is catheterization. However, there are risks with most types of catheterization, including permanent, intermittent, and "condom" catheterization (in men). Permanent catheterization—an indwelling Foley catheter, which consists of a tube inserted through the urethra, or suprapubically, into the bladder to drain urine into an external bag strapped to the leg—is not a good long-term solution. For one thing, in women, the urethra dilates to accommodate the catheter, and eventually will no longer hold it. For another, the risks—of infection and scarring, of rebound pressure to the kidneys, of stones developing in the urinary tract—are simply too high. Most doctors believe that diapering is far better than long-term catheter use for people who are too mentally ill, or physically frail, for any other form of treatment. Although there are risks here, too, if meticulous care is not taken to keep the "diaper area" dry, these are nothing compared to the risks of catheterization.

Intermittent self-catheterization is a far safer approach (although there is still a significant risk of infection), but it requires a certain amount of hand-eye coordination, and must be done every three or four hours. In self-catheterization, the patient inserts a catheter—held in place by an inflated cuff—into the urethra, and drains the bladder into a rubber or strong plastic bag strapped or taped to the leg. The urine collected in the bag must then be emptied into the toilet.

For men with severe incontinence, condom catheters may be better still. These are pouches that slip over the penis and drain into a bag secured on the leg. However, if the bladder does not empty all the way, the risk of infection is significant. Also, there is always the risk that the condom attachment may not fit properly, or that it may leak inappropriately. Skin problems, due to the constant, irritating presence of urine, are also common.

WHAT RESEARCH IS BEING DONE?

Much of the research in this field is geared toward refining surgical procedures, designing better urinary-control devices, and developing medicines targeted toward the bladder and urethra, with few side effects for the rest of the body. Researchers are also working to make existing devices better—even replacing the artificial sphincter with a "real" one, made from a muscle in the thigh. The sphincter operates by electromagnetic energy—an electrode, implanted under the skin, supplies the power to keep the sphincter closed. When they feel an urge to urinate, patients open the sphincter with the help of a special magnet (placed over the skin), which temporarily blocks the electrode, and causes the sphincter to open.

Recently, scientists have also been investigating means of preventing urinary incontinence, and even finding genetic causes for the problem. The idea that something more than the ramifications of an aging body may be at work here is still fairly new. However, scientists have learned that there may be an inherited predisposition to urinary incontinence. For some women, there may also be a link to connective tissue disorders. Genetic linkage studies of large numbers of women and their families may help identify other preventable causes. One possibility is that women prone to urinary incontinence have abnormal collagen expression. Another is that women and men with urge incontinence have a neurochemical imbalance—changes in the nerves that control the internal organs (which may be linked to depression, anxiety disorders, obsessive-compulsive syndromes, irritable bowel, and mitral valve prolapse)—that result in overactive bladder.

WHAT YOU CAN DO NOW

Most of the treatments discussed here are not "instant fixes." It may be months before there is an improvement in urinary control. In the meantime, it is essential to keep the area around the urethra clean, and minimize the risk of infection and irritation. Ask your doctor for a list of "moisture barriers," products designed to keep the skin dry and protect it from the harshness of urine.

There are many other things you can do now that may help. Lifestyle modifications and readily available personal hygiene products can be helpful in reducing incontinence and some of embarrassments it causes.

PERSONAL HYGIENE PRODUCTS

Familiarize yourself with the ever-increasing variety of pads, shields, and other products now available. Look for products that draw moisture away from the skin, keeping the area around the urethra and the perineal area as dry as possible. Some pads are wafer-thin; some take the form of men's briefs. Also available for men are "drip collectors," absorbent pouches that fit around the penis or scrotum. For women with stress incontinence, pads, patches, or shields are available that fit over the opening of the urethra, expanding to create a seal. These tiny pads simply stop urine from coming out. They are not effective in stopping urge incontinence, may shift with exercise, and can't be worn all the time—just a few hours a day. They are not a good option in women who are prone to urinary tract infections. Some women with mild stress incontinence are helped by wearing tampons for a few hours a day. (Postmenopausal women may want to coat the tampons with a lubricant such as Astroglide to avoid discomfort from vaginal dryness.) The tampons compress the urethra, and help it stay closed. Vaginal pessaries—silicone cubes or rings, fitted by a doctor—have a similar effect. They are inserted in the bladder and support the urethra and bladder neck. They must be kept clean, to minimize the risk of infection.

LIFESTYLE MODIFICATIONS

If you never go to bed without a nightly glass of water on the bedside table, change this habit today. Don't drink anything for at least two hours before you go to bed. And pay attention to your dietary fiber: Constipation can add to the pressure in the bladder and pelvis. If you keep your bowel movements regular (and avoid straining), this may help control incontinence, too.

FOOD, DRINKS, AND MEDICATIONS TO AVOID

Some foods and beverages may stimulate the bladder, or make incontinence worse.

- Caffeinated coffee
- Caffeinated tea
- Carbonated drinks
- Alcoholic beverages
- Chocolate (which contains a caffeine-like ingredient)
- Orange juice, grapefruit juice, or any citrus products
- Tomatoes (which, like citrus fruits, are highly acidic and can irritate the urinary tract)
- Spicy foods
- Sweeteners, natural (sugar, corn syrup, honey) and artificial (aspartame or saccharine)

Certain medications also can irritate the bladder and produce more urine or relax the urethra, contributing to incontinence. These include:

- Diuretics (which should be taken early in the day, definitely not after late afternoon)
- Alpha-adrenergic blockers (which can relax the urethra and trigger stress incontinence)

Less common contributors to incontinence include:

- Antidepressants and antipsychotic drugs
- Sedatives and muscle relaxants
- Narcotics
- Antihistamines and decongestants

Certain lifestyle changes that may help, in addition to the pelvic floor exercises described above. One simple tip is to go to the bathroom regularly, even if there is no immediate urge to urinate. Many people—schoolteachers, nurses, mothers of young children, and others with stressful, busy jobs—go for hours without urinating. This is not good for the bladder; in fact, long-term bladder distension may result in damage to the nerves and muscles that make the bladder contract properly. Doctors may recommend that patients go on a "voiding schedule," giving then regular times at which they are supposed to urinate. They will likely be asked to reduce the amount of liquid they drink every day.

But not all lifestyle changes have to be drastic. Some are quite simple. For people with stress incontinence, one solution is so obvious that many people who try it can't believe they haven't thought of it before: When a woman knows she is about to sneeze, cough, or laugh—or do anything that causes urine to leak—she can cross her legs, and keep them crossed until the urine-prompting activity is over. In one study, nearly two thirds of women were able to prevent almost all episodes of incontinence just by crossing their legs ahead of time.

For patients who are prone to urinary tract infections, some experts believe they can be prevented by drinking cranberry juice every day. To reduce the risk of urinary tract infections, some doctors recommend drinking two 8-ounce glasses of 100% cranberry juice per day ("Cranapple" or similar cranberry-and-fruit blends do not count) or taking cranberry essence capsules, available from a health food store. Finally, several other measures are useful to prevent urinary tract infections:

- Urinate after sexual intercourse.
- Avoid long periods of not emptying the bladder. For example, during long car trips or plane rides, stop and/or get up to void.
- For some, a low dose of suppressive urinary tract antibiotic daily is helpful. Consult your health care provider.

ADDITIONAL RESOURCES

The American Foundation for Urologic Disease

1128 North Charles St.

Baltimore, MD 21201

800-242-2383 or 410- 468-1800

www.afud.org

The American Urological Association

www.auanet.org

National Association for Continence (NAFC)

800-BLADDER

www.nafc.org

National Kidney and Urologic Diseases Information Clearinghouse

3 Information Way

Bethesda, MD 20892-3580

800-891-5388

www.niddk.nih.gov

Vision Disorders in Older Adults

By age 65, one of every three Americans will suffer from a vision-reducing eye disease. While many of these conditions are controllable or even correctable, the scope of the problem remains staggering. The nation spends more than $22 billion per year for health care and services for the blind and vision impaired. Vision loss can be among the most debilitating of all diseases, as it robs the elderly of independence and places tremendous burdens on family members and other caregivers. People with vision disorders are at much greater risk for falls and other accidents as well.

Close monitoring remains the best weapon against vision loss. Many disorders, including glaucoma and diabetic retinopathy, can be detected and controlled before they cause significant vision loss. Others, such as cataracts, may be corrected with surgical procedures. Regular vision screenings and monitoring of risk factors can save vision, or at least keep vision loss to a minimum.

WHAT IS IT?

Some vision changes are inevitable. The most common age-related eye change is called presbyopia. This occurs when the eye's lens, which focuses light on the back of the eye, becomes inflexible. Nearly everyone suffers from presbyopia, usually starting in a person's early to mid-40s. Most people notice difficulty focusing on objects at close range, especially when reading. Headaches and eye fatigue are also common. Regular eye exams can detect presbyopia, and reading glasses or contact lenses are usually enough to correct the vision changes. Presbyopia is not considered a disease, but rather a natural part of the aging process.

More serious vision disorders include:

- Age-related macular degeneration
- Glaucoma
- Cataract
- Diabetic retinopathy
- Other eye diseases
- Low vision

AGE-RELATED MACULAR DEGENERATION

Age-related macular degeneration(AMD) is the most common cause of vision loss in people over age 65. It is marked by damage to the retina—thin, flat nerve tissue in the back of the eye that converts light into electrical signals, which are interpreted by the brain as vision. The center of the retina, called the macula, is important for fine visual discrimination; this is the vision people use to read, drive a car, recognize faces, and thread a needle. Without this central vision, people are left only with peripheral vision, the ability to see poorly focused objects to the sides of the person's line of sight.

There are two main types of AMD. The nonexudative, or "dry," form of the disease accounts for about 90% of all cases. Dry AMD is characterized by the buildup of abnormal, yellow-white material, called drusen, in the retina. Drusen can cause mild distortion of central vision, or may lead to no noticeable symptoms. In some dry AMD cases, a more serious problem called geographic atrophy may develop. This happens when the cells responsible for central vision start to die off in patches. In time, these patches may coalesce into larger areas, which can cause more serious loss of vision. Why this happens is incompletely understood. People with geographic atrophy usually have blurred vision. Some parts of the visual scene may be absent. They usually need more light and higher magnification to complete fine visual tasks. This condition generally affects both eyes but may be asymmetric.

The remaining 10% of people with AMD suffer from the "wet," or exudative, version of the disease. Although less common, it is usually far more serious: 80 to

90% of all severe vision loss due to AMD occurs in the wet variety. Exudative AMD is marked by the growth of abnormal blood vessels beneath the retinal tissue. These blood vessels leak fluid, which can damage nerve cells in the retina. The damage is especially serious when it happens near the fovea, the center of the macula.

Experts do not know what causes AMD. Symptoms can be quite subtle. The problems usually start with distortion. A patient may notice that a straight fence may appear somewhat wavy or that picture frames appear to be somewhat irregular at the edges. As the disease progresses and the extent of damage to the nerve cells increases, new blind spots develop. This is sometimes perceived as missing letters in a word when trying to read. If the disease is more advanced, the blind spot may be so large that it is impossible to read or recognize faces. The process is completely painless. In some cases, when damage is occurring in only one eye, it may go unnoticed until the other eye is inadvertently covered and the visual loss detected.

GLAUCOMA

Untreated glaucoma is the world's second-leading cause of vision loss. While that ranking is somewhat lower in the United States, as many as 120,000 living Americans have completely lost their sight because of complications from this group of diseases. Another one million people over the age of 65 have lost part of their sight because of glaucoma.

Glaucoma damages the optic nerve, the link between the eye and the brain. In most cases, unusually high pressure in the fluid that flows through and nourishes the inside of the eye causes the damage. The most common type of glaucoma, open-angle glaucoma, occurs when the eye's natural fluid drain, called the angle, fails to operate properly. Fluid does not drain quickly enough through the angle, causing an increase in pressure. Over time, this can destroy the optic nerve. Open-angle glaucoma causes 10% of all new cases of vision loss in this country each year.

Vision loss from open-angle glaucoma is painless and insidious. Generally, the peripheral vision deteriorates first; this is often not noticed by the person suffering from glaucoma in its early stages. As the disease progresses, tunnel vision develops. In some cases, even this is undetected. Eventually the center of vision is affected and the person will notice blurring. This generally represents an advanced stage of the disease. Unfortunately, damage to the optic nerve by glaucoma is not reversible, although it is usually possible to slow or stop the progression of the visual loss by lowering the eye pressure.

Other types of glaucoma develop faster. Acute-angle closure glaucoma is a medical emergency. The eye's drainage system is closed off by the iris because of an anatomic abnormality. Acute-angle closure glaucoma is sudden in onset, quite painful, often associated with nausea, vomiting, and an immediate drop in vision. Urgent evaluation and treatment are necessary to preserve vision. Some medications such as anticholinergics are contraindicated in persons with untreated narrow-angle glaucoma because they may precipitate closure of the angle.

A less common form of glaucoma, neovascular glaucoma, is sometimes seen in persons who have severe diabetes or a blood clot in the fine vessels of the eye, such as a retinal vein occlusion. This disease presents similarly to acute-angle closure glaucoma and involves very high pressures in the eye, associated with pain, often nausea and vomiting, and generally severe visual loss. It is difficult to treat, typically requiring a combination of extensive laser treatment and surgery. In many cases, vision is severely, irreversibly lost.

CATARACT

Cataract formation is the leading cause of blindness worldwide. As with glaucoma, the condition causes less blindness in the United States, because replacement surgery is more readily available. The prevalence of the disease increases greatly with age. While about 5% of all Americans have cataracts in one or both eyes before age 65, about 50% will develop them by age 75.

Cataract refers to loss of clarity of the eye's lens. The lens is located toward the front of the eye, and focuses light on the retina. To produce a sharp image, the lens must remain clear. But sometimes the lens becomes obscured or unable to flex enough to do its job properly. This usually happens when natural proteins in the lens clump together and interfere with the passage of light.

There are several types of cataracts. Nuclear sclerosis, or hardening and darkening of the lens, can initially improve near vision but ultimately results in loss of sight. The posterior subcapsular cataract is a plaque-like change on the back surface of the lens that more often produces glare from bright lights, but eventually progresses to visual loss as well. This type of cataract is more often seen in younger persons, diabetics, and in persons using steroids such as prednisone. Cortical cataracts are whitish, spoke-like changes that begin in the periphery of the lens and very slowly, over years, migrate toward the center. They cause no symptoms early on, but eventually result in glare and loss of vision, similar to posterior subcapsular cataracts.

Cataracts are painless. The most common symptoms include cloudy or blurred vision, glare from lamps or bright sunlight, poor night vision, double vision, and frequent changes of eyeglass prescriptions.

DIABETIC RETINOPATHY

This disease is marked by damage to the eye's blood vessels. A result of diabetes mellitus, it is the leading cause of new blindness in middle-aged Americans, and a significant cause of vision loss in older Americans as well.

There are two types of diabetic retinopathy. The first is called nonproliferative and is caused by damage to the fine blood vessels in the eye, which can sometimes cause swelling and interfere with normal eyesight. This happens most frequently in the macula, the part of the retina responsible for central vision. The disease can advance to the more serious proliferative stage. At this point, the retina does not receive adequate oxygen and produces factors to promote the growth of new blood vessels. These new blood vessels, however, are abnormal. Instead of growing within the retina tissue they grow on its surface. Traction on these vessels from the vitreous humor can produce severe hemorrhages or retinal detachments and irreversible visual loss.

LOW VISION

Low vision is a catchall category that includes any visual impairment that interferes with daily activities and is not correctable by glasses, surgery, or medication. This can include vision loss from all sources, including glaucoma, diabetic retinopathy, and AMD. In fact, AMD accounts for about 45% of all cases of low vision. About 14 million Americans—one in every 20—suffers from low vision.

OTHER EYE DISEASES

A great number of other conditions can affect vision. Chief among these are complications from vascular disorders like high blood pressure and atherosclerosis.

Blood clots in the eye's arteries and veins can lead to temporary or permanent loss of vision, depending on how long the clots block blood flow to or from the eye.

Retinal detachment is an uncommon (1 in 10,000), but sometimes serious disorder. This occurs when small tears in retinal tissue allow fluid under the retina and separate it from the back of the eye. These tears often follow derangement of the vitreous humor. Retinal detachments also sometimes happen after cataract surgery.

WHO IS AT RISK?

Age is the single biggest risk factor for vision disorders. Nearly every eye disease is more prevalent among those over the age of 65.

Other risk factors include:

For AMD. Family history, high blood pressure, and smoking. Caucasians are at higher risk.

For glaucoma. Family history, high blood pressure, diabetes, and African-American race.

For cataract. Excessive lifetime exposure to ultraviolet light is a possible risk factor as are steroid use and prior intraocular surgery.

For diabetic retinopathy. Diabetes. The risk of retinopathy increases with the length of time a person has diabetes and with poor control of blood sugar and blood pressure.

For low vision. All risk factors for the above diseases. African Americans and Hispanics over the age of 45 are at increased risk because they are more likely to suffer from high blood pressure and diabetes.

HOW IS IT DIAGNOSED?

Eye specialists search for vision problems with a series of tests that check the eye's structural integrity and function. Most of these can be performed by either an ophthalmologist or an optometrist. An ophthalmologist is a doctor of medicine (M.D.) who can perform surgery, prescribe medication, and perform all eye-related tests and procedures. An optometrist is a doctor of optometry (O.D.), who specializes in determining the need for glasses and other vision devices and can screen patients for abnormalities of the eye. Optometrists can prescribe a limited number of medicines.

Eye tests will vary according to the suspected cause of vision problems, but a few basic tests are common to most examinations.

Visual acuity test. The first exam is called the visual acuity test. This involves asking the patient to identify a series of letters or numbers while either standing or seated. The test helps determine how well the person sees at various distances. The results are read as a series of two numbers; 20/20 means that the patient can identify letters from 20 feet away that a person with normal vision can see at the same distance. Vision that is 20/40 means the patient can identify objects at 20 feet that someone with normal vision can discern at 40 feet.

Tonometry. The second procedure is known as tonometry. The main purpose of this exam is to measure the pressure in each eyeball, to test for the presence or progression of glaucoma. While seated, the patient rests his chin in front of a tonometer, which then moves slowly closer to the eyeball. The pressure test can be taken in a number of ways; the most common methods include blowing a small puff of air against the eye to check for resistance or using a blue light and a prism that presses against the eye to measure its pressure. The pressure of the fluid is measured in millimeters of mercury (mm Hg), just like the atmospheric pressure. The normal range for eye pressure is 12 to 21 mm Hg, although glaucoma sometimes may be present even within this band, and a higher pressure than 21 does not necessarily indicate glaucoma.

Pupil response. Doctors also can use a small, hand-held flashlight to test how pupils respond to light changes. The pupils usually constrict when light is bright and expand when less light is available. This controls the amount of light that enters the eye and helps the eye process visual stimuli most effectively. Problems with pupil reaction may indicate damage to the optic nerve or extensive retinal disease. The doctor can move the flashlight and ask the patient to follow its track. This helps the doctor check for the coordination of eye movements.

In addition to the basic eye examination, the doctor can choose from a number of specialized tests to help pinpoint vision problems. One measures the patient's visual field, also known as the peripheral vision. Again, this can be done in several ways. At its simplest, the test involves counting the number of fingers a doctor holds up to the side of the person's head. A computer-assisted device can flash small points of light on an evenly lit background, to test for defects in a person's visual field. This is a common way to monitor the visual status of a person with glaucoma.

Doctors may ask a person to look at an Amsler grid, a piece of paper with a checkerboard pattern and a central dot. While the patient focuses on the dot, he also looks at the lines surrounding it to see if they look straight, crooked or fuzzy. This test can help the doctor identify early cases of macular degeneration, and also measures changes in the visual field of a person who already has the disease. If the doctor suspects "wet" macular degeneration, he also may order a fluorescein angiogram. This test involves injecting a small amount of dye into a vein and tracking the dye as it flows through the blood vessels in the eye. Angiography also is useful in checking for vascular disorders of the eye, such as diabetic retinopathy.

Ophthalmoscopy checks for damage to the retina. The doctor uses a bright, head-mounted light and special magnifying devices to peer into the retina for signs of damage—including leaking blood vessels, swelling or other signs of damage.

Ophthalmologists use other specialized tests as well. If a person is a candidate for cataract surgery, doctors can check how much improvement the procedure may provide with a potential acuity test. This involves projecting a small eye chart onto the retina with a device called a potential acuity meter. The patient is asked to read it, and the results can determine how much the surgery could enhance the person's sight.

Ultrasound tests can help doctors check the structure of an eye when other devices are unable to give a clear picture. This typically happens when blood or scar tissue is present in the eye. In some cases, the eye doctor may order computer-assisted tomography (CAT) scans or magnetic resonance imaging (MRI) tests to check the status of structures behind the eye and in the brain. These help spot tumors that could affect vision, and also can detect the telltale signs of strokes, which sometimes affect the vision.

HOW IS IT TREATED?

MACULAR DEGENERATION

No treatment is available for the nonexudative, or dry, form of the disease. Exudative, or wet, AMD can be treated surgically in some cases. When abnormal blood vessels grow near but not under the center of the retina, laser treatment is usually recommended. The laser destroys the vessels and the overlying retina tissue and helps prevent the disease from progressing, preserving the central vision. When the blood vessels are directly under the center of the retina then standard laser treatment is usually not recommended, as the laser will often do as much damage as the disease.

In these cases a procedure called photodynamic therapy might be recommended. A photosensitizing dye, called verteporfin (Visudyne), is administered intravenously. It accumulates in some types of abnormal blood vessels and can be activated by a very low power laser that does not damage nerve tissue. Once activated, the dye damages these vessels and leads to their closure. In many cases, several treatments are necessary over a course of a year to a year and a half to stabilize the disease. The dye increases sensitivity to light and after receiving it, one must avoid exposure of the skin and eyes to direct sunlight or bright indoor light for a few days.

Operating on the eye to either move the retina or remove abnormal blood vessels involves very delicate microsurgery. It is performed by experienced vitreoretinal surgeons in a clinic or hospital, usually on an outpatient basis. In most cases the patients are taken to the operating room, sedation is administered, and anesthetic injected behind the eyeball. The surgery takes between one and one and half hours and the eye is patched at the end of the case for a day.

GLAUCOMA

In the United States, eyedrops are the most common initial approach to reducing pressure in the eyes. It is worth discussing the types of drops available for the treatment of glaucoma in some detail. One of the oldest medications is Pilocarpine, a parasympathetic drug that constricts the pupil and mechanically opens up the drainage system of the eye to lower the pressure. However, some patients on Pilocarpine develop brow ache and a dimming of the vision as well as increased nearsightedness from side effects of the drug. In addition, chronic use of the drug makes it difficult to dilate the pupil, making it harder to evaluate the optic nerve. Pilocarpine is dosed four times a day. With newer drugs on the market, Pilocarpine has become somewhat less popular.

Beta-blockers are another class of extensively used drugs. The most common of these include timolol (Timoptic) and betaxolol (Betoptic) although a variety of other similar drugs also are in common use. These drops decrease the production of fluid by the eye, lowering the pressure. Beta-blockers are usually well tolerated. Because eyedrops are absorbed into the blood circulation, they can, however, occasionally result in fatigue, a slowed heart rate and sexual dysfunction, and could worsen pre-existing asthma or emphysema. Patients with heart failure, slow heart rates, asthma, or emphysema usually are given these drugs only with caution and close monitoring, or other classes of eyedrops are used. While beta-blockers have a variety of side effects as noted, they are very effective in lowering the eye pressure and decreasing the progression of optic nerve damage in many cases of glaucoma. They are given once or twice a day.

A newer class of drugs, the alpha-adrenergic agonists, such as apraclonidine (Iopidine) and brimonidine (Alphagan), also decrease the production of fluid by the eye, and some of these drugs increase fluid outflow. They have fewer systemic side effects and can be used in patients with pre-existing asthma and heart disease. However, some patients develop an allergy to the topical drops that results in a red, itchy eye and must stop the medication. Some patients experience drowsiness and decreased mental alertness. These drugs are given two or three times a day.

Another class of drugs, the carbonic anhydrase inhibitors, is also effective for lowering the eye pressure. One of these drugs, acetazolamide (Diamox), has been available for many years as a pill. It was initially developed as blood pressure medicine but was found to have greater effect on the eye pressure. The pill, however, has some systemic side effects, including fatigue, diuresis and potassium wasting, and giving a metallic taste to foods. A topical form of this medication, known as dorzolamide (Trusopt), is now available. It does not appear to have the associated systemic side effects. However, carbonic anhydrase inhibitors are sulfa drugs, and must be used cautiously in patients allergic to sulfa. Dosing is two to three times a day for the drop. A new class of drugs, prostaglandins, has recently become available for the treatment of glaucoma. These drugs work by increasing the rate of fluid outflow through the eye through pathways not involving the typical drainage system. The most commonly used prostaglandin is latanoprost (Xalatan). It is convenient to use, since the dosing is once a day. It does not appear to have substantial systemic side effects but can make hazel eyes browner and increase the length of lashes. Some doctors feel that it can exacerbate pre-existing swelling in the retina (known as macular edema), but this continues to be debated.

In many patients, it is necessary to use a combination of these drugs to achieve an adequate reduction in eye pressure. Common combinations involve a beta-blocker and a carbonic anhydrase inhibitor. This is available as a single twice-a-day drop (Cosopt). Another relatively common combination is a beta-blocker and a prostaglandin. It should be borne in mind that elderly patients sometimes have difficulty applying the drops, whether because of limited dexterity, poor vision, or arthritis. These issues should be discussed with the patient and the patient's caregivers before instituting any type of therapy. In some cases laser treatment or surgery might be preferable if it is not possible for the patient to use the eyedrops.

Placing the drops in the eye is relatively easy. First, wash your hands thoroughly. Tilt the head back or lie down and gaze upward. The lower lid is pulled down, exposing the conjunctival sac. A drop can be placed into this sac and the eye closed for a few minutes. Avoid contact of the dropper with the eye, finger, or any surface. Do not rinse the dropper after use. Patients should allow at least five minutes to elapse before applying a second drop of a different medication. This prevents the second medication from washing out the first. Closing the eye for a few minutes or holding the finger over the inner corner of the eye to block the tear duct allows the medication to stay on the eye a bit longer and probably increases its effectiveness.

When medication is not sufficient to control glaucoma, surgery is in order. The most common type of surgery is called trabeculectomy. This procedure involves creating a new drainage hole for the eye. Another procedure, called laser trabeculoplasty, involves using a laser to stretch the drainage meshwork in the eye by creating fifty to one hundred evenly spaced burns on the eye in the angle. This allows fluid to drain more easily. The procedure is done on an outpatient basis, is painless and takes about fifteen minutes to complete.

CATARACT

In its early stage, a cataract does not require treatment. Eyeglasses or other vision aids can help overcome the mild loss of vision and glare problems that accompany the disease. But when the cataract begins to affect everyday tasks—such as driving, reading, or watching television—surgery may be required. This involves removing the clouded natural lens and replacing it with an artificial lens. Cataract removal is the most common procedure covered by Medicare. More than one million procedures are performed each year in the United States.

Modern cataract surgery is done on an outpatient basis. The surgery itself typically takes less than one hour. Removing a cataract involves some type of sedation, followed by an anesthetic given by local injection or topically (eyedrops). A small incision is made either in the cornea or the front of the sclera and a very fine blade is used to enter the anterior chamber of the eye. The lens resides in a thin capsule, commonly referred to as "the bag." A hole is made in the front of this bag and the lens is either removed as one piece or broken into smaller pieces with an ultrasonic device known as a phacoemulsifier.

Replacement lenses are made of either Lucite, acrylic, or silicone. Acrylic and silicone lenses are soft. They can be folded and introduced through very small incisions. Lucite lenses require a larger incision as they are not flexible, but are preferred in some cases. The lens selected for replacing the cataract can correct the vision for either long or near distance, but not both, so it is often necessary to have reading glasses or distance glasses after cataract surgery. There are a few lenses available that simulate bifocals in an effort to eliminate the need for glasses after surgery. However, some surgeons find that patients with these lenses complain of glare. It is worth discussing postoperative visual correction with the doctor before surgery.

After completing the operation, the surgeon closes the incision with one or a few very fine sutures, although some incisions seal without suturing. A patch is typically applied to the eye for a day. Postoperative care involves the use of steroid and antibiotic drops, sometimes used in conjunction with a topical nonsteroidal anti-inflammatory medication for a few weeks.

DIABETIC RETINOPATHY

Leaking blood vessels are sometimes treated by laser surgery, which can help reduce the amount of fluid buildup in the retina. When abnormal blood vessels are actively growing in the eye, heavy laser treatment to the peripheral retina is often necessary. Studies have demonstrated that this can reduce the chance of blindness from diabetes by one half.

Laser treatment for diabetes is similar to that described for glaucoma. The surgeon starts by placing a drop of topical anesthetic in the eye, followed by a contact lens, which helps to focus the laser in the appropriate place. Laser treatments take between five and twenty minutes to apply. The procedure is generally pain-less, although heavy laser applications sometimes sting a bit.

For more advanced cases, vitrectomy surgery may be necessary to remove the vitreous humor from the eye, treat the abnormal blood vessels and scar tissue, and repair any retinal detachment. In many cases, laser treatment is added at the time of surgery. In addition to these ophthalmic procedures, it is critically important that the blood pressure and blood sugar be controlled to help reduce the chance of progression of the disease.

Vitrectomy surgery is usually performed with local anesthesia and sedation. Par-ticularly long operations may require general anesthesia. A typical vitrectomy involves making three small holes into the white part of the eye to allow the passage of a variety of instruments used to remove the vitreous humor and abnormal blood vessels as well as apply laser treatment. As with glaucoma surgery, vitrectomy surgery can make a pre-existing cataract worse and sometimes it is necessary to remove the lens as well with these operations. In some cases, a plastic or acrylic lens is not inserted in the eye but rather saved for a second operation, once the eye heals.

WHAT SHOULD YOU EXPECT?

Surgical techniques and drugs have greatly reduced vision loss in all types of eye disease. About 90% of people who have surgery for cataract removal have better vision afterward. Complications occur only in about 1% of cases. These include the development of glaucoma, bleeding, infection and retinal detachment. In addi-tion, the formation of an after-cataract may develop in a part of the natural lens that is not removed. This must be removed later with outpatient laser surgery.

Glaucoma is not curable, but a combination of drugs and possibly surgery is often successful in reducing eye pressure and keeping the disease in check. Laser surgery on the angle is sometimes effective, but may need to be repeated within five years in about one-half of all patients. Conventional trabeculectomy surgery is about 80 to 90% effective, but also may require a second procedure. In some cases, the surgery will prevent blindness but may result in somewhat worse vision than existed before surgery.

Laser surgery can reduce the risk of severe vision loss by more than 50% in patients with diabetic retinopathy. Successful management of blood sugar and other problems associated with diabetes also helps. Unfortunately, the prognosis for age-related macular degeneration is not always so good. Many people with the less severe dry form of the disease will never suffer severe vision loss. But people with wet AMD do not always fare as well. Laser surgery often is effective, but only a minority of patients are good candidates for the procedure. And despite treatment for wet macular degeneration, there is still a substantial rate of recurrence of the abnormal blood vessels—approximately 50% in the first few years. It's important to reassure people with the condition that AMD does not cause total blindness. People with the disease almost always maintain a degree of peripheral vision.

HOW IS IT PREVENTED?

Researchers believe that, barring disease, eyes should function perfectly well for as long as one hundred and twenty years. The key to keeping eyes in good shape is getting regular, comprehensive eye examinations every one to two years. Eye doctors may want to check a patient's eyes more often if he or she already shows signs of eye disease, or if a risk factor is present for a particular disease.

Glaucoma screenings that include a dilated eye exam should begin by age 40. People who have glaucoma, or are at risk for the disease, should have formal field vision tests periodically. These will provide a benchmark against which to measure progression of the disease. People with diabetes, who are at higher risk for cataracts, glaucoma and diabetic retinopathy, can lower their risk of developing eye troubles by keeping their blood sugar levels and blood pressure under control. This can be done with diet, oral medications, or insulin, depending on the nature and severity of the underlying diabetes.

There's some discussion that a diet high in certain micronutrients might help ward off eye diseases—particularly AMD. Several small-scale studies have found a possible benefit from eating foods rich in carotenoids. These are nutrients that the body converts to vitamin A. It's too early to say for certain whether the link is real; large studies are now under way to help answer this question.

WHAT RESEARCH IS BEING DONE?

Experts are working to refine current treatments for all eye diseases, and to find new methods to reduce the occurrence of vision loss. Clinical trials are now underway for a new procedure designed to reduce the accumulation of abnormal material in the retina in cases of dry macular degeneration. For wet AMD, one possible new treatment, called macular translocation, involves moving the fovea, or center part of the macula, away from abnormal blood vessels before beginning regular laser surgery. Another involves surgically removing the abnormal blood vessels.

Several large trials are now underway to find what benefit, if any, a diet high in carotenoids and antioxidant vitamins A, C, and E, may have on improving vision and preventing eye disease. And researchers have recently discovered a gene responsible for causing a type of early-onset glaucoma—the first proven genetic link with the disease. Experiments on neuroprotection, that is, finding drugs that might protect the optic nerve from damage, are also underway. Long-term research is even exploring replacement parts for the eye, including artificial retinas that may help people whose natural retinas have been destroyed by disease. A series of microchips placed on a damaged retina already have shown promise in restoring rudimentary sight in selected candidates, although true artificial vision could still be a decade or more away.

WHAT YOU CAN DO NOW

When vision cannot be completely restored with medical or surgical intervention, caregivers must help the patient make the most of his or her remaining eyesight. It's vital for people to maintain as much independence as possible. Many low-vision aids can help. These are particularly helpful in persons who have lost their central vision, such as persons with macular degeneration. In some cases, simply adjusting the lighting, by using high-powered halogen lights can help a person to read. Large print books can be helpful, as can a variety of hand held magnifiers, some of which have their own light source. Magnifiers with built in stands can be particularly helpful to persons with arthritis or Parkinson's disease, or others who have difficulty holding a lens.

More sophisticated devices include telescopic lenses that can be built into glasses for seeing objects in the distance, or loupes that magnify text to read. Electronic devices such as closed-circuit televisions, computer scanners, and head-mounted cameras can magnify images and adjust the contrast to allow for improved visual function. While these devices are rather expensive, they can sometimes dramatically improve the quality of life for patients with limited vision.

Caregivers also should pay attention to practical matters, such as shopping, cooking, and moving around the house. When possible, avoiding open gas flames on stoves can be very helpful to elderly patients with limited vision. Labeling pots and pans with brightly colored tape can help these patients distinguish between various pieces of kitchenware. Talking alarm clocks and telephones with extra-large lighted buttons can also help with the general activities of daily living.

Because people with impaired vision are at increased risk for falls, take time to identify and address problem areas. Bright tape or paint lines on the edge of stairs, thresholds, and other uneven surfaces can alert the person to danger. Keeping furniture in predictable, permanent places also can help.

In many cities, special bus services are available for visually handicapped patients to help them get around town without driving. Finally, most major eye institutes have specialized optometrists, known as low vision specialists, who can help optimize the care of these patients.

Eye care coverage often is limited in health insurance packages. But financial assistance may be available for people who cannot afford treatments or low vision aids. See Additional Resources (next page) for a list of resources.

Finally, caregivers should be wary of some advertised "cures" for macular degeneration and other eye diseases. If there is a question regarding the efficacy or safety of a treatment, it is generally best to check with an eye care professional.

ADDITIONAL RESOURCES

ORGANIZATIONS AND WEB SITES

Foundation for Fighting Blindness

www.blindness.org

Macular Degeneration Foundation

www.eyesight.org

National Eye Institute

www.nei.nih.gov

Glaucoma Foundation

www.glaucoma-foundation.org

American Academy of Ophthalmology

www.eyenet.org

Wilmer Eye Institute

/www.wilmer.jhu.edu

FINANCIAL AID SOURCES

Vision USA

Provides free eye care to the uninsured.
800-766-4466.

EyeCare America–National Eye Care Project

Provides free or low-cost exams for people over 65 who have not seen an ophthalmologist for at least three years.

800-222-EYES

Lions Club International

Gives financial aid for eye care through its local clubs.
National office: 630-571-5466

Mission Cataract USA

Provides free cataract surgery for people unable to pay.

800-343-7265

Knights Templar Eye Foundation

Offers financial aid for eye surgery for those unable to pay.

773-205-3838

PART 2

Day-to-Day
Caregiving

Exercise and Physical Rehabilitation

Have you ever experienced a midafternoon slump but then gotten a second wind after you've taken a walk or moved about a little? Or did you ever find yourself feeling more invigorated after doing yard work or engaging in some other physical activity? If you have, you know that movement of your body affects many aspects of your total well-being. Exercise stimulates your various body systems to function at their best, sharpens your mind, and lifts your spirit. Regular physical activity not only offers protection against many diseases, but also plays an important part in keeping persons with chronic conditions from developing unnecessary disability and complications. And regular exercise is equally important for persons who serve as caregivers to loved ones with chronic conditions.

WHAT PREVENTS PEOPLE FROM EXERCISING?

Despite the numerous benefits, getting an ample amount of exercise is a challenge for many people, witnessed by the fact that too few Americans engage in exercise regularly. When people have a chronic condition, the challenge to exercise is even greater.

Physical factors can impair the ability to exercise. Limitations in the ability to freely move all body parts can exist. Coordination may be poor. Pain, shortness of breath, fatigue, and other symptoms can create significant obstacles to overcome.

BENEFITS OF EXERCISE

The fact that exercise is good for one's health is widely understood, but the many benefits of physical activity may not be fully appreciated. Physical activity impacts virtually every body system, every aspect of life. It can help not only to increase the length of life, but also to improve the quality of life.

Here are just of few of the things exercise can do.

- Strengthens and tones the muscles, allowing them to perform more work with less effort
- Improves the ability of the muscles to use available oxygen so that the heart doesn't have to pump as hard to meet the body's circulatory needs
- Raises the blood volume pumped with each contraction (stroke volume), thereby slowing the heart rate
- Lowers blood pressure
- Increases breathing capacity
- Assists in moving respiratory secretions and preventing respiratory infections
- Improves the flexibility of the muscles and joints
- Maintains and promotes strong bones
- Enhances circulation of oxygen to all body tissues, including the brain
- Reduces triglyceride levels (fatty acids) and raises "good" high-density (HDL) cholesterol
- Stimulates the production of red blood cells
- Aids lymphatic circulation
- Improves digestion
- Aids in the elimination of body wastes
- Releases endorphins, which promote relaxation and comfort
- Activates neurotransmitters to improve coordination
- Stimulates metabolism and helps to burn calories, which assists with weight control
- Sharpens mental function
- Elevates mood
- Improves self-esteem

Medications can cause dizziness, drowsiness, or other effects such as low blood pressure and heart rate that can interfere with the ability to exercise.

Even when physical factors are not the reason for inactivity, emotional factors can be a stumbling block to exercising. Depression can cause an individual to have low motivation and interest for exercise. There can be fear and anxiety about worsening one's condition. At times, the burdens imposed by the condition can be so overwhelming that there isn't sufficient emotional or physical energy to even think about, much less perform, exercise.

Psychosocial factors can have an effect on exercise. A person may have non-supportive family members who discourage exercise. Misguided caregivers may believe they are helping by encouraging a person to "take it easy." Sometimes, health care professionals may fail to assess or mention exercise and other lifestyle factors that influence health, and focus more on medications as a means of managing health conditions. There may be little opportunity to take a walk or exercise, or not enough space to engage in other forms of physical activity. Equipment that could be used for exercise may be unavailable. Meeting the demands of taking care of personal needs, health conditions, family, and home may leave little time and energy for exercise. No one may be available to offer companionship or assistance with exercise.

Some special efforts must be taken to overcome these obstacles. Caregivers often make the crucial difference as to whether a person engages in regular exercise or becomes immobile. Be it knowing how to schedule medication administration so that effects will improve tolerance for exercise, providing assistance with movement, or offering encouraging words, caregivers play an important role in maintaining and improving physical activity of the persons whom they help.

WHAT ARE THE PURPOSES OF EXERCISE?

There are many reasons for people being interested in exercising. Often, it is because they have put on a few pounds or find themselves huffing and puffing when they climb a flight of stairs and realize that they are out of shape. In some cases, a health care professional has recommended an exercise program to prevent the onset or progression of a disease. Being bombarded with news and advertisements hyping the latest exercise equipment, gym, or workout routine teases the interest of others. Whatever the motivator, exercise serves the purpose of maintaining or improving physical fitness and function through attention to cardiorespiratory (heart and lung) endurance, flexibility, muscle strengthening, and regaining function.

CARDIORESPIRATORY ENDURANCE

There are many aspects of physical fitness, one of the most important being cardiorespiratory endurance. This refers to the ability of the heart, lungs, and blood vessels to get oxygen into the body and deliver it to every cell, particularly when physical activity is being performed and the demand for oxygen is increased. In order for the cardiorespiratory system to be in the best position to accomplish this, it must be stimulated by physical activity, particularly of the large muscles in the legs, arms, and shoulders. The basic principle of exercise training is that it must challenge the body, thereby causing the body to respond by improving its capacity to meet the challenge. In other words, you must engage in a higher level of physical activity when you exercise than you would normally do in order for improvement to be realized. For cardiac endurance, not only must muscles be exercised, the exercise must be performed long enough to require a continuous supply of oxygen. This requirement for oxygen puts a demand on the cardiorespiratory system and helps to increase its endurance. Exercises that require a continuous supply of oxygen are referred to as aerobic (meaning "with oxygen") and include walking, jogging, cycling, swimming, rowing, tennis, racquetball, and aerobic dancing. Depending on the exercise, it should be done for twenty to sixty minutes (plus warm-up and cool-down times) and at least five times a week (preferably daily).

Aerobic exercises should be individualized. Determining target heart rate can assist in this effort. The heart rate increases during exercise in direct proportion to the amount of exercise that is being done and the oxygen demand that arises. For this reason, the heart rate can be used as a "meter" to provide feedback, similar to the manner in which a car's speedometer offers feedback regarding how fast you're traveling. The target heart rate represents a level of intensity of exercise that raises the heartbeat to a certain range, and it varies depending on age. To estimate your own target heart rate range: find your maximum heart rate by subtracting your age from 220. The target heart rate zone (range) is estimated by taking 60% and 80% of that number. For example, if a person's age is 65:

$220 - 65 \text{ (age)} = 155$ maximum heart rate
$155 \times 0.6 = 93$, the low end of the target zone
$155 \times 0.8 = 124$, the high end of the target zone

While you are performing aerobic exercises, the heart rate (pulse) per minute should fall within the target heart rate zone. If the heart rate during exercise is more than ten beats above the target heart rate, the exercise should be reduced the next time it is done. If it is lower than the target heart rate the exercise should be increased the next time. The American Council on Exercise's Web site provides a chart to help you to quickly calculate your target heart rate in their fact sheet "Monitoring Exercise Intensity Using Heart Rate," which can be accessed at www.acefitness.org.

The heart rate during exercise is monitored by taking the pulse. The correct method for taking the pulse is to:

- place the index and middle fingers on the inside of the wrist, just below the thumb joint;
- apply light pressure until the pulse is felt; then
- count the pulse beats for thirty seconds and multiply by 2 to get the pulse rate per minute.

Heart rate monitors are an alternative to taking one's own pulse. The most convenient heart rate monitors are those strapped around the chest. They detect the heart rate, much like an electrocardiogram (ECG), and transfer this information to a receiver (that looks like a wristwatch) worn on the wrist. People can then check their heart rate at any time just by looking at the device on their wrist. Because the transmitter uses radio signals, certain types of electronic devices (e.g., electric treadmills and monitors used by persons exercising nearby) can interfere with the radio signal, leading to inaccurate readings, so it is best to stay at least 4 feet from other exercisers using these devices. There are devices that clip to the earlobe or fingertip and read the pulse by using an infrared light that beams through the skin to measure the amount of blood being pumped through the vessels. They may cost less than chest monitors, but unfortunately, they also can be less accurate, particularly if there is a lot of movement.

The target heart rate zone may need to be adjusted if certain medications for heart or blood pressure conditions are being taken. For example, a very common class of drugs known as beta-blockers usually prevents the heart rate from going above 110 to 120 beats per minute regardless of the amount of exercise. People who are taking these types of medications and those of advanced age or with heart conditions should consult with their physicians to determine the target heart rate zone that is best for them personally.

FLEXIBILITY

Flexibility, or the ability to move muscles and joints freely through their range of motion, is another part of physical fitness. Good flexibility improves posture and reduces muscle tension, stiffness, and injury. Individuals can show differences in their flexibility; not surprisingly, children tend to be more flexible than adults and women are more flexible than men.

Gentle stretching exercises can keep muscles and joints flexible. Stretching five to ten minutes before and after exercise helps to reduce soreness. To stretch properly, extend as far as possible without pain and hold the stretch for ten to twenty seconds. Don't bounce; instead, hold the stretch.

Range of motion refers to the ability to straighten, bend, and turn a joint. Moving joints through their normal range of motion helps the body to maintain flexibility. Normally, people independently can move their joints within their full range, and when they can, this is called active range-of-motion exercises. There may be times when stroke, multiple sclerosis, or other health conditions impair a person's ability to move independently and assistance may be needed to exercise the joints. In these situations, passive range-of-motion exercises, meaning that the individual depends on others to exercise his or her joints, are necessary to maintain flexibility. There are some points to remember in assisting with range-of-motion exercises.

- Support the limb above and below the joint.
- Avoid moving a joint beyond its normal range of motion or the point of pain.
- Gradually increase movement in joints that have reduced movement.
- Avoid jerking or bouncing as this can cause injury.

Some good stretching exercises that can be done every day are shown in the sidebar on p. 553.

Although they may not be thought of as flexibility exercises per se, deep breathing exercises (also called diaphragmatic breathing, belly breathing, or abdominal breathing exercises) are beneficial in increasing lung activity, encouraging good air exchange, and preventing respiratory infections. Many people with chronic con-

DAILY STRETCHING EXERCISES

Daily stretching exercises, including modified yoga postures, are helpful in maintaining flexibility and muscle strength. A head-to-toe plan for stretching exercises could follow this format:

Face. Raise and lower the eyebrows, squeeze them together as though frowning; open the eyes wide and then close tightly; wrinkle the nose; open the mouth as wide as possible and then purse the lips.

Neck. Turn the head from side to side; bend the head down and then bend it back; pivot (roll) the head as though trying to trace an imaginary halo around it.

Arm and shoulder. Shrug the shoulders to raise them as high as possible; lower them; straighten the arms and raise them straight up and then swing them down behind the back; cross the arms in front of the body and reach for the shoulder blades; stretch the arms to the sides and make circles that get progressively larger.

Trunk. Twist the body from one side to the other at the waist while keeping the hips and legs in place.

Lower back. Lie on the floor on your back, tighten the stomach muscles, and press the small of the back toward the floor.

Hips and knees. While holding on to a sturdy piece of furniture or hand rail, bend and lift a knee straight up; bend and lift the knee toward the side; with the knee straight straighten the leg behind the body; from a seated position straighten the leg in front and then bend under the chair as far as possible; repeat these exercises with the other leg.

Ankle and foot. From a seated position bend the toes toward the head and then point them straight out; pivot the foot on the ankle to make circles with the foot; stretch and separate the toes and then curl them under; repeat for the other foot.

Begin by doing these stretching exercises one to five times daily, and gradually increase until they are done ten to twenty times.

ditions have the risk of reduced respiratory activity due to the symptoms they experience (e.g., pain, fatigue) or the effects of medications. These people need to pay particular attention to keeping their lungs fully expanded. Breathing exercises can help in this effort and consist of:

- inhaling a long breath to the count of 2 through the nose while pushing the stomach out,

- exhaling through the mouth to the count of 4 as the stomach is pulled in, and
- repeating the set of inhalation and expiration five to ten times.

Placing a hand over the stomach can be helpful in guiding the correct movement of the diaphragm during inhalation and expiration. It is useful to perform sets of breathing exercises several times during the day. Playing relaxing music that has a slow beat can help establish a regular rhythm for breathing out and breathing in.

MUSCLE STRENGTH AND ENDURANCE

Exercises for muscular strength and endurance are also a component of physical fitness. Typically, these exercises start by lifting a manageable amount of weight and then, as strength is gained, increasing the working load or resistance on muscles. The muscles must be challenged in order for them to improve. The key elements are resistance and progression. Resistance can be achieved through the use of weight machines, lifting weights (canned goods can substitute for barbells), and using one's own body weight through calisthenics such as push-ups and pull-ups, or isometrics. Progression involves increasing the workload on the muscles (e.g., lifting heavier weights) as the muscles improve their ability to do more work. In other words, to increase strength, the muscles must always be challenged. The American College of Sports Medicine, advises a typical regimen for adults under age 65:

- Exercise a muscle through a set of eight to twelve repetitions. If eight repetitions are difficult, start with fewer and gradually increase.
- Exercise the muscle at least twice each week. It could prove useful to exercise the muscles of the upper extremity on alternative days from the lower extremity muscles.

A well-rounded exercise program should include six to eight exercises that involve the major muscles of the upper and lower body.

EXERCISE TO REGAIN FUNCTION

In addition to their health benefits, exercises can be valuable in helping older people improve their abilities to take care of themselves. Activities of daily living (ADLs) are basic self-care activities and include feeding, toileting, bathing, dress-

EXERCISES FOR ARTHRITIS

Here are some simple exercises that caregivers and their patients can do together to strengthen and increase flexibility in stiff joints.

- Ask the person to hold your hands and squeeze them as hard as possible.
- Point your index finger straight up, move it to different points in front of the person, and ask the person to touch your finger at each position.
- Face the person and while holding hands with him, lift his hands above his head.
- Gather an empty egg carton and Styrofoam peanuts (or similar-sized objects) and have the person put the objects into different sections of the carton, one at a time.
- Place canned goods of several different weights in front of the person and have him lift each one as high as possible, beginning with the lightest and progressing to the heaviest.
- Have the person hold both ends of a rolling pin and roll it along a tabletop.
- Place a checkerboard in front of the person and have him, using his index and middle fingers, "walk" each row of the board, one square at a time.

- Give the person some clay and ask that he form a ball, a snake, a pancake, and other shapes. (Dough can work if you don't have clay.)
- While bracing the person's upper chest with one hand and his lower back with the other, encourage him to straighten his trunk as much as possible.
- Provide a belt that is buckled or a rope tied in a circle and have the person hold it as he places his foot on it and pulls the foot up.
- Play catch with a beach ball.

For the person in bed:

- Ask him to lift his straightened leg and apply gentle resistance to his leg as he does; repeat for the other leg; do the same for the arms.
- While standing at the foot of the bed, gently push the sole of the person's foot and ask him to push against your resistance; repeat for the other foot.
- Stand on one side of the bed and ask the person to remain flat and reach his arm that is farthest from you toward you; do the same for the leg; repeat on the other side.
- Encourage the person to roll from one side to the other.

ing, grooming, personal hygiene, ambulation (walking), and transferring. Instrumental activities of daily living (IADLs) are tasks that normally need to be done to function in the community, such as cooking, shopping, cleaning, doing laundry, managing finances, using the telephone, taking medications, and traveling. Certain health conditions impair the ability to independently perform ADLs and IADLs. This can result in a need for rehabilitation so that lost function can be regained. For example, someone who has had a stroke may need to improve grasp in order to handle objects. Likewise a person who has been on prolonged bed rest may need to restore ample strength and balance in order to walk. Special exercises may prove useful in these circumstances. Usually, rehabilitation specialists such as physical and occupational therapists will plan an exercise program based on the individual's needs and develop a customized exercise program to improve the ability to perform ADLs and IADLs.

As a caregiver to someone with deficits you should follow the prescribed program. However, there are exercises that you can easily incorporate into your daily activities with the impaired person to aid in improving function. Depending on the type of function that needs to be restored, you could assist the individual with some basic exercises. See the sidebars on pp. 553 and 555 for specific activities you can do.

Exercise is especially important in preventing complications to persons of advanced age or who are disabled because of health conditions. Reduced muscle tone and strength contribute to falls. Lack of movement can cause the joints to stiffen and develop contractures (a distorted flexion of the joint due to shrinkage of the muscle or tendon). Insufficient activity and change of position can impair good circulation to the tissues and lead to pressure ulcers (bedsores) and blood clots. Limited activity can decrease expansion of the lungs and increase the opportunity for secretions to remain in the respiratory system, contributing to pneumonia. Appetite can be poor and digestive functions sluggish in inactive people. Constipation is more likely to be a problem when individuals lack regular exercise. When not in the best physical condition, people tend to feel depressed, lack motivation to engage in activities, and have a low self-concept. These problems can compound many of the challenges persons with chronic conditions already face and significantly threaten their health status and the quality of their lives.

TIPS FOR SAFE EXERCISING

While exercise is extremely beneficial, when done improperly it can cause discomfort and injury to the muscles and joints. To avoid this there are some points to keep in mind:

Consult your physician. While most healthy people can start a light to moderate exercise program without medical screening, the American College of Sports Medicine recommends that healthy women over 50 years of age and men over age 40 consult a physician before starting a vigorous exercise program. Likewise, persons of any age should consult with a physician if they have a history of cardiac or respiratory disease, high blood pressure, diabetes, elevated cholesterol levels, or any disease of the muscles, joints, or nervous system. Exercise is one of the best means of improving health and the quality of life for persons with chronic health conditions but careful attention must be paid to assuring it is of the appropriate type, intensity, frequency, and duration to maximize benefits and prevent complications.

Individualize. No single approach to exercise will work for everyone. An exercise program needs to be tailored to the individual's age, condition, abilities, disabilities, and preferences. Getting an individualized exercise prescription from a clinical exercise physiologist or personal trainer is a wise investment.

Dress wisely. The ideal clothing for exercise is made of fabrics that "breathe," such as cotton, and is loose-fitting to allow free movement. (Of course, clothing shouldn't be so loose that pants legs can get caught on a heel or in a bicycle chain and cause a fall.) Wearing several layers of loose-fitting clothing provides good insulation in cool weather because the clothing traps the heat your body generates. This also allows for removing layers as needed to adjust to the temperature. Safe shoes appropriate for the type of exercise (e.g., aerobic shoes, running shoes, walking shoes) can be extremely valuable in preventing discomfort and injury. It's best to shop for shoes after being on your feet for a while to take into account any swelling that occurs as the day progresses. Poor-fitting shoes and socks can cause blisters and irritation.

Consider the environment. Consideration must be given to the environmental temperature. Ideally, the environmental temperature should be between 40 and 75 degrees F and humidity below 65 percent. Exercising in very cold temperatures will constrict blood vessels in the extremities and increase the workload of the heart. People with respiratory conditions may experience bronchospasms when exercising in cold, damp climates; covering the mouth and nose with a scarf can be helpful. On the other hand, exercising in hot, humid climates will dilate the blood vessels, which reduces the blood return to the heart, decreasing blood pressure and raising the heart rate. (Certain medications that dilate the blood vessels,

557

such as nitrates, will increase the risk of heat stress during exercise.) Attention needs to be paid to drinking plenty of fluids when exercising in hot and humid weather to replace the fluids lost through sweating. Air quality is another consideration. Since respirations increase during exercise, more air—and the pollutants it contains—will be inhaled. Avoid exercising near heavy traffic and on days when air pollution levels are high. Carbon monoxide prevents the blood from taking up oxygen, which reduces the amount of oxygen available to the brain, muscles, and other parts of the body.

Warm up and cool down. A warm-up activity prepares the muscles and joints for the more vigorous exercise that is to come by increasing blood flow to the muscles, raising the temperature of tissues, and helping the joints to be more flexible. Five to fifteen minutes of general warm-up exercises should be done before starting to exercise. These exercises begin with a general warming up that moves the large muscle groups, and can be achieved through brisk walking or riding a stationary bike. This helps to prepare the heart for the main exercise. Although stretching is a beneficial exercise, it is not a substitute for a good warm-up activity. Instead, especially for preventing muscle soreness and possible injury, stretching of the muscles that will be used in the main exercise should be done after the general warm-up and as part of the cool-down. After the exercise, five to ten minutes of gradually reducing activity allows the body to cool down. It is not wise to stop abruptly and be still following vigorous exercise. Also keep tabs on the heart rate. (See the discussion of target heart rate above.)

Replace fluids. When the body exercises, the muscles generate heat that raises the person's temperature. Sweating is a mechanism the body uses to dissipate, or release, the heat buildup. As the sweat evaporates, the blood circulating just below the skin cools, and as it circulates, cools the entire body. This wonderful process results in a loss of fluids, so care must be taken to replace those lost fluids to prevent dehydration. Older persons in particular must be alert to this, as they have lower fluid reserves and dehydrate more easily than younger persons. Waiting until you're thirsty doesn't help, because the body can be dehydrated without thirst being present. Unless a health care provider has recommended otherwise, it is useful to drink:

- At least two glasses (16 to 20 ounces) of fluid two hours before exercising
- One glass (8 ounces) of fluid fifteen to thirty minutes before exercising

- About one half glass (4 to 6 ounces) of fluid during exercise
- At least one glass of fluid after exercise

Ideally, fluids lost during exercise should be replaced after exercise. To determine the amount of fluid lost, take a weight measurement before and after exercise; any reduction in weight after exercise indicates fluid loss. Two glasses (16 ounces) of fluid for every pound lost is sufficient to replace lost fluids. Caffeinated beverages can have a diuretic effect (increasing urination), so they aren't the best types of fluids to drink during or after exercising. Under normal exercise conditions, most people don't need to worry about replacing electrolytes by drinking special (and often expensive) sports drinks. Water and diluted juices can meet fluid-replacement needs adequately.

Get adequate rest. It is important to obtain adequate rest between exercise sets, particularly when doing exercises that require a high degree of muscle effort, such as strength training. This is particularly significant for older adults, whose muscles require longer periods of time than those of younger adults to recover from stress.

Know when to stop. Your physician can advise you about specific warning signs to note based on specific medical conditions. Some general signs that should send up a red flag to stop exercise include:

- Chest pain
- Difficulty breathing
- Dizziness
- Lightheadedness
- Extreme fatigue
- Pallor (becoming pale)

CONSIDERATIONS FOR OLDER ADULTS

Some people claim that the ability to exercise declines with age, exercise can be harmful to older adults, and if a person isn't in good physical condition by the time he reaches old age he can't get in condition then. These are misconceptions. Exercise can help people not only live longer, but also have optimum function within those added years. Flabby muscles, increased body fat, slower movements, decreased energy, and some of the other signs that people have traditionally associated with aging are not entirely attributable to the normal process of growing old. Many of these declines are a result of physical inactivity and can be avoided with regular exercise. Not only can exercise prevent many diseases from developing, it can prevent or slow the debilitating effects of existing chronic conditions.

The aging process can cause changes that have an impact on physical activity. The heart's ability to circulate blood diminishes. There is a reduction in the number and size of muscle fibers; muscle strength and endurance decrease. Bone loss begins at middle age and is more pronounced with estrogen deficiencies (e.g., menopause), lowered testosterone levels, hyperthyroidism, deficiencies of vitamin D and calcium, chronic obstructive lung disease, cigarette smoking, alcoholism, and prolonged inactivity. Some medications, such as anticonvulsants, thyroid hormones, aluminum-containing antacids, and glucocorticoids, also can contribute to bone loss. Degenerative changes in the cartilage reduce the cushion between the joints and impair full joint movement. Balance is more difficult to maintain and restore in late life. Slower responses affect the speed of performance and reaction to stimuli. When walking, older adults tend to take slower and shorter steps and have greater variability in the length of steps.

The changes that have been associated with aging are not inevitable, however. More and more research is proving that exercise can minimize the effects of aging and help people to look younger, enjoy high energy levels, have good physical and mental function, and maintain independence. Exercise can help older adults to improve the ability of the heart and lungs to supply oxygen to the muscles, improve the muscles' use of available oxygen in the blood, slow the rate of bone loss, improve posture, increase flexibility and range of motion, decrease body fat, preserve lean body mass, raise the HDL ("good") cholesterol, and improve glucose metabolism. Psychological benefits also can be derived from exercise, including improved self-concept, preserved cognitive function, and relief of symptoms of depression.

A major benefit of exercise for older adults is the prevention of falls. Many factors contribute to the high rate of falls in later years, including medications, drops in blood pressure, environmental hazards, poor vision, altered mental status, and the reduced ability to maintain balance. Age-related changes in the musculoskeletal and nervous systems can cause older persons to lose and have more difficulty regaining balance than younger individuals. Increasing muscle strength and flexibility improves balance and, therefore, is highly beneficial to reducing falls. Older adults who participated in a program of walking, flexibility, and strength exercises three times a week have been shown to achieve improvements in their balance within several months.

Ideally, people will engage in a moderate to vigorous exercise program in their younger life that they will continue in their senior years. Unfortunately, the ideal picture doesn't exist for many people. But that shouldn't discourage any mature adult from beginning an exercise program. Consider that at 70 years of age a person could live several more decades and most probably would prefer to face these years in peak physical and mental condition. Persons in their 80s and 90s have been shown to benefit from endurance and strength training.

Walking. Walking is an excellent aerobic exercise for older adults. It does not require any special equipment or skill, and can be done almost anywhere. Shopping malls have become popular walking sites for senior citizens who can enjoy exercise and socialization in a climate-controlled, safe environment. Older adults can begin walking at least three times per week for twenty minutes, and then increase the intensity by walking inclines or steps. Persons with disabilities or injuries that prevent them from walking can use seated stepping machines and water exercises as alternatives.

Stationary bicycling, dancing, and swimming. These beneficial aerobic exercises are certainly appropriate for older persons. Swimming not only provides a good workout, but also can ease movement for exercise in persons with painful or stiff joints. If it has not been done on a regular basis, jogging may not be the best exercise to initiate in late life because of the stress it can place on the hips, knees, ankles, and lower back.

Resistance training. This is the best mode of exercise for improving muscle strength in older adults. The most common form of resistance training is weight lifting. Researchers have found that weight training conducted twice weekly significantly improved muscle strength in men aged 60 to 75 who had previously been sedentary. In addition to the benefits achieved in muscular strength, these men experienced a reduction in body fat and a significant increase in their peak aerobic capacity. The improvements in muscle strength and flexibility not only can help older adults to look and feel better, but also can help to prevent one of the villains of late life: falls. Regimens for progressive resistance training for older adults should consist of ten to fifteen repetitions using lighter weights to prevent injury. These should be done at least twice each week. Some standing postures with free weights should be included, as they will enhance balance and muscle flexibility.

Chinese movement exercises. Not all beneficial exercises need to cause a sweat to provide benefit. T'ai chi, for example, is an ancient Chinese exercise consisting of a series of flowing, controlled movements resembling a graceful martial arts routine. According to traditional Chinese medicine, t'ai chi stimulates the flow of "qi" (pronounced "chee"), or life energy, through the body to strengthen the organs and prevent illness-causing energy blocks and imbalances. This exercise has been shown to improve strength, balance, and flexibility in older adults. Reasonably priced videos are available that demonstrate t'ai chi exercises, some of which are designed for seniors.

Older persons should consider several things when beginning an exercise program.

• First, and very important, people should consult with their physician before beginning a vigorous exercise program. Be sure to ask if there are any precautions that must be heeded in light of any health conditions that are present or related to any medications being used. Optimum benefit is achieved by an exercise period that increases the heart rate within the target zone for thirty minutes, done preferably daily but at least five times per week. More frequent or higher-intensity exercises carry more risks than benefits.

• Rest after exercising, to afford the muscles a chance to recover from the physical stress (e.g., don't begin another vigorous activity such as housecleaning).

• If beginning an exercise program after being inactive, start with shorter intervals and progressively increase them as endurance builds.

• Follow the Tips for Exercise Success, on p. 571.

Senior citizen centers, community colleges, and health clubs are among the convenient, affordable options for group exercise programs. Also, many hospitals have opened health and wellness centers with special programs for seniors. These can prove highly enjoyable, provide motivation to stick with an exercise program, and offer new avenues for socialization. You can learn what is available by calling local colleges, hospitals, senior centers, and health spas, contacting the agency for aging services in your community, or calling your library for information and referral guidance.

CONSIDERATIONS FOR SPECIFIC CONDITIONS

Exercise not only helps to maintain function, but also can improve many health conditions. In some cases, adjustments must be made to prevent harm and complications. Some considerations for specific medical conditions are discussed below.

HEART DISEASE

Exercise plays an important role not only in preventing cardiac disease and heart attacks, but also in helping patients with cardiac disease to recover from an acute event like a heart attack or coronary bypass graft surgery. The American Heart Association states that patients with heart disease can benefit from a physician-supervised cardiac rehabilitation program. Cardiac rehabilitation usually begins within a few days following a heart attack (myocardial infarction or, as it is commonly referred to, MI) with an evaluation of the patient's exercise capabilities and needs. An interdisciplinary team of health professionals, along with the patient and his or her family and caregivers, develop an exercise plan that is designed for the individual.

Cardiac rehabilitation progresses through several phases, beginning during hospitalization for the acute cardiac illness (e.g., immediately after the heart attack). An evaluation of the patient's exercise capacity, including a treadmill test, may be done in the hospital or a few weeks after discharge. Mild physical activity is begun, gradually progressing to increase the workload on the heart. The patient will be expected to participate in grooming and other self-care activities, perform range-of-motion exercises, and walk short distances. The activity and exercise aid in preventing deconditioning and blood clot formation, which is a risk for anyone who does not get out of bed. This also promotes a sense of well-being and control, and offers encouragement for recovery. Family encouragement during this early phase can be helpful in encouraging the patient to progress without fear. Soon after discharge from the hospital the patient can be enrolled in an outpatient exercise program where he or she is monitored with electrocardiography to evaluate the heart's response to increasing activity levels. Heart rate and blood pressure also are evaluated to determine the reaction to and appropriateness of various exercise levels. As the patient's condition improves and exercise capacity increases, the amount of exercise during the workout also can increase.

Just as a person will be given prescriptions for medications that may differ from other persons with similar diagnoses, he or she also will be prescribed an individualized exercise program. The prescription will describe the following:

- Type of exercise to be done
- How often it is to be performed
- Duration (length of time for which the exercise is done)
- Intensity (the level of demand at which the exercise is performed)
- The manner in which the exercise is to be increased

Typically, exercises that offer sustained, rhythmic activity using the large muscle groups are prescribed. Treadmill walking is the most common type of prescribed exercise; cycling, rowing, and aquatic exercises are among the others that are often recommended. In addition, resistance training—such as weight lifting and elastic bands and tubes—has been incorporated into the exercise prescription for most patients in cardiac rehabilitation. As with any good exercise program, warm-up and cool-down exercises are included.

Cardiac rehabilitation can do wonders to assist in recovering of function after a heart attack. Usual activities can be resumed and few limitations may remain. In fact, having the scare of a heart attack can be the impetus for some people to adopt a new exercise program that causes them to get in better shape than they'd been in for years.

Persons with heart disease shouldn't wait until they have a heart attack to develop an exercise program. Regular exercise is an integral component of both cardiovascular disease prevention and rehabilitation because it increases the HDL ("good") cholesterol, lowers the blood pressure, tones the cardiovascular system, and helps to keep weight within a normal range. Persons with heart conditions should consult with their health care providers or join a cardiac rehabilitation program to develop personalized exercise programs and to review suggestions and precautions that need to be considered. The scheduling of medication administration in relation to exercise is one area that needs to be reviewed with the health care provider. For example, persons with angina may be told to take their nitroglycerin before doing their exercises, prior to symptoms developing.

Hypertension (high blood pressure) is a highly prevalent problem that affects one of every four black Americans and one of every six white Americans. Uncontrolled, hypertension can lead to heart attacks, congestive heart failure, stroke, and kidney failure. These complications can be prevented by conscientious attention to the prescribed treatments, among which will be a plan for exercise. Regular exercise helps to lower the blood pressure and tone the cardiovascular system. Aerobic exercises are emphasized. Except for persons with more severe levels of hypertension, moderate-intensity resistance training usually can be performed to supplement the aerobic workout.

OSTEOARTHRITIS

It can be difficult to think of exercising a joint that is arthritic, yet according to the Arthritis Foundation, an exercise program can be highly beneficial in maintaining joint mobility and strengthening muscles. The key is to develop a plan that balances appropriate exercise and rest of the joints. Range-of-motion exercises are recommended. Swimming and aquatic exercises can be very beneficial to joint health. Of course, exercise also has the benefit of keeping body weight within an ideal range, which can relieve stress on the joint.

Isometric exercises, in which an exercise is done against an unmovable force, also can prove useful for some persons with osteoarthritis. The joint is not moved in isometric exercises, but instead, muscles are contracted against the resistance of a

ISOMETRIC EXERCISES

- Bend the elbows at 90-degree angles and place the palms of the hands together in front of the chest so that the right hand is facing up and the left is down. Keeping elbows bent, begin raising the right hand and use the left hand to offer resistance by pushing the right hand down.
- Join the hands behind the head and push the head against the hands.
- Straighten the legs out in front of the body and tighten the thigh muscles to make the knee move upward. Can be done one leg at a time, or both together.
- Squeeze buttocks as tightly as possible.

565

still object (e.g., a wall or a body part). The contractions are held for three to five seconds and the entire set repeated five times a day.

RHEUMATOID ARTHRITIS

It is important that persons with rheumatoid arthritis consult with their doctor before starting an exercise program to avoid harming the joints. Typically, range-of-motion exercises are recommended, along with some form of strengthening and flexibility exercises. Studies in which people in a moderate phase of rheumatoid arthritis performed moderate exercise (at 50 percent to 70 percent of maximum heart rate) and some resistance training showed that these individuals had less joint stiffness, fewer hospitalizations, and higher levels of physical function than those who participated in physical therapy alone.

Exercise is vital to helping the joint stay flexible and reducing pain; however, strenuous exercise is not recommended during the acute phase, when the joint or joints are inflamed. Planning exercises during times when medications reach their peak effect and during times when symptoms are reduced is helpful. If muscle cramping or pain is experienced during exercises, stop, and massage the muscle.

LOW BACK PAIN

Most people experience low back pain from time to time, but for some, this condition can be long-term and recurring. Low back pain can result from a variety of causes, including injuries, poor posture, psychological stress, arthritis, and being physically unfit. To avoid injury, get a comprehensive diagnostic evaluation to determine the cause of your back pain before beginning an exercise program.

A well-designed exercise program can do wonders for chronic back pain. It can help to make the back muscles more flexible, strengthen the abdominal muscles to improve posture and keep the spine properly aligned, increase circulation to the back muscles, and strengthen back and leg muscles. Range-of-motion exercises can be beneficial, such as slowly bending and straightening the knee before getting out of bed and twisting your trunk from side to side with your arms hanging limp. Walking and swimming increase circulation to the large muscles of the back, which helps to reduce pain. The gentle stretches of yoga and the slow, dance-like movements of t'ai chi offer good back exercises. Specific exercises may be prescribed based on a person's particular condition.

OSTEOPOROSIS

You've probably heard that osteoporosis is associated with the loss of estrogen during menopause. While this is a major risk factor for developing osteoporosis, there are several other ones, including the lack of exercise. For prevention of osteoporosis, exercises, particularly weight-bearing exercises that put mild stress on the bones, such as walking, dancing, and aerobics, as well as weight lifting, serve to increase the rate of bone formation. The National Institutes of Health Osteoporosis and Related Bone Diseases–National Research Center claims that although significant bone loss can occur within a short time when a person is immobile, it can be reversed if mobility and exercise are restored within a few months.

People with osteoporosis will benefit not only from exercises to strengthen the skeleton in general, but also from exercises to strengthen muscles in areas that are common sites for fractures: the hips, spine, and wrists. Strong muscles in these areas help to stabilize the joints. Some good exercises for people with osteoporosis are shown in the sidebar below.

EXERCISES FOR OSTEOPOROSIS

Hip-kick exercises. These exercises can strengthen the bones of the hip. Have the person support herself with one hand on a wall, and keeping it straight, extend her leg behind her and return it to the floor, extend it in front of her and return it to the floor, and raise it to her side and return it to the floor. After doing eight to ten sets of these, repeat the exercise with the other leg. Sporting goods stores have resistance bands resembling large rubber bands that can be placed around the ankles to assist with these exercises.

Spine exercise. To strengthen the spine, have the person lie on her stomach with a pillow under her pelvis. Anchor her feet beneath a strong piece of furniture (or have someone hold them), and have her slowly lift and lower her head and shoulders, keeping her arms straight at her side, as she moves.

Wrist exercise. Have the person stand about 20 inches from a wall with feet apart, putting her hands on the wall at shoulder level. She slowly leans in and lowers herself so that her shoulders touch the wall, then slowly pushes herself back to a standing position. Repeat ten times. Lifting 1- to 2-pound weights or canned goods about ten times is also effective in strengthening the wrists.

Because osteoporotic bones can break very easily, exercises that can stress the bones—and sports such as tennis and bowling—should be approached with caution, and after consulting a physician who can measure the extent of osteoporosis.

ASTHMA AND OTHER CHRONIC PULMONARY DISEASES

In general, aerobic exercises that raise the heart and breathing rates are useful for persons with asthma or other chronic obstructive pulmonary diseases. However, some exercises may be more beneficial than others. Deep breathing exercises, described earlier, are ideal to build into each day and have helped some people with asthma reduce their symptoms and need for medications. Brisk walking in a climate-controlled shopping mall is a good exercise and may be particularly good for persons whose symptoms are triggered by cold air or air pollutants. The inhalation of warm, humid air during swimming can make this a good exercise for persons with respiratory conditions. Yoga can provide a great means of stretching and deep breathing exercises that can improve respiratory function.

The poor gas exchange that accompanies chronic obstructive pulmonary disease can affect energy levels, exercise capacity, and mental status. To combat this and promote physical fitness, exercise needs to be part of the treatment plan. Pulmonary rehabilitation programs are widely available throughout the country. Supervised exercise programs will measure oxygen saturation (the amount of oxygen carried by the blood) during exercise. The rehabilitation staff will establish an appropriate exercise prescription and teach you how to make the best use of supplementary oxygen to assure an adequate blood oxygen level.

An evaluation of the response to exercise is important for the person with asthma. Some forms of exercise will trigger an asthma attack, so it is important to understand the reaction of your respiratory system to various types of exercise. Exercise should be discontinued immediately if any of the following develop: difficulty breathing, dizziness, palpitations, extreme fatigue, wheezing, cramps, or clammy or discolored skin. Health care providers can offer advice on whether and how to use a bronchodilator inhaler before exercise to reduce symptoms.

DIABETES

There are two major types of diabetes and it is essential that an exercise program be based on the type of diabetes and the person's individual profile. Type 1 diabetes is caused by the inability to produce insulin, whereas type 2 diabetes (adult-onset), the most common type, is caused by the inability of the cells of the body to use insulin and uptake glucose. Health care providers will want to evaluate heart, blood pressure, kidney function, and eyes prior to prescribing an exercise program. This is particularly important for those exercises that will elevate the blood pressure to high levels.

According to the American Diabetes Association, exercise can make a significant difference to persons with diabetes. Regular exercise increases the muscles' uptake of glucose and helps to reduce blood glucose levels. As many people with adult-onset diabetes (type 2) have problems using insulin efficiently (known as insulin resistance) because of obesity, weight loss achieved through exercise can do wonders in reducing or even eliminating the need for medications. Stress can increase blood sugars and as exercise helps to control stress, it can be of benefit to persons with diabetes.

It's important for those taking insulin to work closely with their health care provider before beginning an exercise program. As the exercise causes the blood sugar to fall, taking the same amount of insulin that was used when not exercising could cause the blood glucose level to go too low. When the blood glucose is below normal, the brain may not have enough glucose to meet its needs and diabetics may experience confusion, seizures, and other complications. Also, it is best to avoid injecting insulin into a part of the body that will be used during the exercise, as the absorption can be more rapid with increased muscle activity.

Extra precautions during exercise are needed to assure that glucose levels aren't dropping too low. For example, some people may need to drink some fruit juice before and during exercising, or eat a high-carbohydrate snack at intervals. Ask your health care provider to guide you in a plan that is best for balancing insulin and glucose levels. It is wise to measure blood sugar level before and after exercise. Also, be sure proper shoes are worn, to protect the feet during exercise, and always inspect feet after exercising.

Aerobic exercises are well suited for persons with diabetes. While strength training can be beneficial for many persons with diabetes, it should be approached with caution because it raises the blood pressure and can stress the heart and blood vessels of the eye. Again, ask your health care provider for resistance-training guidelines.

DEPRESSION

Studies have shown exercise to be helpful in improving mood in persons with depression. In some persons, exercise may be as effective as antidepressant medications, and in some cases has been shown to have longer-lasting effects. Aerobic exercises and other forms of exercises such as weight training and t'ai chi have proven helpful in relieving depression and improving mood. Some researchers suggest exercise improves mood by increasing the production of chemicals that increase brain cell activity or trigger the release of endorphins and other natural painkilling substances. Others propose that the feeling of accomplishment and self-worth provides an emotional lift.

One of the challenges of depression is getting motivated enough to exercise. Finding an "exercise buddy" who can share the activity might provide the extra incentive needed to walk, bicycle, jog, or engage in other exercises. Tailoring the exercise to a person's personal interests also helps.

DEMENTIA

Dementia includes Alzheimer's disease and other conditions that involve a deterioration of intellectual function. The Alzheimer's Association states that physical activity is important to persons with dementia in helping to reduce some of the problematic behaviors that often accompany this disorder, such as wandering, restlessness, and agitation. As it is common for persons with dementia to confuse daytime and nighttime, physical activity during the daytime hours can help normalize normal day and night schedules and promote sleep. Exercise also is beneficial in preventing pressure sores, contractures (stiffened joints), blood clots, pneumonia, and other complications that are of high risk in persons who are inactive, including those who stay in bed or sit in a chair for prolonged periods of time.

Exercise programs must be individualized based on the capabilities of the individual. As most people who have dementias are of advanced age, physical limitations must be considered. Walking in a supervised area is a good exercise for persons who are able to ambulate safely. Repetitive activities, such as throwing a ball or moving objects from one place to another may be appropriate in light of the limited intellectual function that persons with dementia have. As the condition progresses and the person is limited in mobility, assistance with range-of-motion and resistance exercises is beneficial to build into the caregiving routine.

TIPS FOR EXERCISE SUCCESS

If you are a caregiver for someone with a chronic condition, you can have an important role in helping your loved one develop and stick to a regular exercise program. Your encouragement can motivate the person to exercise at times when he or she is experiencing physical symptoms or doesn't feel in the mood to do anything. Your guidance can assure that benefit rather than injury results from exercise. Your hands-on assistance in performing exercises can enable the person to move body parts that couldn't otherwise be moved.

Most of us are more enthusiastic about performing an activity that matches our interests and capabilities. This principle applies to exercise as well. Your close relationship with the person for whom you care provides you with good insight into tailoring a well-suited exercise program. Consider the following:

What types of activities has the person enjoyed in the past? For someone who despised shopping, a walking program in a shopping mall may not be received as well as walking in a park. A gregarious person may enjoy exercising at a gym or in a group program, while those who don't like working up a sweat with others may prefer a treadmill or bicycle in the privacy of their homes. Modified versions of sports that the person played in the past can be used as a means of exercise; for example, if he enjoyed baseball and is now confined to a wheelchair, catching and throwing a lightweight ball may prove to be an enjoyable form of physical activity.

MEDICATIONS AND EXERCISE

Many persons with chronic conditions are taking medications that can affect or be affected by exercise. This emphasizes the importance for people with chronic health conditions to plan their exercise program with a health care provider and become knowledgeable about the side effects of their medications so that complications can be avoided. For instance:

- Many cardiac, antihypertensive, and chemotherapy drugs can cause fatigue and sleepiness that can reduce the desire and ability to exercise.
- Some diuretics, tranquilizers, and antidepressants can cause overheating during exercise.
- Some antidepressants, antihistamines, tranquilizers, sedatives, and cardiac and antidiabetic drugs can cause dizziness and lightheadedness during exercise.
- The required dosage of antidiabetic drugs may need to be adjusted when a regular exercise program is initiated.

What capabilities and limitations does the person have? Exercise programs need to be realistic in light of what the person is able to do. A person with dementia may be unable to follow the steps of a complex aerobic routine but might do well when given one or two instructions at a time. Likewise, an unsteady gait could prevent safe walking for long distances, but a stationary bike, either upright or recumbent, could prove to be a good alternative.

What is the best schedule for exercising? The time of day that exercises are done does not matter in terms of attaining optimal benefits. The choice should be based on convenience and preference. Someone who becomes progressively more fatigued as the day goes on may do better exercising in the morning, when energy levels are at their peak. A person with osteoarthritis who has joint stiffness in the morning may benefit from morning range-of-motion exercises that promote flexibility. A person with Alzheimer's disease who tends to wander in the midafternoon may have that behavior reduced by being taken for a walk in early afternoon.

Physical and occupational therapists can be great resources for suggestions that could be helpful for the individual patient.

In addition to structured exercise programs, physical movement can be promoted throughout the day in your approach to routine care activities. Other persons in the household may believe that they are doing your loved one a favor by not asking him or her to do any tasks. Sometimes the person takes so much time doing a task or performs it less well than more able-bodied members of the household that family members may feel it is more efficient to just do tasks themselves. However, every task that the person is asked to do is an opportunity for activity that may promote health. Ask your loved one to assist in washing dishes, folding linens, rearranging a cabinet, and other routine activities. In addition to the physical benefits of performing these tasks, the person can derive a sense of purpose and an improved self-concept by knowing he or she is an active participant in household functions.

For many of us, sticking to an exercise program can be a challenge; for the person with a chronic health condition or disability, being physically active can be a major accomplishment. For someone who is experiencing symptoms or feeling overwhelmed by the demands of an illness, staying in bed with the covers pulled over one's head may feel much more desirable than subjecting oneself to a physical workout. Without badgering the person or making him or her feel guilty, offer encouraging words. Be an exercise buddy, engaging in the exercise along with your loved one to help motivate (not to mention to contribute to your own physical fitness!). And by all means, recognize and praise the person's efforts to exercise. The positive reinforcement can make a difference in helping the person stay with his or her exercise program.

EXERCISE BENEFITS THE CAREGIVER, TOO!

If you are providing care to someone with a chronic health condition or disability, it is likely that you are subjected to considerable physical and emotional stress. The person may require hands-on assistance with personal care that can be physically draining; on days when symptoms and discouragement are high, he or she may take out frustrations on you. Observing someone you love experience the consequences of an illness can be emotionally draining for you. Finances may be strained. Other members of the family and friends may accuse you of not paying enough attention to them. Of course, this is added to taking care of your own needs and managing all of the other routines of daily living. Little wonder you may feel stressed!

The body reacts to stress in many ways, such as by tensing the muscles, increasing the heart rate and blood pressure, interfering with digestion, disrupting sleep, reducing the depth of our respirations, decreasing interest in sex, weakening immunity, impairing our thinking, and playing havoc with emotions. These effects can be quite threatening to your health, but there is something you can do to combat them: exercise. If you review the benefits of exercise described at the beginning of this chapter you will see that many of them are antidotes to the effects of stress. Not only can exercise relieve the symptoms of stress, but also it can enable you to cope with stress more effectively so that you will be more resilient to its effects. Taking care of yourself by building exercise into your schedule will not only promote your own good health, but will help you to better provide care to your loved one.

ADDITIONAL RESOURCES

ORGANIZATIONS AND WEB SITES

American Association of Cardiovascular and Pulmonary Rehabilitation

www.aacvpr.org

American Heart Association

www.americanheart.org

The American Lung Association

www.lungusa.org

American Occupational Therapy Association

www.aota.org

The Arthritis Foundation

www.arthritis.org

ARTICLES AND BOOKS

American Council on Exercise. "Strength training 101."

www.acefitness.org

American Diabetes Association. "Clinical practice recommendations: Diabetes and exercise."

www.diabetes.org

Depression.org. "Exercise and depression."

www.depression.org

Exercise: A Guide from the National Institute on Aging.

To order: 800-222-2225. Or write to:

NIAIC

Department US

P.O. Box 8057

Gaithersburg, MD 20898-8057

National Institutes of Health

Osteoporosis and Related Bone Diseases National Resource Center. "Osteoporosis prevention and treatment." www.osteo.org

Falls and Mobility Problems

Have you tried getting out of a bathtub lately? Or reaching for a can of soup on a high shelf, or rising from a low chair? It takes some effort. For elderly adults, these and other simple movements can be especially challenging—and risky.

Every year, about a third of those 65 years and older will fall at least once. For those in nursing homes, who tend to have poor balance and muscle strength, the annual incidence of falls is even higher. In the United States, accidents are the sixth leading cause of death in the elderly, and falls account for the majority of these accidents. Even apart from falls, reductions in strength and mobility often limit the ability of elderly adults to live as fully as they'd like.

If you are caring for an elderly person, you've probably heard him or her say, "I'm just getting older," as though that's reason enough to stop working in the yard, going to the store, or walking up and down stairs. But getting older shouldn't prevent people from doing the things they want to do. When simple physical movements become difficult or painful, there are bound to be underlying health problems that need to be addressed.

Regardless of an older adult's overall health, it's wise to keep moving—that's the key to improving balance, preventing falls, and improving strength and flexibility. If your loved one has fallen recently, he or she might need help recovering strength and confidence. Older persons certainly should be encouraged to do things for themselves whenever possible. Physical therapists having a saying: "If it's physical, it's therapy." Some people have little interest in "formal" exercise such as swimming

575

or bicycling. Even so, there are hundreds of everyday activities that can dramatically improve mobility, and with it the ability to live more independently.

UNDERSTANDING MOBILITY PROBLEMS

We all slow down as we get older. Activities that once seemed easy—walking, lifting groceries, or getting out of bed in the morning—may get increasingly difficult. Muscles get weaker. Joints often ache. There may be pain in the neck or lower back.

Over the years, we naturally make little adjustments to compensate for these and other physical limitations. Older adults may spend more time sitting or lying down, especially if they sometimes get dizzy while standing. If they've ever slipped on the stairs, they may start looking for reasons to avoid going up or down.

These are all natural reactions. But avoiding activity, for whatever reason, rarely makes things better. In most cases, it makes them worse.

Here's what often happens. Suppose your loved one has a flare-up of arthritis. She might curtail her daily activities for a few weeks. In the meantime, the muscles will get weaker from underuse and the tendons and ligaments will shorten. By the time the arthritis pain is gone, your loved one will probably feel weaker and stiffer than ever. So she'll avoid physical activities still more.

Thus can begin a downward cycle, in which decreasing levels of activity contribute to declines in strength, mobility, and balance, which in turn lead to even lower levels of activity. Your loved one may need more help around the house. She might have trouble getting out of bed without assistance. Rather than walking to the kitchen to get a glass of water, she may ask someone to get it for her.

As she becomes more dependent on others, her confidence will decline. She might not trust herself to walk without falling. She may quit leaving the house or visiting with friends. After a while, she'll start feeling isolated or depressed. It's hard to imagine that all of this could begin with a simple arthritis flare-up. But that's what often happens: Small problems with mobility snowball into something much more serious.

WHAT'S NORMAL AND WHAT ISN'T?

Before we discuss the physical problems that can lead to declines in mobility, it's important to understand some of the natural changes that occur over time.

- Elderly adults commonly walk more slowly than young people and they have a shorter stride. A slow, tentative gait makes it difficult to stay balanced, in part because the body lacks the forward momentum of a brisk, confident walker.

- People sway more from side to side as they get older. In young people, the range is about 1 inch. The elderly sway about 50 percent more. When this is combined with an overall loss of muscle strength, older adults' ability to recover from off-balance movements—such as reaching to one side to retrieve a bath towel—is reduced. This can greatly increase the risk of falling.

- Reaction times get slower.

- Muscle strength and mass decrease.

By themselves, none of these changes should have a significant effect on older adults' ability to get around. What often happens, however, is that other physical problems get "superimposed" on these natural, age-related changes. Studies have shown that about half of all falls are caused by underlying medical problems. The ability to move comfortably and maintain balance requires input from nearly every one of the body's systems, from the cardiovascular, musculoskeletal, and central nervous systems to the "balancing system" in the inner ear. Illnesses that disrupt any one of these systems can have a significant impact on mobility and balance.

WHAT YOUR HEALTH CARE PROVIDER WILL LOOK FOR

People often wait months or even years before telling a health care provider that they're having trouble moving around. This is unfortunate, because prompt attention to physical changes will greatly improve the chance for regaining full mobility and balance.

Your health care provider may simply want to watch your loved one as he moves. Is it easy or hard for him to get up from the chair and walk to the examination table? Does he use his hands to steady himself? Can he walk in a straight line without faltering? Can he bend over or turn in a circle without getting dizzy?

If problems with mobility have begun recently, your health care provider will suspect that there may be an acute (sudden onset) condition. Dehydration, for example, can cause drops in blood pressure that result in dizziness. Heart or lung conditions can restrict the flow of blood and oxygen to the brain. Side effects from medications—or interactions between different medications—can also affect balance and mobility.

WHO IS AT RISK?

Dozens of conditions may contribute to falls or mobility problems in the elderly. Some of these disorders disrupt the body's ability to balance or the way the person walks (gait). Others are caused by declines in vision or hearing. Still others reflect avoidable hazards in the home environment, such as wet floors or loose throw rugs. Health care specialists emphasize that most falls do not have one particular cause, but rather may reflect several medical and other conditions that must be understood and treated together.

Experts who specialize in the assessment of elderly adults to minimize their risk of injury through falling do not analyze these persons in terms of particular diseases, however. They use what has been described as a "multifactorial" approach, recognizing that falls and mobility problems are due to multiple conditions and risk factors, which must be treated together.

Following are some of the leading risk categories recognized by geriatric nurses and physical therapists:

Low blood pressure. If the heart isn't able to pump blood with sufficient force, the brain may not get all the blood it needs. This can cause dizziness or a temporary loss of consciousness (syncope), which may result in falls. Some older persons can have low blood pressure without dizziness. The same condition can be caused by rapidly rising from a lying to a standing position, without giving the body time to adjust. Dehydration can also cause low blood pressure. Persons who have a drop in systolic blood pressure of more than 20 mm Hg upon standing, or a reduction in systolic blood pressure to less than 90 mm Hg, are considered to be at risk of falling, although lesser changes may cause problems as well.

Sleeping medications. Persons who are taking sedative-hypnotic drugs, including any benzodiazepines or over-the-counter sleep medication, should consult their health care provider about their risk of falling and should be educated about non-drug-related means of dealing with sleep disturbances.

Polypharmacy. Dozens of over-the-counter and prescription drugs can affect balance. Persons taking four or more drugs at the same time are at increased risk of falling. Medications to control high blood pressure can be a problem, especially if they cause blood pressure to drop too low. Other drugs that may cause dizziness or a loss of balance include antihistamines, antidepressants, and diuretics. Balance, coordination, and mobility problems that result from overmedication may be helped by consulting a health care provider to see if it is safe to lower the dose or change to another medication.

Transfer difficulties. Regardless of underlying cause, any person who has difficulty in moving between a standing and a sitting position—such as moving onto or away from the toilet or the bathtub—is at increased risk of falling.

Impairments in gait or overall strength and flexibility. Regardless of underlying cause, anything that affects the way an elderly person walks (gait) or the strength and flexibility of key joints (ankle, knee, hip, hand, elbow, or shoulder) will pose an increased risk of falling.

Environmental hazards. Finally, many falls result from unsafe conditions in the home. Attention to detail can minimize or prevent many of these common hazards. See "Make Your Home Safer" on p. 586.

Because so many different health problems can interfere with mobility, the specific tests and treatment options will vary widely from person to person. The good news is that conditions that diminish mobility are often reversible.

WHAT CAUSES A FALL?

Many medical problems in the elderly can contribute to falls. Here are some of the more common ones.

- Low blood pressure upon standing—a common condition for seniors rising in the night to go to the bathroom, or getting out of bed first thing in the morning.
- Degenerative changes in the spine, whether in the neck or back, that can be caused by arthritis, osteoporosis, or other rheumatologic conditions.
- Sensory deficits caused by impairment in vision, such as cataracts and macular degeneration, or by inner-ear disturbances resulting in a loss of balance.
- Dizziness, a common symptom that can have one or many contributing causes.
- Neuropathy, or nerve damage in the extremities, especially the feet, which can be caused by conditions including diabetes and alcoholism. This can make the feet numb and interfere with the ability to judge one's position.
- Parkinson's disease, Alzheimer's disease, or other neurologic diseases and conditions.

UNDERSTANDING FALLS

Falls are a major cause of injury for the young as well as the old, representing one of the leading causes of emergency visits to hospitals across all age ranges. However, young people are, by and large, more resilient. As people age, they are more at risk for serious injury, in part due to osteoporosis, a condition in which bones lose calcium and get weak, brittle, and prone to fractures. One in four women will have fallen and fractured a hip by the time she reaches 90. In the United States, the treatment of fractures caused by falls is estimated to cost $10 billion a year.

Even apart from the risk of immediate injury, falls can have devastating consequences. Elderly adults who fall may be too weak or disoriented to get up from the floor or ground without assistance. One study found that the average "lying time" was fifteen minutes; some elderly adults who fall will wait hours for help. The longer they're down, the greater the health risks—from dehydration, pressure sores, or kidney failure caused by drops in blood pressure and breakdown in muscle.

Falls have more subtle consequences, as well. Between 10 percent and 25 percent of those who fall will begin curtailing their normal activities because they're afraid of falling again.

COPING WITH FALLS

Sooner or later your loved one may fall. How you handle the situation—and how you plan for it—will make a big difference in how well she recovers.

• If your loved one starts to slip and you're right next to her, you may be able to hold her up. Otherwise, don't rush forward to try to stop her from falling. You probably won't get there in time, and you may hurt yourself in the process.

• If your loved one has fallen and doesn't appear to be injured, let her sit up for a few minutes to regain her composure. When she feels ready, encourage her to get up using her own strength rather than having others try to pull her up. It isn't always easy for elderly adults to get up once they've fallen. Have your loved one crawl to a heavy piece of furniture such as a sofa and climb up onto it. It's easier to pull up on furniture than to rise straight up from the floor.

• If she isn't able to help herself, rather than trying to lift her yourself, call for emergency help.

• Make an appointment for her to be evaluated for fall risks, even if she doesn't seem to be hurt. It's not uncommon for people with bone fractures or even head injuries to appear to be fine, only to develop symptoms later on. Your health care provider may recommend x-rays or tests to ensure that the fall wasn't caused by an underlying medical condition. For example, many elderly people take diuretics (water pills) that can cause low blood pressure. Getting up and rushing to go to the bathroom at night is a common cause of falls. Your health care provider can evaluate whether a change in medication or the environment can reduce risks. The causes of falls aren't always medical, of course. Perhaps an older person is no longer able to function safely in some aspect of the home environment. For example, your loved one may fall when she rises from a particular chair that is too low. Maybe the solution is getting a chair with a higher, firmer seat. Information about fall patterns can help the health care provider suggest ways to avoid falls.

• Encourage the person to resume normal activity after a fall. It's normal for elderly adults to lose confidence in their abilities after they've fallen. As long as your loved one wasn't seriously hurt, it's essential that she stay active; it's important for her self-confidence to continue getting around on her own. Just as important, she needs to keep her muscles strong and joints flexible.

• Help out as much as necessary—but no more. Family members may inadvertently slow their loved one's recovery by helping too much. You don't want your loved one to become overly dependent. It's important that she continue her daily routine of activities to maintain stamina.

IMPROVING BALANCE, PREVENTING FALLS

An important strategy for preventing falls is to help your loved one develop better balance. Physical activity is often the best way to achieve this. Surveys of elderly adults reveal that those who spent less than four hours a day on their feet had the highest rate of fall-related fractures.

A physical therapist can instruct your loved one about how to keep her balance while doing everyday tasks, such as getting up from a chair, washing dishes, or putting linens on a closet shelf.

Physical therapists put it this way: "The key to improving balance is to safely challenge balance." The therapist will work with a person as she practices "displacement activities" in a controlled, safe way. Most of the exercises are very simple. Note: For someone who has a balance problem, these exercises should only be done at the direction and supervision of a therapist.

For example:

Hip sways. The person stands at the kitchen sink or in front of a counter, using her hands for support. Make a big circle with the hips to the left, then to the right.

Standing on one leg. One of the best balance exercises is to stand on one leg like a stork, holding on to the counter or the kitchen sink. The therapist will stand nearby as the person tries to balance on each leg for about five seconds.

Toe raises. While the person is standing at the sink or a counter and supporting herself with her hands, she'll rise up on her toes as far as she comfortably can. She'll hold the position for a second or two, then lower herself slowly down. This exercise improves balance and also strengthens the ankle and calf muscles, which will make it easier for her to walk and climb hills or stairs.

Seated knee lifts. It's important to practice sitting balance, as well. Seated knee lifts are done while the person is sitting on the side of the bed. Sitting upright, she'll fold her arms across her chest, then lift the left knee up toward the ceiling. She'll slowly lower the knee, then repeat the movement with the other knee. It's important to hold the upper body straight when doing this exercise.

Sit-to-stand transfers. A movement that is difficult for some older adults is rising from a sitting position. Apart from the fact that it requires quite a bit of muscle strength, the body can be off balance during the transition from sitting to standing. Practicing this movement will help improve strength as well as balance. While the person is sitting, she should put one foot slightly in front of the other, then try to stand up in one smooth movement, using her hands and the strength of her arms and legs to push off from the chair. Then she'll slowly lower herself back down in a controlled movement, again using the strength of her arms and legs to prevent drop sitting.

IMPROVING STRENGTH

Men lose about 10% of muscle mass each decade after age 65. Women retain a larger percentage of muscle, but they lose more bone: By age 90, women have about 35 to 50% of the bone mass that they had in their 20s. The combination of declining strength and fragile bones increases the chance of injury if elderly adults fall.

Declines in mobility can also be caused by reduced aerobic capacity. Aerobic capacity is the ability of the heart, lungs, and blood vessels to deliver adequate oxygen to the muscles. Aerobic capacity generally peaks at age 20 and afterward declines at the rate of 1% annually. An 80-year-old may have only half the aerobic capacity that he had at his peak.

Some loss of strength and mobility is inevitable, but research has shown that elderly adults can maintain—or rapidly regain—many of their physical abilities. The secret is to stay physically active.

In one study of elderly adults, participants who performed regular exercise were able to increase their muscle strength more than 110%. Their walking speed increased 12%, and their stair-climbing strength increased 28%.

Even if your loved one hasn't been physically active in the past, a regular exercise regimen can greatly increase strength, balance, and flexibility, and reduce the risk of falls. He'll be better equipped to safely perform routine daily activities with less fatigue. Just as important, he'll be better able to get around on his own without depending on others for help.

GETTING STARTED

The hardest part about exercise is getting started. Muscles and joints that haven't been used a lot get stiff and "lazy." Working up the motivation to go for a walk can be a challenge. But doing simple stretches can be a good way to get started.

The first step may be a meeting with a physical therapist. The therapist will design an exercise program that takes into account the person's limitations and strengths. If she has trouble with balance, for example, the physical therapist may begin by suggesting how to improve her posture and develop exercises that will help her stand, sit, or walk more efficiently. The exercises won't seem like a workout at all. The person may be told to tighten or relax certain muscles while lying in bed. She may be advised to do nothing more difficult than standing up and sitting down a few times. The goal is simply to restore strength and flexibility, a little at a time. Exercises can become more challenging as abilities improve.

Some of the early exercises might include:

Standing. If a person has spent a lot of time sitting or lying down, just standing more often will help improve balance, muscle tone, and circulation. Prolonged sitting is to be discouraged; the person should try to stand and walk every hour.

Toe raises. This is another exercise that can be incorporated into everyday activities. While your loved one is standing at the sink, for example, she can hold on with both hands and strengthen and stretch her leg muscles by raising herself up on her toes, then slowly lowering back down.

Stair climbing. Going up and down stairs is among the best ways to improve leg strength as well as balance. Encourage your loved one to use the stairs as often as she comfortably can. (If you don't have stairs indoors, she can practice on outdoor steps, going up and down a few times.) It is important to move slowly and use the handrail for support.

Standing up and sitting down. It sounds too easy to be exercise, but just going from a sitting to a standing position helps strengthen muscles in the legs and torso. This movement will be most effective when your loved one raises and lowers herself slowly, without jerking upward or dropping the last few inches into the chair.

Arm curls. Your loved one doesn't need to work out with weights in order to increase arm strength. She doesn't even have to set aside extra time. Every time she picks something up—a carton of orange juice from the refrigerator, or a bag of groceries—she should flex her arms up and down a few times.

These little movements may not seem impressive, but every bit of exercise adds up, especially when you consider that even a half-gallon carton of juice weighs several pounds.

THE NEXT STEP

Experts once thought that sustained, vigorous exercise—which was difficult for elderly adults to do—was the only way to increase fitness. Research has shown, however, that people can make substantial gains in strength, flexibility, and balance with small amounts of moderate exercise.

Guidelines from the Centers for Disease Control and Prevention and the American Heart Association call for getting thirty minutes or more of low-to-moderate-intensity exercise on most days of the week.

It isn't necessary to get the exercise all at once. Studies have shown that people who exercise in short bursts—say, walking for five or ten minutes in the morning, raking leaves for ten minutes in the afternoon, and stretching or walking some more in the evening—will get the same benefits as those who exercise for thirty minutes straight.

If an older adult hasn't been physically active in the past, she'll want to talk with her health care provider before starting an exercise program. This is especially important if she has a history of heart or lung disease, or if she's taking medications. Drugs that are used to control high blood pressure and diabetes, for example, may affect the ways in which the body responds to exercise.

Once your loved one has the go-ahead to be more active, try to find enjoyable activities. Some of the most popular activities include:

Walking. The simplicity of walking belies its health benefits: It's among the best exercises for increasing flexibility, strength, endurance, and balance. Encourage walking at least twenty to thirty minutes daily, whether all at once or in three or four shorter sessions throughout the day. The great thing about walking is that it doesn't have to be "formal" exercise. If someone is reluctant to set aside extra time, walking can be incorporated into other daily activities. Walking from one end of a shopping mall to the other, for example, may take fifteen or twenty minutes. Someone riding the bus can get off one stop early and walk the rest of the way. If you're driving, take advantage of the back parking lot. It's easier to find an empty space—and you and your loved one will have the opportunity to walk a little more.

T'ai chi. Many Americans have discovered the benefits of t'ai chi, a type of martial art that involves very slow, dance-like movements. One study found that elderly adults who practiced t'ai chi reduced their risk of falls by about 40%. You can find classes in t'ai chi at many senior centers as well as health clubs.

Water exercise. Water workouts put almost no stress on the joints because water supports the body's weight. A person doesn't have to be a good swimmer to benefit from this exercise. Simply walking through water challenges balance, increases flexibility, and strengthens muscles in the arms and legs.

Lifting weights. This is among the best exercises for people of all ages. Lifting weights strengthens muscles, moves joints through their full range of motion, and may help reverse bone loss caused by osteoporosis. One study found that people who lifted weights three times weekly for up to 10 weeks had strength gains of up to 200%. The one drawback to lifting weights is that it requires instruction. But going to a gym to lift weights can be an advantage, because many people enjoy getting out of the house. Also, an increasing number of health clubs offer weight-training classes geared toward older adults

Yard work. People don't think of gardening or raking leaves as exercise, but yard work provides an excellent workout. It involves a lot of bending, kneeling, and walking that will count toward anyone's exercise "total."

MAKE YOUR HOME SAFER

More than 75% of falls occur at home, often when people are pursuing their usual activities, such as standing, climbing stairs, or walking to the bathroom at night.

The average home probably has hundreds of potential trouble spots. You can minimize the danger of falls by recognizing risky areas and making a few simple adjustments. For example:

• Install low-pile, wall-to-wall carpeting wherever possible. It provides a softer surface if a fall occurs. But don't overpad the carpet, because this may pose a tripping hazard.

• Put nonslip rubber mats in the bathroom, kitchen, and other "wet" areas.

• Route electrical cords behind furniture. In areas where cords have to be exposed, tape them down. You can buy tape that's made for this purpose in hardware stores.

• Make sure there's good lighting in halls, stairwells, and other fall-prone areas. Even if your loved one sees well most of the time, her night vision probably isn't optimal. You don't want an open closet door or an "invisible" step to take her by surprise. It's ideal to have electrical switches at both ends of hallways and at the tops and bottoms of stairs. If this isn't possible, take advantage of nightlights. They only cost a few dollars, and the bulbs typically last six months or longer.

• Few things are more comfortable than an ankle-hugging bathrobe, but the long folds are a

OTHER STRATEGIES FOR PREVENTING FALLS

Good balance is important for preventing falls. But your loved one will also need to ensure that his posture and style of walking (gait) are most efficient and stable.

• Many older adults stoop forward when they walk. This challenges balance and results in smaller steps than usual, which in turn reduces the body's momentum and walking efficiency. The person takes more energy to travel a given distance and faces an increased risk of falling on the hip. Encourage your loved one to stand as straight as he comfortably can. The trick is to tighten the abdominal muscles while slightly pulling the shoulders back.

• If your loved one has musculoskeletal problems, he may find himself taking uneven steps (long steps when his weight is supported on the "good" leg, short steps when he's standing on the "bad" one). This style of walking can be unstable. Your loved one needs to practice putting equal weight on each leg when he

tripping hazard. Choose a robe and sash that stop just below the knee.

• Falls in the kitchen are common. Wet floors are only part of the problem; particularly injurious falls occur when people are standing on chairs or stepladders to reach high shelves. A good preventive strategy is to store frequently used items, such as cans of soup, cereal boxes, or cooking utensils, in easy-to-reach places so they don't require climbing or overhead lifting.

• On stairs, persons should always keep their hands free to hold the railing.

• Rearrange furniture to create wide walking areas. This can be a challenge in small houses and apartments, but it's worth doing because a lot of falls occur when people bump into the protruding corners of end tables or sofas or trip on furniture legs.

• Smooth out rough patches on sidewalks. You can buy small cans of instant cement at hardware stores. The cement can be used to seal cracks in sidewalks and curbs.

• If your loved one spends time in the yard, take a few minutes to look for holes or depressions in the grass, then fill them with soil or gravel.

• If you have children or pets in the house, do a regular patrol for blocks, balls, or other toys that can create a tripping hazard. Keep pet feeding bowls out of places where your loved one walks.

walks. He should also try to keep the stride length equal. If he isn't able to do this, you'll need to ask your health care provider for advice.

• Some elderly adults need canes, but neglect to use them. This is a mistake, because canes and other devices to aid mobility give support and help maintain balance, reducing the risk of falls.

• Remind your loved one to change positions slowly. This helps prevent a condition called postural hypotension, in which blood pressure temporarily drops during changes in position, causing dizziness and sometimes falls. This can occur when people get out of bed first thing in the morning. Your loved one should first swing his legs into a sitting position, rest for a few seconds, and then stand all the way up. He should stand still for a few seconds before starting to walk. This gives blood pressure a chance to normalize between positions.

• Persons taking medications should periodically review them with a health care provider. Start by making a list of all the medications the person is taking, including over-the-counter drugs and supplements. Even when individual medications don't affect balance or mobility, interactions between different drugs may cause dizziness or other side effects.

• Encourage the consumption of calcium-rich foods, such as yogurt and low-fat milk. Calcium is essential for strong bones and reduces the risk of fractures. Elderly women need 1500 milligrams calcium daily; elderly men need 1200 milligrams. An 8-ounce glass of milk has about 350 milligrams of calcium. A half-cup serving of cottage cheese has nearly 340 milligrams, and a cup of plain, low-fat yogurt has more than 400 milligrams.

• Another important strategy is to wear well-fitting shoes with nonskid soles. They provide good traction on slick floors, and they also provide better balance than heels or pumps. Also, remind your loved one not to walk around the house wearing socks, which provide little traction. You may want to get him a pair of comfortable slippers with nonskid soles. Avoid backless slippers.

OVERCOMING THE FEAR OF FALLS

The fear of falling can be almost as disabling as the falls themselves. Many elderly adults are so frightened of falling that they curtail their daily activities unnecessarily. Apart from the fact that this can take a lot of the pleasure out of life, it also results in a sedentary lifestyle, which increases the risk for balance and mobility problems.

If you suspect that fear is causing your loved one to restrict normal activities, it may be helpful to see your health care provider or physical therapist right away. The more sedentary a person becomes, the harder it will be for her to regain full mobility later on. Offer to take your loved one for short walks, and allow her to hold on to her walker or take you by the arm. The same techniques that physical therapists use to improve balance are also used to reduce the fear of falling. When people are given the opportunity to bend, twist, and move in a controlled way under the supervision of a therapist, they begin to regain their strength as well as their confidence. Here are some other helpful techniques.

Talk about previous falls. If your loved one has fallen in the past, encourage her to talk about it. Falls can have an enormous emotional impact. Give your loved one a chance to tell the story. Acknowledge how frightening the experience really was. Talking about fears will go a long way toward helping your loved one overcome them.

Keep phones within easy reach. If someone doubts their ability to get up after a fall, the very idea of losing balance—and lying helpless on the floor until help arrives—can be terrifying. One way to overcome this fear is to put telephones in all the places your loved one is likely to go. That way, she'll be able to call for help if necessary. And be sure to locate the phones in easy-to-reach places. If your loved one falls, she may not be able to reach a phone that's high on a wall or on a tall table.

Consider a personal alarm. A number of companies sell personal emergency response systems that are worn on the wrist or around the neck. Should your loved one fall, she can press a button, which will automatically dial an emergency phone number. There's a good chance she'll never use the alarm, but simply knowing it's there will help her feel more confident and secure. You should practice using this so your loved one is able to use it in the event of an emergency.

Rehearse. Ask your loved one's physical therapist to help him or her practice getting up from the floor.

ASSISTIVE DEVICES

According to national surveys, the one thing that frightens older adults the most—even more than dying—is losing their independence and being a burden on their families. Physical disabilities, however, present formidable obstacles. How can someone live alone if he can't walk more than a few steps or get up from the toilet without assistance? How can he get dressed if his fingers are too stiff to manage buttons, laces, or zippers?

Assistive devices can make the difference between living independently and depending on others. Just as important, these products, which are simply devices that make it easier to perform everyday tasks, can make it possible for many persons to stay active and mobile regardless of physical limitations. Approximately 65% of elderly adults with disabilities own one or more assistive devices. All too often, however, people buy assistive devices, then never take the time to learn how to use them.

Inconvenience is certainly a factor. Using a cane or a walker can seem more cumbersome than walking unassisted. Also, some persons may be embarrassed to use them in front of other people.

Don't let these or other issues prevent your loved one from taking advantage of these very helpful devices. Physical and occupational therapists can recommend products that are efficient and easy to use, and also give advice on the best ways to use them. The potential benefits of these products—the ability to walk farther, go more places, and generally live more safely and independently—will more than offset the initial resistance.

People tend to get overwhelmed when they first start looking at assistive aids. There are probably 20,000 to 30,000 different products to choose from. Most of them, however, fall into a few main categories. You'll find aids for:

• General mobility
• Getting out of bed or chairs
• Dressing
• Eating
• Using the toilet
• Recreation
• Grooming

It would take an entire book to discuss all of these products in detail. In the following pages we'll discuss some of the most popular products and provide advice on the best ways to use them. One more point: Even though assistive aids can be expensive, some of their cost may be covered under Medicare Part B, which will pay 80 percent of the cost for certain specific diagnosis-related aids if they are prescribed by your health care provider.

AIDS FOR MOBILITY

Whether your loved one's disability is temporary or permanent, mobility aids are an excellent investment. But to get the most for your money—and to make sure your loved one is best protected against falls—mobility aids need to be selected and fit by a therapist who can also instruct you and your loved one on their proper use. Aids can actually cause falls, rather than prevent them, if they are not selected and used properly.

Canes. These are the least conspicuous of all the mobility aids, and they're also the least cumbersome. The most popular ones are simply straight canes. They can support about 25% of the body's weight, and they're easy to use in tight or crowded places. If your loved one is frail or has problems with balance, her therapist might recommend a multiple-prong cane, which provides additional balance and support

When selecting canes, consider the handle. The simple curved "candy cane" configuration is comfortable to hold and can be looped over the arm when it's not in use. However, the curved handle may be hard for those with poor wrist or hand strength to grip. Your health care provider may recommend a cane that has a "pistol grip." This style distributes the body's weight more evenly and is generally more comfortable to use.

A common mistake people make is holding the cane on the side of the body that's weak. It should be held in the hand on the unaffected side of the body. The cane and the affected leg should swing and hit the ground together.

When using a cane to go up steps, your loved one should step up with his good leg, then bring up the cane and the affected leg together. Coming down, he should lead with the affected leg and cane, then follow with the good leg. This technique makes it possible for the strong leg to lift and lower the weight of the body.

Walkers. If your loved one is frail or has pain or weakness, a therapist might recommend a walker. Walkers support up to 50% of the body's weight. They're not as maneuverable as canes and can be cumbersome to get in and out of cars. On the other hand, people who use walkers can often stand or walk for a long time without discomfort.

Walkers should be adjusted for your loved one's height and posture. Many walkers have rubber tips on the legs. This style works well if your loved one is physically able to lift the walker and move it forward as he moves.

If the person doesn't have good balance or upper body strength, the therapist might recommend a front-wheeled walker. Rather than lifting the walker when moving forward, all he has to do is push it forward and walk along behind it.

If a person in your home is using a walker, you may need to rearrange furniture or rugs at home in order to provide a clear walking area. It may be necessary to remove doors from narrow doorways, as well. Be sure to measure the doorways before you invest in a walker.

Wheelchairs. If your loved one is too frail to use a cane or other walking aids, a wheelchair can be a great liberator. Some people use wheelchairs only on occasion; others depend on them to get around.

Be sure to consult your loved one's health care provider or therapist before investing in a wheelchair. This will help ensure that you don't spend money on features that the person really doesn't need. Also, he'll learn how to use the wheelchair properly. There are many styles of wheelchairs. The most popular are "manual" chairs with large rear wheels; motorized chairs are only recommended for those who have very little strength or mobility. A chair equipped with "desk arms" makes it easier for the person using it to scoot the chair forward when he's working at a desk or the kitchen table.

When you're buying or leasing a chair, you'll have to find a compromise between comfort and mobility. You want a chair that's small enough to fit easily through doorways and other tight places, but that's wide enough for comfort. For adults, the standard seats are 16 inches or 18 inches wide.

Rope pulls or trapezes. Many elderly adults have difficulty getting out of bed or rising from low chairs. A simple solution is to install an overhead "pull," which will allow your loved one to use her arms as well as her legs when standing up.

Elevated seats. These are among the simplest assistive devices. If your loved one has good mobility overall, but still has trouble rising out of a low chair, you can make things easier by folding a blanket and putting it in the seat of a chair, or under a couch or chair cushion. The boost in height may be all she needs to get out of the chair without assistance. The person's feet should be firmly on the floor, but the sitting area should be raised so that their knees are at a right angle and their bottoms are not lower than their knees.

Hand rails. Hand rails provide a good gripping surface when your loved one needs extra support. It's especially important to install rails in stairways, bathrooms, and in the hall between the bathroom and the bedroom.

AIDS FOR BATHING

The bathroom is probably the most challenging room in the house. The floors get wet and slick. Your loved one may have to balance on one leg while climbing into the tub or shower. She'll have to lower herself to the toilet, and then stand up again—a high-risk movement that causes many elderly adults to get dizzy and lose their balance.

Another danger in the bathroom is simply the isolation. When the door is closed and the water's running, you may not hear your loved one call for help should she slip and fall.

Hundreds of products are available that can make bathrooms safer. Some of the most important include:

Grab bars. Get a therapist's advice about placing them around the tub, shower, and toilet. Your loved one can use the bars as an aid to standing up. Should she get dizzy, a grab bar will allow her to hold herself upright until she recovers.

Nonskid mats or strips. They should interrupt every slick surface—in the shower and tub as well as on tile or linoleum floors.

Tub seats. If your loved one doesn't have enough mobility to settle comfortably into the tub, or if she isn't strong enough to stand in the shower, you may want to get a tub seat, which will allow her to sit down while she's washing. If you do get a tub seat, you'll probably want to install a hand-held shower device as well.

Bath stools. These are similar to tub seats, except they don't have backs. The advantage of stools is that they fit in narrow tubs and are easy to move and store. They don't provide back support, however, which your loved one may need.

Modified bath brushes. If your loved one finds it difficult to move her shoulders or bend her arms, a bath brush with an extra-long handle makes washing much easier. Some models have U-shaped handles, which allow people with limited mobility to wash their backs without assistance.

OTHER HELPFUL PRODUCTS

You can find assistive aids for virtually every type of disability. Consult an occupational therapist for advice and ideas. They are thoroughly familiar with the variety of deficits that people may have and the assistive devices that can help them. Your loved one may need a product that makes it easier to brush her hair. If she cooks, she'll need kitchen utensils that aren't too heavy and are easy to carry. If she has poor hand or finger strength, she'll benefit from products that make it easier to fasten a dress or blouse.

Talk to an occupational therapist about the following possibilities:

Easy-to-fasten garments. They're equipped with Velcro closures, enlarged zipper pulls, or hooks instead of buttons. They come in every size and style imaginable, and your loved one will appreciate being able to dress herself without having to ask for assistance.

Long-handled grabbers. They can help your loved one get what she needs from high shelves. They're also handy for picking up things from the floor, like socks.

Padded handles. If your loved one has arthritis or poor hand strength, padded handles are a must. Made from foam or easy-to-hold plastic, the handles make it much easier to hold cook pots, yard implements, and other household products. You can buy utensils that already have the padded handles. Or you can buy kits that allow you to modify the handles of utensils that you already own.

Oversized grooming aids. It takes a lot of dexterity to handle small objects like toothbrushes and fingernail clippers. Manufacturers now make these products in larger sizes. They generally have foam or rubber handles that are easy to grip.

Electric toothbrushes and razors. These are a real boon for those with limited arm or shoulder strength. They're easy to hold and they work just as well as the "manual" kinds.

ADDITIONAL RESOURCES

ORGANIZATIONS AND WEB SITES

National Institute on Aging
800-222-2225
www.nia.nih.gov

BOOKS AND ARTICLES

Anderson, Bob. *Stretching*. Bolinas, Calif.: Shelter Publications, 1980.

Consumer Product Safety Commission. *Safety For Older Consumers Home Safety Checklist*. CPSC Document #701. Internet on-line. http://www.cpsc.gov/CPSCPUB/PUBS/701.html. July 2002.

Nelson, Miriam. *Strong Women Stay Young*. New York: Bantam Books, 1998.

Rowe, J. W., and R. L. Kahn. *Successful Aging*. New York: Pantheon Books, 1998.

Nutrition, Feeding, and Eating Problems

illions of the country's elderly quietly face a grave concern: They are unable to consume enough food to remain healthy.

A recent government survey shows that 40% of all Americans over age 70 eat less than two-thirds of their recommended daily calorie requirements. This epidemic of undernutrition stems from a wide range of physical, psychological, and social problems. Many older people, facing the high cost of medication and housing, simply do not have the money necessary to purchase nutritious food. Others lose interest in food because of depression, grief, or alcoholism. And for an estimated 16 to 22% of people over the age of 50, disease or injury makes the actual process of feeding or eating difficult or impossible.

Any number of diseases or underlying health conditions can lead to difficulties with feeding and/or eating. Arthritis can make movement in the hands and mouth so painful that people give up and fail to get enough nutrition. Those with Alzheimer's disease, Parkinson's disease, stroke, and other neurologic disorders can lose the muscle coordination needed to bring food to their mouths and eat it. These conditions also are leading causes of dysphagia—the inability to process food and deliver it from the mouth to the stomach. Other causes include cancers in the mouth and esophagus, chronic heartburn, or structural or motility problems that prevent food and liquids from reaching the digestive tract or being properly digested and absorbed. Medications can reduce saliva flow, increase drowsiness, and cause other side effects that make eating harder.

Even those who ingest enough calories may not receive the proper mix of nutrients to maintain healthy body function. Many senior citizens eat foods that are high in fat, sugar, and sodium. They also tend to eat fewer fruits, vegetables, and dairy products, instead favoring processed foods that are easier to prepare and eat, but may be lower in essential nutrients. As a result, many elderly people may be lacking in essential nutrients such as vitamins A, B1, B2, B6, C and D, and minerals such as calcium and zinc.

This type of diet can lead to many maladies. Malnourished older adults are at greater risk for infections, anemia, loss of muscle mass and strength, falls, and decreased cognitive abilities. It has been estimated that about 85 percent of all chronic diseases and physical disabilities among the elderly could be prevented, or at least improved, with proper diet.

Fortunately, certain types of therapy (physical, occupational, and diet) and other interventions can improve a person's ability to obtain an adequate diet. Caregivers and patients both can learn how to create the right environment for eating, one that encourages a person to eat more and to eat better, more nutritious food. Exercises to improve muscle strength and coordination can make the job easier, as can placing the patient in positions that make swallowing and chewing more efficient. Learning how to choose and prepare nutritious, easily digestible foods is also an essential part of a feeding and eating program. And consistent monitoring of a person's food intake, weight, and nutritional status can help prevent or reverse malnutrition and its consequences. It's never too late to detect and correct these problems; researchers have shown that even patients age 85 and older can live significantly longer, healthier lives with the help of improved nutrition.

WHAT CAUSES FEEDING AND EATING PROBLEMS?

AGE-RELATED CHANGES

As men and women age, they usually need fewer calories to maintain proper body functions. On average, senior citizens require about 25% fewer calories than young adults. The Recommended Daily Allowance (RDA) recommends about 2300 calories per day for an average man over the age of 50, and about 1900 calories for women in the same age bracket. These figures are 20 and 15% lower, respectively, than the RDAs for younger adults. The actual needs of individuals may vary greatly from the RDAs, depending on activity levels, metabolism, and other factors, such as illness.

In general, older adults need fewer calories for two reasons. First, because with age comes a decline in metabolic rate associated with a decline in muscle mass; second, because older people tend to be less physically active than younger adults. Studies have found that people who get little exercise lose about 15% of their lean muscle mass between age 20 and age 70. But loss of muscle may not be completely inevitable. Active seniors can often slow the rate of decline with exercise and weight training.

Muscle mass. Changes in muscle mass (and fat tissue) can result in weight loss. Men begin losing weight at an average of 0.5% per year starting at about age 60, while women typically begin the same rate of decline at about age 65. Although weight loss in obese people is usually welcome and healthy, it can be a warning sign in the elderly. Weight loss beyond about 4% in one year (about 5 pounds in a 120-pound person, or about 6 pounds in a 150-pound person) often indicates an underlying health problem.

Nutritional requirements. Although calorie requirements decline over the years, elderly people continue to need about the same intake of micronutrients—vitamins, minerals, and other substances that aid specific body functions. The RDA levels for micronutrients are not significantly different for seniors than for younger adults, although older people more often fail to reach the recommended daily levels. This points out the need for nutrient-dense foods, which pack more micronutrients into fewer overall calories. Daily supplements can help some older people reach their RDA needs for micronutrients. Experts stress, however, that vitamin pills should complement, not replace, nutrients from a balanced diet.

Appetite. Normal, age-related changes in the body can make eating more challenging. Appetite tends to decrease with age, often because the stomach senses fullness earlier in a meal. Older people also tend to have decreased senses of taste and smell, which can make food less appealing. Sweet and salty tastes are usually affected the most; this is why many older people desire increased amounts of sugar and salt in their diets. Seniors also usually have a decreased sense of thirst, which can keep them from drinking as much as they should to keep from becoming dehydrated.

Gastrointestinal function. Most stomach and intestinal functions remain the same as a person ages. But abnormal conditions are common. Atrophic gastritis, an inflammation of the stomach lining, occurs in 20 to 50% of the population. It can cause stomach pain that makes eating unpleasant, and also may interfere with nutrient absorption. Problems in the small intestines often lead to lactose intolerance in older people. Eating milk-based products creates painful side effects, and can keep people from eating for fear of a bad reaction. This can be especially dangerous for elderly people, who need calcium in milk products to ward off osteoporosis.

Dental changes. Tooth loss or replacement of teeth with dentures is another common age-related cause of poor eating. People with dentures must use up to five times as much effort to chew food as those with natural teeth. This can lead to inadequate chewing, which in turn can cause problems with swallowing and digestion. Since chewing activates taste buds and makes food enjoyable, people with dental problems may show a lack of interest in eating. When they do eat, people with chewing troubles often pick soft foods, which tend to be high in calories and refined ingredients and low in nutrients.

DISEASE-RELATED CHANGES

Scores of diseases and conditions can cause eating difficulties in older adults. These range from site-specific problems, such as gastroesophageal reflux (persistent heartburn) and peptic ulcers, to neurologic disorders like Parkinson's disease, stroke, multiple sclerosis, and Alzheimer's disease. In addition, cardiovascular disease, arthritis, and other conditions can rob people of the energy and mobility they need to prepare and eat meals. Following is a brief look at some of the most common conditions that affect eating and/or digesting food.

Oral problems. Gum disease and inflammation can cause pain in the mouth and give food unpleasant taste. Tooth loss is a problem, of course—but so are cavities and other problems such as receding gums that lead to sensitive teeth. In some older adults, salivary glands in the mouth fail to provide enough moisture to process food for easy swallowing and digestion. Bone loss in the jaws can result in tooth loss, difficulty chewing, and the inability to wear dentures. Oral cancers are also a major concern. More than 98% of mouth cancers occur after the age of 40, and the average age for onset is 60. Cancer in the lips, tongue, and other parts of the mouth can destroy a person's ability to chew and swallow.

Gastrointestinal diseases. Peptic ulcers are not more common in older people, although the risk of bleeding ulcers grows greater with age. Diverticulitis, the formation of small, painful pouches in the large intestine, can cause great pain and discourage eating and is much more common in older people. Inflammatory bowel disease, which includes Crohn's disease and ulcerative colitis, can have the same effects. These can also affect the body's ability to absorb nutrients. The incidence of cancers in the gastrointestinal tract—including colon and rectal cancer—also increases greatly with age.

Diabetes. This disease affects the body's ability to process sugar and starches obtained from food. In most people, diabetes can cause unusual changes in thirst and hunger. It also can lead to inadequate saliva production, which in turn can cause cavities and infections in the mouth. People with diabetes must learn to adapt their diets. They must eat smaller, more frequent meals and avoid refined sugar and excess fat. These changes can be difficult for elderly people, who must overcome a lifetime of eating habits while also learning to deal with the other complications of the disease.

Anorexia. Anorexia—a diminished appetite or an aversion to food—affects many older women and men. Women who had the eating disorder of anorexia nervosa in the past may suffer a recurrence of the disease when they are older. Both women and men are at risk for anorexia tardive, a form of the disease that, by definition, begins late in life. This can be triggered by depression and other psychological causes.

Stroke. As many as 700,000 Americans suffer strokes each year. Strokes can have devastating effects on a person's ability to eat. The most common problem is dysphagia, or difficulty with swallowing. This occurs in about 45% of all stroke victims. Strokes can lead to paralysis in the throat or mouth, which can make chewing and swallowing extremely challenging. In some cases, stroke victims develop aphagia, the complete inability to swallow. Even when swallowing seems to be occurring normally, some older people may develop aspiration pneumonia, when some food or secretions enter the trachea instead of the swallowing tube (esophagus). Of course, strokes also can affect a person's mobility and mental capacities, making eating far more difficult.

Parkinson's disease. This nerve-related disease causes swallowing difficulties in about 50% of people with the disease. Symptoms can be mild or severe, and can worsen over time. Many people with Parkinson's disease eventually rely on others to feed them, or need to have feeding tubes inserted to provide adequate nutrition and hydration.

Arthritis. While primarily a disease of the joints, arthritis also can lead to eating problems. In fact, people with arthritis are often poorly nourished. In rheumatoid arthritis, inflammation can occur in the intestinal linings and interfere with the absorption of several nutrients—including vitamins C, D, B6, and B12; iron; magnesium; and others. Some people must take more than the RDA (or normal amounts) of these nutrients, since the body has difficulty absorbing them. In addition, the loss of mobility and depression that often results from arthritis can cause a person to eat less food.

Alzheimer's disease. Dementia resulting from Alzheimer's can destroy a person's desire and ability to eat, or may cause them to choose foods that do not meet their nutritional needs. While specific intakes of nutrients have not been clearly linked to prevention or progression of Alzheimer's, it is vital that patients receive proper, balanced meals. A daily multivitamin with minerals may also be recommended.

SWALLOWING DISORDERS

Swallowing difficulties are the most important eating-related problem facing the elderly. Swallowing is a complex, three-part process that requires no fewer than 50 pairs of muscles and a vast number of nerve inputs to complete. It involves both voluntary and involuntary actions to complete properly. Problems can arise at any point in the process, depending on a patient's underlying condition.

In the first stage of swallowing, the mouth readies food for passage into the stomach. The lips, teeth, tongue, cheeks, and salivary glands work together to form a softened ball of food that is easy to swallow. In the second stage, the tongue pushes the food to the back of the mouth and triggers the involuntary swallowing reflex. The windpipe closes, preventing aspiration of the food or liquid into the lungs. Muscles in the throat then help propel the food downward in a series of contractions called peristalsis. In the third and final stage, the food or liquid passes through the lower portion of the throat, through the swallowing tube (the esophagus), which connects with the upper part of the stomach. Peristalsis continues until the food passes through a muscular gate called the lower esophageal sphincter (also known as the gastroesophageal sphincter) and into the stomach.

Normal aging does not appear to seriously affect the swallowing process. There is some evidence, however, that humans become less efficient at swallowing as they grow older. People take longer to complete the first two swallowing phases, and may leave some food residue in the back of the mouth or top of the throat. But a number of underlying diseases and conditions can lead to more severe swallowing difficulties, a problem called dysphagia. This condition affects at least 7 to 10% of all adults over the age of 50. The number may actually be higher, since many people do not report mild cases to their physicians. People who

COMMON CAUSES OF DYSPHAGIA IN THE ELDERLY

- Stroke (the most common cause)
- Parkinson's disease, Alzheimer's disease, and injury to the brain and/or spinal cord
- Tumors in the esophageal tract
- Scar tissue in the esophagus
- Schatzki's rings (abnormal cords of tissue that constrict the lower esophagus)
- Medications, including certain antibiotics, blood pressure drugs, antihistamines, and painkillers

live in nursing homes are far more likely than others to show signs of dysphagia; estimates show that 30 to 40% of those who live in these settings have trouble swallowing.

Dysphagia can be a dangerous condition, putting people at risk for several serious complications, including ruptures of the esophagus, choking, and aspiration pneumonia. The last condition occurs when food that is being swallowed accidentally ends up in the lungs and causes infection. Of course, people with dysphagia also are at great risk for undernutrition or malnutrition, since they are much less likely to eat a proper diet or consume adequate amounts of food than people who can swallow normally.

Dysphagia usually requires major changes in food selection and preparation, to make swallowing easier. Swallowing therapy also can help, as can a number of physical techniques, such as positioning the patient in ways that enhance the body's limited ability to swallow. In cases of severe dysphagia or aphagia, the patient may require a temporary or permanent feeding tube. These can be placed through the nose and down the esophagus, or directly through the abdominal wall and into the stomach or small intestine.

A final note: Dysphagia should not be confused with a condition called "globus sensation," which is simply a feeling of having a lump in the throat. This condi-

SIGNS OF DYSPHAGIA

Swallowing problems are often predictable when an underlying condition or disease is present. But sometimes the changes are subtle and not easily detected at first. Below are signs of dysphagia that caregivers should be on the alert for.

- Hesitation when swallowing
- Regurgitation of food, through either the nose or the mouth
- Coughing during swallowing
- Drooling
- Repeated throat clearing of a "lump" in the person's throat
- Recurrent bouts of pneumonia
- Noticeable hoarseness or repeated complaints of a sore throat
- Complaints of chest pain when swallowing
- Complaints that food is "sticking" in a person's throat
- A constant need to "wash food down" with liquids
- Loss of interest in food
- Weight loss due to decreased food intake

tion is not related to swallowing, and often occurs when a person is facing a great deal of anxiety or grief.

WHO IS AT RISK?

Because of the large number and variety of health conditions that can cause feeding and eating problems, virtually every older person is at risk. The occurrence increases with advancing age, as might be expected. Older people are more likely to suffer from one or more diseases, and those diseases are more likely to be at an advanced stage. In an ongoing national study of 3000 older Americans, about 4% of those ages 60 to 69 were unable to prepare and eat their own meals, compared with 23% of those over 80 years old.

Living arrangements and socioeconomic status also can play a role. Older people who live alone are more likely to eat poorly, regardless of physical barriers to food preparation and eating. Inadequate nutrition also is more common among the poor. Between 8 percent and 16 percent of older adults don't have consistent access to nutritionally adequate, culturally compatible diets.

HOW ARE EATING PROBLEMS DIAGNOSED?

Feeding and eating difficulties are usually signs of an underlying health condition. Yet elderly people and their caregivers often accept mild swallowing problems, moderate weight loss, and reduced caloric intake as normal parts of aging. Most people only seek medical attention when more pronounced, tangible symptoms appear—dementia, for instance, or slurred speech, painful joints, headaches, or other problems. Small changes in appetite or activities may indicate a need for evaluation.

This is an unfortunate and potentially dangerous scenario. In many ways, poor nutrition can contribute to the severity and scope of diseases. Low intake of vitamin D and calcium, for instance, can hasten the progression of osteoporosis. Inadequate intake of B vitamins has been linked to a number of conditions, from heart disease to anemia. And overall malnutrition can lead to fatigue and diminished mental function.

It is very important for caregivers to monitor a person's eating habits and weight carefully. Elderly people should not lose weight as a matter of course. Any unusual shift in weight—more than 10% in either direction—could be a sign of underlying problems. When weight loss or gain occurs with no readily apparent cause, a visit to a physician is in order.

PHYSICAL EXAM

The first, and often most important, part of making a diagnosis involves taking a history of a patient's symptoms, medications, and previously known health conditions. This can help the doctor narrow the possible causes for the new complaints. The problem may be evident, such as tooth decay or loss of a loved one, or it may be due to an underlying disease. Therefore, doctors may require a number of tests, including x-rays, CAT scans, blood analysis, and more, to determine the cause.

When swallowing difficulties are suspected or observed, doctors may perform other tests to determine the extent and location of the problem. These are usually conducted by, or under the direction of, a specialist known as a speech and language pathologist. A physical examination is usually the first step. The doctor will check the patient's reflexes and look for signs of cognitive impairment that could indicate an underlying neurological disorder. A physical examination of the mouth can show problems. Bad breath or poor coloration in the mouth, for instance, can indicate poor saliva production. Palpation of the mouth, throat, and neck can detect other problems, such as growths on the thyroid gland, esophagus, and larynx.

The doctor also may observe the patient as he drinks and eats. This can help reveal the location of the difficulty, be it in the mouth, pharynx, or esophagus. Touching the throat while the patient swallows can indicate whether the person is able to close off the windpipe during swallowing, or whether food or liquid is slipping into the lungs.

LABORATORY TESTS

Based on the results of the physical examination, the specialist may order several laboratory tests, including blood tests for infections or inflammatory conditions. These initial tests are usually sufficient to identify the nature and extent of a person's swallowing difficulties. But several additional examinations can help confirm the diagnosis and show whether the patient is at risk for aspiration. These tests are usually performed by specialists like radiologists, otolaryngologists, or gastroenterologists.

Nasopharyngoscopy. This test involves using a small, fiber-optic camera to observe the function of the mouth and nasal passages during eating. A small amount of anesthesia is used to ease the insertion of the device through the nose or mouth. The test can identify growths or lesions in the mouth, nose, or upper throat that might be interfering with food chewing and swallowing.

Modified barium swallow study. Also known as videofluoroscopic cineradiography, this test can help doctors observe the transit of food from the mouth through the esophagus. During the test, patients are asked to eat and drink items that have been mixed with barium. As the patient processes the food, a series of x-ray pictures are taken to track the progress of the food. The procedure usually takes about twenty to thirty minutes. It is primarily used to identify the location of the swallowing difficulty. It can be especially useful in pointing out growths and other structural problems that can lead to dysphagia.

Gastroesophageal endoscopy. In some cases, this procedure is used in place of, or in addition to, a barium study. It involves inserting a flexible tube through the mouth into the esophagus to view the area with a small camera. It is considered more accurate than barium studies in many respects. It can show lesions and growths in the esophageal tract, although it does not show overall motility of food as well as barium studies. Doctors are able to perform other tasks while using the endoscope, like taking biopsies of growths found in the esophagus and stretching areas of the esophagus that have been constricted by scarring or other problems. Endoscopies are more expensive to perform than barium studies, so they are performed less frequently.

Manometry. In this test, a probe is inserted into the esophagus that measures the strength and coordination of muscle contractions as food passes down the esophagus and into the stomach. Manometry is usually performed only if endoscopy and barium studies have found no abnormal structures in the esophagus.

Esophageal pH monitoring. Sometimes dysphagia results from scarring in the esophagus caused by escaped stomach acid. This results from acid reflux disease, better known as heartburn. To test for the disorder, doctors will sometimes use a technique called esophageal pH monitoring. A probe is inserted through the nose and into the esophagus. Over a 24-hour period, the probe measures acid levels in the esophagus, to see if stomach fluids are escaping. This test is sometimes combined with manometry to see if acid reflux leads to spasms in the esophagus.

HOW ARE THESE PROBLEMS TREATED?

Once eating difficulties are diagnosed, the goal is to return the patient to as normal a dietary routine as the patient can tolerate. This usually involves a combination of therapy, dietary changes, and, in some cases, surgery and/or medication. The treatments vary widely, depending on the nature of the problem and its underlying cause.

Nutritional therapy. In many cases, doctors will recommend a consultation with a nutritionist, who will help the patient and caregiver design a workable plan for choosing, preparing, and eating nutritious and easily eaten foods. The nutritionist, preferably a registered dietitian (R.D.), will take a number of factors into account, including the patient's food preferences and the consistency of foods. Nutritional supplements such as liquid shakes and vitamin supplements also may be part of the plan. The nutritionist can create specialized eating programs to help with hypertension and heart disease, arthritis, diabetes, and other health conditions common among older persons.

The nutritionist can also provide instruction on how to interpret food labels. These labels, which are printed on almost all packaged foods in the United States, can be a valuable source of information on the nutritional content of food, and can help caregivers make informed decisions about which foods are best for the older patient.

Speech therapy and physical therapy. Specially trained therapists also play a major role. Physical therapists can help with the motor skills needed to prepare, cook, and deliver food to the patient's mouth. This can include training for caregivers of people who are unable to cook or eat on their own. Speech therapists can work with patients to improve chewing and swallowing. Therapists can show caregivers and patients a variety of swallowing techniques and physical positions that make eating easier, and reduce the risk of food going into the lungs. They also can provide exercises to strengthen muscles used in chewing and swallowing. The therapist also may provide advice on creating the proper eating environment, which can help make food more attractive and keep the patient's attention focused on eating.

Medication. At the same time, a physician should review the patient's medications, to see if medicines being taken for underlying conditions may be interfering with feeding or eating. In cases where heartburn affects eating, drugs may be able to help. Over-the-counter antacids can alleviate symptoms of heartburn. In more severe cases, short-acting acid blockers like famotidine (Pepcid AC), cimetidine (Tagamet), and ranitidine (Zantac) can reduce the amount of acid the stomach produces and help prevent heartburn. More powerful, long-acting medicines, called proton pump inhibitors (also called acid pump inhibitors), also work to keep the stomach from producing excess acids. Commonly used drugs include omeprazole (Prilosec) and lansoprazole (Prevacid). Another drug, metoclopramide (Reglan), increases the strength of the sphincter that separates the stomach from the esophagus. This can keep acid from slipping into the esophagus and damaging its lining. The drug also increases muscle action in the stomach, allowing patients to digest food faster and empty the stomach faster. These drugs are available only by prescription.

Surgery: In some cases, surgery may be able to relieve the cause of swallowing difficulty. Obviously, the removal of cancerous and nonmalignant growths in the mouth, throat, or esophagus can clear the passageway and make food easier to swallow. In cases where scarring has narrowed the esophagus, minor surgery can help stretch the opening and permit food to pass more easily. This is typically done with a balloon-like device that is placed in the esophagus and then gently inflated. When heartburn cannot be relieved by medication and dietary changes, surgery can strengthen the esophageal sphincter by wrapping part of the stomach around the lower esophagus. This procedure, called a Nissen fundoplication, is usually done with a minimally invasive technique, using a small camera that guides the surgeon as he uses tiny tools to make the repair. When the sphincter is too tight, a procedure called esophageal myotomy loosens the muscle by creating small incisions in the sphincter. In a growing number of cases, doctors opt for a different treatment: injections of a form of botulinum toxin that weakens the sphincter and allows it to open and close more easily.

Feeding tubes. In grave situations, doctors may decide to use a feeding tube to provide nutrition to a patient who could not otherwise get enough nutrition to survive. These tubes may be inserted either through the nose or through the abdominal wall into the stomach or into a particular area of the small intestine called the jejunum. This is commonly done for patients who have suffered strokes or are recovering from surgery of the mouth, throat, or esophagus. Recent studies show that the tubes inserted through the abdominal wall may provide better overall results. The risk for infection is somewhat higher because a surgical incision is required, but most insertions can be done endoscopically, rather than through open surgery.

The use of feeding tubes in advanced cases of Alzheimer's disease and other neurological disorders has become more controversial in recent years. Some research has shown that using the tubes in people who are no longer able to eat or drink does not enhance the patient's quality of life and may not even significantly extend life.

WHAT SHOULD YOU EXPECT?

The outlook for feeding and eating disorders depends greatly on the underlying disease. When neurologic problems are to blame, as in the case of strokes, improvement is possible over time with proper therapy. Many patients recover quickly in the first few weeks following a stroke, for example. As many as 86% of patients who have stroke-related dysphagia return to normal eating during this initial period. Even in those who remain dysphagic, the use of proper posture and other swallowing techniques can reduce the risk of aspiration by 75 to 80%. All

607

told, about 85% of people who have dysphagia caused by neurologic impairment and malignant growths in the mouth, throat, or esophagus can return to taking nutrients orally. These people may require feeding assistance, however. And in many neurological conditions like amyotrophic lateral sclerosis (Lou Gehrig's disease), Alzheimer's, and Parkinson's, further loss of motor skills is expected as the disease progresses.

Surgical procedures to correct gastroesophageal reflux disease (chronic heartburn) are successful about 90% of the time in people who have not responded to treatment with medications. In about 85% of cases, surgery is not even required; dietary changes, elevation of the head while sleeping, and medication are sufficient to cure the problem.

WHAT RESEARCH IS BEING DONE?

Experts are attacking the issue of feeding and eating difficulties on many levels. Nutritionists are working to reassess the nutritional needs of the elderly; this has resulted in a revision of Recommended Daily Allowance levels for people over the age of 70. Other researchers are looking at new techniques to stimulate swallow reflexes in people with dysphagia. This includes a proposed study of mild electrical stimulation of muscles in the larynx that play a large role in swallowing. New diagnostic techniques are being tested, including the possible use of ultrasound equipment to detect the exact location of swallowing problems. This may someday be used in place of, or along with, tests such as the barium swallow. Other techniques may be used in dysphagia exams, including magnetic resonance imaging (MRI) and computer-assisted tomography (CAT scans). These can help identify structural problems that are not readily seen with endoscopies.

Because feeding and eating problems are secondary to other diseases, research into underlying causes—neurologic disorders, cancers, and other problems—may yield new treatments that are disease-specific.

WHAT YOU CAN DO NOW

Dealing with feeding and eating problems requires a multilevel approach. The first step, diagnosis, is largely in the hands of health care professionals. But the remaining issues often fall to the caregiver to address. A caregiver must work with health care professionals to create a comprehensive plan that addresses all of a patient's needs. This should include nutritional goals; selection and preparation of foods; assistance with feeding; suggestions for improved eating and swallowing; dealing with constipation, incontinence, and voiding issues; securing food sources for the homebound or poor; and knowing how to handle choking.

NUTRITION FOR THE ELDERLY

Most Americans don't know much about specific nutritional needs of the elderly. Simply learning more about what, and how much, an older person should eat can give caregivers a good start on helping a person develop a good diet.

An elderly person's total calorie needs can vary greatly, depending on body size, activity level, and underlying medical conditions. As a general rule, people over the age of 50 need about 30 calories per kilogram of body weight. A kilogram is equal to about 2.2 pounds. Therefore, a 130-pound person (about 60 kg) would need about 1800 calories per day (60 kg times 30 calories) to maintain his or her weight. This figure is usually multiplied by 1.1 to 1.3 to take into account higher levels of activity or disease. Thus, a moderately active 130-pound person may need anywhere from 1980 to 2340 calories per day.

Alcoholic beverages should be limited to no more than one drink per day for women and two drinks per day for men. Wine, especially red wine, is preferable to hard liquor or beer.

Fat content should be kept to no more than 30% of overall calories, and cholesterol intake should not exceed 300 mg per day. In addition, sodium should be limited to 2000 to 3000 mg per day. It's important for elderly people to avoid low-nutrient snacks that are high in sugar, fat, or sodium—potato chips, tortilla chips, and candy bars are prime examples of foods to avoid. They provide empty calories that offer little nutritionally but still take up valuable room in the overall diet.

Below is a review of the United States Dietary Guidelines for Americans over 70 years of age. These are only guidelines; the actual dietary needs of a specific older person must be determined individually. Underlying diseases, such as cancer, diabetes, arthritis, or heart disease, can change nutritional requirements greatly.

Six or more servings of grain products per day. These include bread, rice, cereals, and pasta. One serving equals one slice of bread, 1 ounce of ready-to-eat cereals, or ½ cup of cooked cereals (oatmeal), rice, or pasta. Because older people generally eat less food, it's important to make sure that their diet includes whole-grain products, which contain more nutrients and fiber per serving. Vitamin-fortified foods are also a good choice, as they are more nutrient-dense than other products. Try to limit high-fat or high-salt grain products like biscuits, doughnuts, sweet rolls, and snack crackers.

Three or more servings of vegetables per day. One serving equals 1 cup of raw, leafy vegetables, ½ cup of other vegetables, either cooked or raw, or 6 ounces of vegetable juice. Dark green and yellow vegetables are generally more nutrient-rich than other vegetables. Try to get in at least one serving of raw vegetables per day. Limit deep-fried, highly salted, or pickled vegetables.

Two or more servings of fruit per day. One serving equals a medium-sized apple, orange, or banana; ½ cup of chopped, cooked, or canned fruit; and 6 ounces of fruit juice. As with vegetables, select a variety of fruits and have at least one serving of raw fruit per day. Try to avoid sweetened fruit juices, and high-fat fruits like coconut and avocado.

Three or more servings of dairy products per day. One serving equals 1 cup of milk or yogurt, 1.5 ounces of natural cheese, or 2 ounces of processed cheese. To lower overall fat intake, choose products that are made from skim or 1 percent milk. For lactose-intolerant people, choose from the growing variety of lactose-free dairy products.

Two or more servings of protein-rich foods per day. One serving equals 3 ounces of lean meat, poultry, or fish. Many other foods can replace animal meat for protein needs; try beans, eggs, and nuts. One-half cup of cooked dry beans equals 1 ounce of meat, as does one egg. Two tablespoons of peanut butter and 1/3 cup of nuts also equal 1 ounce of meat. Try to limit fried or fatty meats like sausage and poultry skin.

Fats, oils, and sweets sparingly. While these can enhance the flavor of food, they also can contribute high amounts of fat and minimal nutrition. The best fats are oils and margarines made from corn, cottonseed, olive, sesame, safflower, and canola. Limit butter, lard, and products made with hydrogenated vegetable oil or shortening. Try to choose desserts that are fruit-based and low in fat. Limit sugar-based desserts and whole-milk custards and puddings.

WATER INTAKE

Dietary guidelines call for drinking about two quarts of fluids per day. This is the equivalent of eight 8-ounce glasses of water. Coffee, tea, or other beverages containing caffeine don't count, since they are diuretics that induce urination and can further dehydrate the body. Alcohol has the same effect, and so it, too, doesn't count toward the daily total. People with heart failure or kidney failure should consult their doctor about how much fluid intake is required.

Experts believe that a substantial percentage of America's older population suffers from chronic mild dehydration. Many times, this happens because older people lose much of their ability to detect thirst. They don't drink as much water simply because they don't feel the urge to do so. Others curtail their fluid intake because they're afraid of being incontinent. Unfortunately, this can lead to significant health problems. Even a small water deficit may lead to impaired mental and physical performance.

Dehydration increases the risk of a variety of conditions, including nausea, elevated body temperature, and hypotension (low blood pressure), as well as kidney stones and constipation, which in turn can lead to a reluctance to eat for fear of further constipation.

NUTRITIONAL SUPPLEMENTS

As a rule, vitamins and minerals should be obtained from foods rather than supplements. Nutritional supplements may be helpful and, in some cases, necessary, but they should not be used in place of a balanced intake of a variety of foods. Besides vitamins and minerals, foods (especially fruits and vegetables) contain important nutrients called phytochemicals (such as carotenoids, allicin, and lutein) that may also be important in maintaining good health. But for many older people, especially those with limited food intake, daily supplements may provide some insurance that nutrient intake reaches recommended levels. In fact, studies show that between one-third and three-quarters of older adults already take supplements.

The American Medical Association recommends the use of a daily multivitamin with minerals for older people with reduced food consumption, but the American Dietetic Association recommends that patients consult with their physicians before beginning supplements. For some people, increased intake of certain nutrients can cause health problems. Vitamin and mineral supplements are often thought of as "safe," with little regard to possible adverse effects resulting from their interactions with medications. For example, excess vitamin K may counteract the effects of oral anticoagulants, leading to increased risk of stroke and similar conditions when these medications are being used to thin the blood and prevent abnormal blood clots from forming. Increased amounts of vitamin C may also decrease the effect of anticoagulants like Coumadin. Conversely, reducing the intake of vitamin K below the person's usual intake will tend to increase the effect of oral anticoagulants like Coumadin, and increase the risk of bleeding.

There is some evidence that seniors may benefit from supplementation of a few vitamins and minerals, such as vitamin B12, calcium, and vitamin D. Vitamin B12, found in animal proteins (meats), may become difficult to digest and absorb either because of a disease state, such as pancreatic insufficiency, diseases of the distal small bowel (ileum), and intestinal bacterial overgrowth, or use of medications such as antacids.

Adequate calcium intake may be difficult if there is a decreased intake of milk, cheeses, and yogurt. Recently, more foods have been fortified with calcium, such as juices, bread, and soups, but a daily supplement may be beneficial. Vitamin D is important to aid the absorption of calcium and, as with calcium, it is difficult to get adequate amounts from food. Together, calcium and vitamin D encourage healthy bone maintenance and may reduce the incidence of bone loss (and possibly bone fractures) in older adults.

Before taking a multivitamin supplement, ask a doctor. Typically, daily supplements that provide no more than 100% of RDAs for vitamins and minerals are sufficient and safe. Consider formulas specific to your loved one's stage of life.

In normal, healthy older adults who can consume balanced diets, liquid supplements are not recommended. These often claim to provide nutritional "insurance" to people, but they aren't necessary if a person eats a regular, healthy diet. Further, use of these supplements, which may be high in calories from simple sugars, may dull a person's appetite and keep him or her from eating a normal diet. Of course, when someone is unable to chew or swallow properly, supplements can be quite beneficial. Caregivers should consult with a doctor before giving an elderly patient liquid food supplements.

FEEDING ASSISTANCE

From setting a nice table to using specially designed cutlery, there are many options available to caregivers for helping their loved one get the most out of meals and mealtimes. Here are some suggestions.

Use assistive devices. A variety of assistive devices can make eating easier for people who have trouble bringing food from the plate to their mouths (see sidebar on p. 615).

Focus on the food. It's also important to create an environment that keeps people alert and focused on eating. The dining area should be brightly lit. It usually helps to eat in the same room all the time, to foster the idea that eating is important. The person should always sit in the same chair, and the chair should be placed away from the wall. This will help the caregiver reach behind and assist a person when necessary. It also allows for immediate action if the person should start to choke.

Use solid-colored plates. People with impaired vision usually find it easier to eat from solid-colored plates. Borders and designs can be distracting, and the designs may be mistaken for food. People with feeding difficulties may become frustrated when they repeatedly try to pick up "food" that is actually a design on a plate. To avoid confusion, place only necessary items on the table. For example, do not provide a knife, a spoon, and a fork if a fork is all that's necessary. Salt shakers and condiments also can add to the confusion.

Allow for rest. Because eating can be strenuous, it's a good idea to give an older person plenty of rest before mealtimes. Avoid stressful or tiring activities for one-half hour to two hours before eating. If a person becomes anxious shortly before mealtime, a small amount of exercise (either a brief walk or passive movements of the arms and legs) can help relieve tension. It's usually a bad idea to leave the television playing during mealtime, as this can be distracting. Some people, however, respond well to soft background music—especially familiar tunes that carry fond memories.

Maintain good posture. People with feeding problems should maintain the proper posture during mealtimes. Never give fluids and solid food to a person who is lying down or reclining in a chair—he or she could choke. The person should remain seated in an upright position while eating. Leaning forward slightly and keeping feet on the floor help steady the person. In some cases, a low table that allows the person to put his or her elbows on the table also can increase stability. When your loved one is confined to a bed, make sure he or she is sitting as upright as possible. Use pillows or wedges to position the upper body in a comfortable and stable posture.

The head should always be kept slightly down and pointing forward. If a person finds it difficult to keep his head steady, a caregiver can place the palm of her hand on the person's forehead, or position the patient's hand in the same position. The caregiver should sit directly across the table from the person, where she can observe most closely.

Allow sufficient time. It's important to allow enough time for meals. Many people need one-half hour to a full hour to take in enough food. Caregivers should make sure they clear their schedules to allow for these extended mealtimes. Sometimes, smaller, more frequent meals can keep a person focused on eating and minimize frustration at their slow pace.

Be supportive. Kind words and gentle reminders always help. Compliment your loved one when she or he eats well. Try to keep focus with comments like, "We're eating right now," or "Bring the fork all the way to your mouth." When necessary, caregivers can help a person bring food to her mouth with the hand-over-hand feeding technique. Place the utensil in the person's hand, then gently place your own hand overtop. Slowly bring the utensil to the mouth, letting the patient do as much work as possible. Only use this technique when needed; otherwise, encourage independent feeding as much as possible.

Consider finger food. Sometimes, eating with utensils becomes impossible. This can happen when motor skills decline to the point where handling tools is too difficult, or when cognitive skills erode and the person can no longer remember the purpose of utensils. At this point, it may be time to consider a "finger-food" diet. This involves creating bite-sized pieces of food that can be brought by hand from the plate to the mouth. Foods like cut raw vegetables are easily handled, and pita bread and rolls can carry pieces of meat, gravy, or other items to the mouth. Soups, hot cereals, and other liquids can be served in mugs that are easy to lift and sip from. Finger foods can provide a great opportunity for adequate calorie intake and allow for more independence than caregiver feeding. As with any change in diet, it's best to consult with your doctor. A dietitian will also be able to provide guidelines.

ASSISTIVE DEVICES

A variety of assistive devices can make eating much easier for people who have trouble bringing food from the plate to their mouths. Many of these utensils can be purchased at large retail stores or through specialty pharmacies.

• Use utensils with large handles. These are usually easier for people with reduced motor skills or arthritis to handle. Weighted handles also can reduce the effects of hand tremors. In some cases, placing Velcro straps around the utensils and hands can keep people from dropping food.

• Plate guards or scoop plates help a person pick food off the plate with a utensil. These are extra lips that allow the person to push the food against the edge of the plate and onto the utensil. Nonslip placemats underneath plates also help.

• Double-handled cups help some people pick up beverages with more steadiness. Straws will allow a person to drink easily without picking up the cup at all.

• Small mirrors placed on the table can help people who have trouble finding their mouths with the utensils. They also can help people avoid putting the food between their cheeks and teeth, where it can be difficult to remove.

Encourage social contact. Older people tend to eat more when in the presence of others. Even if a person is independent enough to prepare and eat his or her own meals, caregivers should try to arrange times to dine together to provide this valuable contact.

Consider community assistance. Many cities and states offer programs to deliver foods and prepared meals to homebound older people. Meals on Wheels is a well-known example. Caregivers can contact local social service agencies to inquire about what programs are available in their area.

CONSTIPATION

Constipation affects as many as one-third of all older women and more than one-quarter of all older men. People who have a fear of becoming constipated are less likely to eat enough food. Initially, the best way to deal with constipation is to make sure the person drinks enough fluids. The typical older person should drink about two quarts of water or other liquids per day, not counting caffeine-containing beverages like coffee or tea. A high-fiber diet may also help. Dietary fiber

CARING FOR PEOPLE WITH DYSPHAGIA

Caregivers can offer great assistance to people with swallowing difficulties. Once a diagnosis has been made, a dietitian will be able to create a menu that can be easily eaten and swallowed. This usually involves changing the texture of foods and fluids, making them smoother, more consistent, and thicker. People with severe dysphagia may need to use thickening agents to decrease the risk of liquids slipping into the lungs. These agents are available at drugstores, and usually don't alter the taste of the liquid. Many people need their food (meats, vegetables, and fruit) to be finely chopped or even pureed. Pureed foods are far easier to swallow than small pieces of food.

Caregivers can also use a variety of tech-niques to help a dysphagic person swallow properly.

• Before beginning a meal, offer the person a sip of cold water. This can clear the throat and stimulate proper swallowing reflexes.

• Encourage your loved one to breathe out before he or she places any food in her mouth. This helps avoid problems with aspiration of food. During meals, remind the person with swallowing difficulties to breathe through his or her nose.

• Remind the person not to tilt his or her head or body back while chewing or drinking. They are more likely to aspirate fluids in this position.

• Keep bites small and manageable. Allow your loved one to chew for as long as necessary,

seems to increase the speed with which food passes through the intestines. High-fiber foods include vegetables like peas, potatoes (with skin), broccoli, Brussels sprouts, and beans; fruits like raspberries, oranges, peaches, and apples (with peels); as well as whole-grain and bran cereals.

Many types of medications can cause constipation in the elderly. These range from drugs like verapamil, used for high blood pressure and heart conditions, to painkillers such as codeine and Vicodin; iron supplements; and drugs for central nervous system problems, like levodopa (Sinemet) for Parkinson's disease and tricyclic antidepressants. On average, an older person has five to seven bowel movements per week. If a person falls below that level for more than one or two weeks or the person's normal pattern changes, it's a good idea to consult a doctor or other health care provider. Do not use over-the-counter laxatives without first talking to a physician. They may have marked side effects in the elderly. Stimulant-

then remind him or her to stop breathing before they swallow.

• Do not allow a person with swallowing difficulties to take more food until the previous mouthful is swallowed completely. People with dysphagia sometimes "squirrel" bits of food in the sides of their mouths, which can lead to choking.

• Remind persons with swallowing difficulty to close their lips and keep them closed after inserting food. This helps avoid dribbling and drooling and gives the person better control over the food as it is chewed.

• Avoid placing food on the tip of the tongue, where it is difficult to move. Food should be placed in the middle of the tongue. Conversely, do not allow food to be placed too far back in the mouth; this can trigger a gag reflex.

• Encourage the person to swallow twice between bites. If you are feeding your loved one and notice food remaining in the mouth, place the utensil back in the mouth without food. This can sometimes trigger the person to swallow.

• Don't mix textures in the same mouthful. Many soups, for instance, mix broth and solid pieces like vegetables. This can make swallowing more difficult.

• Alternate between solid food and sips of liquid. This will keep the throat clear.

• The use of flavor enhancers, like monosodium glutamate, can help keep your loved one's eating interest higher. Check with a doctor before using these products.

based laxatives, like castor oil or senna, may decrease the absorption of some nutrients as well as electrolytes. And overuse of bulk laxatives can lead to impaction or diarrhea.

INCONTINENCE

Urinary incontinence is a major concern among the elderly; it affects approximately 10% of all persons aged 65 and over and as many as 50% of all nursing home residents. Unfortunately, fears of incontinence can keep many older people from drinking as much liquid as they should. To help with this situation, caregivers should encourage people to avoid caffeinated drinks like coffee or tea, and encourage urination at regular intervals. Liquids should be avoided prior to bedtime. For more detailed information on this topic, see the Urinary Incontinence chapter on p. 505.

CHOKING AND THE HEIMLICH MANEUVER

People who have trouble feeding themselves and eating properly are at increased risk for choking. This can occur when the person is alone or in the presence of caregivers. It's important to know how to deal with a choking person in order to act quickly and effectively in removing the food blockage. Learn the Heimlich maneuver, which can be life-saving. Ask your doctor or local Red Cross chapter for a detailed demonstration.

A person who is choking almost always moves his hand to his throat. He is unable to speak or breathe. When this happens, it's essential to take quick action.

• Stand the person up and move behind him.
• Place your fist against his abdomen, with the thumb side of your fist touching his abdomen.

• Grab your fist with your other hand and pull up quickly toward the person's chest. Repeat several times if necessary. Do not use this maneuver if the person can cough or talk.
• If the person is lying down, roll him onto his back and press your hands into his abdomen above the navel and below the rib cage. A sharp thrust toward the chest can dislodge the food in the person's throat.

When appropriate, teach a person how to perform a version of this technique on himself, should he begin to choke while alone. The person can lean his abdomen against the back of a chair and thrust quickly into the chair.

Do not attempt to give fluids to a choking person in an attempt to wash the food down. This can only make the person's condition worse.

HEARTBURN

Heartburn is a common complaint among people with feeding and eating problems, and with the elderly in general. In many cases, over-the-counter heartburn remedies can help control the problem. But caregivers should always check with a physician before giving these medicines to an elderly person, and they can interfere with the digestion and absorption of nutrients. Self-medicating may also delay evaluation and proper treatment of the underlying problem.

ORAL HYGIENE

Tooth brushing, flossing, and denture cleaning can help stimulate a person's appetite. Good hygiene habits also keep mouth problems from growing worse and discouraging people from eating because of painful teeth or sores in the mouth. Caregivers should make sure an elderly person gets regular dental exams and cleans his or her teeth at least two times per day.

DRUG INTERACTIONS

Prescription and nonprescription drugs alike can have a great impact on an older person's ability to eat, digest, and absorb nutrients. Some diuretic medications, for instance, can cause the body to excrete nutrients like calcium before they can be used by the body. A few drugs that lower blood cholesterol levels, such as cholestyramine, can interfere with the absorption of vitamins and minerals. Even aspirin and other painkillers can cause nausea and stomach upset that make eating more difficult. Antacids may inhibit digestion of foods and bind some minerals, therefore decreasing their absorption. Because the combination of food and drugs is so important, check with your doctor to make sure that medications are not interfering with either the ability to feed (through fatigue or loss of muscle coordination) or eat. And never give over-the-counter medicines without first checking the label or consulting your pharmacist for possible warnings about food interactions.

NUTRITION AND THE DYING PATIENT

Proper nutrition is essential for all elderly people, even those near death. But for people who are dying, create meal plans with an eye toward enjoyment and comfort. For example, favorite foods may be provided more often. Good nutrition should be encouraged, but a person should not be forced to eat and/or drink. Any vitamin or mineral supplements that are causing constipation, diarrhea, or other gastrointestinal distress might be stopped without complications. A dying patient and her caregiver should also discuss whether artificial feeding measures are desired as disease reaches its end stage. Hospitals and nursing homes require patients to fill out advance directives that include questions about whether feeding and hydration tubes are to be used. This is a personal decision, and wishes vary from person to person.

ADDITIONAL RESOURCES

American Dietetic Association

www.eatright.org

Nutritional Guidelines for Parkinson Patients

www.parkinson.org/nutrguid.htm

Safety in the Home

It is fairly common for us to take special precautions to avoid harm when we are away from our homes. We check for traffic before crossing a street, steer clear of automobile fumes, avoid petting animals that we don't know, try to travel on well-lighted streets, keep our wallets secure in our pockets or pocketbooks, and wouldn't dream of drinking from an unlabeled bottle that we found on a park bench. When we return home we breathe a sigh of relief as we settle into the safety and comfort of our familiar environment. We may believe that once we closed our front doors we removed ourselves from serious threats to our safety and well-being. But we may be deceiving ourselves with a sense of false security because many serious hazards exist within our own homes—hazards that we frequently overlook! We often become so familiar with these hazards that they no longer stand out, like the frayed wires on appliances, the leaking pipe that drips water on the floor, and the temperamental furnace. To make matters worse, in the comfort of our homes we also tend to let our guard down, being less alert to hazards and taking more risks than we would when traveling in our community. For example, we may securely hold the rail of a store escalator to avoid falling, yet come down a flight of stairs in our home with our arms overloaded, with our view obstructed, or without holding the railing.

WHAT CONTRIBUTES TO INJURIES?

In addition to the safety hazards in the home everybody faces, there are added risks when someone in your home is elderly or disabled or both, and dependent on you for caregiving assistance. Risks to safety can arise from common age-related changes such as:

- Reduced ability to read small print, which can affect the ability to read labels and recognize hazards in one's path
- Decreased peripheral vision (ability to see to the sides), which can limit the ability to see items that are not in the central visual field
- Distorted depth perception, which impairs the ability to judge the height of a step or curb
- Cataracts, which cloud the lens of the eye, blur vision, and impair the ability to see in the presence of sunlight and glare
- Decreased responsiveness of the pupil to light, making it hard to see in dim areas and at night
- Slower adaptation of the eyes from dark to light areas
- Age-related progressive hearing loss, which causes sounds (such as alarms and warnings) to be distorted or missed altogether
- Slower reflexes, which slow response to injury or danger

These factors contribute to the reality that accidental injuries rank among the top-ten leading causes of death in persons over age 65. According to the U.S. Census Bureau, injuries and poisoning account for 15.8 annual hospital days for every 1000 men ages 65 to 74 and 20.2 days for every 1000 women in this same age group; those rates more than double for persons over age 75. The consequences of injuries can threaten the length and quality of life for older adults.

And the consequences of those age-related changes listed above can also create a setting for accidents and injuries. Consider:

Health conditions. Both acute and chronic health conditions can impose certain threats to safety. Many conditions cause weakness, fatigue, dizziness, and lightheadedness. Depression, anxiety, and other mental health problems can impair judgment and make people less attentive to their surroundings. Strokes (cerebrovascular accidents) can leave people with paralysis and restrictions in their abilities to sense and respond to hazards in their environment. Neurological conditions, such as Parkinson's disease and multiple sclerosis, can impair balance, coordination, and gait. Alzheimer's disease and other dementias can significantly affect individuals' abilities to protect themselves and lead to hazardous behaviors, such as drinking poisonous liquids or climbing out of a second-story window.

Medications and medical equipment. The treatments and equipment used by persons with chronic health conditions provide additional sources of safety risks. Many persons with chronic health conditions use multiple medications that can affect their ability to protect themselves from danger. For example, some drugs can cause people to become dizzy or sleepy, which can lead to falls. Oxygen, often prescribed to assist persons with respiratory difficulties, supports combustion and can cause a fire when there is a spark from a cigarette or static electricity. Canes and walkers can be tripped over, and wheelchairs can slip away if left unlocked during a transfer or tip over if the occupant reaches over too far. The cords from pumps, electric beds, and other equipment can be a tripping hazard. Medical supplies can add to the clutter and create an obstacle course through which to navigate. Treatment solutions left at the bedside for convenience can be mistakenly ingested.

Finances. Limited finances can contribute to safety hazards in the home. Faulty heating systems, overflowing toilets, leaking roofs, broken windows, and malfunctioning appliances may be unattended to because of the lack of funds. To save money, unskilled hands may attempt to make electrical repairs or patch a roof. Space heaters may be used to reduce heating costs. Food that has been stored well beyond its expiration date may be consumed rather than thrown away.

Caregiver stress. Your burdens as a caregiver also can contribute to accidents and injuries in the home. The multiple demands on you can divert your attention. You may forget you have a pot of food cooking on the stove as you hurry to make a quick run to the supermarket. You may be trying to get from one room to another in a hurry and not pay attention to obstacles that are in your path. You may try to lift your loved one without help and sustain a back injury or both of you may land on the floor as a result. Getting insufficient rest and eating poorly can cause your mind to function less acutely and impair your judgment. Caregiving stresses can cause you to be accident-prone and less attentive to safety risks to your loved one.

Recognizing that there are many factors that contribute to a high risk of accidents, you need to pay particular attention to home safety. Let's examine some of the major areas of concern and what you can do about them.

FIRES AND BURNS

Every year in this country, thousands of people are injured and hundreds die from fires in the home. The National Fire Protection Association (NFPA) advises that the top five causes of home fires, in order of occurrence, are cooking equipment, heating equipment, arson, other household equipment, and electrical systems. According to the NFPA the top five causes of *fatal* home fires are smoking, arson, heating equipment, children playing with fire, and electrical systems. Most of the fires that kill happen at night when people are asleep. Although home fires can expose victims to temperatures that exceed 1000°F, it isn't the heat or burns that are responsible for most fire-related deaths. In fact, the majority of people die from inhaling smoke and poisonous gases. During a fire, the amount of oxygen in the air drastically drops to levels that make it difficult or impossible to breathe. Fire produces deadly carbon monoxide, and some substances produce poisonous gases when burned.

KITCHEN FIRES

Kitchens, where one-fifth of all home fires in the United States start, are a prime area for you to consider in your prevention efforts. Here are some measures to help you reduce the risk of kitchen fires.

- Avoid placing items on the burners when you are not cooking.
- Always stay in the kitchen when you are doing stove top cooking.
- If you must leave the room, set the timer to remind you that something is in the oven or on the burners; carry a timer with you if you are going to an area where you will not be able to hear the stove's timer.
- Do not wear loose clothing, garments with draping sleeves, or sheer materials that can easily catch on fire when cooking.
- When reaching to back burners, do so from the side rather than reaching across the top of another burner.
- Avoid storing spices and other items on the back of the stove, since you could set your clothing on fire when reaching for them.
- Use pot holders that are nonflammable rather than kitchen towels or cloths, and keep them away from burners (dish towels and pot holders

ignite at 400°F while the average electric burner reaches 800°F and gas flames exceed 1000°F).

- Keep the stove and range hood clean and free from grease buildup.
- Have the lids to the pots and pans you are using nearby so that you can use them to cover burning pots and pans.
- Do not heat items in closed containers in the microwave, because they can build up enough pressure to explode. (This applies to eggs, too.)
- Keep a fire extinguisher in the kitchen. Not all fire extinguishers are alike, so read the label to assure it will work on grease and other sources of fire in the kitchen.

Should a fire develop in a pot or pan cover it immediately with a lid to cut off the supply of oxygen that the fire requires to burn. Leave the pot or pan on the stove; carrying it to the sink or outdoors could harm you and cause the fire to spread. Never use water to put out fires in pots and pans, as this could cause the burning liquid to spatter and the fire to flare up, burning you in the process. Call the fire department and get yourself and your loved one out of the area.

If you should accidentally burn yourself, put the burned area in cool water for several minutes. It's important to keep the injured area clean. After cooling the burn for several minutes in cool water, you can apply aloe vera gel, which helps soothe and heal minor burns. You can purchase an aloe vera plant and keep it in the kitchen. When you need some for a burn, break off a leaf and squeeze the liquid gel onto the burn. Never apply butter to a burn.

SCALDING

Fires aren't the only cause of burns. Scalds can easily happen in the average home, not only from boiling water in the kitchen, but also from faucets when hot water temperatures are excessively hot. This can be a particular problem for older adults, since their tactile sensations often are duller, so they are unaware that water is too hot and their slower reactions can delay their ability to rapidly withdraw from the water. For example, an older person may step into a tub of excessively hot water and sit down before he or she begins to feel the burning sensation. By the time the person is able to get out of the tub, significant burns could have occurred. Make sure faucet handles are clearly marked and easy to operate.

The easiest and least expensive way to prevent scalding water from coming from your faucets is to set your water heater no higher than 120°F (which usually is its lowest setting). You can install antiscalding devices in your faucets and showerheads. When the water temperature gets too hot, the internal parts of these devices expand and turn off the flow of hot water. Another helpful device is a pressure-sensitive and/or temperature-limiting valve that replaces the current hot and cold mixing valve on your shower. If there is a sudden change in water pressure (as can happen in some homes if someone flushes the toilet or turns on the cold water in another part of the house), the valve causes an adjustment and ensures that the shower water doesn't become scalding hot. You can have electric-eye faucets installed in your faucets that not only turn water off and on automatically based on motion, but also can deliver water at preset temperatures. You can discuss these options with a local plumber or request catalogs from some of the companies that supply these devices, such as Accent on Living (800-787-8444), AdaptAbility (800-288-9941), American Standard (800-223-0068), Brookstone (800-926-7000), Keeney Manufacturing Company (800-243-0526), and Kohler Company (920-457-4441). There also are nonslip tub mats that not only protect from falls, but change color when the water gets too hot; one company that offers this is Joan Cook (800-935-0971).

ELECTRICAL FIRES

Electrical fire risks can develop so subtly and gradually that you may fail to recognize the hazard. For instance, receptacle adapters may have been used to accommodate new items that have been added to the family room, resulting in a socket intended for two items now supplying electricity to a half-dozen appliances. These overloaded sockets can be a source of fires. Likewise, extension cords running under carpeting and frayed or exposed wires on old appliances may pose risks. It is helpful to schedule a time to check every outlet and appliance wire in your home to detect these types of problems and arrange to have them corrected if they are present. Inspect appliances regularly to assure they are not malfunctioning.

ELECTRIC SHOCK

It is not unusual for persons in poor health to be less attentive to routine precautions in the way they handle common household electrical appliances. In addition to having many distracting concerns on their minds, they may be less alert because of symptoms associated with their medical conditions or caused by their medications. For persons with Alzheimer's disease and other types of mental impairments, the risks of being careless with electrical appliances is compounded.

Scan the environment for appliances that could come in contact with water or wet hands. In the kitchen, this can include electric coffeepots, radios, can openers, blenders, toasters, and breadmakers that are on counters close to the sink. In the bathroom, hair dryers, electric razors, electric toothbrush stands, curling irons, and heaters can be culprits. Even if the appliances are not turned on, they can be dangerous because they are plugged into the electrical outlet. To reduce risks, unplug electrical appliances when not in use. When possible, avoid using appliances near water. For example, establish an area in the bedroom for hair-drying rather than in the bathroom to avoid the risk of contact with water. If you don't already have them, consider having an electrician install ground fault interrupter (GFI) outlets and circuit breakers. You can tell if you have GFI outlets and breakers by looking for a test or reset button either on the breaker itself or on the circuit breaker in the electrical panel. When the button is pressed—or there is a short circuit—the mechanism pops and the electrical outlet is automatically disabled and nothing will work in the outlet until it is reset by pushing the mechanism again. If the button does not make a popping sound, the GFI outlet may no longer be working and will offer no protection. You can use the button to turn off an outlet temporarily, as when your loved one is alone in the bathroom and you are concerned that he or she may attempt to use an electrical appliance unsupervised.

SMOKING-RELATED BURNS

Most fatal home fires are caused by careless smoking. Smoking can pose a serious risk to persons with physical and mental disabilities. Weakness can reduce the ability to safely handle smoking items, resulting in lighted cigarettes, pipes, or cigars being dropped. Dulled sensations, whether from a stroke or some other cause, can prevent the person from feeling the lighted end of a cigarette that is coming in contact with his or her body. Altered mental status can lead a person to forget that a cigarette was lighted and allow it to start a fire.

The ideal approach is to discourage smoking altogether. If this is not possible, allow your loved one to smoke only under supervision. Hiding all smoking products while you are not present can help to reduce unsupervised smoking. Be sure to hide all smoking products, not just matches, as your loved one could attempt to light a cigarette on the stove and burn himself or herself, or create a fire hazard by leaving the stove on.

SPACE HEATER AND CHIMNEY FIRES

Space heaters are used in many homes to reduce heating costs by providing extra warmth in areas where families spend most of their time. Although this approach can save money, it can also cost lives: The use of space heaters is a major cause of home fires.

Several types of space heaters are available. Electric ones are popular because they're easy to use. Some electric space heaters consist of ribbon or quartz heating elements that produce heat in a limited direct path; others have fans that produce sufficient heat to warm an entire room. Only use heaters that have the Underwriters Laboratories (UL) label and that have automatic turn-off features if the machine becomes overheated or tips over. Be sure your home's electrical system can handle the demand imposed by this appliance.

Kerosene heaters are best for outdoor use, for which they originally were intended. Some states have passed legislation banning the use of kerosene heaters indoors. (Contact your local fire department to find out if they are banned in your state.) In addition to the fire risks, kerosene heaters produce significant amounts of pollutants when they burn, necessitating good ventilation to reduce health hazards. If you are going to use one, be sure it has the UL label. Use only K-1 grade, clear kerosene and never use gasoline. Store kerosene outside and refuel the heater outdoors.

Wood-burning stoves produce considerable heat, enough to warm an entire house. Check with your local fire department for guidance as to requirements for permits to allow you to install a wood-burning stove. Hard wood that has been dried for at least six months is the most effective fuel source; never use gasoline, building scraps, or trash within the stove. Clean ashes from the stove's interior regularly and make sure they are disposed of properly.

Keep at least three feet of space clear around heaters so that furniture and objects won't burn. They should not be in use if unattended, when you're asleep, or in areas where an unsupervised disabled person could come in contact with them.

Chimney care is also very important. Creosote, a tar-like substance, can accumulate in the chimney and catch fire. (It ignites at 451°F, which is about the same temperature at which paper will ignite.) Check your chimney every few weeks for these deposits and have your chimney inspected and cleaned by professionals at least once during the heating season. Stainless steel chimney linings are effective in reducing the buildup of creosote in chimneys. If you haven't used the chimney for a while, check it for nests and other obstructions. Installing a wire basket or spark arrestor on the top of the chimney can discourage birds and squirrels from making their nests in the chimney and reduce the risk of sparks from your chimney starting a fire on your roof or on nearby objects. Be sure to keep a fire extinguisher handy for every stove or fireplace; you may want to consider purchasing a special chimney fire extinguisher.

OXYGEN USE

Your loved one may have been prescribed oxygen for home use to assist with breathing. While it is life-sustaining, oxygen also can be life-threatening, as it is highly flammable and supports combustion. Some special precautions are essential to prevent fires. First, be sure to post a sign at the entrance of your house indicating "OXYGEN IN USE. NO SMOKING" so that everyone entering is sensitive to the need for safety. When anyone is using oxygen, keep him or her away from pilot lights, working fireplaces, space heaters, candles, and other sources of flames. Avoid static electricity and the use of electrical devices in your loved one's presence as these can be the source of sparks that can trigger a fire. No grease, oil, or other potentially combustible substance should come in contact with the oxygen equipment. Prevent your loved one from using alcohol, nail polish remover, perfume, or other flammable liquids. Store the oxygen cylinders in a cool place and have a fire extinguisher readily available.

SMOKE DETECTORS AND SPRINKLERS

Your home should be equipped with smoke detectors in key locations. Make sure they are working properly and use them. Develop a system to replace the batteries of smoke detectors at least annually; choosing your birthday as the day to replace the batteries is a useful way to remember this task. Many people replace batteries twice a year when we switch from daylight savings time to standard time.

If safely reaching the smoke detector to replace the battery is a problem for you, ask someone to help or contact your local fire department, which usually will assist. Fire departments often have programs for installing smoke detectors or providing them free of charge; contact your local station for information. A smoke detector system can be installed into your home's electrical system or along with a burglar alarm system. This type of system not only alerts you to the presence of smoke in your home and eliminates the need to worry about battery replacement, but also phones your local fire department to summon help.

Smoke detectors are excellent for alerting you to the presence of a fire, but they do nothing to eliminate the fire. By the time you or your loved one are alerted by the smoke detector, particularly if either of you is a heavy sleeper or has limited hearing, it could be too late for you to escape. A sprinkler system in the home could prove to be life-saving under these conditions. Sprinkler systems contain heat-sensitive elements that detect fire and release water. Systems are made to allow each sprinkler to respond independently, so that a fire in the basement would trigger the sprinklers in that part of your house only. They are more costly than smoke detectors, but not prohibitively so. The most economic route is to have them installed during the construction of a new home; however, they can be easily retrofitted into hallways and kitchens of older homes for a reasonable cost. (An added benefit: Installation of sprinkler systems could reduce your homeowners' insurance; check with your insurer.)

FIRE ESCAPE PLAN

If you do not have one already, you can help your household by developing a fire escape plan and familiarizing everyone in your home with this plan. This plan begins by assuring that you have working smoke alarms and that you pay attention to them when they do go off. A survey done by the National Fire Protection Association found that 81 percent of people who had smoke alarms go off in their homes assumed there was no fire and ignored them. Since smoke alarms reduce the risk of dying in a home fire by half, they need to be taken seriously when they do sound.

Make an escape plan for your home and ensure that all family members understand it fully. Identify two ways out of every room (including windows) and the best route to reach the outdoors quickly. The route through the house should be such that everyone can find his or her way out without the ability to see (which could be the reality if the house was filled with smoke). The bedroom of a person who would have difficulty escaping from a second-story window should be on the first floor if this is at all possible. If your loved one is unable to escape from the home independently, have a plan to assist the person. This could include an understanding that certain members of the household would immediately go to the person's room and help the person to escape if a fire was suspected or an alarm sounded. You also may need to plan on carrying the person outdoors, so practicing this procedure before an actual emergency occurs will prove useful. In fact, the National Fire Protection Association recommends practicing your exit escape plan at least twice a year. If you live alone with a loved one who is disabled, develop a plan in advance with a neighbor, who will know to come to your home and give help in the event of a fire or other emergency.

If a fire should occur or there is smoke in your home, focus on getting yourself and the others out as quickly as possible. Don't worry about dressing or collecting your wallet or other items. Don't stay in the house to phone the fire department; instead, grab a portable phone or a cell phone on your way out or call for a neighbor to alert the fire department after you are safely outdoors.

If you are in a room with a closed door when you are warned of a fire, kneel and touch the door, door frame, and knob with the back of your hand before opening the door. If the door is warm, use another route to escape. If the door is cool, slowly open it, being prepared to quickly slam it shut if you detect smoke or flames on the other side.

If you must escape through a smoke-filled area, crawl on your hands and knees. The lower you are to the ground, the cooler the temperature and the more oxygen will be available.

CHOKING

The risk of choking is particularly high when people have swallowing difficulties or poor control of the muscles of their mouth, tongue, or throat, as is the situation when someone has had a stroke. Persons with Alzheimer's disease and other dementias are at high risk for choking, not only because of their declining neuromuscular function, but also as a result of poor judgment that could cause them to put foreign objects in their mouths, feed themselves inappropriately, or chew food insufficiently before swallowing.

If your loved one is at high risk for choking, preventive measures are crucial. Obtain an evaluation and consultation from a speech therapist if the person has swallowing problems. The therapist can offer an individualized plan for feeding and diet modification, and suggestions for assistive devices that can promote safe swallowing. If your loved one has a dementia, supervise his or her feeding and remove small food items (e.g., nuts, hard candies, popcorn) and objects (e.g., paper clips, coins, parts of plants) that could be placed in the mouth and accidentally enter the breathing passage. Don't overlook getting the person's poor-fitting dentures corrected, since these can slip out of place and block the air passage. For a caregiver, learning the Heimlich maneuver, a series of abdominal thrusts, can be an advantage in providing emergency care to your loved one in the event of choking. (This can be learned along with CPR—cardiopulmonary resuscitation—classes or you can ask your health care provider to demonstrate the technique to you.)

Warning signs that someone is choking include the inability to speak, cough, or breathe; the person may clutch at his or her throat and his or her face may turn blue. If the person is able to talk, the airway is not completely obstructed and you should allow the person to cough and dislodge the obstruction alone. But if the person shows the classic signs of choking, call 911 immediately and assist in dislodging the obstruction by using the Heimlich maneuver. It is important that action be taken immediately. Death or permanent brain damage can occur if the body is deprived of oxygen for four minutes or longer.

POISONING

Many potentially poisonous substances reside within the average home that can pose risks to your loved one, and common household products are among them.

CLEANING SOLUTIONS AND POLISHES

Some cleaning solutions and furniture polishes are lemon-scented and can be mistaken for a beverage, particularly by someone who has a dementia or other cognitive impairment. People with normal mental function but poor vision can mistake these products for a flavoring or drink and accidentally ingest them. A confused person may be at risk for consuming pesticides and insecticides. For example, a box of colorful mouse-killer pellets can be mistaken for candy.

Be sure to keep these products in a safe, specific area rather than on kitchen counters or in kitchen cabinets, so that there is less risk of them being confused with a food product. If your loved one is confused, keep these products in a locked area to reduce the risk of the person being tempted to taste or drink them.

PLANTS AND FLOWERS

Many popular plants are poisonous if parts of them are ingested, including azalea, holly berries, hyacinth, iris, ivy, lily-of-the-valley, mistletoe, rhododendron, tulip, and wisteria. The leaves of some fruit plants are toxic, such as those found on avocado plants, cherry trees, peach trees, and tomato vines. Potato sprouts and apricot and peach kernels are poisonous. Persons with Alzheimer's disease and other types of confusion can eat these items and become sick. Even persons with good mental function may poison themselves with plants by using them inappropriately. This can happen by people thinking it is "healthy" to use plant leaves in salads or to brew them in "natural" teas. If you are concerned that plants in your home environment could be hazardous, you may call your local poison control center for a list of poisonous plants common to your area. Local representatives of the Department of Agriculture also can be resources and may be willing to inspect your property and offer advice. When purchasing plants, ask the nursery if they are poisonous or research the plants yourself at your local library. (In addition to evaluating plants for their poison potential, you also should examine them for the chance that fruits or leaves could fall on the walking path of your loved one and cause a fall.)

PRESCRIPTION AND NONPRESCRIPTION MEDICINES

Most likely, you have at least a few medications in the home for the miscellaneous health problems that arise from time to time. These can be the source of accidental poisoning for anyone in the home in several ways. Your loved one may mistake one medication for another, take an incorrect dose, or, forgetting that a medication already had been taken, overdose. Tablets that look like candy can be consumed as such and cause overdosage. It is important to develop a medication administration system that can help your loved one (and you!) remember if a drug was taken at a specific time. Your local pharmacy should have medication systems with boxes designated for different times and days that enable you to keep track of what was taken and when. Developing a charting system can prove helpful also. If your loved one is confused, keep all medications locked—and don't overlook vitamins and herbs that also can be toxic in high doses. Locking medicine cabinets are available or you may find that a small lockbox, available at most office supply stores, could do the trick as well. Remember also that proper disposal of used medication patches, syringes and needles, and other drug-related items is important. Topical medication patches are commonly prescribed, and used discarded patches contain enough residual drugs that they have caused poisonings when chewed or ingested by children or pets. Also, it is wise to discard medications, both prescription and over-the-counter, that are no longer needed so as not to accumulate pill bottles.

CARBON MONOXIDE

Some poisons that lurk in the home environment are less obvious than others. For instance, poor ventilation coupled with improperly used or malfunctioning equipment can lead to carbon monoxide poisoning. The Consumer Product Safety Commission (CPSC) reports that approximately 200 people each year are killed and an additional 5000 people injured by accidental carbon monoxide poisoning. Carbon monoxide is a colorless, odorless, tasteless, and toxic gas produced as a by-product of combustion. Dangerous levels of carbon monoxide gas can be produced by any fuel burning appliance, vehicles, or tool, and fuel-fired furnaces, gas water heaters, fireplaces, wood burning stoves, charcoal grills, and gas dryers and stoves. Carbon monoxide reduces the amount of oxygen carried in the blood, leading to headaches, nausea, loss of consciousness, and eventually death if uncorrected. You should suspect carbon monoxide poisoning if you or your loved one have chronic flu-like symptoms. You can take some steps to prevent carbon monoxide from escaping into your home; these include promptly repairing malfunctioning furnaces and water heaters, keeping chimneys unblocked and clean, avoiding the use of charcoal grills and gas-powered machines near open windows or air vents into your home, and not leaving your automobile running in a closed garage. Consider having a heating contractor install a fresh air takeup system in your home. You can purchase carbon monoxide detectors from major hardware stores (buy only UL-listed alarms) and install them near the ceiling. The CPSC recommends a detector on each floor of a home, particularly on each floor where there are bedrooms. If the alarm goes off, call 911, leave the house immediately, and get to an area where you can breathe fresh air. You can obtain government publications on carbon monoxide by searching the CPSC's Web site.

RADON

Another poisonous gas that could possibly be present in your home is radon. The Environmental Protection Agency (EPA) estimates that as many as 8 million homes throughout the country have elevated levels of radon. Radon is a radioactive gas that cannot be seen, smelled, or tasted. It seeps into homes from the surrounding soil through cracks and other openings in the foundation. Breathing radon increases your chance of lung cancer; in fact, the Surgeon General has warned that radon is the second leading cause of lung cancer in the U.S. today. The risk is especially high if a person is a smoker and lives in a home with high radon levels. The EPA, the Surgeon General's Office, the American Lung Association, the American Medical Association, and the National Safety Council have urged widespread testing for radon. There are no symptoms warning you of elevated radon exposure, which emphasizes the importance of testing your home for the presence of this gas. Radon testing kits are available in major hardware stores. Elevated radon levels usually can be reduced without significant cost.

LEAD

Although lead poisoning primarily is a health problem affecting children, there can be health concerns for you and your loved one as well. Lead is a heavy metal used in many materials and products. When absorbed into the body, it is highly toxic to many organs and systems. Lead paint is a major source of poisoning. Homes built before 1950 typically used lead paint; at that time this type of paint was considered of higher quality. Lead pipes and solder can cause lead to get into drinking water. Persons who work in construction, demolition, painting, radiator repair, and other jobs in which they come in regular contact with lead particles could carry lead particles home on their clothing. Some ceramics and leaded crystal are other sources of lead. There is little that you can do to treat lead poisoning once it occurs, so prevention is important. Be sure to remove old paint and renovate carefully. Have your drinking water checked for lead and, if you can, replace lead pipes with safe ones. If members of your household work in occupations in which there is a risk of lead particles being carried home, have them remove work clothes before coming into the home.

DROWNING

Swimming pools and hot tubs can be deadly for persons with disabilities. While in the water, people can become dizzy, develop cramps, become too weak to get out, or lose their balance and slip underwater. While walking alongside pools, the elderly or disabled can fall into the water or fall on a slippery surface. It is important to limit access to a pool or hot tub, if you have one, by installing fencing and locks. You can install alarms that will sound if the gate or door to a pool or hot tub area is opened; there also are pool alarms that sound if the water is disturbed so that you can be alerted to your loved one being in the water. Your local pool or spa supply dealer can help you locate these products. You also can obtain useful government publications on pool and spa safety by visiting the CPSC Web site.

Bathtubs pose a potential risk for drowning. An older person can slip underwater and not be able to sit up quickly enough. The effects of medications and symptoms associated with diseases can cause drowsiness, dizziness, and weakness that can contribute to drowning. (Keep in mind that when someone is sitting in warm water the blood pressure drops, which in itself can make a person weak and dizzy.) Provide adequate assistance and supervision during bathing to reduce the risk of drowning. Be sure to have adequate grab bars alongside the tub or shower that can be reached easily.

If you find your loved one with his or her head submerged in water and not breathing, call for help immediately and begin CPR. It may be that you don't witness it, yet you suspect that your loved one's head had been submerged in water. This is referred to as near-drowning, in which the person survives after suffocating underwater. Signs and symptoms include difficulty breathing, wheezes, rapid pulse, chest pain, confusion, seizures, bluish color around the mouth, paleness, and a cough with pink frothy sputum. Call for emergency assistance and provide CPR.

FALLS

Falls in the home are a significant hazard to older adults and persons with disabilities. Studies have indicated that one-third of persons aged 75 years and older experience a fall each year. Most of these falls occur in the home, and half of these people experience multiple falls. The consequences of falls are serious: 20% of the hospital and 40% of the nursing home admissions of older adults are related to the consequences of falls. Even if people do not sustain injuries from a fall, they may be so fearful of falling again that they unnecessarily restrict their function and become more dependent than they need to.

Many factors increase the risk of falling in the elderly or disabled:

- Age-related changes: poor vision, less lifting of the foot during stepping, tendency for balance to be lost more easily, slower responses
- Effects of medications: diuretics that cause frequent urination, antihypertensives that can cause dizziness when rising from a chair or bed, sedatives and tranquilizers that can cause drowsiness
- Unsafe clothing: pants legs that drag the floor, poor-fitting shoes and socks
- Improper size or use of canes, walkers, and wheelchairs
- Environmental hazards: wet floors, poor lighting, clutter
- Symptoms related to diseases: dizziness, weakness, confusion, incontinence

Because of these serious consequences, active prevention of falls needs to be one of your top priorities. Consider using some of these helpful strategies.

- Provide adequate lighting in all areas used by your loved one: Make sure light switches are within easy reach of the person. Motion-sensitive lamps and lamps that can be turned on by clapping the hands may be beneficial. Use nightlights in bedrooms and bathrooms, and keep a flashlight on each person's nightstand to provide a quick source of light in a dark room.
- Use contrasting colors between chairs and floor coverings: If the seat cushion of the chair is the same color as the rug, the person may misjudge the location of the edge of the chair and fall. This is a particular problem for older adults who have difficulty discriminating shades in the same color family.
- Eliminate clutter and obstacles in pathways: Remove throw rugs, and secure area rugs with nonslip backing. Do not leave items on stairways or in hallways.

• Provide safe furniture for your loved one: Make sure chairs are of a proper height and have arm rests to assist the person in getting in and out of them easily. Check the stability of tables so they won't tip over if someone leans against them. If your loved one's bed has wheels, lock them securely.

• Check carpeting for uneven or torn areas: Secure the ends of carpeting to prevent tripping. Low-pile carpeting is preferable to thick, plush carpeting for ease in walking and wheelchair mobility.

• Keep floors clean and dry: Do not wax floors. Prevent lighting and direct sunlight from causing glare on the floors, as this can distort the appearance of the walking surface and contribute to falls.

• Reduce risks in the bathroom: Install grab bars near the toilet and tub or shower stall. Place nonslip strips or a rubber mat in the bottom of the tub or stall. Provide a tub seat or bathtub transfer seat if mobility in the tub is a problem. Install an elevated toilet seat to enable your loved one to safely transfer on and off the toilet. Make sure it is easy for your loved one to reach the toilet paper from the toilet. Wall-to-wall carpeting can reduce the risk of slipping on a wet floor and cushion a fall. Cushioned tub and shower stall walls are available to minimize injury if anyone should fall; some companies that supply these are International Cushioned Products (800-882-7638) and KidKusions (800-845-9236).

• Install strong railings at all stairways: Installing railings on both sides of the stairs is beneficial, particularly if your loved one is weak on one side, as he or she can hold a railing with the stronger arm when going up or down. If your loved one wanders or is confused because of dementia, place a gate at the top and bottom of the stairs to limit access. Install slip-resistant stair treads. Placing a different color tread or warning strip on the bottom and top step can alert the person to the change in level. If your loved one is unsteady or has limited ability to climb stairs, consider installing a stair lift. This device consists of a motorized seat, attached to the existing staircase, which moves slowly up and down the staircase with the push of a button. Information on stair lifts can be obtained from Access Industries (800-925-3100), Elevators Etc. (800-785-8585), and Whitakers (800-445-4387).

• Install an awning over patios and porches to reduce slippery surfaces caused by rain or snow. Check the safety and functionality of outdoor furniture.

• If your loved one walks outdoors, keep paths clear of leaves, fallen branches, stones, hoses, and other items that can be potential sources of falls. Have slippery moss removed from walking areas.

- Place an intercom or monitoring device in your loved one's bedroom and bathroom so that you can hear calls for help.

- If your loved one attempts to get out of a chair or bed without necessary assistance, use a fall-prevention monitor. They come in a variety of styles, including a pressure-sensitive pad that sounds an alarm if the person moves off of it and a string/tab type in which one end of the string is attached to the person's clothing and the other to a device that sounds an alarm if the person tries to get up. Some companies that supply these fall-prevention devices are Alert Care (800-826-7444), American Health Care Supply (800-677-7180), Posey Health care (800-447-6739), and Senior Technologies WanderGuard (800-235-8085). There also are pressure-sensitive floor mats that sound a remote alarm when stepped on that can be used to alert you of your loved one's movements. Padded undergarments also are available to cushion the impact on the hips in the event of a fall.

- If your loved one spends periods of time alone, give him a portable phone or a cell phone to wear on a belt so that he can summon help in case he falls.

Yet falls may happen despite your best preventive measures. If your loved one does fall, don't move or lift the person until you are certain there is no injury. It is best to err on the safe side and have your loved one examined if there is any suspicion of an injury. Keep in mind that some fractures are not readily apparent immediately after the fall; it may be only when the person attempts to resume normal activity that the injured bone becomes misaligned. Also, areas other than the direct point of impact may be injured in the fall—for instance, a person may have fallen on the knee, but the force of the fall may have placed enough stress on the hip to fracture the hip.

For a more extensive discussion of falls and how to avoid them, see the Falls and Mobility Problems chapter on p. 575.

FOOD HANDLING

Unsafe handling and storage of food can cause food poisoning. Food poisoning is a term used to describe nausea, vomiting, diarrhea, abdominal pain, and other gastrointestinal symptoms caused by eating contaminated food. Bacteria that can cause food poisoning include:

- Salmonella from eggs (such as the raw eggs used in a Caesar salad) and improperly cooked poultry, pork, beef, and lamb.
- Clostridia from improperly canned or preserved food (e.g., home-preserved tomatoes) that can cause botulism. Other sources of possible *Clostridium* infection are meat or poultry dishes that have been cooked at low temperatures.
- Toxin-producing strains of Staphylococci contaminating improperly refrigerated or stored prepared dishes, meat, milk, and bakery products; transmitted from the skin and respiratory tract of persons who handle food (e.g., handling meat when you have a staphylococcal skin infection).
- *Escherichia coli* (*E. coli*) from contaminated beef (e.g., undercooked beef, meat from an unsanitary butcher shop) and from contaminated, unpasteurized fruit juices.

As mentioned, food poisoning causes gastrointestinal symptoms. In addition, botulism can affect the central nervous system, causing headache, dizziness, inability to talk and swallow, breathing difficulties, confusion, paralysis, and other symptoms. Seek medical attention promptly if you suspect food poisoning.

Food poisoning can cause distressing symptoms for most people, but for your loved one who already has compromised health, the effects can be deadly. This emphasizes the importance of safely handling and storing food. Some points to remember include:

- Wash your hands before handling food. Use soap, scrub your hands vigorously for fifteen seconds, and rinse them under running water.
- Use paper towels rather than a cloth towel to dry your hands or clean countertops.
- Refrigerate items promptly upon bringing them home from the grocery store or after using them for meals.
- Keep your refrigerator temperature no higher than 40°F and your freezer at 0°F or below.
- Avoid using any refrigerated, frozen, or canned foods after their expiration dates.
- Thoroughly wash all fruits and vegetables before eating or refrigerating them.
- Freeze meat and poultry if not using it within two to three days; freeze seafood if not using it within a day.

- Do not consume cracked eggs or raw eggs, oysters, clams, or shellfish.
- Cook meat at oven temperatures greater than 300°F.
- Use a meat thermometer to make sure meats and fish are completely cooked.
- Refrigerate leftovers within two hours after they have been cooked.
- Use proper techniques for canning foods.
- When refrigerating raw meat, poultry, or fish, place it in a dish or plastic wrap so that the juices won't come in contact with other foods.
- Check your refrigerator contents weekly and discard leftovers or opened containers that have been there for more than a week. If you are in doubt about the amount of time a food has been in the refrigerator or whether it remains safe to eat, throw it out.
- Wash lids of food cans and necks of bottles before opening them.
- Discard canned foods if the contents bubble or spray when opened.
- Wash dishes in hot water and allow them to air-dry.
- Do not reuse dishes and utensils for eating meals that have been in contact with raw meat or poultry unless you wash them first.
- Disinfect the kitchen countertops after meal preparation. Plain soap and water will not kill germs. In addition to commercial products, you can make your own disinfectant by mixing 1 teaspoon of chlorine bleach with 1 liter of water (this will lose its strength in about a week).
- Regularly disinfect cutting boards, sponges, and handles on cabinets and appliances.

ANIMAL BITES

Many households have resident pets who bring considerable joy to their owners' lives. For persons who are elderly or who have disabilities, pets can be very therapeutic and improve health and the quality of life. But even the most loving animal can be provoked to bite.

Although dogs are responsible for a majority of the incidents of animal bites, cats, ferrets, and farm animals also do significant damage when they bite. Cat bites have a great potential for causing infections, because a cat's teeth are more pointed and sharp and are more likely to reach tendons and joint capsules. Cats' claws and teeth often carry the bacteria of the rodents with which they come in contact. The risk of infection from these bites is especially high in older adults, persons with diabetes, and those with depressed immune systems.

There are some safeguards you can take to reduce the risk of your pet biting:

- Make sure your pet is in good health and well groomed; cats or dogs who are not feeling well or who have matted hair may be irritable and uncomfortable and snap when touched.
- If your loved one is confused and inappropriate in his or her behavior toward the pet, restrict the contact between the two.
- Obedience training is helpful to both dog and master. Train your dog and ensure that all family members are consistent in their treatment of the animal.
- Nip aggressive behavior in the bud and do not teach your dog to attack or fight.
- Spay or neuter pets to decrease aggression and other behavioral problems.
- Keep your pet's inoculations up to date.

First aid to a bite wound is important. Another significant action is to determine if the animal has been immunized with a rabies vaccine. You should keep your pet's immunizations current and maintain a record of them. If the bite was from someone else's pet, ask for proof of current immunizations. If the bite was from an unfamiliar animal, call your local animal control authority so they can track the animal's owner or take the animal into their care for observation to make sure it does not have rabies. If the biting animal cannot be found or is suspected to carry rabies, the person who was bitten may need to receive immunization against rabies.

THE SPECIAL CHALLENGES OF DEMENTIA

There are special concerns when your loved one has Alzheimer's disease or some other type of dementia. Persons with dementia lack proper judgment, which could cause them to take hazardous actions, such as starting a fire in their closets or attempting to climb out a second-story window. They often wander, which could lead them into a busy street or nearby body of water. Their memory impairment can cause them to forget they left food cooking on the top of a stove or can cause them to leave a lighted cigarette where it could fall and start a fire. They may consume spoiled food that they have hoarded. As the illness progresses, they may become stiff, incontinent, and have poor balance and coordination, which significantly increases their risk of falling. They may eat plastic or paper objects because they are unable to differentiate them from food and choke as a result. Their ability to feed themselves safely may decline, causing them to stuff large quantities of food into their mouths and to swallow foods unchewed. Awakening at night often is a problem and could heighten the risk of falls. Their misidentification of people could cause them to invite strangers into their home who may burglarize or harm them. Caring for a loved one who has a dementia is a difficult challenge. In addition to the suggestions offered throughout this guide there are some additional thoughts to keep in mind:

Keep the environment simple. Remove objects that are unnecessary and that could be distracting or cause injury. For example, you may want to store your collection of antique porcelain plates to prevent breakage and cuts. If mirrors contribute to disorientation and agitation, remove them. Prevent overstimulation by having only one radio or television set operating at a time, using nonglare lighting, and maintaining a stable room temperature (about 75°F).

Keep items in the same location. Keep clothing, grooming aids, eating utensils, and other commonly used items in the same location. In addition to making it easier for your loved one to use these items, it minimizes the risk that she will rummage for them in other locations and find something that could get her in trouble.

Limit areas of unsupervised access. Designate certain rooms of the house as "off limits" by locking their doors or putting a cloth tape across the entrance (you can secure the ends to the frame and use Velcro to attach the strips). Sometimes, a "Stop" sign at the entrance to an area will discourage the person from entering.

Remove potentially harmful items. Look at your home with an eye to everything that could possibly lead to a problem. For example, remove candles so that your loved one won't be tempted to light them, lock up power tools, keep knives in a locked cabinet, avoid having peanuts and other small objects on which they could choke easily accessible, and do not leave car keys in areas where your loved one could take them and use them to drive the car.

643

Look for potential hazards. Normal household items could prove to be a danger to someone with a dementia. For example, your loved one may stick a metal object in an electric outlet, choke on peanuts, or get tangled in a clothesline. Remove such items or keep them locked away. Consider safeguarding your home with the child-proof devices that are available for drawers, doorknobs, refrigerator doors, electrical outlets, stove knobs, cabinets, and windows. Baby supply and hardware stores carry many of these devices.

Reevaluate periodically. Typically, persons with Alzheimer's disease and other dementias will have a progressive worsening of their conditions. The environment and approaches you use will need to change to accommodate this and assure ongoing safety. Be sure that your loved one wears a bracelet that has his or her name and your phone number engraved on it in case the person wanders from home or becomes unconscious. Also, keep a recent photograph available to help identify your loved one if he or she becomes lost. Support groups can provide a means for you to meet other family caregivers who are living with problems similar to yours. The members, many of whom are caregivers, can offer valuable advice and share resources that they've found within your community.

ASSESSING CAUSE AFTER AN ACCIDENT

After experiencing an accident and taking care of its immediate consequences, you may want to give some thought to the factors that contributed to the mishap. Often, it is an unusual or isolated situation, such as a burn from a cup of tea that slipped from your loved one's hand or a fall that resulted from melted ice cubes that made the floor slippery. However, there could be other reasons. Your loved one's health status and level of function may be changing, causing the person to be less able to manage independently. Perhaps a new medication has caused the person to have an unsteady gait or impaired memory. Malnourishment or an undiagnosed infection may be contributing to weakness or confusion. Perhaps you are being more careless and creating hazards in your home because you are stressed and fatigued.

Identifying the underlying reasons for the accidents is essential to reducing safety risks. You may find that additional modifications need to be made to

HOME SAFETY CHECKLIST

Below is a checklist of items for you to use in evaluating the safety of your home:

❏ House numbers large enough to be visible from the street for emergency help to easily locate you

❏ Readily available phone numbers of local police, fire department, poison control center, physician, and neighbor. Poison control centers recommend that these phone numbers be taped to your phone

❏ Smoke detectors on each level of home

❏ Carbon monoxide detector on every level of home

❏ Radon testing done within past year

❏ Telephone on every level of home

❏ Fire extinguisher on every level of home

❏ Vented heating system

❏ No clutter

❏ Properly functioning appliances

❏ Refrigerator set at 40°F or lower

❏ Freezer set at 0°F

❏ Safe stove with burner control on front

❏ No foods stored beyond expiration date

❏ Adequately lighted hallways and stairways

❏ Handrails on all stairs

❏ Nonslip stair treads

❏ Floor surface even, easy to clean, requiring no wax, free of loose scatter rugs and deep-pile carpets

❏ Doorways unobstructed, painted a contrasting color from wall

❏ Bathtub or shower with nonslip surface, safety rails, no electrical outlets nearby

❏ Hot water temperature less than 120°F

❏ Windows screened, easy to reach and to open

❏ Secure locks on windows and doors

❏ Ample number of safe electrical outlets, not overloaded

❏ Shelves within easy reach, sturdy

❏ Faucet handles easy to operate, clearly marked hot and cold

❏ Proper storage of medications, no outdated prescriptions

❏ Proper storage of cleaning solutions, paints, poisonous substances

❏ No peeling paint

❏ Covered trash container

❏ Outdoor stairs and walking surfaces free of ice, moss, and tripping hazards

❏ Railings on outdoor stairs

accommodate your loved one's declining status. Perhaps the person needs to be evaluated for a new health problem or a change in medication. It could be that you need to obtain help to preserve your health. Consider the subtle message that the accident may be offering.

GENERAL SAFETY MEASURES

You may not be able to change the risks imposed by your loved one's illness or disability, but you can make adjustments in your home environment and practices to minimize many safety risks.

- Be prepared for emergencies by taking a CPR class (often available through local community colleges and local chapters of the American Red Cross) and know how to administer it.
- At least quarterly, review emergency plans with those in your household.
- Regularly inspect your home for potential hazards and correct them promptly. The AARP (formerly known as the American Association of Retired Persons) has a useful section in their Web site that reviews home modifications to promote safety; this can be accessed at http://www.aarp.org/universalhome. For financial assistance and low-cost loans to pay for the cost of making structural changes to increase the safety and functionality of your home you can contact the local offices of the Department of Housing and Urban Development (HUD), the Veterans Administration (VA), the Farmers Home Administration (FmHA), and the Department of Aging.

ADDITIONAL RESOURCES

ORGANIZATIONS AND WEB SITES

Alzheimer's Association
800-272-3900
www.alz.org

American Association of Poison Control Centers
www.aapcc.org

Consumer Product Safety Commission
www.cpsc.gov

National Fire Protection Association
www.nfpa.org

Radon Information Center
www.radon.com

BOOKS

Adamec, C. *The Unofficial Guide to Eldercare.* New York: Macmillan, 1999.

Horan, M., and R. A. Little. *Injury in the Aging.* New York: Cambridge University Press, 1998.

Kaufman, D. L. *Injuries and Illness in the Elderly.* St. Louis, Mo.: Mosby, 1997.

Mace, N. L., and P. V. Rabins. *The 36-Hour Day. A Family Guide to Caring for Persons with Alzheimer Disease, Related Dementing Illnesses, and Memory Loss in Later Life*, 3rd ed. Baltimore: Johns Hopkins University Press, 1999.

Morse, J. M. *Preventing Patient Falls.* Thousand Oaks, Calif.: Sage Books, 1997.

Pynoos, J. *Home Modification Resource Guide*, 2nd ed. Los Angeles: Andrus Gerontology Center, University of Southern California, 1996.

Tideiksaar, R. *Falls in Older Persons: Prevention and Management*, 2nd ed. Baltimore: Health Professions Press, 1998.

Visiting Nurse Association of America. *Caregiver's Handbook: A Complete Guide to Home Health Care.* New York: DK Publishing, 1998.

Warner, M. L. *The Complete Guide to Alzheimer's Proofing Your Home.* West Lafayette, Ind.: Purdue University Press, 1998.

PART 3
Treatment and Treatment Options

Complementary and Alternative Medicine

Complementary and alternative medicine (CAM) refers to practices that are not typically included in mainstream or "conventional" medicine as we know it in the United States. Some CAM therapies may appear strange, yet most people probably have used some of them within their own families without giving it much thought. For instance, comforting a child by rubbing his injured knee, burning a scented candle to create a mood, or comforting yourself with chicken soup when you have the flu are all forms of complementary medicine. Many of the folk medicine practices that once were viewed as having no place in a progressive health care system now are gaining widespread acceptance and being scientifically proven to be effective. Today, more than four out of every ten Americans have visited an alternative health practitioner and most are paying for these services out of their own pockets. The significance of the interest in CAM further is evidenced by the fact that in 1992 Congress established an Office of Alternative Medicine, now called the National Center for Complementary and Alternative Medicine, as a branch of the National Institutes of Health to represent this area of health care.

WHY THE INTEREST IN CAM?

Rather than our health care system introducing CAM to consumers as an improved means to promote wellness and treat diseases, it has been the groundswell from consumers that has sparked interest. There are a variety of reasons for this:

Medicine can replace body organs but not cure a common cold. Medical advancements have been profound in past decades. Damaged hearts can be repaired, women approaching their senior years can be aided to become pregnant, and mangled bodies can be reconstructed. Yet many people find that conventional medicine offers little to relieve them of chronic headaches, fatigue, indigestion, and other basic symptoms that affect the quality of their daily lives. On the other hand, suggestions for lifestyle modifications and nonconventional treatments offered by CAM sometimes prove successful in managing these problems.

People are less willing to "grin and bear" the consequences of health conditions. Previous generations were unlikely to challenge assumptions that they had to learn to live with the unpleasant consequences of diseases. But that has changed. Today's consumers want to look and feel their best and are demanding care to assist them in doing so, even if that care reflects practices outside mainstream medicine.

Blind obedience is being replaced by active participation. The passive compliance that health care consumers once demonstrated is diminishing as people assume increasing responsibility for their own health care. They are becoming informed about their health conditions, exploring the Internet for innovative approaches, and requesting that their doctors order certain tests and treatments, including those considered alternative therapies.

Evidence and experience with CAM are growing. It is the rare person who doesn't know someone who has benefited by taking an herb, getting acupuncture, or having a treatment from a chiropractor. Frequently, glowing testimonials stimulate interest in giving these therapies a try. The media regularly highlights the latest research that supports various CAM therapies.

Using CAM is often more pleasant than using conventional medicine. Unless you've lived in a cave for the past decade, you're probably familiar with the growing dissatisfaction with the health care system. The cost of drugs is skyrocketing. Many consumers have no say in selecting their physicians. Care has become impersonal. Health care providers typically spend an average of ten to fifteen minutes with clients and don't take the time to listen, explain, or individualize services. Contrast this to consumers' experiences with CAM, in which practitioners take the time to know their clients, offer comforting therapies, and partner with clients to develop lifestyle practices to improve the quality of their lives.

COMPLEMENTARY AND ALTERNATIVE THERAPIES

The National Center for Complementary and Alternative Medicine has organized the hundreds of various complementary and alternative therapies into seven fields of practice. These are listed below, along with examples of therapies that fall into each category. Some of these therapies may be more familiar to you than others. Some, like acupuncture, have existed for centuries; others are relatively new.

Mind/body interventions
- Aromatherapy
- Art therapy
- Biofeedback
- Hypnosis
- Imagery
- Meditation
- Music therapy
- Relaxation
- T'ai chi
- Yoga

Alternative systems of healing
- Acupuncture
- Ayurvedic medicine
- Environmental medicine
- Homeopathy
- Naturopathy
- Traditional Oriental medicine

Diet and nutrition
- Cultural diets (e.g., Mediterranean, Native American)
- Supplements

Manual healing methods
- Chiropractic medicine
- Energy work (e.g., therapeutic touch, Reiki)
- Massage
- Herbal medicine

Pharmacologic and biologic treatments
- Bee venom
- Cartilage products
- Hoxsey method

Bioelectromagnetic applications
- Electroacupuncture
- Magnet therapy

Strong research exists supporting the effectiveness of some alternative therapies, whereas others lack scientific proof and rely only on subjective experiences. The fact that a complementary or alternative therapy lacks scientific evidence to prove that it is effective doesn't necessarily mean that it's ineffective. It could very well be that the therapy has not been proven to be effective yet!

WHY USE CAM THERAPIES?

Despite the differences among the various types of alternative therapies, they do share some common principles, the most basic being that healing comes from within a person. Many conventional treatments, like medications, work by attacking the illness. For example, an infection is treated by taking a drug that kills the bacteria causing the infection. But the body has a tremendous capacity to heal itself. Although this is quite obvious when a cut on the skin grows new tissue and closes, many examples not easily seen with the naked eye take place in the body every day. Many alternative therapies work by strengthening the body's own abilities to resist and fight illnesses. In the case of an infection, herbs can be used that stimulate the body's immunity and enable the body to fight the bacteria on its own.

In the past, it was common for people to look to their physicians to solve their health problems. Patients passively received treatments that were prescribed or performed by the physician. Alternative therapies demand a different role for clients, an active one in which clients are active participants in promoting their health and managing illnesses. Rather than a subservient role, patients are partners with their health care providers.

Complementary and alternative medicine recognizes that health and healing are related to the status and harmony of body, mind, and spirit. A physical symptom, for instance, would not be viewed separate from a person's emotional or spiritual states. All aspects of an individual's makeup are considered and addressed in the treatment plan.

Another important principle of most alternative therapies is that positive health practices must be present to promote health and care for illnesses. Many people visit their physicians for medications and other means to treat symptoms. They may take their prescribed treatments but continue lifestyle practices that are counter to good health. For example, a person with high blood pressure may take the antihypertensive drug that his doctor ordered, yet continue to eat high-sodium junk food, use tobacco, manage stress poorly, and get little or no exercise. Complementary and alternative approaches emphasize the importance of improving health habits in general (e.g., nutritious diet, adequate rest, regular exercise, effective stress management, fresh air, good elimination patterns, frequent interaction with nature, development of a positive attitude, avoiding contact with hazardous substances).

A very important principle to keep in mind when using alternative therapies is this: Care is optimized when alternative therapies are *integrated* with conventional treatments. Despite their value, alternative therapies are not intended to replace conventional medicine. Indeed, it would be like throwing the baby out with the bathwater to suggest turning your back on conventional medicine and only use alternative remedies. Alternative therapies can be highly beneficial in improving overall health and managing symptoms; sometimes medications can be reduced or avoided by using an alternative therapy. But there are times when modern medicine is essential. Using the best of both worlds is the ideal approach.

A SURVEY OF POPULAR CAM THERAPIES

As mentioned earlier, some alternative therapies are well established and supported by sound research, whereas others are new or based on theories alone. In this section are some of the most popular alternative therapies, what they are used for, and specific precautions to keep in mind.

Of course, there are scores of other alternative therapies aside from those listed below, and new ones are appearing with regularity. Some of these may have merit but may be as yet unproven. Some may be advanced by persons attempting to sell a related product. The fact that printed matter or an impressive Web site exists doesn't necessarily mean that a therapy or product will do what it claims. Consumer discretion is warranted. For some assistance in gaining objective information about alternative therapies, contact the National Center for Complementary and Alternative Medicine.

ACUPUNCTURE

Although it didn't become popular in the United States until the 1970s, acupuncture has been used in China for over two thousand years. This technique is part of Traditional Chinese Medicine and is based on the belief that there are invisible channels called meridians throughout the body in which vital energy known, as qi (pronounced "chee"), flows. A blockage or imbalance in this energy flow produces disease and symptoms; an insufficient flow of qi can cause fatigue. Acupuncture helps to restore the proper flow of qi by stimulating acupuncture points on the meridians. The treatment, performed by a trained acupuncturist, consists of placing special needles under the skin at acupoints. Not only is the site at which the needles are placed important, but the angle and depth of needle insertion as well.

Typically the acupuncturist conducts an assessment during the initial visit, which consists of taking a history, examining the tongue, and evaluating pulses in both wrists. This assessment assists in making a diagnosis, which can be very different from the type of diagnosis in a conventional medical office. For example, rather than state that a particular organ is not functioning well, the acupuncturist is more likely to talk about imbalances. The acupuncturist places needles at the appropriate points, which may have no correlation to the area of the body experiencing symptoms. Sometimes the acupuncturist applies heat to the acupoints by burning a dried herb in the top of the needle or on the skin to energize the effect of the needle treatment, a procedure known as moxibustion. Other means of stimulating points might also be used, such as electroacupuncture, in which a small current of electricity is applied to the tip of the needle.

Of the many uses for acupuncture, the most common is for pain relief. The National Institutes of Health Consensus Panel on Acupuncture also has identified other areas in which research has shown benefits of this procedure, such as for dental pain and chemotherapy-induced nausea and vomiting. Additionally, some popular uses for acupuncture are for back pain, nicotine withdrawal, stroke rehabilitation, carpal tunnel syndrome, asthma, and hives.

Some people feel very relaxed after a treatment, so it would be wise for someone undergoing their first acupuncture treatment to have someone drive them home, in case they have any symptoms that could interfere with their ability to drive home. Many people report an increased sense of well-being after a treatment. Because acupuncturists use disposable needles the risk of infection is low. Complications from acupuncture treatment are rare.

Initial appointments with an acupuncturist can take one to two hours; follow-up appointments range thirty minutes to one hour. Growing numbers of medical insurance companies are paying for acupuncture treatments.

AYURVEDA

Ayurveda is perhaps the oldest of all medical systems, existing in India for over five thousand years. The term *Ayurveda* means "science of life." This system of care promotes spiritual, mental, and physical balance. Approaches to achieve balance are noninvasive and include yoga, massage, vegetarian diet, purification regimens, breathing exercises, meditation, and herbs.

In Ayurveda, people are described as having body types called doshas, which are categorized as vata, pitta, and kapha. The body type determines the treatments used to restore balance; therefore, Ayurvedic treatments are highly individualized.

The first visit to an Ayurvedic practitioner can take about one hour. The practitioner will take the patient's history, examine the tongue, take the pulse in several places, and learn about the patient's habits. The practitioner may then prescribe a special diet, exercises, herbs, and a daily routine to follow. Costs vary depending on the type of treatments provided, and at this time health insurance generally does not cover the services of an Ayurvedic practitioner.

Meditation, yoga, herbal remedies, dietary modifications, and other approaches used by the Ayurvedic practitioner can benefit health in general. As is the case in the use of any supplement, discuss with your physician any herbal supplements prescribed by the Ayurvedic practitioner before using it to assure there will not be drug-herb interactions or other adverse effects. There has been concern that herbs imported from India could be contaminated with heavy metals, which further emphasizes the importance of consulting with your physician before using these products. Purification treatments (e.g., purging, laxatives, cleansing enemas) to remove toxins may be used by Ayurvedic practitioners; be aware that they can increase the risk for dehydration or affect other health conditions (e.g., diabetes, heart disease), so check with your physician first.

There is no process for certifying Ayurvedic practitioners in the United States, so you need to be cautious when selecting a practitioner.

BIOFEEDBACK

Biofeedback is a technique in which people are taught to control or bring about changes in certain bodily functions, such as blood pressure, heart rate, respiration, and skin temperature. Machinery is used to measure body functions (e.g., pulse, blood pressure) while the person uses relaxation techniques, images, and mental exercises to change those functions. The machine gives feedback on the body's response. In time, the person learns how to bring about the response and no longer needs to rely on the equipment.

Biofeedback can prove helpful for a variety of conditions, including Raynaud's syndrome, urinary incontinence, cardiac arrhythmias, headache, back pain, and irritable bowel syndrome. Studies have found that biofeedback training can help persons who have had a stroke to improve their gait, grasp, and grip.

CHIROPRACTIC MEDICINE

Chiropractic medicine is a popular alternative therapy in the United States, where it was developed in the latter part of the nineteenth century. Chiropractors are licensed in every state, and an estimated one in three people with lower back pain has been treated by one.

Chiropractic medicine is based on the belief that misalignments of the spine, known as subluxations, can put pressure on the nerves, leading to pain and disruption of normal body function. The chiropractic treatment consists of the chiropractor using his or her hands to manipulate or adjust the spine.

Most people seek chiropractic treatment for relief of pain, a use for which research has supported its benefit. Although these areas have not been well researched, many people find benefit from chiropractic treatment to improve breathing with asthma, relieve gastrointestinal disorders, and prevent tension headache.

At the first visit the chiropractor will take a detailed medical history, perform a physical examination, and perhaps order x-rays (or review those already done). The chiropractor performs the treatment by moving and stretching the joints and applying pressure to specific areas. Often, exercises and dietary and lifestyle changes are recommended.

Most of the reported complications associated with chiropractic treatments have involved cervical (neck) manipulations that caused fracture, blood clots to the brain, and injury to the trachea (windpipe); these complications are rare. The risk of these complications is reduced when treatments are given by an experienced chiropractor. The risk of injury from a chiropractic treatment can be lessened by informing the chiropractor of any history of osteoporosis, spinal problems, blood clots, or stroke. Be sure the chiropractor asks if the patient is taking a blood thinner (anticoagulant), because treatments can increase the risk of bleeding and bruising.

The length and cost of visits to a chiropractor vary. Most major medical insurance companies will pay for chiropractic treatments, so you may want to check with your insurer to see if chiropractic treatments are covered.

DIETARY SUPPLEMENTS

There are some legitimate reasons for taking dietary supplements. With the growing numbers of people depending on fast foods, there is a strong likelihood that many people fail to consistently eat healthy, well-balanced meals. Unlike our ancestors, who had ready access to fresh fruits and vegetables, our "fresh" foods may have been in transit or sitting in the produce section of the supermarket for days before they reach our homes and may have lost some of their nutritional value, since vitamins and minerals break down in the process. People are under so much stress these days that we may need higher levels of vitamins and minerals to provide adequate protection. Research is growing that demonstrates the role of high doses of certain vitamins and minerals in preventing and improving many diseases.

The Johns Hopkins Medical Institutions offer the following advice to older adults regarding dietary supplements:

- Take a basic multivitamin supplement daily.
- Get a total of 1500 mg of calcium each day. (If taking this in a supplement, split it into three doses of 500 mg each, the maximum the body can absorb at one time.)
- If a person isn't exposed to much sunlight, take 400 IU of vitamin D to help with the absorption of calcium. Take an extra 1 mg of vitamin B12 to assure that excessive folate (folic acid) consumption doesn't mask deficiencies of B12.
- Use the natural form of vitamin E, because it is absorbed about twice as well as the synthetic form.
- Take supplements with food.
- Avoid supplements that supply more than 100% of the recommended daily allowances for vitamin A and iron; the body needs less of these nutrients with age. Be aware that not all calcium supplements are alike. Some people absorb calcium citrate better than calcium carbonate. Ask your health care provider which form is best for you or your loved one.

Taking high doses of vitamins and minerals can be risky business. For example:

- More than 2500 mg of calcium daily can cause kidney stones and impair the body's ability to absorb other minerals.

- Vitamin D taken in levels above 2000 IU daily is toxic and can cause nausea, poor appetite, weakness, and calcium deposits in the blood vessels and kidneys.
- High doses of folic acid can mask a vitamin B12 deficiency, which can cause dementia.
- Excess vitamin K can interfere with the action of anticoagulants (blood thinners) and lead to blood clots in patients taking anticoagulation therapy.
- High doses of beta-carotene could increase the risk of developing lung cancer in smokers.
- High levels of vitamins A and E could interfere with chemotherapy. Other possible side effects from high levels of vitamin A include fatigue, malaise, lethargy, psychiatric changes, anorexia, sweating, and skin changes.

It is important to read labels carefully to know the supplements you are taking and their dosage. Tell your health care provider what supplements you are taking and learn about the side effects and adverse effects that can occur. It is particularly important to ask about potential interactions with prescription medications you are taking before you begin to take dietary supplements. Other considerations include discontinuing certain supplements before elective surgery. It is therefore very important to tell your physician what you are taking.

HERBS

Herbs are plants that are used for medicines or as seasoning. Every culture in the world has used herbs for healing purposes. Although opinions vary as to the number of Americans who currently use herbs, a national survey on trends in the use of alternative medicine published in the *Journal of the American Medical Association* reported that in the United States there has been a 380 percent increase in the use of herbal remedies between 1990 and 1997, and that over $5 billion is spent annually for these products. This survey also revealed that about one in five persons took herbal remedies and/or high-dose vitamins with prescription drugs, subjecting themselves to serious adverse effects with the mixing of these substances. It is therefore recommended that you talk with your physician or pharmacist before starting any herbal remedies or dietary supplements. Be cautious about the use of herbal supplements prior to any surgery and discuss this issue with your physician or pharmacist.

Herbs can be used in a variety of forms: capsules, tablets, tinctures, teas, syrups, soaks, oils, and ointments. Aromatherapy is a branch of herbal medicine that uses the scents of essential oils of plants to produce therapeutic results. Not only does each herb have a unique action, but different parts of the same herb can have different actions. In dandelions, for example, the leaf has a diuretic (urine-producing) effect, but the root acts as a laxative (stimulates bowel movements).

Well over twenty thousand herbs can be consumed, so you can imagine that staying informed about most of them could be a full-time job. There are, however, a small number that tend to be highly popular or particularly useful, including:

Echinacea. Commonly referred to as a natural antibiotic, this herb stimulates the body's immune system to fight infectious agents. It has no serious side effects, although it does cause an upset stomach and gas in some people. Some persons with environmental allergies (e.g., ragweed) may not tolerate echinacea well and could experience severe reactions. It is best to limit echinacea to short-term use (i.e., less than two months).

Chamomile. Many people have discovered that a cup of chamomile tea at bedtime can get them in the mood to sleep. This herb does have a sedative effect. Chamomile also can calm an upset digestive tract and relieve symptoms of diarrhea with cramping. As there is some thought that chamomile can affect bleeding time, anyone taking an anticoagulant or blood-thinning drug, such as warfarin (Coumadin), aspirin, and nonsteroidal anti-inflammatory drugs (NSAIDs), should discuss this with their doctor.

Garlic. This highly popular herb is beneficial for a variety of purposes, including lowering blood pressure, reducing "bad cholesterol" levels, protecting against infection, and boosting the immune system. There are deodorized forms to avoid the breath odors commonly associated with garlic. Some people experience an upset stomach when taking garlic. Garlic can prolong bleeding time, so people who are taking drugs that could thin the blood (e.g., an anticoagulant such as warfarin [Coumadin], aspirin, and NSAIDs) should discuss this with their doctors.

Ginger. Sipping ginger ale has long been known to settle an upset stomach. That's because of this herb's antinausea effects. It is as effective as over-the-counter

661

motion sickness and antinausea medications without the side effect of drowsiness. Because this herb can prolong bleeding time, anyone taking drugs that could thin the blood (e.g., an anticoagulant such as warfarin [Coumadin], aspirin, and NSAIDs) should discuss using ginger with their doctor.

Ginkgo biloba. This herb has become popular lately for its ability to improve cognitive performance in persons with Alzheimer's disease and other dementias. In addition, it has some benefit in the treatment of dizziness and tinnitus (ringing in the ears). Ginkgo can prolong bleeding time, so anyone taking drugs that could thin the blood (e.g., an anticoagulant such as warfarin [Coumadin], aspirin, and NSAIDs) should discuss using ginkgo with their doctor.

Ginseng. Ginseng serves as an energy booster and offers protection against the ill effects of stress. Its stimulant effects can cause insomnia (which is a reason for not taking it in the evening), headache, nosebleeds, palpitations, and a rise in blood pressure. Ginseng should not be used in those who have high blood pressure or who are taking drugs that could thin the blood. Ginseng can also lower glucose (sugar) levels, so it is important for patients with diabetes mellitus to discuss taking this herbal supplement with their doctor.

Green tea. Many people drink green tea as a cancer preventive, for stomach disorders, to control diarrhea, and to promote overall wellness. It contains a small amount of caffeine and acts as a stimulant, which can cause dizziness, restlessness, insomnia, loss of appetite, diarrhea, and headache. Decaffeinated varieties are available. Because of the effect of green tea on blood platelets, discuss its use with your physician.

Hawthorn. Blood pressure can be lowered with the use of this herb. In fact, blood pressure can drop so profoundly that dizziness and lightheadedness leading to falls can occur. When using hawthorn, it is wise to rise slowly from lying or sitting positions to reduce the risk of falling. Hawthorn also can be useful in mild cardiac disease in improving the function of the heart. Hawthorn may increase the effects of the medication digoxin and could profoundly reduce blood pressure when taken with a prescription antihypertensive drug, so discuss its use with your physician.

Saw palmetto. This herb has gained wide popularity for treatment of benign prostatic hyperplasia (enlarged prostate gland). Although at this point there is no evidence that it reduces the size of enlarged prostate glands, saw palmetto

THE ST. JOHN'S WORT DEBATE

The sales of St. John's wort in the United States significantly increased in the 1990s as its value in improving depression and anxiety were discovered. But in 2001, several major studies found that St. John's wort was no more effective than a placebo for treating certain types of depression. Despite these results, St. John's wort remains one of the top-selling herbal supplements in this country.

There are some things to keep in mind if you decide to use this herb. Like prescription antidepressant drugs, St. John's wort's effects in relieving depression can take four to six weeks to be apparent. Some people have experienced a sensitivity to sunlight, increased blood pressure, drowsiness, and rashes when using this herb. St. John's wort can interact with several prescription drugs, including oral contraceptives, the asthma medication theophylline, the heart medication digoxin, the immunosuppressant cyclosporine, the HIV drug indinavir, and the blood thinner warfarin (Coumadin). It is best to avoid taking it with mood-altering drugs, such as prescription antidepressants. Therefore, discuss its use with your physician.

improves urine flow and some of the symptoms associated with this problem, making it a useful herb for prostate complaints. It also has benefit in treating urinary tract infections. Men should have a prostate exam and laboratory studies (a prostate-specific antigen [PSA] test) to rule out cancer before using saw palmetto for symptoms of benign prostatic hyperplasia. Some people experience an upset stomach when taking saw palmetto, but this can be reduced by taking the herb with meals. It is best to avoid taking saw palmetto in combination with hormones, such as estrogen.

Valerian. This herb is used as a natural sedative (sleep inducer) and tranquilizer. Other than occasional stomach upset, it is not known to have any adverse effects, so it can be safely used. Do not take valerian while using tranquilizers or alcohol.

Herbal products are not regulated by the FDA, although in 1994 Congress passed the Dietary Supplement and Health Education Act, which prevents manufacturers and distributors of herbal supplements from making unproven claims, such as promising a cure, and requires that the active ingredients be listed. It is the manufacturer's responsibility to ensure that its products are safe and are properly labeled prior to marketing. However, labels are not required to list potential toxic effects and interactions with drugs. Also, there is no guarantee that the amount of active ingredient stated on the label is actually in the product that you buy. These general guidelines apply also to the increasingly popular Chinese herbs, which were once consumed primarily as teas and are now being marketed in capsules and other forms. This can create some challenges for consumers, because quality and potency can vary from batch to batch.

Consumers must take special precautions to ensure they are using herbal supplements safely. Do not exceed the recommended doses for the herbs. "More" does not mean "better results," and serious complications could develop. Avoid using an herb on a long-term basis without the guidance of a health care provider who can supervise and monitor the effects. Treat herbal remedies with the same caution that you would apply to pharmaceutical drugs, and become knowledgeable about the herbs you use. Be aware that herbs from India and China may be contaminated with heavy metals, or may include pharmaceutical agents used in the herb preparation. In addition to the growing number of books in libraries and bookstores, there are some useful resources on the Internet for seeking information about herbs.

HOMEOPATHIC REMEDIES

Homeopathy is a branch of medicine developed by Samuel Hahnemann in the late eighteenth century. In the 1990s, Americans' interest in homeopathy began to soar, evidenced by skyrocketing sales of homeopathic remedies.

Homeopathy is derived from the Greek words *homios*, meaning "similar," and *pathos*, meaning suffering. This sheds light on the basic foundation of homeopathy, which is the Law of Similars, meaning that remedies are prescribed that produce symptoms similar to those of the illness being treated. This may sound strange until you consider that people who suffer from allergies are given injections of the suspected allergens to increase their tolerance to the responsible allergen and that trace amounts of disease-causing pathogens are administered through vaccines when you are immunized against a disease. An extract of a plant or other biologic material that is known to produce a particular symptom is made into a tincture by being soaked in alcohol. This tincture is then diluted many times, to the point that there is only a trace of the original substance. The more dilute the preparation is, the higher its potency. The final solution is added to a sugar tablet or powder to be taken orally, or to a lotion or ointment for external use.

It is believed by practitioners that homeopathic medicines stimulate the body's ability to fight the disease. In the classical practice, a homeopath (the practitioner of homeopathic medicine) observes the symptoms and develops a customized prescription based on many unique characteristics of the individual. The homeopath evaluates the person's healing based on the Law of Cure, which claims that if the remedy is effective, symptoms will travel from vital to less vital organs of the body, move from within the body outward, and disappear in reverse order of appearance. If symptoms fail to respond to the Law of Cure, additional treatment is given or a new remedy is prescribed. Often, a worsening of symptoms after the homeopathic remedy is given is considered a positive step in the healing process.

Homeopathic remedies have been shown to be effective for a wide range of conditions such as hay fever, rheumatoid arthritis, influenza symptoms, headache, and vertigo.

Although the ideal method of using homeopathic remedies is under the direction of a homeopath, homeopathic remedies are available over the counter for various ailments, ranging from ear infections to arthritis pain.

HYPNOTHERAPY

Hypnosis refers to an induced trance-like state, which causes a person to be receptive to suggestion. The therapist starts by guiding the person into a relaxed state and then creating an image that focuses attention on a specific area or problem. The therapist then gives suggestions for the person to follow after the session. Suggestions will not be followed if the person is hypnotized superficially; posthypnotic suggestions will be accepted only when the person is in a deep state of hypnosis. Successful hypnosis depends upon the willingness of the person to be hypnotized, the amount of trust in the therapist, and the control of environmental interferences.

Popular uses for hypnosis include weight control and smoking cessation, but it also has proven beneficial in a wide range of conditions, including chronic pain, migraines, asthma, nausea, irritable bowel syndrome, and behavioral disorders. The World Health Organization advises against the use of hypnosis in persons with psychosis, antisocial personality disorders, and other psychiatric conditions.

IMAGERY

Imagery is growing in popularity, most likely because it is easy to learn and do. As the name implies, imagery is a process of creating an image in the mind that can cause a specific response in the body. Although imagery is used in hypnosis, it differs in that in hypnosis an image is offered by the practitioner, whereas in imagery the person creates his or her own image.

Typically, imagery begins by identifying the problem that needs to be addressed or the desired goal. For example, the problem may be the presence of cancer. The person works toward achieving a state of deep relaxation. (Progressive relaxation exercises can be useful for this purpose.) When fully relaxed, the person develops an image that portrays the desired outcome, being the destruction of the cancer cells. Possible images could include viewing the cancer cells as dots and imagining an eraser wiping them away or seeing the cancer as specks and imagining a vacuum cleaner traveling through the body and removing them. Learning and mastering imagery requires clear thinking and practice, so it may not be appropriate for someone with Alzheimer's disease or other forms of mental impairment.

Imagery has been shown to be effective in pain control and stress management, and is believed to play a role in boosting immunity.

MAGNET THERAPY

Magnet therapy has enjoyed popularity in Japan and Germany for some time but only recently has been accepted in the United States. Although the manner in which magnets work is not completely understood, some theories attempt to explain their effects. Magnets are believed to relieve pain by creating a slight electrical current that stimulates the nervous system and consequently blocks pain sensations. The theory behind magnets' ability to speed the healing process has to do with the magnets attracting and repelling charged particles in the blood, a process that dilates blood vessels and increases circulation. In addition to pain management and wound healing, some people wear magnets to boost their energy and for a variety of other purposes. Many of the suggested uses for magnets come from testimonials, but research on magnets is increasing. For example, research on the benefits of magnet therapy is being conducted at Baylor College of Medicine for use in postpolio syndrome, at Tufts University School of Medicine for fibromyalgia pain, and at New York Medical College for foot pain in persons with diabetes.

Magnets come in a variety of forms, including coin-sized disks that can be strapped on specific areas of the body, pads, seat cushions, blankets, insoles, and mattresses. Magnets differ in strength and price. The strength of magnets is measured in units called gauss and the most effective magnets for therapeutic purposes should have at least 500 gauss. (For comparison, those little refrigerator magnets typically have a gauss of 60.)

Without a full understanding of the dynamics of how magnets work it is difficult to determine all of the precautions and complications that could be associated with this therapy. Some general guidelines, however, are to avoid using magnets if wearing a pacemaker and not to apply them to the abdomen if it's possible the person is pregnant.

A search on the Internet using the term "magnet therapy" will display many Web sites of manufacturers and distributors of magnetic products that offer information about magnets in addition to promoting their specific merchandise. Consumers should be cautious about the claims made on Internet sites that are intended to promote sales of magnets and not provide accurate scientific information.

MASSAGE AND BODYWORK

Massage for healing purposes has been used, literally, for thousands of years, as a preventive health measure to keep people healthy. Massage is the manipulation of soft tissue by using rubbing, pressing, rolling, slapping, and tapping movements. In recent years, energy balancing, movement awareness, and deep tissue manipulation has been combined with massage and is described by the term *bodywork*. Some of the common types of massage and bodywork are listed below.

Swedish (European) massage. Massage consists of long strokes, kneading, and friction movements.

Pressure application. Pressure is applied to unblock meridians and allow energy to flow freely. Acupressure, shiatsu, and Jin Shin Do are examples of this.

Reflexology. This is a form of pressure point application, in which the practitioner applies pressure to specific areas of a person's hands or feet that correspond to various parts of the body.

Movement integration. This system rebalances and teaches new ways to move the body. The Alexander technique and the Feldenkrais method are examples.

Therapeutic touch. Here the touching is not directly on the body, but on the person's energy field, which extends a few inches outside the body. The practitioner draws upon a universal field of energy and by moving his or her hands in a purposeful manner directs that energy on the person being treated to mobilize the person's inner healing resources. The flowing energy unblocks the person's obstructed energy.

In addition to promoting relaxation and reducing stress, massage can be useful for reducing edema (swelling from fluid retention); promoting circulation, breathing, and elimination; and relieving pain, anxiety, and depression. It may be best to avoid massages if blood clots or skin infections are present.

MEDITATION AND PROGRESSIVE RELAXATION

Meditation is the practice of calming the mind and focusing on the present. Other parts of the world have used meditation for centuries, but it wasn't until the 1970s, when Harvard Medical School cardiologist Herbert Benson discovered that after people meditated for twenty minutes, physiologic signs of relaxation appeared, such as decreases in heart rate, blood pressure, and respirations. This opened the path for meditation to be used for reduction of stress, anxiety, pain, seizure activity, and high blood pressure, and to boost immune function. Persons who meditate tend to have improved self-esteem and higher levels of mental function.

There are several approaches to meditation, including:

Concentrative meditation. The focus is on breathing, an image, or a sound, such as a mantra or chant.

Mindfulness meditation. Attention is paid to sensations, sounds, scents, thoughts, and feelings that are being experienced. The person is aware, but does not control or judge the experiences, which promotes a calm state of mind.

Transcendental meditation. Introduced by Maharishi Mahesh Yogi, this form of meditation involves having the body reach a level of profound relaxation while the mind becomes more alert.

Progressive relaxation. This is another means to calm the body and mind. Typically, a person learns to guide himself or herself through a series of exercises that relax the body. The person may tighten the muscles in one arm and then relax them, make a tight fist and then open the hand, repeat these exercises on the other arm and hand, tighten the muscles on one leg and then relax them, and so on. Progressive relaxation has the same benefits as meditation, and as it is a great stress reducer, it is a helpful practice for caregivers to build into their schedules.

Audiotapes are available in bookstores and many health food stores. The tapes have scripts for guiding meditation and progressive relaxation exercises.

NATUROPATHY

As the name implies, naturopathy involves using natural approaches to enhance health and treat illnesses. Naturopathic doctors (N.D.s) help their clients identify unhealthy practices; educate them about healthy living habits; encourage a balanced diet, exercise, and rest; and counsel them in the management of health problems. They may treat illnesses with herbs, dietary supplements, diet modifications, homeopathic remedies, hydrotherapy (the therapeutic use of water), and other natural approaches. Some N.D.s are trained to do minor suturing, acupuncture, and other procedures. Most N.D.s will refer clients to conventional physicians for conditions that are beyond their scope of practice. For chronic health conditions, however, N.D.s can offer considerable help in learning about lifestyle practices and natural remedies that can help.

Not all N.D.s are the same. Some gained their experience by working with other N.D.s; others may have taken a variety of educational programs to prepare them to educate and counsel people about health. There are a limited number of accredited naturopathic medical schools, such as Bastyr University (www.bastyr.edu), Southwest College of Naturopathic Medicine and Health Sciences (www.scnm.edu), and National College of Naturopathic Medicine (www.ncnm.edu). A limited number of states (Alaska, Arizona, Connecticut, Hawaii, Maine, Montana, New Hampshire, Oregon, Utah, Vermont, and Washington) license naturopaths and require that N.D.s must have graduated from a school accredited by the Council on Naturopathic Medical Education. However, naturopaths do practice in other states; some of these have licenses in other fields (e.g., acupuncture or nursing) and have training from schools not accredited by the Council on Naturopathic Medical Education.

Fees for naturopathic care vary. Typically, the first visit to an N.D. consists of an assessment that can take approximately one hour with a cost ranging from

$100 to $200. Shorter follow-up visits can range from $50 to $75. Some insurance companies cover visits to N.D.s and it is best to check with your individual insurer to learn about coverage.

PRAYER AND FAITH

According to Gallup polls, 95% of Americans believe in God or some higher power, 76% pray on a regular basis, and 79% believe faith can influence a recovery from illness. So faith and prayer can hardly be viewed as "alternative therapies" in the United States. However, we have recently seen a new emphasis on the role of faith in health and healing, and research to support that positive relationship. The accumulation of hundreds of well-done studies reveals that:

- People who profess a faith and attend regular religious services are healthier than those who do not.
- Caregivers of persons with cancer and Alzheimer's disease who had a strong faith had a healthier emotional state than caregivers without faith.
- Older adults who attended religious services lived longer and had lower rates of disability than those who did not, even when they had chronic health conditions.
- Hospitalization rates and lengths of stay are lower in people who attend church regularly.
- People with a religious faith had lower rates of depression and recovered faster when they did experience depression.

In addition to those and other studies that show a positive relationship between people's faith and their health status, research has demonstrated the value of distant, intercessory prayer. The International Center for the Integration of Health & Spirituality (www.nihr.org) has published a summary of scientific research done and advances education and research in the area of spirituality and health.

Praying with or for a person who has an illness and is open to prayer certainly cannot harm and could do considerable good. Likewise, caregivers could benefit from praying and asking others to pray for them. Neither you nor the person you care for should be forced into prayer or religious practices that are contrary to personal beliefs. It is important that prayers for cures that are not answered with the desired outcome not cause you to feel as though you have failed or that God has failed you. Also, be wary of spiritual organizations or persons who offer "guarantees of cure" or are willing to pray only if given large amounts of money.

T'AI CHI

T'ai chi is a combination of exercise and energy work that gives the appearance of a slow, graceful dance using continuous, controlled arm and leg movements. This is another Traditional Chinese Medicine practice that is used to balance and stimulate the flow of qi, the life energy discussed earlier under "Acupuncture."

The Arthritis Foundation recommends the value of t'ai chi to persons with arthritis, particularly rheumatoid arthritis. The *Journal of the American Medical Association*, in an article on exercise and elderly individuals, described a study in which older adults who practiced t'ai chi experienced an increase in muscle endurance and a 25 percent reduction in falls. T'ai chi exercise videos are available, but attending a class may be more helpful.

A publication called *Qi: The Journal of Traditional Eastern Health & Fitness* (www.qi-journal.com) offers articles on t'ai chi, a list of practitioners, and an animated demonstration of t'ai chi movements.

YOGA

Although yoga originated more than five thousand years ago as a mystical Hindu form of worship, it now commonly refers to a system of exercises involving various postures, meditation, and deep breathing. The word *yoga* means "union," which appropriately describes the connection of body, mind, and spirit achieved during this practice. Yoga has been found helpful for pain, anxiety, stress, fatigue, high blood pressure, poor circulation, and respiratory and digestive disorders.

Some of the yoga postures and stretches can be difficult for older adults or persons with restricted movement. However, modifications can be done and stretching the body to a person's own limits, even if not to the full postures typically done in yoga exercises, could prove helpful. Yoga videos and yoga classes are available in most communities.

HOW TO USE CAM WISELY

People with chronic conditions can integrate CAM with conventional therapies to use the best of both worlds. CAM provides additional options for persons with chronic health conditions that can assist in relieving symptoms, improving health status, and lowering health care costs. Using CAM doesn't imply that the medications and other treatments that conventional medicine offers should be rejected. Rather, it means that people assume responsibility for improving their health, adopt positive health habits, and develop a plan with their physicians to integrate safe, effective CAM therapies into their care. CAM also offers practices and therapies that can assist you as a caregiver to take care of your own health and minimize the effects of caregiving stress.

However, used indiscriminately, CAM therapies can have more negative than positive effects and create a new host of problems. To be sure you are maximizing the benefits of using alternative therapies while minimizing risks, consider the following advice:

Know the conditions you are dealing with. Before using CAM for your loved one, be sure that he or she has been properly evaluated by a conventional health care practitioner. Symptoms such as pain or insomnia that could be managed with an alternative therapy could be associated with a serious health condition. Masking or reducing the symptom without addressing its cause could postpone the person's receiving essential care and cause the condition to worsen, leading to serious complications. Be sure that a complete physical examination and lab tests have been done and that a diagnosis has been established or ruled out.

Do your homework. Learn about alternative therapies that could prove useful for your loved one's health conditions. The Web sites of associations that address specific health concerns (e.g., Arthritis Foundation, American Heart Association) may provide information about both conventional and alternative treatments. A search of Web sites related to a specific disease (e.g., multiple sclerosis, Alzheimer's disease) could lead you to alternative therapy products that could prove useful, but be aware that you need to use discretion to assure claims made are based on sound evidence rather than the opinion of the person selling the product. Likewise, you may learn of potentially helpful alternative therapy products from friends and family, but ask for articles or other proof that supports claims and make sure those articles or fact sheets are from reputable sources and not merely the distributor of the product. As mentioned earlier, the National Center for Complementary and Alternative Medicine is an excellent resource for checking out claims and getting objective information. Associations related to specific alternative therapies and their practitioners, such as the ones provided under the discussion of various therapies in this chapter, can be good sources of information. Members of support groups also may be able to share useful information that they have gathered.

Consult with your physician or other conventional health care provider. Ask your health care provider about alternative therapies that may be beneficial for the conditions being treated. Share information that you have gathered through your search and ask your health care provider for advice about the usefulness of these therapies for your loved one's specific condition. If your health care provider approves or recommends an alternative therapy, find out if your loved one's health insurance covers it (as may be the case with acupuncture and chiropractic treatment) and if so, ask your health care provider for a prescription or referral. If your health care provider flatly refuses to consider an alternative therapy, ask for an explanation. And do not discontinue a medication or other conventional treatment without consulting with your health care provider.

Give the therapy time to work. Many alternative therapies need time to work because they are bringing about changes within the body rather than just reducing the symptom. Be patient and don't expect miracles after one treatment or dose. (Here again, doing your homework can assist in helping you to understand results you can expect and the time frame in which you can expect them.)

Inform all health care providers of all the CAM therapies and practices being used. You most likely have helped your loved one develop a list of all medications being used that accompanies him or her to every visit to a health care provider. To this list add all herbs, dietary supplements, special diets, and other remedies being used. It is a wise practice to have a few copies of this record: one that the person keeps in his or her wallet, one that is kept in an easily accessible place, and one for you to keep.

Don't postpone diagnosis and treatment. CAM therapies should not be a substitute for good medical care. For example, it may be fine to use acupressure or an herb to assist with an occasional headache, but a chronic headache could indicate an anemia, high blood pressure, or another health problem that needs attention.

Easing the symptoms by using an alternative remedy could postpone having the problem diagnosed and treated. Avoid "playing doctor" and treating symptoms yourself.

Promote good health practices. Neither conventional nor alternative therapies should be viewed as substitutes for good health practices. For example, it makes little sense for a person to use a medication or herb to treat indigestion if he or she continues to eat junk foods that trigger symptoms or fails to modify a stressful lifestyle. A balanced diet, regular exercise, effective stress management, and adequate sleep and rest are among the basic healthy practices that need to be at the core of any treatment plan. Help your loved one to develop healthy practices to promote his or her health and maximize the benefits of all therapies.

Consider using CAM yourself. As a caregiver, you are subjected to many stresses and there is the potential that you may not properly eat, sleep, or otherwise meet your basic health needs. Your own health can suffer as a result. Promote your own health by building some CAM practices into your life. Consider taking a daily multivitamin and mineral supplement, doing a progressive relaxation session daily, bathing in lavender-scented water, treating yourself to a massage, building t'ai chi or yoga exercises into your daily routine, and sipping on herbal teas rather than caffeinated beverages throughout the day. And don't overlook the benefits of improving your own basic health habits to protect yourself from the effects of the stresses of caregiving and to be able to offer your best to the person for whom you care.

ADDITIONAL RESOURCES

ORGANIZATIONS AND WEB SITES
National Center for Complementary and Alternative Medicine

888-644-6226

www.nccam.nih.gov

ACUPUNCTURE
The American Academy of Medical Acupuncture

www.medicalacupuncture.org

The National Commission for the Certification of Acupuncturists

www.acupuncture.com

The Ayurveda Holistic Center

www.ayurvedahc.com

AYURVEDA
The Ayurvedic Institute

www.ayurveda.com

The Maharishi College of Vedic Medicine

www.maharishi-medical.com

The National Institute of Ayurvedic Medicine

www.niam.com

BIOFEEDBACK

Association for Applied Psychophysiology and Biofeedback

www.aapb.org

The Biofeedback Certification Institute of America

www.bcia.org

Biofeedback Webzine

www.webideas.com/biofeedback

CHIROPRACTIC

The American Chiropractic Association

www.amerchiro.org

International Chiropractors Association

www.chiropractic.org

DIETARY SUPPLEMENTS

National Institutes of Health Office of Dietary Supplements

www.dietary-supplements.info.nih.gov

The American Nutraceutical Association

www.americanutra.com

Food and Drug Administration (FDA) Guide to Dietary Supplements

www.vm.cfsan.fda.gov

HERBS

The American Botanical Council

www.herbs.org

Consumer Labs

www.consumerlabs.com

Food and Drug Administration (FDA)

http://vm.cfsan.fda.gov

HerbNet

www.herbnet.com

HOMEOPATHY

The National Center for Homeopathy

www.healthy.net/clinic/therapy/homeopat

HYPNOTHERAPY

The American Institute of Hypnotherapy

www.hypnosis.com

The American Society of Clinical Hypnosis

www.asch.net

The International Medical and Dental Hypnotherapy Association

www.infinityinst.com

The National Guild of Hypnotists

www.ngh.net

GUIDED IMAGERY

The Academy for Guided Imagery

www.healthy.net/agi

Exceptional Cancer Patients

www.hmt.com/cyp/nonprof/ecap

The Simonton Cancer Center

www.simontoncenter.com

MASSAGE

The American Massage Therapy Association

www.amtamassage.org

The Association of Reflexology

www.reflexology.org

Feldenkrais Guild

www.feldenkrais.com

Nurse Healers Professional Associates

www.therapeutic-touch.org

Healing Touch International

www.healingtouch.net

MEDITATION

Mind/Body Health Sciences

www.healthy.net/wellness/mindbody.htm

Maharishi University of Management

www.mum.edu

NATUROPATHY

Council on Naturopathic Medical Education.

www.cnme.org

American Association of Naturopathic Physicians

703-610-9037

www.naturopathic.org

YOGA

The American Yoga Association

www.americanyogaassociation.org

The Himalayan Institute of Yoga, Science and Philosophy

www.himalayaninstitute.org

The Yoga Site

www.yogasite.com

BOOKS AND ARTICLES

American Chiropractic Association. *The Art of Healthy Living: The Consumer's Guide to Chiropractic Care.* Brochure series. Arlington, Va.: American Chiropractic Association. (Free. To order a set, call 800-986-4636.)

Cummings, S., and D. Ullman. *Everybody's Guide to Homeopathic Medicines: Remedies for You and Your Family.* New York: Putnam Publishing, 1997.

Davis, C., ed. *Complementary Therapies in Rehabilitation: Holistic Approaches for Prevention and Wellness.* Thorofare, N.J.: Slack, 1997.

Dossey, L. *Prayer Is Good Medicine.* New York: Harper Collins, 1997.

Eliopoulos, C. *Integrating Conventional and Alternative Therapies: Holistic Care for Chronic Conditions.* St. Louis: Mosby, 1999.

Fontanarosa, P. B., ed. *Alternative Medicine. An Objective Assessment.* Chicago: American Medical Association, 2000.

Francina, S. *The New Yoga for People Over 50.* Health Communications, 1997.

Garrison, R. H., and E. Somer. *The Nutrition Desk Reference,* 3rd ed. New Canaan, Ct.: Keats Publishing, 1997.

Jwing-Ming, Y. *Arthritis: The Chinese Way of Healing and Prevention.* Roslindale, Mass.: YMAA Publishing Center, 1997.

Larson, D. B., J. P. Sawyers, and M. E. McCullough. *Scientific Research on Spirituality and Health: A Consensus Report.* Rockville, Md.: National Institute for Healthcare Research, 1997.

Matthews, D. A. *The Faith Factor: Proof of the Healing Power of Prayer.* New York: Viking-Penguin, 1999.

Matthews, D. A., D. B. Larson, and C. P. Barry. *The Faith Factor: An Annotated Bibliography of Clinical Research on Spiritual Subjects.* Rockville, Md.: National Institute for Healthcare Research, 1993.

Mount Sinai School of Medicine. Eating healthy after 50. *Focus on Healthy Aging* 3 (2000): 7.

NIH Consensus Development Panel on Acupuncture. Acupuncture. *Journal of the American Medical Association.* 280 (1998): 1518-1524.

PDR for Herbal Medicines. 2nd ed. Montvale, N.J.: Medical Economics Co., 2000.

Medication Management

In the United States today, roughly 90 million people—nearly one-third of the total population—suffer from chronic disease. One of the principal forms of treating and managing disease is medication. Why? In addition to behavioral and lifestyle modifications, medications are one of the most cost-effective, safe, and least invasive means of treating and managing chronic disease, playing a crucial role in helping people feel better and live longer.

Unfortunately, chronic disease is both undertreated and overtreated in the United States. In some cases, patients are not properly diagnosed, or once they are diagnosed, they're not adequately educated about how to manage their disease. In other cases, patients are overmedicated, prescribed multiple drugs unnecessarily, leading to unnecessary expenses and adverse health effects.

Medications can and should be a vital component of medical treatment. But in order to be so, they must be managed. That's why medication management is a critical issue—especially for caregivers, who are often charged with the task.

WHAT IS MEDICATION MANAGEMENT?

Perhaps no one has said it more simply than former Surgeon General C. Everett Koop: "Drugs don't work if people won't take them." Drugs also don't work if people don't take the correct dosage, at the correct time, in the correct manner, and for the correct duration. Worse, drugs can have very harmful—and even life-threatening—effects if not carefully monitored. To reap the full benefits of medications, receive their therapeutic effects, and avoid unintentional toxicities, it's critical that patients take their drugs, and take them properly.

Unfortunately, despite occasionally dire consequences, medication nonadherence (failure to take prescribed medications, or to take them correctly) is a great problem in the United States, resulting in enormous health-related and financial costs. Current estimates place nonadherence levels at 50%, with 30% to 40% of patients adhering only partially to their medication regimens and 10% failing to take their medication entirely.

There's another critical issue facing patients and caregivers today: medication safety. In 1999, the Institute of Medicine published a report highlighting this problem. The study estimated that each year, over 770,000 people suffer injuries from adverse drug events and medication errors. In addition, 7,000 deaths are caused each year by medication errors, a number higher than deaths due to workplace injuries. Still other studies estimate this number to be even higher, placing adverse reactions to drugs among the top ten leading causes of deaths in the United States.

But there is hopeful news. Many of these drug reactions and deaths can be prevented through education, communication, advocacy, and careful medication management. When knowledgeable consumers (including caregivers) ask appropriate questions about their prescriptions, and when they provide their doctors with complete information about their medical conditions, medications, and allergies, they help ensure that their medications are safe.

Without a doubt, caregivers play a crucial role in medication management. People over the age of 65 take more drugs than members of any other age group; at any given time, the average older American takes four or five prescription drugs and two over-the-counter (OTC) drugs. In many cases, the caregiver is charged with a number of medication responsibilities:

- Discussing the prescription with the doctor and pharmacist.
- Understanding the medication's benefits and adverse effects (including when to seek medical attention).
- Being aware of all drugs the patient is taking, prescription and OTC.
- Checking for interactions among drugs.
- Filling prescriptions and obtaining refills before the supply runs out.
- Administering the medications throughout the day.

Even if you're not involved with all of these tasks, it's important to be informed about your care recipient's medication regimen. That way, in the event of a medical emergency, you can educate her health care providers.

A CAREGIVER'S CHALLENGES

As a caregiver, you may face special challenges regarding medication management:

MONITORING ADHERENCE

Challenges to medication adherence can be different as people age. Older people take many more medications than younger people, so schedules for taking drugs can become complicated. Older people may be more likely to forget to take their medication, or they may be more easily confused. Many drugs can cause mental fogginess in older people, which makes adherence still trickier.

As a caregiver, you may find that monitoring your care recipient's medication adherence is simply a matter of checking in once a week to make sure that she's taking her medications as prescribed. On the other hand, for people dealing with patients suffering from dementia, it can be considerably more labor-intensive. Some caregivers create a daily chart, administer medications at prescribed times, and check off medications as they're taken. Later in this chapter you'll find strategies for how to best manage your care recipient's medications.

PREVENTING UNDERTREATMENT

Chronically ill patients often go undertreated in the United States—not because health care professionals harbor malicious intent but because patients are not always informed about all of the treatment options available. Pharmaceutical research has made dramatic strides in recent years, and many new drugs—and old drugs in new forms—are available.

As a caregiver, becoming aware of and knowledgeable about treatment options for your care recipient may fall to you. When your care recipient receives a diagnosis, you have the power to request information and conduct research. Your resources include doctors, nurses, pharmacists, peers, patients (especially in online forums), disease-oriented organizations and advocacy groups, books, magazines, and the Internet. See the Additional Resources at the end of this chapter for resources specifically geared to medication management.

PREVENTING POLYPHARMACY

Just as some patients go undertreated, still others suffer from overtreatment, particularly in the form of polypharmacy, or the administration of multiple drugs at the same time. While polypharmacy is generally a necessity for people who suffer from more than one illness, there are plenty of instances in which drugs are prescribed unnecessarily.

For instance, some patients self-medicate with OTC drugs, taking medications for age-related ailments that might be better served by lifestyle changes. Alternatively, sometimes doctors prescribe supplementary medications to counteract adverse effects from primary drugs, when a better solution might be to try a different type of drug to treat the primary condition.

Sometimes, a specialist prescribing a drug may not be aware of what other health care providers have been prescribing for the same patient. In this case, the problem is a lack of communication. As a caregiver, you can prevent this form of overprescription by carrying a complete and up-to-date medications list to every medical appointment.

Your role as caregiver may entail advocating with your care recipient's health care team to be certain that every drug prescribed is medically necessary. An in-depth discussion of polypharmacy (and how to prevent it) follows in this chapter.

SEEKING FINANCIAL REIMBURSEMENT

Recent political attention to a prescription drug benefit for Medicare has called national attention to what most of us already know: Medications can be expensive. And as the caregiver, dealing with the financial issues surrounding your care recipient's medications may be your responsibility.

Depending on your care recipient's insurance plan, you may have to do some footwork to get certain medications covered. At the same time, you may want to look into ways of reducing the costs of medications—such as requesting generic drugs (when appropriate), getting samples from doctors, and appealing directly to pharmaceutical companies. Later in this chapter, we'll provide specific information about the high costs of medications, including strategies for lowering these costs.

GETTING ANSWERS FROM MEDICAL PROFESSIONALS

Crucial to every medication-related decision is knowledge. Because patients can be overwhelmed with the physical and emotional demands of being ill, caregivers are often tasked with doing the research—and asking the questions—to learn as much as possible about the prescriptions. And that means talking to health care professionals—including doctors, nurses, and pharmacists. Getting the information you need involves knowing what to ask, when to ask, and whom to ask. Later in this chapter, we'll provide a list of questions to ask about each medication.

MEDICATION AND THE ELDERLY

People age 65 and older take more medications than any other age group. In fact, older adults take one-quarter of all drugs prescribed in the United States. At the same time, elderly people are more susceptible than their juniors to the adverse effects of medications. Clearly, as a caregiver monitoring medications for an elderly care recipient, you have special concerns.

POLYPHARMACY

Not only do older people suffer from more chronic conditions than younger people, but they also tend to suffer from more than one at a time, leading to polypharmacy—the consumption of several different drugs at once. Of Americans ages 65 to 84, 61% receive three or more prescriptions in a year, 37% receive five or more, and 19% receive seven or more.

In some cases, polypharmacy is an unfortunate result of overprescription, particularly when some drugs produce adverse effects. For example, beta-blockers such as metoprolol or propranolol are used to treat high blood pressure. Some people who take these drugs experience side effects such as difficulty sleeping, nightmares, and, occasionally, depression. If these symptoms are not recognized as possible drug side effects, additional drugs—such as sleeping pills or antidepressants—may be added unnecessarily.

In other cases, polypharmacy may result from an attempt to deal with the normal aches and pains of aging. For instance, rather than exercise and/or lose weight to reduce joint pain, a patient might self-medicate with OTC drugs such as ibuprofen (Advil) or acetaminophen (Tylenol). Overprescription might also result from a lack of communication and coordination among multiple doctors treating the same patient.

Often, however, because many older adults can suffer from multiple chronic conditions, polypharmacy is a simple fact of life for senior citizens.

Polypharmacy presents some very specific risks to the elderly:

More adverse effects. Because of the multiple physiologic changes that occur as we age, aging bodies process drugs differently and more slowly than younger bodies do. Therefore, the elderly are much more likely to suffer adverse effects from drugs, and the more drugs they take, the more adverse effects. Seniors have twice as many adverse reactions to medications as younger adults.

Negative drug-drug interactions. Polypharmacy greatly increases the likelihood of negative interactions between drugs. Sometimes, one drug can blunt the effects of another, preventing a medication from properly doing its job. Equally dangerous, some drugs actually enhance the effects of others, leading to undesired effects and severe and unintended physical symptoms.

As a caregiver, how can you handle polypharmacy?

Make sure all prescriptions are medically necessary. Assemble a list of all of your care recipient's medications, including a detailed description of what each medication is intended to do. Be sure to include OTC drugs as well as vitamins and other dietary supplements. Then review this list with at least two members of the health care team—a doctor or physician's assistant or nurse and the pharmacist—to determine that each drug is medically necessary. In addition, it's helpful to bring the pill bottles to the office, especially for the first visit. You may want to organize the information into a chart (see p. 684).

Check for drug-drug interactions. When you review the list of medications with the health care professionals, ask them to check for possible drug-drug inter-actions. In addition, check the warning labels on the prescriptions to make sure that there are no conflicts. You can also use published guides to check for drug interactions at various Web sites like www.medscape.com and www.webmd.com.

Streamline the regimen. With multiple medications to manage, adherence becomes a greater challenge. To make sure that your care recipient takes all of her medications at the right times, in the right way, in the correct dosage, and for the correct duration, you may want to create a medication calendar (see p. 684).

PROPER DOSAGES

Unfortunately, one in five elderly adults has experienced an adverse reaction to a prescription medicine. The incidence among older adults is twice as high as it is for younger adults because as people age, they become more sensitive to the effects of medication:

- As we get older, the amount of water in the body typically declines, which means drugs aren't diluted as much.
- Older bodies have proportionately less muscle and more fat. Because some drugs dissolve in fat, the body may retain more of the drug for a longer period.
- Like all organs, the kidneys and liver decline in efficiency as we age, so it takes longer for some drugs to be broken down and eliminated from the body.

In fact, the increased effect of medication on the elderly is so pronounced that in the mid-1980s, the Food and Drug Administration established guidelines for drug manufacturers to include elderly adults in their studies of new drugs. (Previously, the elderly had not been isolated as a group in drug trials.) Today, new prescription drugs are generally required to include information on the labels about their use in the elderly.

Because elderly adults are more sensitive to the effects of medication, it's crucial that the dosages they're prescribed be adjusted. The "usual" doses prescribed to adults are often too high for the elderly. As a caregiver, you can remind your care recipient's physician to "start low and go slow," beginning with the smallest dose that might be effective and increasing it only if necessary. In addition, increases must be made slowly to give the recipient time to adjust to the drug's effects.

COMMON ADVERSE EFFECTS

Certain side effects are more common or more problematic in the elderly than in younger people. For instance, the elderly are particularly vulnerable to drugs that may cause lightheadedness, confusion, and impaired coordination. In the first place, aging bodies are more susceptible to these kinds of reactions; in the second, these reactions are more dangerous in the elderly, because older people are at a much higher risk of falling and fracturing a bone.

KEEPING UPDATED RECORDS: THE CAREGIVER'S ROLE

As a caregiver, you're in the ideal position to keep an updated medication list—including a list of your care recipient's allergies and a history of drug toxicities and failures. While there may be some labor involved initially, once you've completed the record, you'll save yourself a lot of time—and you could save your care recipient's life. At the very least, you'll be contributing a great deal to ensure that your care recipient gets the most appropriate medical treatment. Many caregivers elect to record this information in chart form, where it's easily accessible. Here are some examples.

1. Medications chart

	Drug #1	Drug #2	Drug #3	Drug #4
• Name of Drug				
• Date Prescribed				
• Purpose				
• Strength of Each Pill				
• Dose (# of Pills or Amount of Liquid)				
• Times per Day				
• Time of Day				
• Special Instructions				
• Duration				
• Avoid (Foods or Activities)				
• Side Effects Experienced				
• Other Concerns				

Other adverse effects common and problematic in the elderly include:

Delirium and sedation. Disorientation, confusion, irritability, and "sundowning" (worsening confusion and agitation in the evening; awake at night and sleeping during the day) may be due to a newly added medication. Some antihistamines (diphenhydramine, Benadryl), narcotic pain relievers, and other drugs with anticholinergic properties can cause delirium in the elderly. In addition, be watchful

2. Drug allergies chart

Drug/Substance	Date of Reaction	Reaction	Action Taken

3. Medication calendar

Time	Drug /Dose	How Many	Sun	Mon	Tues	Weds	Thurs	Fri	Sat

4. Drug toxicities or failures chart for previous medications

A list of past medications is extremely helpful to health care providers. When a doctor knows which drugs have been tried and didn't work, or which caused intolerable side effects, she can issue new prescriptions more effectively. That is, she can avoid prescribing the medications on the list (or similar drugs in the same class). Or, she may evaluate the cause of the failure and restart the drug in a different manner.

Name of Drug	Date Prescribed	Purpose	Reaction or Problem	Action Taken

of sedation, "morning hangover," and lethargy due to medications. These adverse effects may indicate the need for either a different choice of medication, a reduced dosage, or slower titration, or any combination of these. Or they may simply indicate that the drug should be administered at bedtime rather than during the day.

Urinary retention. Difficulty in voiding experienced by older men with benign prostatic hypertrophy (an irregular enlargement of the prostate that constricts the urethra and interferes with urination) can be aggravated by some drugs. These include some tranquilizers, antidepressants, and antihistamines. Ask about this side effect, and avoid medications that produce it.

Constipation. Constipation is both a frequent problem in the elderly and a common side effect of drugs such as codeine, Vicodin, and verapamil (Calan, Isoptin). Preventive measures include adding bulk and more fluids to the diet and using natural laxatives (prune juice) or OTC stool softeners (docusate, DSS). (For more information in this area, see the Constipation section in the Gastrointestinal Disorders chapter on p. 270.)

It's important to monitor adverse effects caused by medications. When a drug is prescribed, learn what side effects are common and expected, and ask what you can do to prevent or minimize these problems. While some side effects are an unfortunate companion to the benefits of a drug, in many cases adverse effects are a sign that the medication needs to be adjusted. If your care recipient experiences any of the following conditions, call her health care provider immediately:

- Dizziness, lightheadedness
- Sleep changes
- Diarrhea
- Incontinence
- Blurred vision
- Mood changes
- Confusion
- Rash, hives, itching
- Wheezing, shortness of breath

ALTERNATIVE DOSAGE FORMS

Some medical conditions make swallowing very difficult, so having to take a great number of pills may be a source of stress for elderly patients, not to mention an ineffective delivery system. Fortunately, many medications are available in more than one form; others can be crushed and taken in juice or soft foods, such as applesauce. If your care recipient has trouble swallowing, discuss alternative dosage forms with her health care providers:

- Capsules
- Liquids
- Powders and granules
- Inhalers
- Topical patches
- Suppositories
- Long-acting injections
- Nasal sprays

SAFE MEDICATION STORAGE

All medicines need to be stored safely—away from moisture, heat, light, pets, and children. If your care recipient is depressed or forgetful, or has dementia, it's also very important to store her medications where she doesn't have ready access to them.

Store medications in a high, locked cabinet—not under the bathroom sink or behind the bathroom mirror, where toothpaste and other items are stored. In addition, avoid storing drugs in a kitchen cabinet, where they could be confused with vitamins or food. Finally, keep medications stored in their original bottles, with the prescription label and child-resistant caps.

HELP FOR THE VISUALLY OR PHYSICALLY IMPAIRED

If your care recipient is visually or physically impaired, you can request special bottles for her medication. Pharmacists will readily supply oversized, easy-to-open bottles with larger labels bearing larger, bolder print. It might be helpful to keep a magnifying glass in the medication cabinet for added aid.

THE BASICS OF MEDICATION MANAGEMENT

In medication management, as in every aspect of health care, the more you know, the more powerful you are—and the better informed your decisions and actions. Below is a list of questions to ask your care recipient's doctor and pharmacist.

Why is this drug prescribed? When a drug is prescribed, ask your care recipient's doctor why. What does the drug do, and what is it expected to do for your care recipient? It's also important to ask how you can tell whether or not the drug is working. What specific changes should you see? In addition, ask what the doctor will check for (e.g., blood pressure, lung tests, walking distance) to determine the effectiveness of the treatment.

Finally, ask what laboratory tests the doctor will run to see if the drug is working—and that a correct dose was prescribed and taken. For example, a blood cholesterol test would measure whether a cholesterol-lowering drug dose was adequate, and a bone density study would evaluate the effectiveness of a treatment intended to prevent or treat osteoporosis. With some drugs, a blood sample is taken to make sure that the drug concentration in the bloodstream is both adequate and below the toxic level.

What are the various names for the drug? Every drug has several names. First, it has a chemical name, used by researchers who need to refer to its chemical structure. Next, it has a generic name, used by the FDA and manufacturers once the drug enters the medication pipeline. Finally, it has brand names—the names that different pharmaceutical companies assign to it when they market it. (That's why it's possible to be taking double dosages of the same drug without knowing it—for instance, both Motrin and Advil are brand names for ibuprofen.)

When the doctor prescribes a new medication for your care recipient, ask for the generic and brand names, including abbreviations, and learn the correct spellings and pronunciations.

How is the drug taken? Drug administration includes the strength of each pill, how many are taken at a time, when they're taken (time of day), how often they're taken (times per day), and how they're taken (with or without food, with or apart from other medications, etc.). It's also important to learn how long the drug therapy will last (its duration).

What side effects can be expected, and what should you do about them? Almost every drug can have side effects—alternately called "adverse effects," to emphasize their undesirability. Some side effects are medically harmless; others can be very harmful indeed. It's important to ask the doctor to discern between these two types and to tell you what to do in the event of any side effect. Find out if there are preventive steps you can take to avoid or minimize these side effects.

Will this drug react with other medications? When the doctor prescribes a new medication, share the list of medications that your care recipient is currently taking. Ask the doctor or pharmacist to confirm that the new medication will not react with any of the other medications on the list. Be sure that your list is complete, including OTC drugs as well as vitamins and other dietary supplements.

How should this drug be administered? In general, pills should be swallowed, but find out whether a pill can be split or crushed and mixed with food, in case your care recipient has trouble swallowing. In addition, it's crucial that you learn how to administer drugs that come in other forms—eyedrops, eardrops, pulmonary inhalers, topical patches, injections, and suppositories, for example.

How should this drug be stored and disposed? Although most medications follow the same rules for storage (i.e., they should be kept away from heat, light, moisture, pets, and children), some come with special instructions—refrigeration, for example, or cleaning instructions for inhalers and dropper bottles. It's also important to ask what to do with unused pills. If the medication is administered in a patch or an inhaler, learn how to dispose of these items once they've been used. (Used delivery devices can contain residual amounts of the drug and may be harmful to children or pets.)

What kind of records should you keep for your next visit? As the caregiver, it's often up to you to note changes in your care recipient's health and/or behavior and to report these to the doctor. When a new drug is prescribed, ask what signs, symptoms, or behaviors you should monitor and what kind of information to record for the next visit.

MEDICATION ADHERENCE

Medication adherence is "the taking of medication by patients as intended by the prescriber." That means taking pills correctly as prescribed, or taking:

1. The right drug,
2. At the right dose,
3. At the right time,
4. In the correct manner (e.g., with or without food), and
5. For the correct duration.

Conversely, nonadherence is "not taking doses, or taking doses incorrectly, jeopardizing the intended therapeutic outcome" (as defined by the National Community Pharmacists Association). Total nonadherence is not filling the prescription or not taking the prescribed drug at all. Other forms of medication non-adherence include skipping doses, ending medication too soon, taking more or less than prescribed, and taking doses erratically or at improper intervals.

Medication nonadherence is widespread, and health care experts have recognized it as a major public health problem. Its prevalence generally is estimated at 40 percent to 50 percent of all people prescribed medications, but some surveys have documented it as high as 75 percent. Another way to size up the problem is with "the rule of thirds." Some studies reveal that approximately one-third of patients always take their pills correctly, one-third sometimes adhere to their prescriptions, and one-third never follow their regimens.

Because medications can be so effective, the consequences of nonadherence can be staggering. One dramatic example is transplant recipients. Transplant patients are prone to nonadherence, because their drug regimen is not merely complex, it's lifelong. And indeed, many studies have documented a rate of 20 percent to 47 percent of nonadherence to antirejection medications. But when transplant patients don't adhere to their medication regimen, the consequences can be severe, including loss of the transplanted organ and even death.

REASONS FOR NONADHERENCE

Here are some of the more common reasons that people don't take their medications as prescribed.

Forgetting. Forgetting to take or administer pills is very common. In fact, some studies indicate that forgetting accounts for the majority of instances of medication nonadherence. Many of us lead very busy lives, and caregivers are particularly challenged with hectic schedules. It's difficult to remember to take or administer pills multiple times each day. In addition, some people have cognitive impairments or psychiatric disabilities that make medication management more difficult.

Intolerance to side effects. Patients who don't take their prescribed medications often cite intolerable side effects. For them, the treatment is worse than the disease. For example, many people find it unacceptable that the pills that lower their blood pressure cause impotence and other forms of sexual dysfunction, daytime drowsiness or insomnia, depression and fatigue, and/or a constant dry cough. Instead of discussing side effects with their physician or pharmacist, many (24 percent, in one study) simply stop taking the offending drugs.

Lack of perceived benefits. Taking drugs several times a day is particularly challenging for people with an asymptomatic condition, such as high blood pressure. Many people don't understand the need for daily pills when they feel fine. However, the benefits of treatment are well documented.

Lack of understanding of the drug regimen prescribed. Sometimes, medication nonadherence is due to miscommunication and a misunderstanding of the regimen prescribed. One frequent error is discontinued use of a prescription after completing the initial supply, or once a condition appears to clear up. Even for short-term conditions, it's important to finish all the doses prescribed, even if the patient feels better.

Sometimes, the instructions are inadequate; sometimes a patient or caregiver forgets them. Some drugs should be taken at specific times or in a specific manner (such as with food or on an empty stomach). Nonadherence to these instructions can greatly diminish the effectiveness of certain antibiotics in eradicating infections.

Occasionally, medication nonadherence stems from taking *too much* of a medication—the same drug is mistakenly taken twice because of different (brand) names on the prescription vials. Underdosing also occurs frequently when administering drugs that are difficult to deliver. Prime examples are metered-dose inhalers used in asthma and emphysema and eyedrops that treat ophthalmic disorders (such as glaucoma).

Costs and affordability of prescriptions. Unfortunately, many people can't afford their prescription medications. They may forgo filling their prescriptions or skip doses to stretch their budget. (For more detailed information, see Financial Concerns, below.)

Lack of motivation or lack of belief in the drug's effectiveness and safety. Some people deliberately refuse to take their pills. Research has unearthed a variety of reasons why this happens.

- Fear and mistrust of the prescribed therapy
- Denial of the illness
- Lack of readiness for intervention and change
- A battle for autonomy and control
- Stress and depression (leading to lack of motivation)
- A choice to be "sick" and evade responsibilities
- Lack of family and social support, or even discouragement

As you can see, there are plenty of reasons that people don't adhere to their prescribed medication therapy, despite demonstrable benefits. Perhaps you've identified ones that apply to you or that apply in your role as caregiver. Or maybe you recognize factors that are present in your family member.

HELPING YOUR CARE RECIPIENT ADHERE TO MEDICATIONS

In the light of current statistics and the multitude of reasons for nonadherence, minding a medication regimen can truly be a challenge. The good news is that there are plenty of strategies to aid you and your care recipient with medication adherence:

Open communication with the health care team and joint decision-making. People are much more likely to adhere to their medication regimen when they've had a part in the decision-making process. Ask your care recipient's provider to approach the treatment plan as a joint decision, laying out the options and allowing your care recipient to have her say. It's also important to establish ongoing, two-way communication with the doctor, so that your care recipient can relay concerns as they arise. Finally, try to work with medical professionals who openly express concern for your care recipient. Studies have shown that if the patient believes that the doctor cares whether or not she adheres to her medication, she'll be much more likely to take her prescriptions as directed.

Simple regimens. Adherence is much more difficult with complex medication regimens. But you can attempt to simplify the regimen by working with your care recipient's doctor and pharmacist:

- Try to decrease the number of drugs and the number of daily doses
- If possible, synchronize the dose times to three or fewer each day (e.g., morning, dinnertime, and bedtime)
- Find out which medications can be taken together
- Use more long-acting drugs, which are dosed less frequently

Reminder systems. Whether you choose to use a daily medication chart, a watch alarm, or products designed especially to remind people to take their pills, devise a system for minding the medication regimen each day. Products currently available include containers that beep when it's time for a dose, computerized drug organizer-dispensers, and caps designed to count openings of the bottle to determine whether or not today's dose was taken.

Positive feedback. It's simple but all too easy to forget—and positive feedback works wonders. When your care recipient adheres properly to her medication regimen, congratulate her for her diligence. You may want to point to specific positive health consequences that are a result of her adherence, so she can make the connection between her behavior and her health.

Timely medication refills. Prescriptions can run out when you least expect it, and pharmacies usually need time to refill them, especially over the weekend. Mind the medications as you use them, and always order refills at least a week before you need them. You may want to calculate how many pills are used a day and mark your calendar with the refill date accordingly.

Disease management programs. In recent years, medical professionals have developed comprehensive disease management programs for people with chronic illnesses such as heart failure, diabetes, kidney failure, and asthma. These programs offer reminders, phone callback systems, compliance surveillance, and other strategies to improve medication adherence. Because they work in tandem with the patient's physician, your care recipient would receive the benefit of a multidisciplinary health care team as well as the information technology tools that make collaboration easier and more efficient.

Ask your care provider about these programs. You may find them offered through the local hospital, Medicaid, health insurance plans, and some pharmaceutical companies. Commercial services are also available, and you can locate these on the Internet. You may want to start at a general disease management site, such as the Disease Management Association of America (www.dmaa.org) or Medicaid Disease Management and Health Outcomes (www.dmnow.org).

The American Heart Association runs One of a Kind, a program designed to help people lower their risk of heart attack and stroke. For patients who already suffer from heart disease, the association offers a compliance management program, available online at http://www.americanheart.org/cap/patient/con_tctools.html.

WORKING WITH A "DIFFICULT" PATIENT

Sometimes, patients aren't cooperative about taking their medications—whether because of stubbornness, lack of good judgment, or dementia. In these cases, it's important to understand and honor the wishes of your care recipient. Try the following tactics to encourage medication adherence:

• Set mutually acceptable goals, and create a step-by-step plan to achieve these goals. Give your care recipient as much control and autonomy as possible. In addition, a written document with signatures (including the physician's) may strengthen the commitment.

• Always emphasize the health benefits of adherence. At the same time, help your care recipient to understand the health consequences of nonadherence. You may strengthen your case by stressing how much you care about your care recipient, and mentioning the burden that nonadherence imposes on you, the caregiver.

• Home help may be invaluable. Sometimes, "prescriptions" from an authority figure such as a registered nurse are more readily accepted. Mental health experts and geriatric case managers can also be helpful.

WORKING WITH THE PROFESSIONALS

For the benefit of both you and your care recipient, it's important that you get the most out of your interactions with medical professionals and it helps if you're organized and informed. Here's what to do:

Be prepared. Arrive at appointments with a full medication list, a list of questions, and a list of doctors currently treating your care recipient. You may even want to conduct research about your care recipient's conditions ahead of time, by doing an Internet search or connecting with other patients on message boards or through disease-oriented organizations.

Centralize the medical records. Individual specialists treating the same patient aren't always able to talk with each other, so they're not always aware of each other's activities. Therefore, it's up to you and your care recipient to keep up-to-date files about her treatment and care. Bring these files to every appointment.

Consult with the pharmacist. With every new prescription, the pharmacist is required to provide a consultation. Use this resource to learn everything possible about the new medication.

FINANCIAL CONCERNS

It's the sobering and dangerous truth: Many Americans simply cannot afford to buy the medications they need. Each year, the average senior citizen fills thirty prescriptions (including refills), and that number continues to increase.

Surveys show that nearly half of elderly Americans have no prescription drug coverage. One-third of Medicare beneficiaries pay for medications out of pocket. In an effort to save money, elderly citizens have been known to not fill prescriptions, take fewer doses than prescribed, use the others' medications to treat themselves, and even to buy less expensive veterinary medications. And seniors without drug benefits are more likely to report both poor health and disabilities—both of which might be greatly improved with prescription medications.

No matter what the financial situation, everyone worries about the high costs of medications. And wanting to save money is not a sign of stinginess—rather, it's a way of making the most of your care recipient's resources. If you or your care recipient is facing a dilemma about medication costs, don't forget that medications often reduce overall health care costs by decreasing expensive hospitalizations and surgeries—along with improving quality of life. But there are indeed ways to get the medications you need less expensively.

HOW CAN YOU LOWER YOUR DRUG EXPENSES?

There are plenty of things that you can do to lower drug costs. The following is a list of strategies for getting your medications at lower prices.

Begin at home. Always be sure to take advantage of the professional expertise of your personal pharmacist or doctor to resolve drug cost problems. Ask the pharmacist about discounts. Many drugstores offer senior discounts, and many participate in savings card programs. In addition, the doctor may be able to provide you with free samples that she receives from pharmaceutical companies. (In this case, the doctor's office must label the sample properly, as though it were a prescription label.)

Choose the drugs on the plan. If your care recipient has a prescription drug benefit plan, find out which medications are on that plan's formulary, or list of approved medications, and ask the doctor to prescribe those drugs. Most plans have a three-tiered structure:

- First-tier items, involving the lowest co-pay, are usually approved medications on the plan's formulary
- Second-tier items, requiring a higher co-payment, are usually alternative brand products for which your plan has negotiated a discount in return for volume purchasing
- Third-tier items are usually not covered at all

Encourage your doctor to prescribe from the first two groups to keep down your costs.

Use generic drugs. Ask your care recipient's doctor to prescribe generic drugs whenever possible—the savings are substantial. For most medical conditions, several drug treatment options are available. Newer, brand-name drugs are usually more expensive; older drugs often become available as generic formulations. These generic formulations are manufactured both by generic drug companies and by brand manufacturers.

Generic drugs require testing and approval by the FDA. They are considered "therapeutically equivalent" to brand-name products if tests show that they reach equal blood levels after an oral dose. Doctors and pharmacists agree that FDA-approved generic drugs are less costly yet equally effective.

Choose lower-cost drugs in the same therapeutic category. Some medical conditions are treatable with a great variety of drugs. In these cases, drugs are grouped into therapeutic categories based on how they work. For instance, therapeutic categories for medications used to treat high blood pressure include diuretics ("water pills"), ACE inhibitors, beta-blockers, and calcium channel blockers. Each category of drugs acts upon a different part of the biologic system to lower blood pressure.

Drugs within a therapeutic category are chemically similar, and they all use the same pharmacological action to produce the benefit. But within the category, there are cost differences, so ask your doctor or pharmacist whether there is a less expensive drug available in the same therapeutic category. At the same time, ask whether there's a trade-off for the cost savings. For example, you may need to take a cheaper pill more often.

Choose lower-cost drugs in a different therapeutic category. Just as there are significant cost differences among drugs within a single therapeutic category, so are there differences among categories. For example, with medications used to treat high blood pressure, a diuretic may be less expensive than a calcium channel blocker or a beta-blocker. If you can't afford the prescribed medication, it's worth asking about medications in other categories.

Of course, your care recipient's doctor will need to consider the overall picture—which requires an expert combination of drug knowledge and an assessment of your care recipient's medical situation. Sometimes, the cheapest alternative may not be the best. Finally, remember to ask about trade-offs when switching from one therapeutic category to another.

Choose combination products. Often, you can save money with a combination product—a product including two drugs from different categories. For example, there are products that combine an ACE inhibitor with a diuretic or a calcium channel blocker to treat high blood pressure. Part of the savings comes from buying just one prescription rather than two.

Split pills. Many people split pills to take half tablets, and some insurance plans actually require it. Often, for a particular drug, the cost for a higher-strength tablet is the same or just a bit higher than for a lower-strength tablet (drug manufacturers don't want to penalize patients whose conditions require higher doses). As consumers, we can take advantage of this pricing by splitting higher-strength tablets if the lower dose is appropriate.

Be sure to ask your care recipient's pharmacist and doctor whether this practice is safe and advantageous for the prescribed medications. Some long-acting pills should never be split, since cutting through their slow-release coating lets too much of the drug enter the body at once, which can cause an overdose. If you have trouble splitting pills, you can buy a pill-splitter to do the job for you.

Buy in bulk. Ask the doctor to prescribe a larger quantity for medications taken continuously, such as a three-month supply. That way, you'll save on the pharmacy fee applied to each prescription.

Comparison shop. Prices can vary substantially among pharmacies, even in one community. A survey conducted by the nonprofit International Patient Advocacy Association showed wide price ranges for some fairly common prescription drugs. Prices for the same prescription dose and amount could vary as much as 132%. You can do research on prices by phone or through online pharmacies.

Use drug company–sponsored prescription drug assistance programs. Most drug companies offer prescription cost relief in several ways. In addition to providing free drug samples to doctors, they provide vouchers for patients to obtain drugs from the pharmacy at no cost. If your care recipient has been prescribed a new medication, both of these approaches allow her to take the drug on a trial basis, to see if it's effective and doesn't cause significant adverse effects.

These programs are not just for low-income people. Your care recipient may qualify because she doesn't have health insurance, or doesn't have prescription

MEDICARE, MEDICAID, MEDIGAP, AND PRIVATE INSURANCE

Medicare

Medicare is a U. S. government health insurance program for people 65 years of age and older, some disabled people under 65 years of age, and people with end-stage renal disease (permanent kidney failure treated with dialysis or a transplant). Administered by The Centers for Medicare & Medicaid Services branch of the federal government, Medicare is the nation's largest health insurance program, providing medical coverage for nearly 40 million Americans.

In general, Medicare does not cover outpatient prescription drugs. The few exceptions to this rule include the following:

- Organ transplant antirejection medications (if the transplant was paid for by Medicare)

- Some drugs associated with kidney dialysis
- Some oral drugs for cancer treatment

For people with diabetes, Medicare does pay for supplies needed to test blood sugar at home, but it doesn't cover insulin, insulin syringes, or oral antidiabetic pills. Vaccinations against flu, pneumonia, and hepatitis B are preventive health services covered by Medicare Part B. To read more about Medicare's drug coverage, visit the Medicare Web site.

Medicaid

Medicaid is a jointly funded, federal/state government health insurance program for certain low-income and needy people. It covers approximately 36 million individuals including

benefits, or because her medical costs are high. Talk to her doctor about them, as the doctor must apply to these programs for you. A volunteer organization such as The Medicine Program (www.themedicineprogram.com) or NeedyMeds (www.needymeds.com) can offer help in the application process. For a list of prescription drug assistance programs, visit www.phrma.org/patients.

Use state-sponsored assistance programs. Many states have appropriated state funds for medication assistance programs. At last count, 24 states have established or are implementing such plans. And 60 to 70% of America's elderly live in these states, which include California, Florida, Illinois, Kansas, Maine, Maryland, Massachusetts, Missouri, New Hampshire, New Jersey, New York, Rhode Island, and South Carolina.

children, the aged, blind, and/or disabled, and people who are eligible to receive federally assisted income maintenance payments.

Prescription benefits vary among states' Medicaid programs. If you have Medicaid, ask your physician and pharmacist about the program's drug formulary (list of covered medications). To decrease your out-of-pocket expenses, have your doctor prescribe medications that are on the formulary. To read more about Medicaid's drug coverage, visit the Medicaid Web site.

Medigap

Medigap policies supplement benefits provided by Medicare. These policies are standardized into ten different plans, three of which offer prescription benefits. Visit the Medicare Web site to find more information about Medigap coverage. In addition, you can use an interactive tool designed to locate insurance companies that sell Medigap in your state.

Private insurance plans

Private health insurance plans typically provide prescription benefits. As noted earlier, each plan has an approved list of drugs on its formulary. These drugs have the lowest co-payment amount, because the plan provider has negotiated a volume discount price for its members.

These programs usually subsidize a portion of the prescription costs for low-income seniors. Some have negotiated lower prices with drug manufacturers and provide seniors with access to these discounts. Contact your state legislative representative for information about state assistance programs.

THE VA AND OTHER ORGANIZATIONS

You can check eligibility for veterans' prescription drug benefits at www.va.gov/health. Your care recipient may also be entitled to prescription benefits or discounts through various senior organizations, many of which have leveraged their membership's buying power to provide a prescription program or drug discounts. Search the Internet or ask your local reference librarian for help finding these programs.

HERBAL AND NUTRITIONAL SUPPLEMENTS

(For a thorough discussion of herbal and nutritional supplements, see the Complementary and Alternative Medicine chapter on p. 651.)

HERBAL PRODUCTS

In recent years in the United States, herbal products have seen an explosion in popularity. Today, one in three Americans uses some type of herbal product. And while many people have seen undeniable benefits from these substances, there can be profound medical risks associated with taking them. Briefly, they are:

Unproven efficacy. Because herbal remedies are not subject to the research and strict approval process that prescription drugs must endure, in many cases their efficacy has not been scientifically proven. Therefore, you may end up investing time, money, and hope in a substance that has no beneficial effect.

Adverse effects and/or interactions with other substances. Worse than having no effect, herbal substances can produce very harmful physical reactions, by themselves and when they interact with other substances. Patients are particularly vulnerable to these effects when they don't share information with their health care providers, who may unknowingly prescribe a medication that interacts adversely with a certain herbal substance. To keep abreast of safety alerts and product recalls, use the FDA's MedWatch program at www.fda.gov/medwatch.

Delayed treatment. Patients who use herbal products have a tendency to self-diagnose. In some cases, that means delaying seeking professional medical attention, which can be quite dangerous.

Lack of regulation. Herbal products do not require evaluation and approval by the FDA. That means that information regarding side effects, drug interactions, and product consistency is limited. In addition, there are no standards for the testing of ingredients, the quantity of active compounds, or toxic impurities. And proper "dosage" remains unknown. Those are a lot of unknowns to contend with when ingesting powerful substances that have a direct effect on health.

NUTRITIONAL SUPPLEMENTS

Unlike herbal products, nutritional supplements (vitamins and minerals) are substances that every body needs for growth, function, and health. Like herbal supplements, nutritional supplements are not regulated by the FDA, so it's important to take care with the supplements you select.

The best way to get vitamins and minerals is through eating a balanced diet. As a caregiver, your efforts toward meeting your care recipient's nutritional requirements would be best placed in providing healthful meals. However, it's not always possible to get all of the vitamins and minerals we need through food, especially if we have digestive problems or a condition that is alleviated or ameliorated with the intake of certain nutrients. In addition, nutritional supplements can be very helpful where there are deficiencies due to a poor diet or alcoholism.

In most cases, the best way to get vitamins and minerals is by eating whole foods (fruits, vegetables, grains, lean meats, and dairy products). Whole foods contain not merely one vitamin or mineral, but many. For example, when you drink a glass of milk, you get not merely calcium but also protein, vitamin D, riboflavin, phosphorus, and magnesium. In addition, whole foods provide dietary fiber, which helps the human body digest—and which may help prevent heart disease and bowel cancer.

USING HERBAL AND NUTRITIONAL SUPPLEMENTS WISELY

While there are several profound dangers associated with taking herbal products, it is possible to use them in a responsible, health-promoting way, particularly when you do so with the knowledge of your care recipient's health care provider. With nutritional supplements, remember that they are exactly that—supplements to a healthy diet, way of life, and routine medical care. They can't replace any of these things, but they can enhance health and fitness when used in conjunction with them. If your care recipient has decided to use herbal products or nutritional supplements, follow these guidelines:

Consult with the doctor. Never administer supplements to your care recipient without first consulting with her doctor. When you ask whether a certain substance might be helpful and appropriate, let the doctor view her entire medication list to check for interactions. Ask how the supplement should be dosed, taken, and stored. If the doctor does approve of an herbal or nutritional supplement, add it to the medication list and show it at all subsequent visits. Then, note reactions as the supplement is taken, and report any unusual experiences to the doctor or pharmacist.

Get educated. Learn about herbal products and nutritional supplements just as you learn about prescription drugs—including the name, what it's intended to do, proper dosage and duration, adverse effects, interactions, etc.

Dose properly. Never administer more than the recommended amount listed on the label. (To that end, don't choose a product that doesn't have dosing recommendations on the label.)

Choose reputable brands. Buy only products that list the manufacturer's name, address, and telephone number. Don't buy a supplement that doesn't carry a lot number or an expiration date, and avoid products without an expiration date at least one year from the date of purchase. Two indicators that can help you select reputable brands are the letters USP (United States Pharmacopeia) and NF (National Formulary). USP indicates that the supplement's manufacturer abided by the standards set by the United States Pharmacopeia (an organization dedicated to ensure that our medicines and other health care products are safe and of the highest quality). That is, the herb has specific uses and a dosage range, and the company manufactured it according to the USP's standards and tested it for quality and purity. NF means that the herb doesn't have an USP-labeled use, but it has been produced according to USP's standards of quality and purity.

Store products safely. Just as you take care with the storage of prescription medications, store herbal supplements away from heat, light, moisture, pets, and children. Never store medications in the bathroom medicine cabinet or automobile glove compartment.

Don't mix herbs and supplements with alcohol. Unless you're certain about the safety of drinking alcohol while taking the herb or supplement, don't allow your care recipients to do it.

Maintain a healthy lifestyle. Don't use herbal or nutritional supplements as a substitute for proper rest and nutrition. Make sure your care recipient eats a balanced diet and gets regular exercise, if practical.

Complement, don't replace. Despite their value, alternative therapies are not intended to replace conventional medicine. Alternative therapies can be highly beneficial in improving general health and managing symptoms; sometimes medications can be reduced or avoided by using an alternative therapy. But there are times when modern medicine is essential. Using the best of both worlds is the ideal approach.

DRUG INTERACTIONS

Sometimes, the drugs that a patient takes may interact with each other, or with food or alcohol, in a way that causes undesired results.

There are three basic kinds of drug interactions:

- Drug-drug (between two prescription drugs, two OTC drugs, or one of each)
- Drug-food
- Drug-alcohol

Drug interactions can be favorable. For instance, your care recipient may be instructed to take a medication with food to increase the drug's absorption and hence its effectiveness. In some cases, two drugs interact to yield a benefit that can be exploited. For example, after receiving a kidney or heart transplant, a patient must take cyclosporine for the rest of his life to prevent rejection. Doctors often add a drug called diltiazem, which has two benefits. First, diltiazem interferes with liver metabolism and the body's elimination of cyclosporine. This interaction allows a lower dosage of cyclosporine to have a greater effect—and hence significantly reduces the patient's drug bill. Second, diltiazem treats high blood pressure, a side effect of cyclosporine.

But many drug interactions are unfavorable, and some are dangerous. Unfavorable interactions occur when one substance blunts the effectiveness of another, when one substance enhances the effectiveness of another to a dangerous extreme, and when the two combine to create undesirable and sometimes dangerous toxicities. Some drug interactions occur frequently and/or are predictable; others are uncommon and unpredictable. Some are minor and cause little harm. Others are severe, and the drug combination that causes them should be avoided if other drugs can be used.

PREVENTING HARMFUL DRUG INTERACTIONS

When drugs interact, either with food, alcohol, or each other, they can produce a wide range of side effects. After a new medication is started, if your care recipient experiences severe and exaggerated known side effects or an unusual change, contact her physician immediately. Ask about the possibility of a drug interaction.

Harmful drug interactions may be frightening, but most can be prevented when you proceed with caution. Information is readily available in more than one source. To avoid harmful drug interactions, use the following guidelines:

Consult with the doctor and pharmacist. When your care recipient's doctor prescribes a new medication, review the list of medications she's already taking. Ask the doctor and the pharmacist whether the new medication might react with any of the other medications currently in your care recipient's regimen—or whether it will react with alcohol or any specific foods. In addition, ask how you will know whether a harmful interaction is taking place.

Start low and go slow. Encourage the doctor to begin dosage as low as possible and increase it slowly and only if medically necessary.

Keep track of reactions and report them. Record any and all reactions your care recipient has after starting her new medication. If the reaction is serious, consult a health care professional immediately. If the reaction is routine and doesn't present a danger, make a record every time it occurs, and report it to the doctor at the next visit.

Get educated. The more you know about your care recipient's medications, the better you can help her stay safe. There is a wealth of pharmacological information available to consumers. Basic sources include the National Drug Data File, accessible online at www.medscape.com/misc/formdrugs.html and PubMed, at www4.ncbi.nlm.nih.gov/PubMed/. (Additional sources of information are listed below.)

Avoid polypharmacy. The more medications your care recipient takes, the more it's likely that an interaction will occur. Consult with the doctor and pharmacist to ask whether you can streamline your care recipient's regimen. In many cases, regimens can be adjusted so that fewer medications—perhaps used in combination with lifestyle modifications—produce the same benefit.

WHAT RESEARCH IS BEING DONE?

The future for medications is extremely bright. Researchers are constantly making new medication discoveries through new computer modeling and intelligence technologies and new automated screening systems. Discoveries now move more quickly and efficiently through the research, development, and regulatory pipelines, becoming available sooner to benefit patients and their caregivers. Laboratory testing is faster than ever before, because scientists have developed test models that return results more quickly. And the FDA has reorganized the drug approval process to fast-track new drugs that provide significant advances and gains.

In addition to discovering new drugs, researchers are modifying the old ones— so we benefit more from their therapeutic powers and suffer less from their side effects. For example, a new, long-acting insulin recently became available. Glargine is a form of human insulin that is released over 24 hours after injection. Many diabetics will be able to reduce their insulin shots to one a day and achieve even greater control of their blood sugar.

We're also getting better at tailoring drug use and dosage to specific populations. Although in the past most drugs were tested on groups of men, manufacturers are now expanding their research to include elderly people, women, and children. We're also developing new ways to take drugs.

The topical patch—a small, adhesive skin patch (like a Band-Aid)—releases medication in a controlled, safe way and is being used to deliver a variety of medications, such as nitroglycerin, nicotine, male and female hormones, narcotic pain relievers, and scopolamine, for motion sickness. Another exciting method of drug delivery is inhalation. In the future, some diabetics may be able to breathe in their insulin doses rather than take shots. Caregivers may find it easier to give medications as a patch or an inhalant, especially to loved ones who have difficulty swallowing. And many other new drug-delivery methods are in research and development. Some of these technologies will deliver drugs directly to the diseased body organ. For example, specialized carrier compounds can transport cancer chemotherapy drugs in the bloodstream directly to the tumor—yielding better results and fewer side effects.

And finally, a recent trend in medication management has been the shift in classification from prescription to OTC drugs. Over the last fifteen years, the FDA has made many former prescription drugs available over the counter without a doctor's prescription, and they will continue to do so. OTC drugs tend to be less expensive, and they're certainly easier to come by. However, they do bring added responsibility for self-care to the patient and medication management to the caregiver.

RESOURCES FOR MEDICATION MANAGEMENT

When facing a complicated medication regimen, you're far from alone. For one thing, you can consult with all of the medical professionals in your care recipient's heath care team—doctors, nurses, and pharmacists—for information and advice. Also, there is a wealth of published, consumer-oriented pharmaceutical information available to you, often free. The following is a list of resources for you to tap as you manage your care recipient's medications:

Doctors, nurses, and pharmacists. Start with the people who are directly involved with your care recipient. In addition to a complete list of medications and OTC drugs, bring a written list of questions to all visits and consultations, and advocate on behalf of your care recipient to make sure that all medications are safe and medically necessary. If you're interested in doing more in-depth research about your care recipient's medications, you might ask her care providers where to start.

PubMed. A service of the National Library of Medicine, PubMed is an online search engine providing access to over 11 million medical citations (www.ncbi.nlm.nih.gov/PubMed).

MedLine Plus. The National Library of Medicine and National Institutes of Health run a joint Web site with excellent information on medications at www.nlm.nih.gov/medlineplus.

Drug information offices at local medical centers. Most medical centers and hospitals have drug information centers or patient medical libraries, where you can learn more about the medications prescribed by your care recipient's doctor. The next time you accompany your care recipient to the doctor, ask for the nearest drug information office. Additionally, you can call the nearby medical center's pharmacy department or the closest school of pharmacy.

Regional poison control centers. Post the number of your regional poison center prominently near your telephones. Use www.aapcc.org to locate this resource.

The U. S. Food and Drug Administration. The FDA is a rich resource for information about medications, including the FDA's important role in the approval process. Visit their Web site or call their Information Hotline at 1-888-INFO-FDA (1-888-463-6332).

Consumers' information desk at drug manufacturers and Web sites. Pharmaceutical companies often have consumer information desks, accessible by calling the manufacturer or visiting their Web site.

ADDITIONAL RESOURCES

ORGANIZATIONS AND WEB SITES

Agency for Healthcare Research and Quality
www.ahcpr.gov

The American Heart Association
www.americanheart.org

The American Pharmaceutical Association, National Professional Society of Pharmacists
www.aphanet.org

The Center for Proper Medication Use
www.cpmu.org

Food and Drug Administration
www.fda.gov

Intelihealth
www.intelihealth.com

The Mayo Clinic
www.mayoclinic.com

Medicaid
www.hcfa.gov/medicaid

Medicare
www.hcfa.gov/medicare

MedLine Plus
www.nlm.nih.gov/medlineplus

The Merck Manual Home Edition
www.merck.com/pubs

National Institute on Aging
www.nih.gov/nia

Safemedication.com
www.safemedication.com

WebMD
www.webmd.lycos.com

BOOKS AND ARTICLES

Margolis, Simeon, ed. *The Johns Hopkins Complete Home Encyclopedia of Drugs.* New York: Medletter Associates, 1998, 8-15.

American Heart Association. *How Do I Manage My Medicine?* (pamphlet). Dallas, Tex.: American Heart Association Pharmaceutical Roundtable, 1998.

Pain
Management

P ain starts as nothing more than a warning signal from the body—and ends
as nothing less than a $100 billion-a-year epidemic that can cause despair,
desperation, and constant suffering for those who must endure it.

Pain affects everyone to some extent. For some, it's an occasional nuisance, the
consequence of a headache, sunburn, or pulled muscle. But for an estimated 50
million Americans, chronic pain is an everyday burden. Whether caused by arthritis, diabetes, cancer, or other disease—or, as in a great many cases, with no apparent cause at all—chronic pain limits a person's ability to function. A recent study
of 50,000 nursing home residents found that those with chronic pain were 2.5
times more likely to have reduced activity levels than similar residents who did
not suffer pain on a daily basis. The same residents were also nearly 1.7 times
more likely to suffer from depression—presumably as a consequence of dealing
with their constant pain.

Unfortunately, pain is often poorly treated. The American Pain Society estimates that only one of every four people who suffer from pain receives proper
treatment. Pain is especially common among the elderly, who are both more likely
to experience pain and less likely to seek proper treatment for the condition.

While pain can be a constant nemesis, it does not have to dominate a person's
life. A wide variety of treatment options are available, from simple analgesics like
Tylenol to surgical procedures that may help block even the most intense pain.
The key is to work with medical professionals to develop a workable pain management program.

The caregiver's role in this process can be especially important. Many people
with chronic pain are unable to treat themselves, and also may be reluctant to

admit how much pain they're feeling. Family caregivers can learn how to interpret a person's pain and when to take appropriate steps to relieve this discomfort. Caregivers also should act as advocates for those who are not getting the proper level of pain management. While pain can be intense and difficult to treat, there's always hope for at least partial relief. Neither patients nor caregivers should simply accept pain as an inevitable part of disease or aging.

WHAT IS PAIN?

While everyone instinctively understands pain, creating a clinical description for it has taken centuries. The International Association for the Study of Pain (IASP) currently defines pain as:

An unpleasant sensory and emotional experience associated with actual or potential tissue damage, or described in terms of such damage.

By this definition, pain is more than a simple biochemical response to harmful or dangerous occurrences. It also includes a broad range of intellectual, emotional, and behavioral reactions. All of these factors—from fear and anxiety to increased heart rate and dilated pupils to concerns about how loved ones will react to complaints about pain—help a person interpret the type, location, and severity of the pain. In other words, they make up the entire pain experience.

Doctors divide most types of pain into two categories: acute and chronic. Acute pain is caused by a known event, such as a broken bone, bruise, kidney stone, infection, or other injury. The pain is often sharp, and serves a clear purpose; it tells patients that something is wrong with their bodies and forces them to deal with the injuries. Pain from a broken toe, for example, keeps a person from walking and allows time for the wound to heal. Acute pain usually disappears after the wound or infection has cleared.

Chronic pain, however, is useless to the body. It is usually defined as pain that lasts for a period of more than six months. Other researchers use a different definition: Pain that persists beyond the normal healing period, or pain associated with a progressive, noncancer disease. The pain can appear suddenly, or may slowly build in intensity. Finally, the pain has no apparent or predictable end. Chronic pain may have a known cause, such as a joint that has been ravaged by arthritis or nerve damage caused by injury or disease in the nervous system. But it also can appear for no apparent reason. Many people with chronic back pain, for instance, have suffered no apparent injury. Chronic pain can last for months or even years, and its effects can go far beyond the physical. It's a leading cause of depression and can rob people of mobility and feelings of independence. While acute pain is often viewed as a symptom of an injury or disease, doctors often treat chronic pain as a disease unto itself. But sadly, even today, doctors are not exactly sure what causes chronic pain, or why some people develop the condition and others don't.

Although some doctors consider cancer pain a subset of chronic pain, other experts make it a category unto itself. An estimated 50 to 80% of people who develop cancer will feel pain from the disease, although it is usually controllable. The pain can come from a number of different sources. The most common are the growth of malignant tumors that invade or apply pressure to another internal structure, or the side effects of chemotherapy and radiation. Some anticancer drugs, for instance, are designed to stop the spread of cancer cells, but also can cause changes in the nervous system that make patients more sensitive to pain.

PAIN IN THE ELDERLY

The question of whether elderly people actually feel pain more acutely than younger people remains controversial. Studies have come to radically different conclusions. For example, some have found that older people, on the whole, are about 20% less sensitive to pain stimuli from heat sources than younger people. But others have found just the opposite. There appears to be a wide variation in pain sensation among the elderly; some feel pain more strongly as they age, others feel it less.

What is certain is that the elderly face more diseases than their younger counterparts. And they are more likely to have advanced stages of arthritis, angina (chest pain), diabetes, cancer, and other conditions known to cause chronic pain. Whether they feel pain more or less acutely, then, is much less important than the total amount of pain stimuli they are subjected to on a daily basis.

Women, on the whole, tend to feel more acute and chronic pain than men. They are more likely to suffer from migraine headaches, fibromyalgia, irritable bowel syndrome, and other conditions that cause chronic pain. And when pain-free women are subjected to pain stimuli in a laboratory setting, they generally prove more sensitive to pain than similar men.

Chronic pain can have a massive effect on a person's quality of life. A survey of nursing home residents, for example, found that pain caused 54% of respondents to curtail enjoyable activities. At the same time, 53% had difficulty walking, nearly half said their posture was impaired, 45% reported trouble sleeping, nearly one-third said they were depressed and had trouble sleeping and 14% said their appetites were impaired by pain.

The National Pain Foundation and the American Pain Foundation report that the total toll from chronic pain in the United States is staggering:

- One-third of all Americans lose more than 20 hours of sleep each month because of pain.
- Pain causes as many as 50 million lost workdays each year.
- All told, pain causes $100 billion in medical treatment, lost wages, and other financial costs each year in America.
- More than 50 million Americans suffer chronic pain, while nearly 25 million others will experience significant acute pain from injury or surgery.

Tragically, much of this damage need not occur. A recent Roper poll found that more than 40% of Americans who felt moderate to severe chronic pain felt that their symptoms were out of control. Doctors believe that the number of people with truly uncontrollable pain is far, far lower than this figure—leading to the conclusion that people simply are not getting the best treatment possible for chronic pain. The American Pain Foundation, in fact, estimates that only about one of every four people suffering from pain receives proper treatment.

HOW IS PAIN DIAGNOSED?

Proper pain management begins with an accurate diagnosis. This can prove difficult, since patients—particularly elderly ones—often find it difficult to describe the type, intensity, and frequency of their pain. Elderly patients are also likely to understate their pain, feeling that they are being bothersome or that they should simply expect a certain level of pain at their age. In diagnosis of pain, the role of the family caregiver is vital. Because they are able to view the patient on a regular and intimate basis, caregivers often are able to give a doctor a more objective sense of the pain than the patients themselves.

The purpose of a doctor's evaluation is fourfold.

- First, doctors want to understand the severity and nature of the pain;
- Second, they want to search for the underlying causes of the pain;
- Third, doctors want to use the information they have gathered to develop a pain-management program that works; and
- Fourth, doctors want to follow the course of treatment and ensure that the patient continues to make progress.

During an office visit, doctors usually start by asking patients to describe their pain. Because pain is a subjective experience, patients often have trouble relaying their feelings. To help with this process, researchers have developed several tools to aid patients. The most common is a simple pain scale. Patients are asked to rate their pain on a scale of 0 to 10, with 10 being the most intense pain imaginable. Doctors will ask when the pain is most severe—whether, for example, it hurts most in the morning, or after performing certain household tasks. Doctors also usually ask patients to describe the nature of the pain: Is it sharp or dull, aching or burning? Of course, physicians also want to know the location of the pain, whether it is confined to a part of the body, such as the chest, or whether the patient feels pain in multiple locations. During this process, the caregiver can provide additional details or descriptions to the doctor when appropriate.

Many times, doctors can pick up nonverbal clues about the extent of a patient's pain. They may look at a person's face, for example, to see if the patient has a relaxed expression or is frowning or clenching his or her jaw. Legs drawn close to the chest, or constantly kicking, are often a sign of severe pain. Caregivers also can share their observations, such as whether patients frequently cry or are inconsolable, or whether their activity levels appear curtailed because of pain.

After this initial discussion, doctors usually will take a medical history. Does the patient have a history of arthritis, high blood pressure, heart disease, or diabetes? Are there other, more rare, conditions that could be the underlying cause of the pain? Does the patient have a history of depression or other psychological disorders? Is the patient losing sleep because of pain?

A physical examination is also performed during the visit. Doctors typically check blood pressure, temperature, and pulse rate. It's important to note, however, that people with chronic pain often have normal results to these basic tests. While acute pain can cause higher heart rates and other high-alert physiologic changes in the body, chronic pain does not usually have the same effects. Physicians also will check for signs of inflammation and spots on the body that trigger pain responses. These could indicate problems like tendonitis, muscle strain, or nerve irritation.

If an underlying cause for pain seems apparent and straightforward—osteoarthritis, for example—the physician may at this point prescribe analgesics such as aspirin or acetaminophen in over-the-counter or prescription dosages. He may also suggest other possible treatments, from physical therapy to acupuncture.

Unfortunately, the root causes of pain are numerous and often difficult to pinpoint. Any number of diseases, from rheumatoid arthritis to fibromyalgia to cancer, can cause unremitting pain. Depending on the findings from the initial examination, doctors may refer patients to specialists ranging from psychologists to arthritis experts to neurologists. The process can be daunting, as patients must sometimes endure a number of tests, ranging from MRIs and CAT scans to blood work to x-rays and psychologic assessments. As a caregiver, it's vital to keep things in perspective for the patient. The dizzying array of tests are designed to locate the exact cause of the patient's pain. Until that cause is uncovered, pain may continue unabated.

In some cases, patients may be referred to pain clinics. These practices are devoted solely to pain relief, and include experts in a number of pain-related disciplines, including anesthesiology, rheumatology, psychology, physical therapy, and neurology. The specialists work together to formulate an individual pain-management strategy for each patient. Patients and caregivers may find that pain clinics are able to address their needs in a more coordinated fashion. Unfortunately, pain clinics are not covered under all forms of insurance and are not available in all parts of the country.

MANAGING PAIN

The goal of pain management is to improve the patient's quality of life. This means increasing activity levels, reducing psychological effects like depression, improving sleeping and eating patterns, and, if applicable, returning to work. With proper care, pain ceases to be the dominant focus of a patient's life and becomes a formidable, but manageable, problem.

Pain is a remarkably complex problem. It shouldn't be surprising, then, that managing pain usually requires blending a number of techniques into an effective, personalized plan. Because pain responses involve biology, emotions, and even learned behavior, doctors now treat pain with a multidisciplinary approach.

Acute pain can almost always be treated effectively using aspirin-like drugs or more powerful, centrally acting painkillers, plus physical therapy, ice/heat combinations, and other nonmedicinal methods. By definition, acute pain disappears when the injury or disease that causes the pain resolves—usually within a period of weeks or months.

The prognosis for chronic pain is not always so bright. While doctors have an array of pain-fighting tools available, including time-proven painkilling medications, electric stimulation, physical therapy and exercise, surgery to block nerve impulses, psychological counseling, and even biofeedback, patients rarely achieve complete, total, and permanent relief from their condition. Many diseases lead to permanent changes in the nervous system, changes that make complete pain remission nearly impossible. Doctors and caregivers both should emphasize these facts to patients. In many cases, unrealistic expectations can make matters worse for pain sufferers. Expecting, and then failing to achieve, total relief from pain can lead to a cycle of depression and increasing pain.

It's vital for patients and caregivers to stay in contact with doctors, nurses, and other health care providers. This way, the patient's pain-management strategy can be changed when necessary to offer maximum relief.

Here are the main tools used in pain management:

ANALGESICS

Analgesics are a broad class of painkilling drugs that includes both over-the-counter and prescription formulas.

Nonsteroidal anti-inflammatory agents

The drugs of first choice for relief of mild to moderate pain are usually nonsteroidal anti-inflammatory drugs, or NSAIDs. Aspirin is the oldest and best-known NSAID, although many similar drugs are now available. Scientists are still not completely sure how NSAIDs relieve pain. Most of the benefit seems to come from their ability to block the body's production of prostaglandin, a fatty acid that controls inflammation and sensitivity around the site of an injury. Prostaglandin production is a normal part of the pain reflex. By making the injured area more sensitive, it discourages people from touching or moving it and possibly causing more damage.

The World Health Organisation (WHO) has set dosage guidelines for the use of many NSAIDs in managing chronic pain, including:

Ibuprofen (common brands include Motrin, Nuprin, and Advil). Can be taken in doses of 200, 400, 600, or 800 mg three to four times daily. Maximum daily dose is 3200 mg.

Naproxen (Naprosyn, Aleve). Can be taken in doses of 250, 375, or 500 mg twice daily. Maximum daily dose is 1250 mg.

Indomethacin (Indocin). Can be taken in 25 or 50 mg capsules or 50 mg rectal suppositories, two to four times daily. Also available in a 75 mg sustained-release formula that can be taken twice daily. Maximum daily dose is 200 mg.

Salsalate (Disalcid, Salflex). Can be taken in 500 mg doses two to three times per day, with a maximum daily dose of 3000 mg.

Unfortunately, NSAIDs come with side effects and limitations. They generally are not effective against severe pain. NSAIDs also can cause stomach ulcers and gastrointestinal discomfort. Another drug, acetaminophen (Tylenol), does not carry the same side effects as NSAIDs. It relieves pain but does not have the anti-inflammatory action of NSAIDs. The WHO guidelines recommend taking acetaminophen in 650 mg doses every four to six hours, or in the form of two 500 mg tablets every six hours. The maximum daily dose is 4000 mg. Acetaminophen also has side effects; it has been shown to cause kidney and liver damage when high doses are taken for prolonged periods.

New NSAIDs, called COX-2 inhibitors, have become available to pain sufferers since 1998 and are now the leading prescription analgesics in the United States. Their main benefit is supposed to be the ability to block only that prostaglandin which is involved in the pain and inflammation responses. Prostaglandin is also used to regulate stomach functions, which is why NSAIDs cause ulcers and other digestive system problems. The COX-2 inhibitors (Celebrex, Vioxx) do not appear to be more effective at pain relief than their predecessors, but appear to carry fewer side effects. Studies demonstrate that they cause a lower incidence of stomach ulcers and bleeding. Many physicians prescribe these newer NSAIDs for people at high risk for gastrointestinal bleeding, such as patients with a previous history of ulcers and those on aspirin, warfarin (Coumadin), and other blood thinners. Their effect on chronic pain remains to be fully tested.

Opioid analgesics

The next class of analgesics are known as opioid analgesics, or narcotic analgesics. These are more powerful drugs than NSAIDs or acetaminophen, and do their work in the brain and spinal cord. Opioids include morphine, codeine, meperidine (Demerol), fentanyl, hydromorphone (Dilaudid), and other compounds. With the exception of methadone, opioids ease pain for a short duration, usually two to six hours, and must be dosed several times a day. However, many of these drugs have been formulated in sustained-release products that provide pain relief for more than eight to twelve hours.

Traditionally, opioid analgesics have been used mainly to treat severe acute pain, such as postoperative pain. They also have been used in cancer pain and in terminally ill patients nearing the end of their lives. Research also has shown that opioids can be effectively used in some cases of chronic pain caused by nerve diseases. Elderly patients seem to respond especially well to the pain-relieving properties of opioids.

Doctors have been hesitant to use the drugs in many pain cases, however, because of real and perceived side effects. Opioids can be addictive in a very small percentage of cases, and they can suppress respiratory function and cause severe drowsiness. Constipation almost always accompanies opioid use, and usually requires additional medical treatment to control. With prolonged use, patients also may become tolerant of the drugs, requiring larger doses to achieve the same amount of pain relief.

Long-term opioid use in cases of chronic pain remains controversial. But sentiment may be turning in its favor—in part because of the recognition that chronic pain remains poorly treated in this country. Many specialists view opioids as a means to provide greater pain relief to patients who have been unable to find help through more traditional methods. The American Pain Society and the American

Academy of Pain Management have issued joint guidelines that encourage doctors to at least consider the use of opioids in some cases of chronic pain. The guidelines strongly suggest that doctors seek the advice of pain-management specialists before prescribing the drugs, however.

In any case, opioids should be viewed as a possible additional tool against chronic pain—not as a replacement for other, time-tested treatment methods. They may be considered in cases where patients have been clearly diagnosed, are in constant pain, and have overused NSAIDs or other analgesics. It's important to note that no long-term studies have been conducted on the effectiveness of opioids for chronic pain not caused by cancer. Opioids are only available with a prescription.

While opioids are usually available in pill or capsule form, the medicine is sometimes delivered intravenously. In some cases of acute pain and cancer pain, patient-controlled analgesia pumps are used. Patients have control of dosing by pressing a button that can release painkilling levels of the drugs on demand. The buttons allow a controlled amount of the drug to flow through the intravenous tubing and into the bloodstream. It is not possible to overdose using this system, since the pump is programmed to release only a certain amount of the drug in a given period. (There have been rare, inadvertent overdoses with pump malfunctioning or human error due to the pump's being programmed incorrectly.) This system does allow the patient the freedom to take the medication when necessary, without waiting for permission from nurses or doctors. And patients given this control end up using less opioid medication. Studies of this method have found that it is effective for both younger and elderly patients, despite fears that older patients may be hesitant to self-administer the medication.

Another effective way of opioid delivery is through the use of topical drug patches applied to the skin. Fentanyl, a potent painkiller, is available as Duragesic transdermal patches, which are changed and applied every three days.

Four types of narcotics are most frequently prescribed in the United States: oxycodone, controlled release (OxyContin); fentanyl (transdermal Duragesic patch); sustained release morphine (MS Contin); and methadone. All of these drugs offer the comparative advantage of staying in the bloodstream over a period of time and avoiding the peaks and valleys of pain relief that characterize other analgesics. All four narcotics are potent painkillers effective for severe pain. "Breakthrough" episodes of pain can be managed with additional rapid-onset narcotics such as oxycodone or morphine in an oral solution or morphine in soluble tablets.

Common side effects of the opioids include sedation and confusion, constipation, nausea, vomiting, and respiratory depression. Patients usually develop tolerance to the sedation and confusion within a few days, so patients taking stable opioid doses can be alert and able to carry out their normal activities. However, management of constipation is important and often requires stool softeners and stimulant laxatives. Nondrug measures often help; these include drinking more fluid and exercising regularly, as well as adding prune juice and bran to the diet. Nausea and vomiting can be managed with medication.

Patients and family caregivers often confuse physical dependence on narcotics with addiction. Physical dependence happens when a narcotic is used regularly for more than a few days. Addiction (a craving for, and overuse and abuse of, the drug) is extremely rare when narcotics are used to treat pain.

Adjuvant analgesic drugs

These are drugs that were not designed as pain-relieving agents but nevertheless can ease pain in many patients. Antidepressants play a major role in many cases of chronic pain. In many cases, depression accompanies pain and may even make it more prevalent. Antidepressants can help improve a patient's mood, improve sleep habits, and reduce anxiety. In addition, tricyclic antidepressants may help control pain in cases of herpes zoster (shingles), nerve pain caused by diabetes, and other nerve disorders. Commonly prescribed antidepressants include trazodone (Desyrel), imipramine (Tofranil), and amitriptyline (Elavil). Anticonvulsant medications such as phenytoin (Dilantin) and gabapentin (Neurontin) often provide similar relief.

Tramadol (Ultram) mimics both opioids and antidepressants. It works by binding to receptors in the nervous system and encouraging the body to keep two neurotransmitters—serotonin and norepinephrine—active in the body. The net result is pain relief. It is often as effective as opioids, and is sometimes used instead. Tramadol can cause nausea, drowsiness, headaches, and constipation in some users. Doctors also may prescribe tranquilizers or mild sedatives to help patients deal with anxiety and sleep disruption brought on by their constant pain.

Other analgesic medicines

Medicines that work specifically against certain painful diseases also play a major role in pain relief. Common examples include sumatriptan (Imitrex), which constricts blood vessels in the head and works to combat migraine headaches, and corticosteroids such as prednisone, which are frequently used to combat swelling in arthritic joints. Topical medications used for pain include capsaicin (Capsin, Zostrix), a cream made from extract of red peppers. Capsaicin has a broad application; it's often useful against headaches, arthritis, diabetic neuropathy, and shingles. It takes three to four weeks of topical use before pain relief occurs.

NONDRUG THERAPIES

Doctors and patients have a number of other tools at their disposal in the fight against pain. Typically, these are used in combination with painkilling drugs to achieve greater relief and increased daily function. It is vital for caregivers to reassure patients that nondrug therapies are not meant to replace pain-relieving drugs. Many patients, especially older ones, may fear that they will be taken off medications if the therapies show even moderate success. Again, the goal is to find the right mix of treatments that deliver maximum pain relief with minimal side effects.

It's also important to understand that much trial and error is involved. Sometimes, even pain experts cannot predict how patients will respond to individual therapies. Patients and caregivers should be careful not to abandon a therapy before it has a chance to work. Because these treatments are noninvasive, caregivers and patients should take the approach that whatever does not hurt probably helps. The role of the placebo effect—the body's ability to kill pain simply by believing that something is working—cannot be overstated. Research shows that virtually everyone is able to benefit from the power of suggestion in relieving the symptoms of pain, with placebos typically producing a response rate of about 60 percent. While it is unethical to lie to patients about the treatment they are receiving, it is nonetheless true that many forms of successful treatment for pain depend on the underlying mechanism of the placebo.

Relaxation therapies. Such therapies, including yoga and meditation, can serve to ease muscle tension and reduce anxiety—both of which can contribute to headaches and other types of pain. Meditation can help patients change their mental focus from pain to another, more pleasant topic. These techniques need not be formal in nature. Depending on a person's background and beliefs, other methods like prayer can be substituted. Listening to music also can serve to distract patients from pain, as can the introduction of a new hobby or group activity.

Psychotherapy. Counseling or psychotherapy can address underlying amplifiers of pain, such as depression. Therapy also can help patients learn to develop new behavior and thought patterns that can divert attention away from pain and toward more productive outlets. Therapy can be accomplished in individual or group settings. Family therapy can provide help for family members, including caregivers, who also suffer because of a loved one's battle with pain.

Biofeedback. Biofeedback teaches patients to become aware of physiologic states that can influence pain. Using monitors, patients can see how autonomic functions—breathing rate, pulse, blood pressure, and skin temperature—increase during pain flares. Many people are able, with training, to achieve pain relief by controlling these functions to some extent.

Hypnosis. Hypnosis can be surprisingly effective for some people with chronic pain. Trained therapists are often able to use the power of imagery and suggestion to help patients to change their focus away from pain. This can offer immediate pain relief during therapy. But more important, posthypnotic suggestion can enable people to remain in a less painful state after hypnotherapy is complete. While hypnosis has been the subject of much derision over the years, the National Institutes of Health have stated that the therapy can reduce the perception of pain in some cases.

Hypnosis, biofeedback, behavioral therapy, and similar methods do have limits. Many patients, for example, no longer have the cognitive ability to understand and take advantage of the techniques. They may be better served by methods that require less concentration.

Physical therapy. Work with a trained physical therapist can help people regain function lost to pain, and can even reduce pain through increased range of motion and exercise. In fact, exercise can help on a variety of fronts. In addition to building strength and confidence in pain patients, it also can improve sleep patterns, elevate mood, and encourage the patient's body to release its natural store of painkillers.

Occupational therapy. By focusing on regaining physical skills that are important to a person's everyday work and home lives, occupational therapy offers some patients ways to compensate for painful movements. Caregivers should reassure patients undergoing these treatments that therapy is not intended to cause additional pain; in fact, it can slowly break the cycle of pain and inactivity that plagues many chronic pain sufferers.

Transcutaneous electrical nerve stimulation. Also known as TENS, this technique uses small amounts of electrical current to stimulate certain nerve endings located in the skin. These nerves are not responsible for causing pain, but rather for sensing touch, temperature, and other nondangerous stimuli. Stimulating these nerves may block pain messages from the pain receptors in the skin. Technicians place electrodes on parts of the skin, and the electrodes then emit small electrical pulses. TENS has proven successful in a number of chronic pain cases, including those involving elderly patients. It may work for shoulder pain or bursitis, broken ribs, and in some cases of diabetic neuropathy. Not everyone receives benefit, however, and sometimes the patient's response to the stimulation treatments declines over a period of weeks or months. One recent study, in fact, found that the pain relief from TENS may actually have been a result of the placebo effect—that is, the body was fooled into thinking something was going to relieve pain and therefore released its own store of painkilling chemicals. While this does not make the pain relief any less real, it does bring the TENS method's effectiveness into question.

INVASIVE METHODS

When patients do not find adequate pain relief from medicines and nondrug therapies, doctors sometimes turn to more complicated methods. These involve surgeries to alter nerve pathways or the implantation of devices that can deliver painkilling medicines directly to the central nervous system. All of these therapies involve the usual risks of surgery, including complications from anesthesia and possible infection.

Anatomic surgeries. Anatomic surgeries include procedures that attempt to fix conditions that may be causing pain, such as herniated disks in the back or compressed nerves that lead to carpal tunnel syndrome. Nerve blocks are also a common type of anatomic surgery. As the name suggests, this procedure involves disabling a nerve that is sending unnecessary pain signals to the brain. These can be short-acting—as in the case of the epidural block that is commonly given to women during childbirth—or long-lasting. The short-term blocks usually involve injecting the patient with an anesthetic that numbs the nerve for a period of hours. In long-term cases, a steroid is added to the injection. This can take a period of days to become effective, and may need to be repeated several times to ensure long-term relief. Nerve blocks can be used to help diagnose the causes of pain as well. Numbing a particular nerve, for instance, may help doctors pinpoint the parts of the nervous system that are responsible for sending the pain signals to the brain. While they rarely cure pain permanently, nerve blocks can allow patients to resume greater activity levels. This can result in more range of motion in joints and allow for increased exercise, both of which can help with pain relief by themselves.

Ablative surgeries. Ablative surgeries are designed to permanently sever nerves from the spinal cord. But this procedure is being done less and less often, because it does not always address the causes of underlying pain. Chronic pain often involves changes to the central nervous system itself, not just one particular nerve. Cutting one nerve, in fact, can sometimes cause additional pain in areas that were previously unaffected. And pain will sometimes return after a period of six months to a year. The surgery is still useful in some cases of cancer pain, however, and when nerve damage appears confined to a particular peripheral nerve. Even when effective, nerve-cutting surgeries may leave people without the ability to sense temperature changes in the affected area.

Augmentative surgeries. Here devices are implanted in the body to help relieve pain by stimulating nerves or by blocking their signals. Electrical devices similar to TENS units can be placed under the skin to deliver low-level electrical stimulation to the spinal cord or peripheral nerves. This procedure allows for constant treatment, unlike the TENS system. It is widely used in the United States for certain types of chronic back pain.

Medication implants. Pain medication also can be delivered through devices placed under the skin. The medicine is usually stored in a reservoir or catheter that is implanted along with a small pump. The pump delivers medicine from the reservoir to the spinal cord in a steady, controlled dosage. Technicians can refill the reservoir when needed (typically every week or two) by injecting the medicine directly through the skin and through a rubber stopper. The unit is usually about as large as a hockey puck. The patient usually can feel the device through the skin, but it is not painful.

723

Implants are usually reserved for patients who do not achieve pain relief through traditional delivery of medicine. They appear to be well tolerated; research shows that more than 90 percent of patients were satisfied with the implants. Still, not everyone gets relief from these systems. Anywhere from five percent to 35 percent of people with the implants still report intolerable levels of pain.

ALTERNATIVE AND COMPLEMENTARY THERAPIES

Because so many patients fail to achieve pain relief, interest in alternative treatments continues to grow. These include magnet therapy for back and neck pain, acupuncture, copper bracelets, aromatherapy, herbal remedies, massage, and manipulation techniques. To date, scientific research has not been able to prove conclusively that any of these methods bring about effective pain relief. In pain management, the power of the placebo cannot be understated; about one in three people will feel genuine relief from a fake treatment or medication if they believe that it will help them. This may help explain why alternative treatments often boast great anecdotal evidence of people who are "cured" by their use. Until alternative therapies are shown to be effective, it's far more helpful for patients to aggressively pursue pain relief through more traditional routes. (For more information, see the Complementary and Alternative Medicine chapter on p. 651.)

THE CAREGIVER'S ROLE IN PAIN MANAGEMENT

Pain can sometimes be more frightening than death itself. A recent study, in fact, found that two-thirds of all cancer patients would choose physician-assisted suicide over unrelieved chronic pain. This highlights the importance of working with doctors, nurses, and other health professionals to create a working pain management plan. While curing an underlying disease remains vital, addressing a patient's pain simply cannot be ignored.

Patients have a right to as much pain relief as possible. While this does not mean complete relief in all cases, it does mean that no patient should be forced to live with pain until every logical option has been explored. The responsibility for proper pain management often falls to family caregivers. Patients may hesitate to discuss their pain, feeling that they are being a "bad patient" or a burden on their families. Others simply accept their pain as an inevitable part of aging. And many elderly patients are unable to communicate their feelings because of disease or mental impairment.

Doctors, too, often fail to pursue the course of pain relief to its full extent. Sometimes this is due to ignorance of the options available. Some doctors also report that they're afraid to prescribe narcotics because of scrutiny from government agencies. In many more cases, doctors undertreat pain because they are unable to perceive the amount of pain a patient actually feels.

The caregiver's role, then, is multifaceted. The first, and most important, step is to work with patients and medical professionals to create a pain-management plan. Second, the caregiver must implement this plan—dispensing medications, tracking the progress of pain relief, and persuading reluctant patients to do their part. Finally, the caregiver must provide the social and spiritual support that only family can offer. Gentle massage, a kind word, or a listening ear can be just as important as medication in effective pain management.

DEVELOPING A PLAN

It is crucial for caregivers to serve as advocates for patients in pain from the very beginning of treatment. Make sure that doctors pay attention to a patient's complaints of pain; remember that pain relief is sometimes the most immediate concern of many patients, even above curing disease itself.

Explain to the doctor that you and the patient would like to create a comprehensive plan that includes physical rehabilitation, medication, alternate pain-control methods, counseling, and other methods when appropriate. Goal setting should be part of the plan. The point of pain management is not always simply pain relief, but rather an improvement of the patient's quality of life. For example, a patient may set a long-term goal of being able to return to a favorite activity, such as gardening. This may require short-term goals, such as pain-free bending, walking, and light lifting. Insist on follow-up visits with the doctor to discuss and modify plans.

It's also important for doctors to perform a thorough physical examination to look for underlying causes of pain. Back pain, for instance, may be caused by something other than osteoarthritis, ruptured disks, or other problems that show up on an x-ray; weakened muscles, poor posture, or bad gait could also contribute to the problem, and all can be addressed.

Most importantly, make sure that you and the patient understand everything the doctor says. If something is unclear, ask for an explanation. Also ask for written materials and visual aids that can help clarify treatments. While being belligerent will not help matters, being insistent and firm about getting answers is sometimes necessary.

If the patient's doctor has been unable to control pain through medication or other methods, consider consulting a specialized pain care center. Such clinics exist in most urban areas and an increasing number of other locations. Typically, the pain clinic is headed by a physician—typically an anesthesiologist—who is well versed in pain-relief techniques. The clinic usually has physical therapists, nurses, and other health professionals who are dedicated solely to pain relief. The clinic sometimes has its own pharmacist on staff as well.

Depending on the patient's health care coverage, a referral from the primary care physician may be necessary. When discussing the referral with the doctor, caregivers should take care to explain that the patient has not found satisfactory pain relief and simply wants to pursue the issue with specialists.

Pain care centers should be multidisciplinary; that is, they should offer a variety of treatment options. Many places that call themselves pain clinics offer only one modality—acupuncture, perhaps, or possibly massage therapy. While these single treatments may be useful, the best approach is to find a center that has a variety of options available.

KEEPING A PAIN DIARY

To help patients and caregivers learn more about dealing with pain, most experts recommend keeping a pain diary. By discovering when a person's pain is at its highest and lowest levels during the day, and what combination of medicine and activities leads to pain relief, it is often possible to achieve greater pain relief and a better quality of life.

The diary may at first cause the patient and caregiver to focus more closely on pain. This can sometimes make the pain seem worse. But over time, the diary may give patients a feeling of control over their pain. It can also allow them to take steps to avoid pain, instead of simply reacting to it when it occurs.

Diaries can be tailored to meet each patient and caregiver's needs. But most should be updated several times per day, while information remains fresh in the mind. Diaries should include the following information:

- When and where pain occurs.
- A description of the intensity of pain. It's often helpful to use a scale of 0 to 10, with 0 being no pain and 10 being the worst pain imaginable. In patients with diminished mental capacity, using colors, faces, or other scales may help. These are available from a doctor or nurse. It's also useful to note the sensation of pain: burning, stabbing, dull, etc.
- How long the pain lasts.
- When medications were administered, and how long it takes them to be effective.
- With each medication dose, the amount of pain relief. Have the patient use the 0 to 10 pain scale and rate the pain after the dose when the medication is working maximally.
- How long the relief lasts with each medication dose. Is the pain controlled until the next scheduled pain-medication dose?
- The patient's state of mind, e.g., stress, confusion, or anger.
- What food has been consumed, and when.
- What activities the patient has undertaken, such as exercise, reading, grooming, or group activities.
- Other, more subjective observations by the caregiver and/or patient. These can include any thoughts about what may have caused the pain to emerge or subside.

It's helpful to review the diary at the end of each day. After a while, patterns may emerge. A person may feel more pain in the morning, or the pain may grow in intensity as the day progresses. Certain actions may trigger reactions or provide relief. All this information can lead to more effective pain relief. Activities can be scheduled during periods that are normally pain-free. Medication may be given at times when it proves most effective. And exercise routines can be altered to take advantage of the ebb and flow of pain.

Share the information with nurses and doctors during each visit. They may have additional insights to share.

HANDLING PAIN MEDICATIONS

Caregivers are often asked to take on responsibilities that they feel unprepared to handle, including how and when to dispense pain medication. This area causes more concern on the part of caregivers than any other role in pain management. Studies show that many caregivers undermedicate their loved ones because they are unsure how to proceed and have unfounded fears about the medicine itself.

It is essential to keep in communication with health care professionals. Ask them for guidance about giving medication, including written instructions. Make sure you have answers to the following questions:

- How much medication should be given, and when?
- Will these drugs react poorly with other medication the patient is currently taking?
- Should this medicine be taken with food?
- What happens when a dose is skipped accidentally?
- What side effects are possible, and what can be done when they occur?
- What reactions should cause concern? When should a doctor be notified?

Many patients and caregivers—not to mention nurses and even doctors—are hesitant to deliver opioid painkillers for fear that the patient will become addicted to them. This is extremely rare. A patient may become physically dependent on the drugs after a period, meaning that the dosages must be tapered off slowly when the medicine is no longer needed. It's also possible that a patient may become tolerant of a drug, meaning that higher doses will be needed to deliver pain relief. Neither of these factors should keep caregivers or patients from using medication.

Caregivers should work to convince patients that taking medication is not a sign of weakness. Many patients are embarrassed about their pain, or feel that they burden family members by complaining about pain. Caregivers need to explain that pain relief is extremely important to recovery and improved quality of life. Giving medication, in fact, often gives caregivers a feeling of involvement and empowerment. Rather than watching helplessly as an obviously distressed patient denies feeling pain, a caregiver can take positive steps to help a loved one rest easier.

Side effects are a common occurrence with pain medication. While they vary widely, constipation is the most frequent complaint. Drinking water and other liquids—as many as eight 8-ounce glasses per day—often keeps bowels moving.

Exercise is useful for this also, as is a high-fiber diet. Most patients on chronic analgesics will also require over-the-counter or prescription constipation aids.

HELPING IN OTHER WAYS

Emotional support is extremely important to people in pain. Family caregivers are in a unique position to help with this, since they usually have a bond with patients that no health professional can match.

Be sure to use the power of touch. A gentle arm around the shoulder can help reassure a person in pain. Light massage of the neck and shoulders often helps relieve tension. Ice packs or heat can often take the edge off pain; be sure to ask whether these are appropriate for the patient. Adjusting pillows, providing blankets, and offering a warm drink can make people comfortable and less frightened. While these things usually come naturally, caregivers often overlook them in the rush to give medication and provide other day-to-day services.

Encouragement and motivation are just as vital. Patients should be reminded of their goals, be they simply walking up a flight of stairs or returning to work. Caregivers need to tell patients that exercise may cause short-term discomfort in the form of sore joints or muscles, but will yield long-term improvements. And it's important to reinforce the notion that talking about pain is all right; denying pain will not help it go away.

TAKING CARE OF THE CAREGIVER

Today's health care system places enormous responsibility on family caregivers. This can often prove overwhelming, especially in the case of chronic or severe pain. A recent survey found that caregivers often feel as much pain and distress, or more, as do patients. Researchers looked at 85 cancer patients who reported pain. The patients were asked to rate their level of pain from 0 to 100, with 100 being the most intense pain imaginable. The patients rated their pain at a median level of 45, while the caregiver estimated the patient's pain at a median of 70. More importantly, the caregivers reported that they themselves felt distress at a median level of 77. This suggests that caregivers are especially sensitive to pain in loved ones.

This added stress can exact a toll on caregivers. That's why experts remind caregivers to take care of themselves first and foremost. That means getting proper amounts of sleep, eating well, and looking after one's own social and emotional needs. A caregiver is of no use to a patient if he or she is unable to function. Because of the severe emotional stress caregivers must endure, experts recommend family or individual counseling. Far from a sign of weakness, going to counseling sessions shows a commitment to providing the proper care to the patient and also to the caregiver himself or herself. By working together, patients, family caregivers, and professionals can provide the optimum pain relief and quality of life that is possible to achieve in each individual set of circumstances.

WHAT RESEARCH IS BEING DONE?

The future of pain relief lies with specialization. Instead of treating pain as a side effect of disease, medical experts are beginning to view pain management as a field unto itself. Most believe that pain medicine will become a subspecialty, like cardiology, obstetrics, and other fields. Pain specialists will become well versed in every aspect of pain management, including drugs, surgery, and other treatments. Because of their expertise, pain doctors may be able to offer treatment options that other doctors miss.

Scientists are quickly learning more about the causes, diagnosis, and treatment of pain. Researchers are focusing on several main topics.

PAIN MEDICATION

Hundreds of analgesics are already available, but all have side effects and contraindications that can limit their use. This will probably be the case with new medications, too. While it's unlikely any one drug will be able to stop pain in all cases, every new drug gives doctors a better chance of creating tailor-made treatment plans that work for individual patients.

Ziconotide is a promising unique new drug that may be able to help people with intractable chronic pain. The drug is a synthetic version of the venom used by an ocean-dwelling cone snail. The snail paralyzes fish by injecting its venom through a harpoon-like tube. The venom is extremely powerful, and so is ziconotide; tests have shown the drug to be 100 times more potent than morphine. The drug works by blocking pain-delivering signals in the dorsal horn of the spinal cord through a different mechanism, by blocking neuronal calcium channels that transmit pain sensations. It appears to be more specific than opioids that are currently in use, and therefore may have fewer side effects. Tests have shown it to be effective in many patients who either get no relief from opioids or cannot use them because of side effects. The drug's manufacturer has recently received an approvable letter from the federal Food and Drug Administration, and the drug could soon be available to doctors. The drug is administered directly into the fluid that surrounds the spinal cord, usually through the use of an implanted pump. Early results show that tolerance does not develop to this drug.

Researchers in America are also looking at the drug neurotrophin, which has been used in Japan to treat pain from chronic regional pain syndrome. This nerve-based disease affects people who suffer chronic pain following an injury, surgery, or similar event. Tests also are being conducted to see if the drug helps relieve acute pain following dental surgery.

Tests are also under way on a class of drugs called AMPA receptor blockers. These drugs block nerve receptors that can trigger pain. When injury occurs, several types of amino acids bind to the receptors and activate the pain response. The drugs may keep the amino acids from binding and signaling pain to the brain. Research remains in the preliminary stages.

Doctors and researchers are also working to refine the uses of current analgesics, such as the new COX-2 inhibitors and other drugs. Clinical trials should help doctors understand which medicines, which doses, and which combinations of drugs will be most effective in a variety of pain types. New delivery methods, such as skin patches, may offer patients better control and less concern about missed dosages.

CAUSES OF PAIN

Tests are under way to see what role genetics may play in pain. Pain perception and sensitivity vary widely from person to person—and finding a genetic link may help scientists discover the reasons for these differences. Researchers also are trying to better understand the pathways and triggers for pain, in hopes that the information may lead to more effective drug treatments.

DIAGNOSTIC TOOLS

Pain is very subjective, and doctors often have difficulty treating it because they cannot properly judge how much pain a person feels—or where the pain is originating. Even though the standard 0 to 10 scale is helpful in measuring pain, researchers are working to develop new tools that can help patients more clearly describe the extent and nature of their suffering. One national study is using volunteers to rate clinically induced pain sensations on various scales before and after taking an opioid painkiller or a placebo.

Scientists also are learning to use MRI machines, positron emission tomography (PET) scanners, and other tools as "magnifying glasses" to pinpoint pain sources. With these machines, doctors can see how blood flow and other body functions change as a person feels pain. This can help isolate sources of pain and help doctors create treatment plans that are tailored to a patient's needs.

ADDITIONAL RESOURCES

ORGANIZATIONS AND WEB SITES

American Academy of Pain Medicine
www.painmed.org

American College of Physicians
www.acponline.org/public

American Pain Society
www.ampainsoc.org

American Pain Foundation
www.painfoundation.org

American Society of Anesthesiologists
www.asahq.org/PublicEducation

City of Hope Pain/Palliative Care Resource Center
www.prc.coh.org

International Association for the Study of Pain (IASP Secretariat)
www.iasp-pain.org

National Institute of Neurological Disorders and Stroke
www.ninds.nih.gov

PART 4
Holding On and Letting Go

Self-Care
for the Caregiver

If you are currently taking care of an older adult—a parent, a spouse, a sibling, a friend—you probably have less time for yourself than you once had. For that matter, you probably have less time to even think about yourself. But now, take a minute or two to ask yourself the following questions.

Do you regularly

- Get a good night's rest?
- Exercise or take long, brisk walks?
- Eat breakfast every day?
- Get the medical attention you need, including such preventive heath care as routine physical examinations; cholesterol checks; flu shots; blood pressure checks; gynecologic, prostate, and colorectal exams; and mammograms?
- Talk to someone—a friend, relative, member of the clergy, therapist, or support group—about your feelings, worries, and questions concerning your caregiving responsibilities and relationships?

Have you, in the last two to three weeks

- Engaged in an activity or hobby that you truly enjoy?
- Asked a relative, neighbor, or friend to relieve you from your caregiving responsibilities for a portion of the day?
- Used any community resource—a home health care attendant, adult day-care program, house cleaner, Meals-on-Wheels—to lighten your load?

If you answered No to more than three of these questions, you could be at risk for caregiver burnout. In addition, engaging in any of the following increases your risk for health problems dramatically:

- Frequent overeating
- Alcohol or recreational drug use
- Smoking cigarettes
- A sedentary lifestyle

Not an easy quiz, is it? The questions are not meant to raise the hairs on the back of your neck or stir up decades of guilt. Rather, they're meant to remind you that however easy it might seem to ignore your own needs, it is crucial both now and later that you pay attention to the person doling out the care—yourself.

Of course, asking people who take care of others whether they are currently taking care of themselves is a bit tricky. For one, caregiving responsibilities vary greatly depending on the situation. For some it means arranging for and supervising an ailing father's care services from a distance. For others it means living with and tending to, twenty-four hours a day, a wife whose Alzheimer's disease has rendered her increasingly forgetful and dependent. But almost invariably, caregivers find one thing to be true—that taking care of a loved one is an important, mostly rewarding, but absolutely demanding and time-consuming job. So to urge every caregiver to carve out the time from an already overbooked schedule and find the energy to enroll in a health club, get eight hours of sleep, eat three nutritious meals a day, and visit a health care provider for routine health care may be a little much. Also, the truth is that not everyone is conscientious about self-care with or without the additional tasks involved in caregiving. It may be too much to ask that, on top of everything else, you change your self-care habits. Indeed, at the end of the day, having to think about yourself may feel like just one more burden. Nevertheless, making time when you don't have it, pushing yourself slightly when you're sure you have no energy left, and taking care of yourself, even in small ways, can make a world of difference.

So no matter how you answered the quiz above, read on. Learning about self-care will increase the likelihood that you will feel better and be healthier as you go about your job(s). And taking care of yourself can mean that you will be able to take care of your loved one more effectively and with greater pleasure in the long run.

CAREGIVING TRENDS

According to a recent government report we are living longer, healthier lives. The study, put together by the Interagency Forum on Aging-Related Statistics, estimates that approximately 13% of today's population is 65 or older; that's a tenfold increase since 1900. People 85 and older now make up the fastest-growing segment of our society. Today, we live in a time of remarkable medical and technologic strides. As a society, we embrace healthier lifestyles and view aging in a more positive light. All this translates into living longer and feeling better about getting older.

As the report indicates, most elderly people believe that they are in reasonably good health. Nevertheless, advancing age can bring illness and disability. At some time or other, every older adult will need some kind of supportive care. And more likely than not, it will be a family member—a wife or husband, daughter or son, sister or brother—or a friend who will provide that care.

Except for those people currently living in nursing or health-related facilities, the majority of caregiving is provided informally. Even when people are no longer able to manage all aspects of their daily life and personal care, they are more likely to rely on family members or friends than on a paid or formal help arrangement. Eighty percent of all long-term care is provided by family members and friends. According to the 1997 "Family Caregiving in the U.S." study conducted by the National Alliance for Caregiving and the AARP (formerly called the American Association of Retired Persons), someone in over 22 million households is currently caring for an adult who is 50 or older. In almost 25% of all American households, at least one person aged 18 or above is caring for or has cared for an older relative or friend.

Most people who take on caregiving responsibilities choose to do so. And the rewards are many. Caring for a loved one reflects individual values and beliefs—to be loving, caring, responsible, involved human beings, many times in the face of difficult circumstances and minimal support. In addition, it is often the case that whenever family members are actively involved in caring for an older adult, he or she is able to stay at home longer, usually to the delight of both the family and the individual.

Depending on the circumstances, the need for care can arise gradually or suddenly. You watch as your mother's arthritis gets worse and makes it harder for her to dress herself. Your father is suddenly wandering off alone late at night, and you fear for his safety. The stroke has left your husband housebound, unable to do all that used to give him pleasure. And there you are—ready or not—assuming the role of caregiver.

And though so many people find themselves caring for an older adult, few caregivers have the training, information, or resources they need. Yet they do it. Few have reserves of spare time on their hands. Yet they find time. Caregivers often wear, at different times, the hat of nurse, attendant, mechanic, accountant, therapist, advocate, companion, educator, housekeeper, chauffeur, social worker, insurance appraiser, and diagnostician, to name a few. Although this job is unpaid, time-consuming, and often exhausting, people find the wherewithal to do it. In the long run, family or informal caregivers can provide the support and assistance that allow older people to stay comfortably in their own homes longer. In return, caregivers are afforded the opportunity to be with their loved ones and to know, deep in their hearts, that they are doing a good and loving deed.

WHO IS THE TYPICAL CAREGIVER?

Most caregivers are relatives—spouses taking care of spouses, children taking care of parents, siblings taking care of siblings. Results from the Family Caregiving study were revealing:

- Almost three-fourths of all caregivers are women.
- About one in five is younger than 35, and more than one in three are 50 or older.
- Most people who care informally for older adults are between the ages of 35 and 49.
- Sixty-six percent of all caregivers are married and 41% have one or more children under the age of 18 living at home.
- Most caregivers provide care for an average of 4½ years.

Typically, the caregiver is a woman in her mid-40s with a high school degree, who is married, works full-time, and has an annual household income of $35,000. In other words, most caregivers have full lives that don't come to a stop once they take on the care of an elderly person.

WHO IS THE TYPICAL CARE RECIPIENT?

On the receiving end, the Family Caregiving survey found that:

- About 85% of caregivers take care of a family member, while 15% take care of a friend or neighbor.
- Care recipients are often female relatives: 31% are the caregiver's own mother, 12% are their grandmother, and 9% are their mother-in-law.
- More than one in five of all caregivers (about 22%) are responsible for a person suffering from Alzheimer's disease, dementia, confusion, or forgetfulness.
- About one-fifth of all recipients of care live with their caregiver. About half of all care recipients live alone, but most are within twenty minutes of their caregiver, and 94% live no more than two hours away.

SPOUSES AND OLDER CAREGIVERS

Increasing numbers of older adults are providing care to a spouse, sibling, or family member. According to the Family Caregiving study, about one-eighth of all caregivers (12.4%) are 65 or older. And nearly one-quarter of those older caregivers (23%) are taking care of a spouse. Spouses tend to supply the most comprehensive care, living with the person, providing round-the-clock care. As a group, husbands and wives typically take care of the most disabled individuals and maintain the role of caregiver for a longer period time than other caregivers.

Compared to other family caregivers, husbands and wives caring for their spouses may face special health challenges. For one, the fact that they tend to be older themselves puts them at particular risk. Many older adults have at least one chronic illness that can render them less capable of combating the stress and strain of caregiving. In addition, they are more likely to have their own health problems that may be linked to the demands of full-time caregiving, such as heart, stomach, and back problems, sleep and weight difficulties, stress-related symptoms, and depression and anxiety.

Spouses taking care of spouses with dementia are particularly vulnerable to health problems. People who suffer from dementia can gradually become more forgetful and less functional in their day-to-day lives, and thus more dependent. They may wander off and have problems sleeping, which can cause considerable disruption in the household. At the same time, they often lose their capacity for loving and intimate relationships. In many cases, they progressively lose their sense of self and can seem completely unrecognizable. If someone you love has dementia, taking care of him or her can truly leave you physically and emotionally drained.

WHAT KIND OF CARE IS TYPICALLY PROVIDED?

The types of care vary tremendously, depending on the situation. Responsibilities can range from very modest and nontaxing care to heavy-duty, round-the-clock care. Caregivers provide transportation, go grocery shopping, do household chores and laundry, prepare meals, and manage finances. Some caregivers monitor medications. Others supervise outside services. Sometimes caregiving entails intimate personal care: helping a person get in and out of chairs, dress, bathe, and eat. Sometimes it means assisting with toileting and tending to incontinence and diapers. And often caregiving means visiting on a regular basis, providing companionship to a loved one.

COMPLICATIONS OF CAREGIVING

Taking care of another person is a demanding responsibility that can complicate an already complicated schedule. The added responsibilities can push their way into the caregiver's family life, leisure time, work, finances, and, in some cases, physical and mental health. Most caregivers find that as a result of their caregiving responsibilities, they have less time for other family members—not to mention for vacations, hobbies, and other personal interests. Not surprisingly, the more time a person invests in taking care of another adult, the more those responsibilities can interfere with other parts of her life. Caregivers who have to split their time between young children and an aging parent, for example, often feel that they can do neither justice. And those caring for someone with dementia are even less likely to have time for other people or interests in their lives.

Finances. Taking care of another adult can bring financial hardships. Even when the care recipient is not a spouse, caregiving usually means extra out-of-pocket expenses. And the higher level of care or the lower the income to begin with, the greater the hardship.

Work. Since the majority of caregivers are employed, and about half work full-time, taking care of another person usually has considerable impact on work life. Most caregivers find that they have to modify their work schedule; they frequently go in to work late, leave early, or take time off during the day to accommodate their caregiving responsibilities. Sometimes it becomes necessary to shift from full-time to part-time work, or to change jobs altogether so that work is less demanding, allows for more flexibility, or is perhaps closer to home. Within the past several years, however, many major corporations have created and implemented eldercare for their employees. Employees who are the main caregivers for aging parents or other relatives can utilize these programs, which offer care for dependent adults during working hours. Caregivers, care recipients, and the employer all benefit from this arrangement.

Social life. Caregiving can drain away the time and energy needed to maintain one's social networks. People who have significant caregiving responsibilities are more likely to experience troubled family relationships. Their social life and leisure time often undergo changes, and many find that they cannot attend church or synagogue as often as they once did.

Physical and mental stress. The degree of physical and mental stress reported by caregivers increases with the age of the caregiver and the intensity of care that the caregiver is required to provide. The burden of caring for an elderly adult can impose a heavy physical and emotional cost on the caregiver. And many times, the resulting physical and emotional stress is likely to hinder the quality of care provided, which in turn increases the need to place an older adult in a nursing home prematurely.

On the whole, women appear to be more likely than men to experience physical or mental health problems as a result of caregiving. Caregivers who do not work outside of the house may be more vulnerable than working caregivers to such problems. Other factors that seem to heighten physical and emotional stress include caring for a person with Alzheimer's disease or other forms of dementia, living in the same household as the person being cared for, and carrying the primary responsibility for caregiving. People who take care of others for a long period of time and who invest a great deal of time and energy in their caregiving are more prone to significant health problems. Caring for someone who requires a great deal of hands-on attention—someone with progressive dementia, for example, or a chronic, disabling physical condition—increases your risk. And the older a caregiver is, the more susceptible he or she is.

The greater the extent of caregiving and the older the caregiver, the greater the risk for developing or worsening such health problems as arthritis, heart, and back conditions. Caregivers who are largely responsible for the day-to-day care of older adults report more stress-related problems, such as migraines and colitis, as well as higher rates of depression and other psychologic symptoms, than noncaregivers.

Not only are caregivers more susceptible to physical and emotional problems, but they appear to be less likely than the general population to practice certain health behaviors that might otherwise help buffer them against such problems. In other words, the emotional, behavioral, and logistical demands of providing care seem to interfere with such self-care habits as exercising, getting enough rest and sleep, eating properly, and obtaining necessary and preventive health care, such as getting flu shots and annual physical examinations. And these very same demands can trigger high-risk health behaviors such as sedentary lifestyle, overeating, smoking, and alcohol and drug use.

Nevertheless, there are things you can do to combat these statistics, ways you can take care of yourself and lower your risk for illness and depression, as well as caregiver's burnout.

Family dynamics. Not surprisingly, family dynamics and conflict can add to the stress of caregiving. Some families pull together during times of crisis—for example, when an older member becomes sick or increasingly disabled, thus needing special care. Other families fall apart. It is not uncommon for one person in the family to take on the responsibility of providing care, yet others in the family may be quite vocal with their objections or disagreement. Sometimes, it can feel that everyone has an opinion about what should be done and how things should be handled, yet few want to do it.

The way individual family members respond to the challenges of caregiving often reflects the larger family dynamics and history. When there is a history of family conflict, the stress of taking care of an older member can exacerbate strain and divisiveness. Yet, some families find this an opportunity to rework the quality of relationships, and a new sense of cooperation, support, and kinship can blossom.

PREVENTING CAREGIVER BURNOUT

As we've noted, more and more people are finding themselves in the role of caregiver. Yet many caregivers, especially those who fail to take care of themselves in specific ways, risk depression, physical illness, and strained personal relationships. In addition, by not engaging in thoughtful self-care, caregivers are more likely to consider placing their loved ones in a nursing home, sooner rather than later. Nevertheless, people who learn how to take care of themselves fare much better, as do the people they are caring for. Broadly speaking, there are four ways of taking care of yourself, so that you can take better care of another:

- Take advantage of assistance so that you free up time for yourself.
- Make a point of understanding your loved one's specific needs and conditions; use this understanding to anticipate and plan for his or her evolving care needs.
- Take care of your own health.
- Actively seek out support and information to help you cope with the emotional toll of caregiving.

Let's take a closer look at each of these options.

TAKE ADVANTAGE OF OUTSIDE ASSISTANCE

For your own well-being, and thus the well-being of the person for whom you are caring, create breathing space for yourself. Ease your direct obligation and carve out time for yourself by reaching out to others for help and support. Caregivers who line up secondary support—relief pitchers, so to speak—do better than those who play out the game alone. They tend to feel better about, take satisfaction in— even enjoy—their responsibilities much more than people who don't. And, perhaps more telling, those who make use of family and community resources are less likely to experience caregiver burnout and therefore less likely to place their loved ones prematurely in alternative housing because they are feeling overwhelmed by the responsibility.

Perhaps another family member, friend, or neighbor can relieve you from time to time. Perhaps someone can help for extended periods of time while you take a vacation or spend time with other family members. Or maybe someone else in the family can take over the finances or driving the person to the doctor's office. Not only does enlisting the help of others relieve you of some of the direct responsibility, but it can enhance your loved one's social connections.

All too often, disability brought on by physical illness or dementia can limit an elderly adult's comings and goings. Aging for some can bring diminished contact with the outside world. In turn, the social and physical responsibility of caring for a housebound adult can settle heavily on the shoulders of the primary caregiver. By asking others to help with your loved one's care, you provide broader opportunities for your loved one to interact with others. And you will get the respite every caregiver needs. Nevertheless, surprisingly few caregivers take advantage of other family or community resources. Rather, many seek the help of others only as a last resort—when they are already at their wits' end.

As you consider what care arrangement would work for your loved one, you, and your family, keep in mind that all families and all situations are unique. Any care arrangement you develop should reflect your unique needs. And know that your caregiving needs will likely change over time. Add to this mix the fact that each community offers its own range of services and resources. Therefore, when you begin to consider what resources would suit your particular needs, ask yourself the following questions:

- What services are available in your community?
- What kinds of services does the care recipient need or want?
- What kinds of care are you happy to give, and what kinds would you be happy to see someone else do?
- What financial resources are available?

Then, you may need to do a little bit of research. Start by calling the National Association of Area Agencies on Aging's Eldercare Locator, at 800-677-1116. The Eldercare Locator offers information on a wide range of community services, and will most likely be able to provide you with a list of resources in your area. Other government and community organizations can guide you as well. In all likelihood, there is an agency on aging in your area; look for the local Office or Council on Aging or Office of Elder Affairs. Otherwise call your local health department, community hospital, nursing home, senior center, or Department of Veterans Affairs.

There is no question that being familiar with and utilizing community services and resources can provide a crucial safety net for you, the caregiver, and the person you care for. Many types of supportive resources are available to caregivers. A little thought and research will uncover just what's out there in your community. Following are some of the types of assistance that are available in many communities:

Senior centers. These community centers provide a range of social opportunities and activities for older adults. Many offer classes, field trips, support groups, entertainment both in and out of the center, occupational therapy, volunteer opportunities, and meals. Very often, senior centers provide transportation.

Adult day-care programs. These public or private programs generally furnish health care, physical and occupational therapy, psychiatric assessment, and counseling, along with social activities and meals, at a central location. Like senior centers, some provide transportation.

Home health care. Nursing care and help with activities of daily living at home are available. Visiting nurses and nurses' aides render a range of treatments and therapies, including physical, occupational, and speech therapy. Home health aides can assist with bathing, feeding, dressing, monitoring medications, and the like. Most agencies supply and help with the use of assistive devices such as walkers, portable oxygen tanks, wheelchairs, and catheters. Home health care workers can usually be employed privately, through an agency, or as part of a government program. In addition to nurses and home health care aides, some health care agencies provide a range of home care services, including physicians, therapists, social workers, homemakers, durable medical equipment supplies, and companions.

Visitation or companion programs. These are usually staffed by volunteers who visit the housebound or isolated elderly in their homes. Such programs offer additional opportunities to spend time with a peer or another adult.

Physical therapists. Therapists can use massage and exercises to help a person regain movement and strength in certain areas of the body. They provide help in using special equipment or managing daily activities, such as getting in and out of chairs or a bathtub safely and more efficiently.

Occupational therapists. Occupational therapists use exercises and activities with the person to strengthen his or her ability to manage typical daily activities, such as eating, putting on clothes, and handling a brush, and they can adapt the person's environment to make navigating easier and safer.

Speech and language pathologists. These specialists offer support and use exercises to help a person strengthen and recover speech skills—after a stroke, for example.

Telephone monitoring services. Volunteers check up by phone on housebound or isolated seniors. Regular, predictable phone calls provide the opportunity to talk as well as monitor a person's well-being.

Home maintenance and repair services. These agencies provide people to perform a number of needed household repairs and practical chores including yard work, electric work, plumbing, etc.

Meal services, such as Meals-on-Wheels. You can arrange for delivery of meals that typically comply with specified dietary needs, along with mealtime companionship.

Homemakers and housekeeping agencies. These agencies can provide workers to assist with both everyday tasks such as meal preparation, cleaning, and grocery shopping and personal care tasks like bathing and dressing.

Gatekeeper/home observation programs. These are sometimes offered as a community service by local utility companies or the postal service. People who regularly visit the home to deliver mail, for example, or read the meter are trained to be on the lookout for and report any indication that something could be wrong inside the home.

Transportation services. These agencies have dedicated buses or vans to shuttle the elderly to and from the doctor's office, grocery store, senior center, etc.

Personal Emergency Response Systems (PERS). These are alert devices that enable a person to call for help should she fall, have an accident at home, or find she cannot move. Once the mechanical device is triggered, a call goes out to an emergency service, relative, or neighbor.

Professional resources. Many professions have established specialty areas in geriatrics and gerontology. These include geriatric social workers, geriatric care managers, geriatric physicians, psychologists, nurse practitioners, special financial advisors, and elder law attorneys.

Respite care. Most respite care is offered through community organizations or residential facilities, such as adult day services. Programs are designed to provide substitute short-term care so that caregivers can take a break from their responsibilities. However, there are also agencies that provide in-home care. Most respite care workers will assume caregiving responsibilities for a day, a weekend, or longer.

ANTICIPATE AND RESPOND TO CHANGING NEEDS

Although there are currently millions of adults caring for millions of older adults in the United States, each older adult is unique, as is each caregiving arrangement. And the more you can individualize your arrangement, the easier it will be for you to manage effectively. That means getting to know your specific situation:

- What exactly are your loved one's needs?
- What is the current state of his or her health?
- Are there specific medical and/or psychiatric conditions that need to be monitored and treated?
- How are those conditions likely to progress?
- What are your own specific needs?
- Do you tend to small children as well?
- Do you work outside of the home?
- What are your other responsibilities?

As you come to appreciate your special situation, you can evolve a care arrangement that works well for all involved: your loved one, other family members, yourself.

In addition, it is important to remember that care needs change over time. Self-care means being ready and anticipating changes in your loved one's health needs and related health care. Think in terms of a continuum of health care needs with independent living at home at one end and total care in a nursing home setting at the other. As the person's needs or competence or ability to function changes, so should the resources in his or her environment.

As your loved one requires greater attention and assistance with day-to-day activities, you may want to explore supplemental or alternative types of care. This is best done, though, before such care is actually required. Rather than waiting for a crisis such as a stroke to force you to look into other arrangements, anticipate possible changes in your loved one's needs. That way, you have the time to collect information and understand your options. Being pressed into making a decision by circumstances without feeling prepared only adds to the stress. On the other hand, if, for example, you notice that your father's health continues to deteriorate, you may want to explore and weigh options in advance. Looking at a number of nursing homes, interviewing the staff, and placing your name on a waiting list in advance will likely lift considerable weight off your shoulder, before it becomes necessary to make the move.

When to consider alternative housing arrangements

Sooner or later, many family caregivers give serious thought to the possibility of moving their loved ones out of the home and into another setting—whether to a retirement community, assisted living facility, or nursing home. Often the need to make other living arrangements is prompted when the older person requires greater, more constant, or more immediate care than can be administered at home. No matter how much you may want to keep your parent, spouse, or sibling at home, a combination of factors may make it a less than practical or workable option. For each family, deciding to place the care of a loved one into institutional hands is a very personal and often difficult matter. Usually, cultural, financial, medical, emotional, and legal considerations enter into the timing of such a decision. Sometimes it becomes apparent that nursing home placement, for example, is in the best interest of the family; at other times, moving into a nursing home is clearly best for the older individual. In the best circumstances, placement is without a doubt preferable for all concerned.

When the time comes that the family or caregiver realizes they are no longer capable of properly caring for their loved one in their own home, they will find that a great variety of housing alternatives are available. Housing alternatives for the elderly include continuing care retirement communities, assisted living apartments, residences, and group homes, Elder Cottage Housing Opportunity (ECHO) housing, and house sharing. Such alternative housing arrangements typically offer various levels of assistance with medical, physical, and social needs. Each type corresponds, more or less, with the level of care that's needed.

Among the more common types of alternative or residential care facilities:

Retirement housing. Residents have their own apartments or rooms, usually with cooking facilities. In most cases, this type of housing provides only minimal caregiving staff. As a result, retirement housing usually suits those adults who, although they may have difficulties managing an entire house, can still live alone safely and care adequately for themselves.

Assisted living residences. Assisted living generally allows for both independence and assistance. In addition to housing, these types of residences can offer supportive, personalized assistance as well as some health care services.

Continuum care retirement communities (CCRC). This campus-like housing allows the levels of assistance and care to increase as a person's need for care progresses. In many such communities, the residents move from one building to another to receive different services or levels of care.

Nursing facilities (nursing homes). These are typically large institutional residences that provide twenty-four-hour medical and supervised nursing care along with assistance with everyday activities. In most nursing facilities, there are different levels of care to accommodate different levels of health and disability.

Subacute care. This is a level of care within a nursing facility that utilizes sophisticated hospital technology to reduce the cost of services while maintaining quality of care. Sections of a nursing facility are dedicated to providing acute treatment to a seriously ill patient, so that it is not always necessary to transfer a resident to a hospital when such care is needed.

Hospice care. This provides comprehensive care for the terminally ill. Medical, emotional, and spiritual care, for the individual and the family, can be delivered in the home or in a community hospice setting. At the heart of hospice is a philosophy that promotes comfort and care at the end of a person's life while refraining from heroic lifesaving measures. Hospice care may also provide related medications, medical supplies, and equipment. Hospice service is generally available through local hospice organizations and some home care agencies, hospitals, and nursing homes. Trained hospice workers are usually available day and night to help the family in caring for the individual, to keep him or her as comfortable and free from pain as possible, and to ensure that the individual's wishes are honored.

If it becomes apparent to you and your family that nursing home placement is called for, you may experience feelings of guilt or failure. Taking care of an older adult inevitably stirs up a wide range of feelings. Those feelings are shaped not only by the current caregiving relationship, but also by the nature and history of the relationship. Children may well have feelings about tending to an increasingly dependent parent. Siblings will perhaps see their own mortality and frailty reflected back in their sibling's eyes. A wife who finds herself taking care of a sick husband may feel particularly abandoned if the marriage has been satisfying or resentful if it's always been depriving. Generally speaking, spouses are more likely to feel that they signed on to long-term care—in sickness and in health. Therefore, wives and husbands tend to be more reluctant to institutionalize than are children.

And while you may feel guilty at the thought of placing a parent, spouse, or sibling in a nursing home, you may be pleasantly surprised by the result. Because a nursing home is set up to provide consistent and vigilant medical and psychiatric care as well as social stimulation, many older people thrive in nursing homes once they get settled. This is especially true with people who are extremely housebound or who have dementia or depression. Many older adults rally and indeed seem more active, more alert, and less lethargic shortly after settling into the nursing home.

In the meantime, as you explore nursing homes, go through the process of placement, and even as your caregiving responsibilities and relationship change once your loved one has made the transition to the home, continue to take care of yourself. Most nursing homes have social workers to help you adjust to the transition and sort through the very mixed and often confusing feelings you may be experiencing. Over time, you may experience peace of mind, knowing that as before, your loved one is being well cared for.

TAKE CARE OF YOURSELF

The very nature of caring for another person means that you will be subject to physical and mental strain from time to time. However, that strain can become worse when you wrap yourself up in taking care of another person's needs and neglect your own. And indeed, some people have called caregivers the "hidden patients."

When caregivers don't take care of themselves, they put themselves at greater risk for depression and physical problems. In turn, even periodic depressions can cause people to feel less interested in or motivated to do those things that sustain good health. Furthermore, the more depressed people feel, the less likely they are to manage any illnesses and chronic conditions they may have. Over time, they have less physical strength and fewer internal resources to care for another. When people actively take care of themselves, on the other hand, they tend to reap the benefits in terms of their physical health, emotional well-being, and pleasure in their tasks. Taking care of yourself involves a variety of health measures. Here's a good checklist to keep in mind:

- Get enough sleep.
- Eat sufficient amounts of varied and healthy foods. Don't skip meals,

and do make a special effort to eat a healthful breakfast every day.

- Maintain a healthy weight.
- Exercise and engage in physical activities like walking, bicycling, swimming, tennis, yoga, and gardening.
- See your own health care provider for routine, preventive, and needed health care. Make sure your health care plan covers such preventive measure as mammograms, EKGs, cholesterol and blood pressure readings, stool blood tests, Pap smears, and rectal exams, as well as immunizations for influenza, pneumonia, or tetanus. Be sure your health care provider knows that you are responsible for the care of your spouse or parent. If you are taking care of your spouse, it may be a good idea to be evaluated as partners, in terms of both your health and the caregiving demands that exist in the home.
- Take prescribed medications.
- Take the time you need to slow down and get rest whenever you get sick so that you can recuperate completely.
- Avoid smoking. Try to quit, if you can.
- If you drink, drink alcohol in moderation (i.e., two or fewer drinks per day).

Finally, continue to do those activities and spend time with those people that give you pleasure. While it may seem that you just don't have an extra minute in your day, make an active effort to carve out time regularly for those activities and people that remind you who you are and what you love, and who support you in your efforts.

FIND SPIRITUAL AND EMOTIONAL SUPPORT

Studies show that a person's attitude—just how burdened she feels about caring for another—is an important factor in how well she copes in general. Studies suggest that caregiving can act to lower a person's sense of control. You perform tasks because another person requires them, even when you don't particularly feel like it. You may feel that you have little control over your own time, and cannot always do what you want to do when you want to do it.

Besides the physical and practical demands of caregiving, worrying about another person's health and well-being can take its toll. Nor is easy to watch a love one's health and sometimes his mind deteriorate. And possibly, the person you care for is not always appreciative; in fact, care recipients have been known to be uncooperative and demanding. Indeed, if you are caring for someone with Alzheimer's disease, you may run up against hostile and confusing responses to your most caring gestures.

On the other hand, you may experience the rewards that come with ensuring caring attention for your loved one. You may feel a deep sense of personal satisfaction, knowing that you are acting in a loving and responsible manner. The person you care for may also recognize and appreciate all you're doing—and let you know it. You may be in a position to watch the care recipient's health improve, as well as enjoy the time you spend in the company of an older adult. Many people who take care of a family member feel gratified that they have the chance to give back or to fulfill family obligations.

Caregivers who have their own social support networks fare much better than those who do not. If you are lucky enough to have a strong support system, you are more likely to get occasional relief from your caregiving duties, thus sufficient rest. Plus, having family members and friends to talk to about all the feelings and questions that get stirred up can be an enormous help.

Thus far, you've been urged to tend to your physical, emotional, and social needs, but for many, it's crucial that their spiritual needs not go unheeded at this complicated time. People find spiritual sustenance and support in various ways, whether it's through attending church or synagogue regularly, speaking with a member of the clergy, individual prayer and meditation, or religious retreat. For many, turning to religion or a sense of spiritual connection helps them deal with adversity and reinforces the fundamental values that underlie providing care.

Be sure that you actively seek out the support and information you need to help you cope with the emotional distress and toll of caregiving. And whether or not you can turn to your family and friends for support, it might be a good idea to participate in a caregiver support group. Run either by trained professionals or peers, caregiver support groups provide a venue for families who are caring for loved ones to interact with others in the same situation. More than just venting or complaining about problems, these groups can offer the opportunity to share practical ways of dealing with the jumble of feelings that inevitably arise. In these groups, people evolve very real solutions to the day-to-day problems they encounter and try out more effective coping skills with the help of others. Studies show that involvement in support groups goes a long way in keeping a loved on at home and out of nursing homes and can reduce the stress or depression that can result from caregiving burnout.

Finally, for some, especially those who expend large amounts of time providing daily and extensive care, counseling or short-term psychotherapy can be extremely helpful.

ADDITIONAL RESOURCES

ORGANIZATIONS AND WEB SITES

National Alliance for Caregiving

www.caregiving.org/

BOOKS

Berman, Claire. *Caring for Yourself While Caring for Your Aging Parents: How to help, How to Survive.* New York: Henry Holt, 1997.

Brandt, Avrene L., *Caregiver's Reprieve: A Guide to Emotional Survival When You're Caring for Someone You Love.* The Working Caregiver Series. Atascadero, Calif.: Impact Publishers, 1997.

Carter, Rosalynn, and Susan Golant. *Helping Yourself Help Others: A Book for Caregivers.* New York: Times Books, 1996.

Caruso, Ellen. *Keeping Them Healthy, Keeping Them Home: How to Care for Your Loved Ones at Home.* Los Angeles, Calif.: Health Information Press, 1998.

Dolan, J. Michael. *How to Care for Your Aging Parents... and Still Have a Life of Your Own!* Studio City, Calif.: Mulholland Pacific, 1992.

Mace, Nancy L., and Peter V. Rabins. *The 36-Hour Day: A Family Guide to Caring for Persons with Alzheimer's Disease, Related Dementing Illnesses, and Memory Loss in Later Life.* Baltimore: Johns Hopkins University Press, 1999.

Meyer, Maria M., and Paula Derr. *The Comfort of Home: An Illustrated Step-by-Step Guide for Caregivers.* Portland, Ore.: CareTrust Publications, 1998.

Visiting Nurses Association of America. *The Caregiver's Handbook.* New York: DK Publishers, 1998.

End-of-Life
Issues

From the moment each of us is born, we are dying. Yet, until circumstances force the idea upon us, death is not a fact we like to dwell on. But eventually, each and every one of us is compelled to face more than just the thought of death; sooner or later we will all confront the experience of death, as someone close to us dies and, finally, as we approach our own death.

WHAT IS DEATH?

According to the Oxford English Dictionary, "death" is defined as "the act or fact of dying, the end of life, the final cessation of the vital functions of an animal or plant or individual." But however we define it or picture it, death is an event that interweaves physical, spiritual, psychological, emotional, communal, and family experiences. The event originates with the person who is dying and emanates to all those around him, in varying ways. As such, death resembles all other rites of passage in a person's life, including birth, graduation, marriage, childbirth, the first job, and retirement. The difference is that with dying, it is the culmination of a life, the final passage, and we cannot know—at least with any certainty—just where the passage leads. And of course, the passage is irreversible.

Dying is not something that happens only to the very old, yet dying in old age corresponds to our sense of a natural order: a person lives a life, grows old, and dies. Of the 2.3 million deaths each year in this country, about 1.73 million are persons over the age of 65.

APPROACHING THE SUBJECT OF DEATH

The prospect and process of dying bring with them a host of emotional and physical challenges. The best way to deal with the feelings and fears, the logistics and obligations associated with dying is by anticipating them. However self-evident that may seem, it is certainly no easy task. Anticipating and planning for death mean raising the subject with the person who is dying.

Yet the best time to explore end-of-life care preferences and options is before someone becomes seriously ill. When conversation is begun early, long before a crisis, the person's wishes and preferences can be discussed and factored into comprehensive decision making about the final phase of life. Because people tend to get overwhelmed during the dying process—by illness, by anxiety, by denial and the hope that they'll get better—many people have trouble making decisions in such intense circumstances. In the long run, talking about dying before it becomes a real issue is the only way to ensure that the end of life has been carefully considered.

Of course, it is impossible to know what one will feel when one has a terminal diagnosis, and the best-laid plans can be meaningless when one is faced with real decisions about dying. As a result, planning and thinking about death can be helpful, but it is equally important to remain flexible and responsive to changing needs. Start by asking the person simple questions, such as: What do you fear the most? What is it that you want most in the final phase of life? Once you have the responses to these questions, share these thoughts with family and friends so that they may respond and act in accordance with the dying person's wishes if ever they are called upon to make decisions on their behalf.

TERMINAL ILLNESS: BREAKING THE NEWS

How a person receives the news that she is terminally ill and will die sets the stage both for how this individual privately confronts her mortality and how she deals with family and close friends about approaching death. Often, people suspect or know that they are dying well before doctors and nurses or family members broach the subject; in such cases, an open conversation about dying can come as a relief to the ill individual.

Generally, doctors and nurses are the ones who tell patients that they are dying. In giving such news, these professionals are taught to be direct yet compassionate, truthful, and always respectful of the patient and family. The news should be presented in language that the patient and family can understand—excessive medical jargon that cloaks the truth will only create confusion or false hope. Patient and family should be given opportunities in the hours and days following this conversation to talk with and ask questions of a knowledgeable professional—often, a nurse directly involved in the patient's care can serve this important role. Physicians and nurses sometimes prefer to tell the patient in the presence of the family, while in other cases they may talk first to the patient alone; sometimes, especially in instances where the patient is seriously ill or mentally incapacitated, they may speak first with the family and then enlist the family's help in determining when and in whose presence the patient is given the news.

Interestingly, research has shown that doctors are often uncomfortable giving bad news to patients, especially patients they know well; some doctors confess that they fear taking away all hope and so may be unrealistically optimistic when talking with patients and families about serious illness and impending death. Knowing this, patients and families can help make these conversations less difficult for everyone by encouraging their doctors to be candid about the diagnosis and prognosis and also by asking the professionals to help the family determine what might realistically be hoped for in the patients' last months or weeks.

DYING A "GOOD DEATH"

Discussions of death in America today often include the phrase a "good death," but the meaning of this phrase is not clear. What each of us means by a good death may be highly individualized. Some people want to die in their sleep, peacefully and without pain. Some insist on "death with dignity." Many say they would prefer to die suddenly without the agony of saying goodbye. The truth is that only 10% of people die suddenly. More often, especially in people over 65, death comes as a result of serious acute or prolonged illness, often with gradual organ or system failure.

Many Americans express distaste for institutional deaths and a distinct preference for dying at home, in familiar surroundings. In a *Time Magazine*-CNN poll of 1200 adults, 73% of Americans said they would prefer to die at home, while only 13% would choose to die in a hospital. When asked if their preference would change if they knew that they were going to die within six months, 80% said that they would rather die at home. Most said that they would prefer being tended to at home, with the help of professional care and medication, rather than being taken to the hospital, where conventional lifesaving interventions would be administered. While that is the wish, the truth is that fully three-quarters of Americans die in medical institutions (hospitals or nursing homes), and a third of those spend at least ten days in an intensive care unit. And despite their expressed wishes to die a painless, dignified death, many Americans are kept alive by aggressive and prolonged medical treatment, sometimes in considerable discomfort, long after the body has seemed ready to shut down.

Whatever the conditions of one's eventual dying and death, perhaps the more pertinent questions address our greatest fears and expectations about dying. Many people fear being alone, becoming dependent, dying among strangers or away from home, abandoning family or friends who need them, bankrupting the family, suffering pain, or lacking sufficient time to put things right with their loved ones or with their god. Questioning a person about her greatest fears can open the door to a deeper understanding of the experience, and indeed may help the person develop a sense of death as the natural ending to her life.

Similarly, asking a person to define what she considers a good death can prompt careful thought about how that individual might wish to guide her dying. When invited to think about how one's dying could or should be, many people will have preferences about many aspects of their dying, including type of care through their last illness, place of dying, activities to be pursued before they become too ill, events to celebrate, and people to see.

CARING FOR THE DYING PERSON'S NEEDS

If we look at dying as an isolated, unnatural event, unrelated to the life that preceded it, we will likely assume that the dying person has uncommon physical, spiritual, psychological, and emotional needs. Even if we see a person's dying as an integral part of his life's continuum, a last expression of his character, many issues arise at the end of life that the individual and his family have never before faced. These issues require a unique approach to care of the terminally ill.

The approach people take to the fact that their life is about to end differs, and reflects individual attitudes, temperaments, and tastes. When death is imminent, some people feel compelled to take charge and get on with the practical business of dying in a thoughtful and methodical fashion. They may make sure their affairs are in order and try to spend as much time as possible with loved ones. Some people throw themselves into finishing last projects. Some people deny that death is approaching and may persist in pursuing aggressive care aimed at a cure, even when medical experts say cure is not possible. Others may retreat—into depression, anger, grief, isolation from family and friends, prayer, or spiritual questioning—until they can absorb and come to terms with what is happening to them. Many people reflect on the course of their life, try to make some sense of it, and come to terms with their mistakes, accomplishments, regrets, and joys.

Feelings of loss. Dying is loss writ large: loss of control over our bodies, loss of strength and agility, loss of health, loss of independence, loss of the illusion of immortality. As the dying person begins to let go of all he knows of this world, he may experience deep grief at all that is passing.

Even as a person is dying, though, he can reinforce connections to loved ones and remain involved as much as possible in the everyday routine and the pleasures and passions of his life. This phase brings the opportunity to review life—a review that may bring a sense of satisfaction and completeness, or sadness and regret. Saying goodbye to beloved people and places, to life itself, is inevitably sorrowful. However, while sadness and grief are natural emotional responses to this phase of life, depression is not an inevitable part of dying.

Depression. It is important to differentiate between sadness and depression. Deep sadness and grieving about approaching death are natural and to be expected. Depression is a clinical condition with clinical features, including persistent sadness not easily linked to specific circumstances, lack of motivation, and problems with eating and sleeping. Depression may be, and often is, experienced by dying persons, but it is not an inevitable part of dying and need not be tolerated simply because a person is terminally ill. Depression can be treated and reversed, often with a combination of antidepressant medication and "talk therapy" with a mental health professional. If a dying person is depressed, her condition should be evaluated and addressed by a mental health professional. There are additional reasons for seeking professional advice about depression: untreated depression can interfere with the body's ability to benefit from pain medications, and certain antidepressant medications actually help to relieve pain.

Anxiety. A person who is dying will naturally feel anxious at times. Despite literature that maps the stages of dying, each person's experience is unique, and it is little wonder that dying is fraught with fear and anxiety. Anxiety can make pain worse, and, conversely, when people are in pain, they often feel anxious.

In most cases, anxiety can be handled by discussing the person's fears and expectations early in the dying process. Some anxiety may stem from concern that things will be left undone after death. Helping the person sort through and put his affairs in order can soothe much of the uneasiness. In addition, some apprehension fades away as the dying person comes to trust the people involved in his care. To this end, establishing a strong and reliable therapeutic alliance with health care providers goes a long way. Therefore, as early as possible in the person's illness, before things progress too far, discuss with your loved one his fears, wishes, and expectations. What are the dying person's greatest fears? How does he want the dying process managed? What should be the doctor's role? The nurse's role? The social worker's role? The chaplain or minister's role? The family's role? Then ask what it is that the person wants at this point in his life.

Sometimes, just encouraging a dying person to talk through his fears can ease anxiety. Such a conversation can also guide family members and health care professionals as they try to respond to the various situations that arise during this time. And while not all wishes can be accomplished, and some may change along the way, having a candid and compassionate conversation about the person's wishes, fears, and expectations can go a long way toward easing his anxiety.

For family and friends as well as for the dying person, when emotional distress gets in the way of tending to the business of dying, it may be a good idea to talk with a mental health professional (who can arrange for appropriate medication) or to talk with a bereavement counselor. Persons who maintain reasonable emotional balance can better attend to the deeper issues involved in dying and in the care of someone who is dying.

THE STAGES OF DYING

In most cases, it is hard to know with any certainty that someone is dying and when precisely the death will occur. Despite the person having received from a physician a terminal diagnosis and a likely time frame for dying, the course and rapidity of the dying process will still likely be unpredictable.

Even when death is imminent, it is sometimes hard to know this, because the appearance of dying is different in different people and varies also with different illnesses and conditions. There are a host of diseases that can cause a sudden decline and take a person quickly, such as a sudden heart attack or massive stroke. Caregivers and loved ones can be caught off guard by such a rapid decline. On the other hand, in older people with long-term chronic illnesses, it is often not possible to know for sure that they are dying. A person may look well one day, then awful the next. This is typical of the end stages of diseases such as lung disease and congestive heart failure.

Although changes in the way a person functions can occur abruptly or they may be gradual, there may be certain telltale signs to alert others that a person is nearing death. It may be that family members or friends involved in direct care of the dying person, and thus very familiar with that person's behavior and bodily habits, will note small but significant changes that a visiting health professional may miss.

Although there is a lot of variability in the death process, there are some specific symptoms that indicate pending death. For example, many people may withdraw from the world and the people around them when death is imminent. For some, spiritual concerns become more central. Other changes common to the final stages of life are described below.

Physical changes. As death draws closer, the dying person's blood pressure may drop and the body temperature may fluctuate between fever and chills. Skin color may shift with temperature changes, ranging from flushed to bluish to a yellowish pallor, outward signs of the dramatic changes occurring internally. Breathing changes also signal the approach of death—usually breathing becomes progressively slower and irregular, and there can be times when breathing seems to stop altogether, for up to a minute. Paradoxically, toward the very end of life, some people experience a surge of energy and speak very clearly even if they had previously been disoriented or apparently unconscious.

Some people nearing the end of life will spend a lot of time with their eyes closed or asleep, and may even enter a coma-like state or experience extreme drowsiness. Despite this drowsiness, it is likely dying people can hear all that is being said around them.

Mental changes. At the very end of life, many patients will experience a change in their mental state, which has been called terminal delirium. Patients with terminal delirium may be confused, disoriented, picking, restless, or talking to or seeing people who are not there. In severe cases they may become very agitated: trying to get out of bed, shouting, or even hitting caregivers. These symptoms may be caused by many things, including medications, kidney or liver failure, cancer that has spread (metastasized) to the brain, electrolyte disturbances, and lack of oxygen. Agitation can be caused or worsened by pain and anxiety. When a terminally ill patient suddenly becomes delirious, it is important to determine if there are any reversible causes for this condition. If this change in condition coincides with addition of a new medication, it is wise to stop that medication. If brain swelling from metastatic cancer is present, steroids may reduce the swelling and improve mental functioning. Some electrolyte imbalances (high calcium or low sodium, for example) can be corrected, and this will occasionally improve the delirium. Many times, however, terminal delirium is caused by the irreversible changes of the dying process.

Even when the delirium cannot be reversed there are many ways to help calm the patient. If the patient is in pain, this should be treated. Keeping the patient in a quiet place, reducing stimulation by limiting visitors, talking in a low, soothing voice, and keeping a calm atmosphere around the person can help. Frequently, delirious patients will need medications such as Haldol or Ativan to keep them relaxed and calm. Severely agitated patients, especially those who are acting in ways dangerous to themselves or others, may need to be heavily sedated.

Disease-related changes. Many of the changes involved in dying, while not inevitable, correspond to individual disease processes. Labored breathing is usually a symptom of lung diseases like emphysema, and becomes more pronounced as the disease gets worse. People dying of cancer typically experience increasing pain as the illness progresses. Cancer and cancer treatments frequently alter digestive patterns and appetite. Digestive changes can occur at the end stage of a number of other diseases as the body shuts down. With cancer, for example, the malignancy leads to a form of bodily wasting called cachexia. As a result, the patient loses her appetite, experiences significant weight loss and muscle atrophy, and begins to look as if she is wasting away. While in the early stages of cancer, when a person is going through chemotherapy, it might be important to boost her appetite; at the end stage, this is seldom necessary.

Loss of appetite. Some persons become unwilling or unable to eat and drink in their last days, when the body has a dramatically decreased need for physical sustenance. While refusing liquids can cause dehydration, studies show that when a person resists or altogether stops consuming food and drink, brain chemicals called endorphins are released, which serve a soothing function.

Many patients lose the ability to swallow as they near death and have no taste for foods they formerly loved. In addition, force-feeding may cause the person to gag. There are no indications that good nutrition serves any real purpose at the very end of life; it neither enhances the quality nor prolongs the length of life. Yet, in part because of the enormous symbolic value of food in human social relations and family life, family members may still feel the need to feed their loved one. It is very difficult to accept that it is natural for a dying person to stop eating. No understanding of disease processes will help families feel good about this shift, but it is important to respect the wishes of the terminally ill patient who no longer feels a need for or can no longer tolerate physical nourishment.

MANAGING PAIN

Dying does not necessarily mean lying in bed, awaiting death. But in order to continue to participate as fully as possible in life, a person must be sufficiently pain- and symptom-free to move around, to stay involved with family and friends, and, possibly, even to work.

And it is indeed possible to manage pain well. A painful death no longer needs to be the norm. For a detailed discussion of the advances in managing pain, medications and treatment for pain, and suggestions for caregivers, please see the Pain Management chapter on p. 709.

Yet at the very end of life, managing pain takes on a different intent. On occasion, especially at the very end of life or when pain is very intense, pain cannot be controlled without sedating the patient. Stimulating drugs, such as Ritalin, can sometimes help the patient stay awake while taking high doses of pain medications. Sometimes less sedating medications can be used in place of more sedating medications. However, if this doesn't work, the physician, family, and patient must balance the need for pain control with the patient's desire to stay alert. Some patients may prefer to have more pain and be more alert, while others may be willing to be sleepy or confused rather than be in severe pain.

Another fear that patients and families have is that pain medication will make the patient so groggy all the time that she will not be able to enjoy life. They may even fear that pain medication will hasten the patient's death. While initially pain medications may make some patients very sleepy, when used correctly this side effect will soon diminish. Most patients will be able to experience good pain control and still be alert. Moreover, strong pain medications have never been shown to shorten life. In fact, using effective pain medication tends to prolong as well as improve the quality of life. If pain is eased, a person might be able to get out of bed, move around, and perhaps even exercise. Even the smallest amount of physical activity will translate into better appetite and healthier digestion. There is no question that when pain is controlled, a person can stay more involved in her life, work, and relationships.

On the other hand, when a person is old and ill, the systemic effects of any narcotic can be intensified. In some instances, strong pain medications can cause confusion or make the person groggy. Depending on the intensity, some people may find the pain more tolerable than the sleepiness and confusion. However, when medication is carefully monitored or when the patient can control the dosage in response to varying levels of pain, adverse effects of the drug can be held to a minimum. Also with time and continued use, many of the side effects of narcotics diminish.

Palliative care. As a rule, the type of medical care offered at the end of life is palliative care. The word "palliative" comes from the Latin word *pallis*, meaning cloak or cover. Palliative care seeks to cover the discomfort as people are dying, to envelop and protect their humanity. Clinically speaking, palliative care is a type of care that attempts to relieve or alleviate symptoms and suffering, rather than to cure the underlying causes of the patient's symptoms.

Therefore, the type of care typically administered at the end of life attends to more than medical issues. Controlling a person's physical symptoms is essential but only a small part of end-of-life care. When you are caring for people who are dying, time—or lack of it—is at issue. The end of the work of palliative care is in sight at the moment it begins. When palliative care works at its best, it helps to make the dying person sufficiently comfortable, physically and emotionally, so that he or she may focus on whatever issues are most important—physical, emotional, spiritual, familial. Pain, anxiety, and distress are managed in a way that the person can continue to live, to connect with people and things that still matter, and to undertake the awesome business of dying. "Only now do I realize what was really important in life," dying persons commonly say. And indeed the person who has this kind of epiphany at this point in his life is truly lucky.

Hospice care. Hospice is a specialized approach to compassionate end-of-life care, intended to provide comfort and care to patients who have fewer than six months to live. Hospice services are the most common resource for supporting patients and families in the home. At the heart of hospice philosophy is the conviction that each person is entitled to die with dignity, free of pain. The spirit of hospice care is to offer community and comfort, a place to go, a place to belong, all the while ministering to the person's fear, anxiety, exhaustion, pain, loneliness, and estrangement. To this end, hospice care is based on a multidisciplinary approach to care that embraces emotional, spiritual, and family support as well as symptom management. A multidisciplinary hospice team shapes treatment around the patient's particular needs and wishes, and around the needs and wishes of the family.

Indeed, hospice services aim to care, not to cure. In fact, people who utilize hospice care are usually asked to waive their rights to curative treatments relating to the terminal illness. However, if other conditions arise, causing discomfort or significant complications, such as an infection or a broken leg, these will be treated. For reimbursement purposes, hospice care is also limited in scope, with persons eligible only if they are expected to die within six months.

Although hospice care can be provided in special residences, nursing homes, and hospitals, in most cases, care occurs in the home, typically anchored by the family caregivers. Hospice workers oversee the care and seek to provide the expertise and support by which families are able to provide front-line care. Typically, in a hospice setting:

- physicians oversee the medical care and medications;
- nurses visit regularly to monitor the patient's condition;
- home health aides provide more practical help with daily tasks;
- volunteers take care of light housekeeping tasks and errands;
- counselors and chaplains offer spiritual and emotional counseling.

767

Hospice care offers a means to obtain medical equipment and supplies as well as medications to control symptoms and relieve pain. In addition, many hospice organizations offer physical, speech, and occupational therapy to bolster functioning.

There is no mistaking the tremendous physical, emotional, and spiritual effort required of the family caregivers, and for this reason strong volunteer support for the family as well as for the patient is a critical part of the hospice philosophy.

Finally, hospice organizations offer bereavement counseling, support groups, and follow-up sessions for family and other caregivers for one year after death.

WHERE TO DIE

Even though most persons who die in the United States do so in hospitals or nursing homes, it is often possible for a person to live out his days and die at home. Whether dying is best done at home, with one's family, or in a hospital or nursing facility where the dying person can be attended by health professionals, depends on the home environment:

- What resources are available at home?
- What is the physical setup?
- Are there a bedroom and a bathroom that would be convenient for both the person and the rest of the family?
- What support services are available in the home community?
- What can the family afford financially?
- What does the medical team overseeing the patient's illness suggest?
- What would the patient prefer?
- What is the family structure?
- Who is available, and when, to provide care?

CARING FOR THE CAREGIVER

It should come as no surprise that people who take care of a loved one with substantial care needs are at higher risk for depression and other health problems than people who care for a loved one with low care needs. In fact, caregivers are twice as likely to experience depression as the person who is dying. Whether you're caring for a dying spouse, parent, sibling, or friend, all sorts of feelings get stirred up.

In addition, the burden of caring for another adult brings with it a higher risk for isolation, fatigue, and feelings of being trapped and overwhelmed. Caregiving responsibilities can interfere with other family relationships as well as with work and income.

Hospice, respite care, and volunteer support can provide much-needed breaks for caregivers, but the work of attending to the dying brings many challenges. It is essential that family members and caregivers distinguish between their needs and those of the person leaving this world. As you tend to a dying person, it is critically important that you remind yourself, however consumed you are in tending to your loved one, that it is not you who is dying. It can feel as though a large part of you is dying, but remember that while your loved one will pass on, you will remain behind. Try to maintain some sense of yourself and your needs during this time, even though it may well be necessary to put your loved one's needs first. His needs are the greatest and the most pressing, but this is true only for a while. Once the person has passed on, you will grieve over the loss, but at the same time, you will need to tend to your own very real and important needs. Eventually your grief will subside and you will need to move on.

There are things you as a caregiver can do to take care of yourself:

- Give thought to what you can and cannot do for your loved one. Remember: You cannot save her or stop the dying process.
- While you may need to put your own feelings and needs on the back burner for a while, resist the temptation to ignore your needs altogether.
- Reach out for help. When people offer to help, let them. Ask them to do specific tasks, such as providing a meal, cleaning your house, doing the grocery shopping, or visiting with your loved one.
- Find time to stay involved with the people and activities that give you joy.
- Steer clear of people who make you feel guilty or make you feel that you are not compassionate or patient enough.

Keep in mind that your task is enormous. You are dealing with your own feelings of loss, anger, and grief, as well as taking care of a dying person who may be in pain and frightened. This is a tall order. Remember to cut yourself some slack; be easy on yourself.

There are a number of support groups for family caregivers offered, for example, by hospice organizations, community hospitals, and specific organizations such as the Alzheimer's Association or the American Cancer Society. If religion or faith plays a part in your life, reach out to your community or spiritual leader for solace and support.

SUPPORT RESOURCES

By the end of life, most patients will be bed-bound and require someone with them all the time. The job of the hospice staff is to relieve the patient's pain and other symptoms, and to provide emotional and spiritual support for patient and family. But it is the family caregivers who are there twenty-four hours a day, seven days a week, feeding the person, helping with toileting and dressing, and giving medications. When possible, caregiver stress can be lessened by having other family members or friends share the burden by working in shifts and regularly relieving one another. Volunteers from the neighborhood, churches, or other community agencies can sometimes supplement hospice volunteers. If the financial resources are available, the family can hire caregivers for part or all of the day (but this is very expensive).

RESPITE CARE

Very often, family caregivers need temporary emotional and physical relief from their responsibilities. Respite care provides the opportunity to place a loved one in a hospital or nursing home for brief stays or provides alternative caregivers who take over the home care while the primary caregivers take some time off. Respite care can be especially welcomed when caregivers are at risk for extreme fatigue or burnout, due to the length or to the stressfulness of care. Taking a break from the physical and emotional burdens of caregiving can be an absolute necessity.

In addition, just because a loved one is dying does not mean that life stops. Other emergencies or needs within the family can and do present themselves and may require emotional energy and resources that are already being spent elsewhere. For these and other reasons, respite care can offer a physically and spiritually renewing break for people ministering to a dying loved one. Respite care is covered by the hospice benefits and can be requested through hospice agencies.

SAYING GOODBYE

It is never easy to say goodbye, in any situation, so it comes as little surprise that saying goodbye to someone who is dying can be emotionally wrenching. In addition to a natural reluctance, our ability to say goodbye is usually colored by the nature and quality of our relationship with that person. Nevertheless, it is important to find a way of bidding farewell. Studies show that family members and friends are able to experience greater closure and perhaps internal peace over time if they have said "goodbye."

In his book *Dying Well*, hospice physician Ira Byock identifies five steps in saying goodbye to a person who is dying:

1. I forgive you. It is often tempting, as a person struggles with illness and slips away, to idealize him. But in reality, it is impossible to live a full life without regrets. Nor is it possible to be a parent or a spouse without feeling some remorse about things done within relationships. Everyone is unkind from time to time; everyone is selfish or neglectful; all people cause pain, sometimes intentionally, mostly unintentionally. At some point in the dying process, it is important to forgive the dying person for his mistakes and any pain caused, and to absolve him; to say, in essence, Whatever you did to me is not important. I forgive you.

2. Please forgive me. It is also inevitable that a dying person's loved ones—children, spouse, siblings, friends—will have regrets about the way they behaved in the relationship. For this reason, ask the dying person for her forgiveness.

3. I'm going to be okay. Death is part of the natural order of things. Living on after a loved one dies is also part of the natural order. Yet, the dying person may be hesitant to let go because he fears that the people left behind will get stuck, stumble, and be unable to go on. By assuring your loved one that you'll be okay, you release him, allowing him to let go, knowing that while you will miss him and feel sorrow and grief, you will be able to move on in your own life.

4. I love you. In some way, you must find expression for the human connection between the two of you. Even in cultures where the words are not said, there are ways of expressing your love to the dying person. Sit with the person. Hold her hand. Stroke her face. Sing. Tell stories. Read to her. Say the words "I love you" out loud.

5. Goodbye. In the end, it's essential that you say goodbye in order to bring closure to your relationship. Odd as it may seem, many dying persons hold on until they receive permission to let go. As the person who will be left behind, it will be easier for you to let go if you say goodbye and thus bless the dying person's passage.

LEGAL CONSIDERATIONS

In legal matters related to death and dying, as with emotional and physical matters, the best way to avoid being knocked off-center is to anticipate as much as you can and to take methodical steps to address issues and problems.

HEALTH DIRECTIVES

It used to be that when a person was dying, there was little to do but let nature take its course. Today, nature's course is not always clear. In the last fifty years, technology has changed the face of death and altered the course of dying. Thanks to sophisticated surgeries, powerful pharmaceuticals, dialysis, defibrillation, feeding tubes, and ventilators, the loss of vital organ function does not necessarily mean the person will die. Many patients and families have benefited greatly from these technologies, and yet they can bring great suffering when used to prolong life despite the inevitability of death.

Indeed, while medical technology can extend life, it can also prolong dying. If a person is taken to the hospital for a medical emergency, the medical staff is obligated to begin resuscitative measures and continue treatment until the patient's wishes can be determined. This may mean waiting to contact a family member or other individual with a close relationship to the patient. Once a medical emergency occurs and a loved one is taken to the hospital, it may be too late for that person or the family to make thoughtful, well-considered choices. This can add to the family's pain, uncertainty, and guilt. When the attending physician believes that life-sustaining methods are of little use, she will consult with the family, other health care professionals, and perhaps an ethics specialist. In all instances, the patient or family should have some say concerning the nature and extent of treatment.

In the best of all possible situations, the patient and the family will have long ago anticipated and discussed the possibility that a medical crisis might occur, and have arranged to have their agreed-upon wishes appropriately noted. Some persons formally designate a surrogate decision maker, who will be responsible for making medical decisions if the patient is incapacitated; appropriately appointed, a surrogate decision maker, for instance, has the legal authority to stop aggressive medical interventions. Some persons write out their general or specific preferences, deciding certain things beforehand, and thus sparing family members the need to decide whether or not to use aggressive measures to sustain life. Families who have the courage and the foresight to designate surrogates and draw up advance directives may sidestep unnecessary problems and pain at the end of a loved one's life.

"Do Not Resuscitate" and "Do Not Intubate" orders. A "DNR" (Do Not Resuscitate) order is a physician's written instruction forbidding the use of CPR in the event a patient's heart or lungs fail. A "DNI" (Do Not Intubate) order is similar, prohibiting use of an endotracheal tube in a patient's airway if the patient should stop breathing. These orders require the informed consent of the patient or of the person who holds medical power of attorney and is the patient's designated surrogate decision maker.

Advance directives. In 1967, an organization called Choice In Dying crafted a document that allowed a person to delineate her wishes for end-of-life care. It specifically addressed when life-sustaining interventions should be started or continued and when they should be stopped, and was intended to be used when the person was incapable of participating in her own health care decision making. In 1976, the parents of Karen Ann Quinlan fought in the courts to disconnect their daughter, who had lain for months in a coma, from a respirator. This very public case gave new urgency to the need for people to prepare clearly defined health care directives.

When asked, many people state that they want control at the end of their lives. While some people do not want to be subjected unnecessarily to life-sustaining procedures and equipment, other people want their health care team to try every possible intervention to sustain life. Despite many people's strong preferences about end-of-life care, only 30 percent to 35 percent of Americans actually write out advance directives.

There are two kinds of advance directives:

• A living will. This is a legal document that details what kind of treatment is desired or acceptable if a person becomes so ill that recovery is unlikely. Laws governing living wills vary by state. Some states require that for a living will to be legally binding, it must follow a particular form. Other states honor a person's directive, no

FIVE WISHES

In 1997, the Florida Commission on Aging With Dignity drew up a type of living will called "Five Wishes." Five Wishes uses straightforward language to guide conversations about end-of-life issues, including durable power of attorney for health care and other significant care instructions. Considered legally binding in thirty-four states, this format can also be useful for people in the other sixteen states; however, once residents of those sixteen states are ready to write up the directive, they need to follow the form mandated by their state. The five wishes are:

• Who do I want to make care decisions for me when I can't?

• What kind of medical treatment do I want at the end of my life?
• How comfortable do I want to be and what kinds of measures would be acceptable to ensure that level of comfort?
• How do I want people to treat me?
• What do I want my loved ones to know?

You can obtain a copy of Five Wishes, written in simple, straightforward language, in either English or Spanish, by sending $5, check or money order, to Aging With Dignity, P.O. Box 1661, Tallahassee, FL 32302, or visit their Web site (www.agingwithdignity.org).

matter the form. In some states, a living will cannot take effect until one or more physicians declare that the patient is terminally ill and expected to die within six months. Rarely is a living will sufficient on its own, primarily because medical circumstances and needs change. Also, it is next to impossible to anticipate all the contingencies that future medical emergencies could bring. A living will works best when a health care proxy or surrogate decision maker has also been named.

• Durable health care power of attorney. This is a legal instrument that empowers someone to make health-related decisions when an individual can no longer speak for himself. This decision maker is called a surrogate, attorney-in-fact, or health care proxy. Typically, a person names someone she trusts to explore options and make thoughtful decisions that are within the spirit of her wishes. Naming a surrogate is especially important when a family is fractured or when there is no spouse or significant other.

Some people begin to think about an advance directive only when their doctor introduces the subject. Other people draw up an advance directive at the time they draw up their will. Your attorney, the state department of health, or the admitting office in the hospital can tell you if your state requires a special form. It is essential, once an advance directive is drawn up, that it be located easily when needed. Therefore, be sure that there are multiple copies of the document, and that the doctor, hospital, and surrogate all have copies.

You can register a living will and durable power of attorney through an organization called U.S. Living Will Registry. This free, nationwide registry stores the advance directive electronically and makes it available by telephone and/or fax twenty-four hours a day to hospitals throughout the country. By limiting access to hospitals, this service promises privacy and confidentiality. The American Bar Association, the AARP, and the American Medical Association also offer guidance on preparing advance directives.

Organ donation. If your loved one dies in a hospital setting, you may want to consider donating his organs. Many people sign their driver's licenses or other documents indicating their desire to be an organ donor, but physicians will not honor these requests unless endorsed by the family. Thus it is essential that you share your desire to be an organ donor with your family, and ask them to agree to honor your wishes. In some states, the medical team attending a dying person must ask if families want to donate their loved one's organs or tissue. In other states, the family must broach the issue with the health care team. However, the knowledge that a heart, liver, or kidney can save a life, that a cornea will help another person see, and that a skin graft can help a burn patient heal often gives a person and the family a sense of comfort in the knowledge that they will ease the suffering of another family.

Anatomic gift. Many medical schools are perennially in need of cadavers for research and teaching purposes. Generally speaking, though, they welcome only whole-body donations, that is, bodies that have not been autopsied and from which no organs have been removed. There may also be other requirements for donation of bodies for the teaching of anatomy (for instance, a body may not be excessively emaciated). Generally, if a body is accepted for medical research or education, the remains are cremated following use and, if the family so desires, the ashes are returned to the family for burial. If you or a loved one is interested in pursuing this possibility, you may contact the nearest medical school for information or call the National Anatomical Service toll-free at 800-727-0700.

Autopsy. In most hospitals, when a person dies, the family will be asked if they would like to have an autopsy performed. Autopsy, which involves the internal examination of the body and its organs by trained medical pathologists, can be especially informative if the specific cause of death is unclear or if there are questions about conditions the patient had that may also affect other family members. Also, even though medicine has sophisticated diagnostic testing and imaging technologies, autopsy can be a powerful educational tool for physicians and medical students, answering important questions postmortem about a patient's condition, course of illness, and response to treatment. The autopsy is usually conducted within hours of death, with the results compiled and provided to the family within a few weeks. Neither families nor insurance companies are billed for autopsies—hospitals pay these costs. Following autopsy, the body is closed and then transported to the funeral service of the family's choice for preparation for burial. Autopsy does not delay funeral planning nor does it render the appearance of the body unfit for viewing. However, autopsy does render a body unfit for donation for purposes of medical research or education.

Assisted suicide. The issue of physician-assisted suicide or euthanasia is tremendously controversial. At this time, in the United States, assisted suicide is legal only in Oregon, and there only in accord with very stringent guidelines.

There is a vital difference between what is allowed by law in most states—that is, withdrawing life support or life-sustaining treatment, including food and water—and actively ending life. Most physicians will terminate life-sustaining measures when the patient and the family have made a clear and direct request, usually in the form of an advance directive. Few doctors will knowingly provide medications by which the patient can intentionally end his life. In short, while the patient or surrogate can request that life support be withheld or discontinued, when anyone actively takes a hand in directly ending someone's life or in assisting someone to commit suicide, he or she can be charged with homicide.

WILLS AND ESTATE PLANNING

By taking care of legal and financial considerations early on, you may be able to avoid discord in the family after death. When wills and estate plans are well thought out and detailed, a dying person can attend to other, more important matters without worrying that she is leaving a mess behind. All valuable items in a person's estate—whether they have financial or emotional worth—should be included in the overall legacy. Beneficiaries—people and organizations to whom the dying person wishes to leave property—should be clearly designated, and distribution plans should be spelled out. If at all possible, the terms of the will should be discussed with all concerned when it is being drawn up. Otherwise, surprises after death can fan sibling and family squabbles and either obscure or amplify the real emotional impact of the loss. On the other hand, if the family is able to talk openly about the will before a final illness sets in, it may lead to constructive negotiations and healing family discussions and avert later conflict.

FINANCIAL CONSIDERATIONS

THE COST OF DYING

The cost of dying in the United States varies greatly, depending on a range of factors. First and foremost, the bottom line will be shaped by time and location—where end-of-life care is administered, and for how long. The bill can run anywhere from $100 per day for hospice care (which may be covered by Medicare, Medicaid, and private insurance, with the exception of small copays and some drug charges) to well beyond $1000 per day in a hospital. People 65 and older, as well as people suffering from end-stage renal disease or certain disabilities, are generally eligible for Medicare.

Paying for end-of-life care is often done through a complex patchwork of public and private funding. Just who pays for what, and how much each payer pays, is based on the patient's age, income, diagnosis, and where the care is administered. Medicare and Medicaid pick up the bulk of most acute medical care, including hospitalization, symptom management, doctor and nurse costs. However, nonhospice care that does not require the direct involvement of a doctor tends to fall between the cracks. For example, when a person chooses to remain in the home, coverage can be a bit spotty and peculiar, and often must be paid for out of pocket. Medication administered and monitored at home, visiting nurses, home health aides, and help with activities of daily living are generally not covered, unless the patient and family have been signed onto a hospice benefit with Medicare, Medicaid, or a private insurance company.

Typically, if a person is eligible, regular Medicare will cover approximately 50% of the cost of direct medical care. Regular Medicaid will pay for another 15%. The patient is responsible for the remaining amount. Many people rely on private insurance to pick up a small percentage of the costs. Some charitable organizations will also pick up a small percentage of the costs. By signing onto the Medicare, Medicaid, or private insurance hospice benefit, patients and families receive 100% coverage for durable medical equipment, medications, and home visitation by nurses, social workers, chaplains, physical therapists, and physicians.

MEDICARE

Medicare is a federal insurance program designed to cover health care services for people age 65 and older. In some cases, people with disabilities and end-stage kidney disease can also tap Medicare to cover a percentage of medical costs. Patients who use Medicare are responsible for a deductible and copayment. Medicare is divided into two sections.

- Medicare Part A is the hospital insurance. It covers inpatient care in hospitals, skilled nursing facility care, hospice, and some home health care.
- Medicare Part B is an optional rider that covers outpatient doctor fees, tests, and other outpatient medical services. People enroll in this type of coverage through the local Social Security office.
- Medicare does not cover most outpatient medication, long-term nonacute care, and support services.
- Medicare, most private health insurance plans, and Medicaid (in forty-four states) cover the cost of hospice care for patients who meet eligibility criteria. Patients may be responsible for small copays and prescription drug charges. Coverage is guaranteed by the Medicare Hospice Benefit, a

special funding mechanism designed to meet the needs of terminally ill patients. It includes support and services not otherwise covered under other policies or plans.

MEDICAID

Medicaid is a program supported by both state and federal funds that covers health care services for low-income patients. Eligibility, means tests, and benefits vary from state to state.

PRIVATE INSURANCE

Many people use their private insurance policies to bridge the gaps left by Medicare. Some private policies cover Medicare deductibles and copayments, as well as other health care services, medical supplies, and outpatient medications.

LONG-TERM CARE INSURANCE

Almost half of all people over age 65 will need long-term health care at home or in a nursing facility. However, Medicare generally does not provide extensive coverage for long-term health care. For this, people can purchase private long-term care insurance. This may be especially important for people who have large assets that they do not wish to see consumed at a nursing facility or by comprehensive home care. Such insurance pays for skilled nursing care and nonmedical services, such as home health aides. Depending on the age and extent of coverage, the cost of this type of insurance can range from $500 to more than $8000 a year. People with pre-existing conditions such as Alzheimer's disease or diabetes may not be able to purchase such a policy.

MAKING ARRANGEMENTS AFTER DEATH

The best way to deal with the reality of death is to know what to anticipate. If the person is expected to die at home, ask the physician or nurse or hospice worker to explain in some detail what you should expect. The more informed you are, the more you will be able to stay calm and be present and supportive during your loved one's last hours and passing.

The adage "Don't just do something, stand there" can apply to the first moments after death. Right after death, do nothing. If you can, look upon the face of your loved one. There is nothing ugly or spooky about your loved one's body. In fact, death usually brings a countenance of peace to the earthly body. Spend time with the body. Look at it, touch it; some people kiss the person goodbye after death or bathe the body one last time.

People of faith or from certain cultures find guidance and comfort in their heritage and traditions. For some, a prayer ritual helps them in the transition. For others, an elaborate ritual process of washing the body allows them to acknowledge the departure of the person's spirit from the body and moves them into mourning.

If you need to call someone, do. If family members, friends, a member of the clergy, or hospice workers are not already present, you may wish to summon them. Laws about who can pronounce a person dead vary from state to state. If you are receiving support from a hospice program, they can tell you whom to call when your loved one dies. If hospice is not involved with your loved one's care, you can call your local hospital, physician, or the hospice program for information about the laws in your state.

If the death of your loved one was expected, and if you are certain that he or she really is dead, you should be aware that if you call 911 or the emergency squad, the body will be transported to the local emergency room. There, unless an advance health care directive is available instructing otherwise, or if a DNR/DNI order has not been written by a physician and made available to the hospital staff, efforts at resuscitation will be made before your loved one is declared legally dead. At the hospital, grieving family members may find their privacy breached or they may feel shut out, as emergency room staff goes about their work. In short, be advised that a hospital emergency room is not a serene place in which to have a loved one declared dead or to begin your grieving process.

DOCUMENTING DEATH

Most paperwork following a death can be taken care of relatively quickly. You have approximately forty-eight hours to place the death notice in the newspaper; most newspapers regularly list telephone numbers and addresses for filing death notices, and many now accept death notices and obituaries submitted via fax. If the deceased person was a Social Security beneficiary, you must promptly notify the Social Security Administration of her death by calling 1-800-772-1213. Do not cash or deposit any checks sent to the beneficiary for the month in which the death occurred or the months following; all such checks must be returned to Social Security.

The death certificate. A death certificate listing the time and cause of the person's death must be signed by a doctor—usually the attending physician—and filed with the proper legal authorities. You can expect your funeral director to handle these important details. If you are the administrator of your loved one's estate, you are likely to need up to ten certified copies of the death certificate for insurance, banking, and Social Security purposes. You should be able to obtain these copies from the funeral director, your local health department, or, later, your state's department of vital statistics. Precise requirements and costs vary from state to state.

The obituary. Writing the obituary can be the last way to give public voice to your loved one. It is a way of presenting one last image of the deceased person to the world. But how do you encapsulate a life in a few paragraphs? An obituary can be just a name and some factual biographical details or it can be an elaborate word portrait of the person and her life. Some obituaries reflect the person, while some reflect the family's wishes—what they want the world to see. Consider drafting the obituary beforehand. Perhaps your loved one will want a hand in preparing it. There is nothing morbid in writing the obituary before death. Instead, it offers an opportunity to review and celebrate a life, and possibly with your loved one.

PLANNING THE FUNERAL OR MEMORIAL SERVICE

When someone in our society dies, we customarily observe this landmark event by holding a ritual ceremony—a funeral, which focuses on the passing of the individual from this life; a memorial service, which celebrates the life of the deceased person; and a burial or disposition of ashes, which commits the deceased person's remains (body or ashes from cremation) to the ground or elements.

Planning any event that marks a significant life transition involves juggling all sorts of details. Like weddings, funerals, memorial services, and burials can be tremendously expensive, and the choices overwhelming. There are many factors that shape a funeral or memorial service, including religious and community considerations, cultural customs, location, personal experience, and family tradition. There are innumerable decisions to make and factors to consider:

- What kind of funeral or memorial service? Simple or elaborate? Public or private? Religious or nonreligious?
- Which funeral home?
- To bury, cremate, or donate the body to science?
- Does the family wish religious or cultural rituals that prepare the body for burial?
- Will there be a wake (a vigil for the deceased, with or without the body present)?
- Will the body be present at the funeral?
- Will there be viewing of the body or visitation? An open or closed casket?
- Which cemetery for burial of the body or ashes?
- What are the local laws governing funerals and burials?
- How much will everything cost?
- Will there be a reception following the funeral, memorial service, or burial at which the family will receive friends and relatives?

Despite all the planning a funeral or memorial service requires, people tend to avoid talking about dying, and few families have prepared themselves beforehand to make such decisions when the time comes. Clearly, in the long run, early planning can ensure that you have the opportunity to weigh your options, that the final ritual is celebratory, loving, and perhaps less hectic—and the costs can be curbed. Some people plan their own funerals or memorial services in advance and stipulate every last detail—including where the service will be held, whether to be cremated or interred, who will give the eulogy, the kinds of flowers and casket, and who will prepare the meal or host the reception afterward, if there is to be such a gathering.

Get to know the chaplain at the hospital or discuss the family's wishes with your minister, priest, rabbi, or religious leader. They can help you sort through a number of family and religious considerations. A member of the clergy or director of the funeral home can guide you on issues such as who will officiate at a service, who should speak, and whether ceremonies will be held in a church, a funeral home chapel, and/or at the burial site. They may also help you navigate any special family issues that arise with extended family, reconstituted families, former spouses, stepchildren, religious differences, and the like.

According to government figures, every year Americans arrange more than 2 million funerals and spend billions of dollars. In fact, a funeral can be one of the most expensive purchases a person will make. According to the National Funeral Directors Association 2001 General Price List survey, the average cost for an adult funeral is $5180. Plans and costs vary widely, however, so check specific costs and charges with the funeral home you choose to work with.

One last word on planning a funeral. It is never easy to find words to express feelings about a loved one who has died. Consequently, many people try to express themselves in these last acts. However public or elaborate a funeral may be, it can never communicate fully the truth and depth of your feelings or your relationship with the deceased. Nor will the amount of money you spend on a funeral be an accurate or sufficient representation of your affection and sense of loss.

CHOOSING A FUNERAL HOME

While there is no law that says you have to use a funeral home to plan and conduct a funeral, most people find that using one makes this difficult time a bit easier. Generally, people rely on a funeral home or cemetery that is nearby, is affiliated with a church or synagogue, has served family members in the past, or comes recommended by someone close to the family.

Most funeral homes offer a number of packages, and prices for these packages depend on the extent of services. When comparing prices, look at the entire package including general services and all specific items, including caskets, outer burial containers, and other items. Please note that you do not have to buy the entire package. Instead, it is your right to pick and choose. According to the federal Funeral Rule, which is enforced by the Federal Trade Commission (FTC):

- You have the right to choose the funeral goods and services you want (with some exceptions).
- The funeral provider must state this right in writing on the general price list.
- If state or local law requires you to buy any particular item, the funeral provider must disclose it on the price list, with a reference to the specific law.
- The funeral provider may not refuse, or charge a fee, to handle a casket you bought elsewhere.
- A funeral provider that offers cremations must make alternative containers available.

(The funeral industry is heavily regulated. If you have serious complaints against a funeral home, you can contact the FTC. If you have a complaint against a cemetery, contact the North American Cemetery Regulators Association or the International Cemetery and Funeral Association. [See the Additional Resources section at the end of this chapter.])

Preneed planning

More and more, people are making funeral arrangements for their loved ones and for themselves in advance. Funeral planning thus becomes an extension of will and estate planning. Preneed planning, making arrangements before there is an actual need, allows consumers to compare prices and services so that when the time comes, the funeral is a less stressful and more meaningful experience for all involved.

Given enough time, you can start by contacting a funeral planning or memorial society, a nonprofit clearinghouse that offers information about funerals. Or you can visit or call more than one funeral service provider and one or more cemeteries. If you intend to have the body cremated, you will have to decide whether to keep the ashes, where to inter them, or where to have them scattered.

Prepaying

In many cases, funeral and burial arrangements can be made in advance but paid for later. You and your family will have to weigh the advantages and disadvantages of this, since prices can go up or down over time, and funeral businesses can close or change hands. Many states have laws that govern prepayment of funeral goods and services; some offer substantial protection to the consumer, and some less protection. According to some state laws, the funeral home or cemetery must put a percentage of the funds in a state-regulated trust or invest the money in a life insurance policy with the death benefits going to the funeral home or cemetery.

The FTC advises that you ask the following question when you consider a prepayment plan:

- What are you paying for? Are you buying only merchandise, like a casket and vault, or are you purchasing funeral services as well?
- What happens to the money you have prepaid? States have different requirements for handling funds paid for prearranged funeral services.

- What happens to the interest income on money that is prepaid and put into a trust account?
- Are you protected if the firm you have dealt with goes out of business?
- Can you cancel the contract and get a full refund if you change your mind?
- What happens if you move to a different area or die while away from home? Some prepaid funeral plans can be transferred, but often at an added cost.

Once you have made your decisions, write them down and tell others close to you what arrangements have been made. Your attorney should have a copy, kept separate from the will, since this information will be needed before the will is read. If you decide to pay in advance, make sure that other family members are aware of this and that your contract is easily accessible. Whatever you decide, be sure to review your arrangements periodically.

BURIAL OPTIONS

Whether to bury or cremate is a very personal decision, determined by a number of factors, such as:

- What is the dying person's desire?
- What is the family tradition or the family's desire?
- Are there religious practices and religious and cultural preferences to take into account?
- Will there be a wake, and does the body need to be there?
- Does the family expect to see a casket lowered into the ground?

If a body turns up at the morgue of the public hospital with no family to pay for its disposition, it will be cremated and, if there is any family at all, they will be given the remains. This is known as a pauper's funeral. Otherwise, the options for burial include:

Direct burial. Direct or immediate burial involves immediate burial without embalming, usually in a plain container.

Direct cremation. Typically, funeral homes offer a cremation package, which includes the funeral director's fee, and transportation and preparation of the body. The body is cremated soon after death, and therefore does not need embalming.

Traditional funeral. A traditional funeral is usually a full-service funeral and as such is typically the most expensive type of funeral. For a "consumer guide" to funerals, including more information on each type of funeral and the associated costs, see the FTC Web site.

Caskets, vaults, and urns

If you opt for direct burial or cremation, or if you donate your loved one's body to science, there is no need to buy a casket. If you choose to have your loved one cremated, you may be able to rent a casket from the funeral home for use during visitation and the service. If there will be no viewing or ceremony, the funeral home is required to provide an inexpensive box or container to be cremated with the body. According to the Funeral Rule, a funeral director cannot insist on a casket for direct cremations and rather must provide an unfinished box or other alternative container.

If you choose a traditional funeral and burial, however, the casket will probably be the single most expensive purchase. According to the FTC, the average cost is slightly more than $2,000. Some caskets sell for as much as $10,000, specifically those made of mahogany, bronze, or copper. No matter what kind of casket you buy or how much you spend, it will not preserve the body forever. Even the most protective or tightly sealed container serves to keep water out or prevent rust and decay only for a limited time.

A grave liner or vault is a container that encases the casket in the grave. While use of such a container is not a federal, state, or local mandate, many cemeteries require them. They prevent the ground from sagging when and if the casket finally crumbles or collapses. Typically made of bronze, copper, marble, or concrete, with a variety of inner liners, protective seals, and decorative features, burial liners and vaults usually cost between $500 and $3000. The cost of cremation urns depends on the material and decoration. Urns come in wood, marble, porcelain, bronze, or cloisonné and can cost as little as $30 on up to $1000.

Cemetery plots and mausoleums

Generally, people purchase cemetery plots based on location and on family or religious considerations. Cemetery plots can be expensive. This is especially true in larger, urban areas. Some cemeteries include perpetual care in the price, but not all. It is therefore important that you ask about this before you sign a contract. If care is not included, find out about contracting maintenance and groundskeeping services and make financial arrangements for that as well.

Veterans and their spouses and dependents are entitled to free burial and a grave marker in a national cemetery. Some civilians connected to military-related services and some Public Health Service personnel are also entitled to such benefits. Benefits include opening and closing the grave, vault or liner, and marker in a national cemetery. Cremated remains also qualify. For more information, call the Department of Veterans Affairs or refer to their Web site.

Headstones and markers

Headstones are usually made of granite or marble, while flat grave markers are usually made of bronze. The size and style (for instance, flat as compared with upright) may be dictated by the cemetery you choose. Indeed, you or your loved one's wishes for a memorial may be one factor in choosing the place of burial. For more information contact the Monument Builders of North America.

COPING WITH GRIEF AND BEREAVEMENT

Grief is the process by which we learn to live with loss. Grief involves detaching gradually from the person, not forgetting the person, but untangling the threads of emotion that tie you to the person and to the past so that you can go on and eventually reattach to people and occupations in the present.

Grieving begins before the person passes away—when, for example, a person receives a terminal diagnosis or after a first serious bout with illness. (Sudden death can be so hard because there can be no anticipatory grieving.) Even before the loved one dies, family members manifest their grief in various ways. They begin to rehearse in their minds what it will be like after the person is gone. They may help the dying person clean out areas of her home—the garage, for example, or the sewing room. They may help the person give things away. Caregivers may begin to think about the future, about what they're going to do with their time when the person is gone. Family members often talk among themselves about their loved one and her illness and dying. They thus prepare themselves and younger family members, and all practice saying goodbye. All this is part of the grieving process.

Bereavement is the condition that, following the death of a loved one, sometimes presents symptoms otherwise characteristic of a major depressive episode, including feelings of sadness, difficulty sleeping and eating, and weight loss. In most cases, these symptoms, even when quite disabling, are considered normal and appropriate; they may vary in their duration according to one's personality, family traditions, and cultural and religious background. However, when severe symptoms last two months beyond the loss, they may indicate the presence of a major depression. Symptoms that go beyond normal grief include preoccupation with the survivor's own feelings of guilt and worthlessness, continued thoughts about death, and significant impairment in daily functioning.

Nevertheless, there is some controversy about what constitutes normal bereavement as opposed to pathologic bereavement. While some of the psychiatric literature suggests that grief that lasts beyond six months and impairs functioning is pathologic, many who write about and work with the dying insist that the process of grieving, like the process of dying, takes its own time and occupies its own space. Just how long it takes to grieve depends on the person grieving and the person who is being grieved over. Both the length and the intensity vary. Some people liken grief to a succession of waves—sometimes they are knocked over, sometimes they feel that they will drown, sometimes the waves ebb, and sometimes they gently wash over them.

In addition, just what the grieving process looks like depends largely on what came before—what the relationship was like between the deceased person and the grieving survivor—and the emotional resources the bereaved person has. People who have not experienced significant losses before, for example, may be hit particularly hard by grief over the death of someone close to them.

DEATH OF A SPOUSE OR PARTNER

There are few more stressful events than the death of a spouse or partner. The transition from wife to widow, husband to widower, is inevitably a difficult and profoundly painful one. When you lose your spouse or partner, you lose your life's companion, often a best friend and a mainstay in your life. Also, when you lose such a close companion, you lose an essential role of your own: that is, you stop being a wife or a husband and become a widow or a widower. Once widowed, you are forced, like it or not, to redefine yourself.

When a spouse or partner dies, the surviving partner must adjust to living alone and taking care of his or her own affairs. This process of adjustment involves other, less visible losses. If, for example, the husband was the primary income earner, saw to all repairs around the house, or took care of the finances, his widow must now find ways to manage those tasks. If the wife did all the cooking, maintained the couple's social ties, or shopped for clothes, her surviving husband must now assume these responsibilities. Learning new skills is never easy, but learning them in the later years and learning them while actively grieving can be especially daunting.

Nevertheless, after a spouse or partner dies, it is probable that with time and support, courage, and effort the pain will ease. If you allow yourself to grieve and find expression for your pain, fear, and confusion, eventually you will come to see that life goes on. And while it may be tempting to jump into activities to keep the pain at bay, sooner or later, you will have to grieve. The longer you put it off, the more intense or confusing the grieving process can be.

There is no real order to the grieving process, nor do the feelings evolve in a methodical way. Among the feelings you are likely to experience at first are shock, numbness, and a sense of disbelief. As time passes you might feel intense pain, loneliness, and yearning. You might have dreams in which your loved one comes to you, speaks to you. After years of being together, you might continue to feel your partner's proximity, and even see or seem to touch them.

Not all the feelings you'll experience will be loving. You may feel anger at being abandoned—anger at the person, anger at circumstances, anger at the doctors who could not save your partner, anger that your loved one did not take better care of herself or leave things in better financial shape. You may feel rage at the living, rage at those who do not know the pain of loss, rage at those who still have spouses and partners to come home to. These feelings are as normal as loving feelings. At the same time, you may feel guilty about feeling that way. If the marriage or relationship was not so satisfying, you may resent what you never had, and feel doubly deprived by the loss.

And you may feel anxiety, because your companion's death brings you face to face with your own mortality. As you realize over time that your partner is irrevocably gone, you may feel deeply sad. As you begin to move on in your life and feel moments of true pleasure or joy again, you might feel guilty. While common wisdom suggests that it takes two to four years to adapt to the death of a spouse, it is just not true that grief ends. But it does get more tolerable. Over time, the pain becomes less acute and constant. Years later, a picture, a song, a place, a story, a smell can inspire tears and that feeling of emptiness at the pit of your stomach, but the feelings no longer paralyze you.

Family and friends wish to offer comfort and support, but people can do this in awkward and, to you, painful ways. It is hard for people to witness others' expressions of deep emotional pain and grief—it makes them feel helpless, sad, and frightened—and frequently they do not know what to say or do. Certainly, other persons close to you, who knew your deceased loved one well, will also be grieving this person's loss for themselves. In such cases, family members and close friends will mirror each other's grief, and mutual support will feel at times like common bereavement.

It is important to remember that death touches people differently, and their responses will differ. Each person you know will have his or her own reactions to your loss and to your grief. Sometimes, it can feel that others around you are going on with their lives, leaving you behind, and you may then feel more isolated with your sadness. And, in some instances, persons around you will be more preoccupied with their own reactions to your grieving than with your needs. If, for example, you feel your children or closest friends are not doing enough, ask them to do more. Because people so often do not seem to know what to do or say to be helpful to someone who is grieving, and would seem to welcome some guidance, you may want to be specific with them about what you need. It may also be wise for you to reach beyond your immediate circle of family and friends to other sources for help in dealing with your loss and grief.

DEATH OF A PARENT

The death of a parent is a major loss. No matter how old you are when your parent dies, even when that parent's advanced age or illness has prepared you for his or her demise, the death itself can be a painful and disconcerting experience. Loss of a parent will affect you like no other loss.

Outliving our parents is along the natural order of things, and we all assume that our parents will die before us. By the time we become adults, we no longer need our parents for our survival, nor, in all likelihood, do we have an intensely interdependent relationship with them. So when a parent dies, we don't necessarily have to reinvent ourselves, as when a spouse or life partner dies, nor do we necessarily have to pick up tasks and responsibilities that someone else did. Yet the impact will nonetheless be deeply felt.

For one, there is the real loss of a loved one and a relationship. Chances are that while you no longer depend on your parents for full emotional and economic support, you rely on them for a sense of continuity, a sense of history, in your life and in the life of the family. In most cases, they are the people who know you best, who knew you at infancy and know you now in adulthood. In addition, when a parent dies, adult children must confront their own mortality—they are, after all, the next in line. Finally, relationships between parents and children are complex and multifaceted. If the relationship was always strained or troubled, that can complicate the grieving process.

When a parent dies, you will no doubt experience a range of feelings—from sadness at the passing to relief that suffering is over and the burden of caregiving is lifted, from anger to denial to regret. It is important, even if you are now taking care of a bereaved parent, that you also take care of yourself.

SUPPORT AND HELP IN GRIEVING

As you go through the grieving process, it is important to lean on other family members or friends who have had similar experiences. Most hospice programs offer follow-up bereavement programs and groups. For some, returning to work and routine soon after the death helps them cope, at least in the short run. For others, counselors can help them sort out the feelings they experience along the way of grieving.

Many local agencies and organizations offer bereavement support programs. Contact the ones that might sponsor bereavement groups in your area, such as:

- Local hospices (many offer bereavement services to anyone, regardless of whether the loved one died under their care)

HELPING A LOVED ONE GRIEVE

It's often hard to watch someone you care for go through the pain of loss, grief, and bereavement, and the slow return to normal. Here are some suggestions for helping those you love.

- Stay in frequent contact with your loved one. Your presence and continual involvement is the most helpful thing you can offer.
- Actively offer and provide both emotional support and practical help. Don't wait to be asked.
- Don't worry about doing or saying the "right" thing. Being there, caring, listening, and tolerating your loved one's grief are the best things you can do. On the other hand, avoid urging her to "cheer up" or "get on with things." Despite good intentions, such advice will only sound dismissive.
- Talk about the person who has died. Reminisce together. Don't avoid referring to the dead person by name.
- Offer practical help. Invite your loved one to dinner. Do the marketing and the laundry. Screen phone calls. Help sort through and pay bills.
- When your loved one is ready, help her sort through and dispose of the dead person's clothing and personal things. (It might be helpful, though, to collect in one place special keepsakes—clippings, photographs, clothing, jewelry, cherished items.) Sometimes, it can be healing for the surviving partner to make gifts of certain special belongings to persons who especially loved the deceased person.
- Help your loved one find practical solutions to fears and concerns. Your loved one may fret about her own health, or be nervous about sleeping alone. Your loved one may resist the idea of making decisions alone. Help her make a plan.
- Discourage your loved one from making irreversible decisions in the first year after the person's death, such as selling the family home, moving, or remarrying.
- Find ways to encourage your loved one to be independent and to take on those tasks that the dead person always handled.
- Gently encourage your loved one to socialize when she is ready. Accept her new friends.
- If your loved one seems to be stuck, encourage her to reach out to a bereavement program. If religion or faith plays a part in her life, reach out to a rabbi, minister, priest, or other member of her spiritual community.
- When your loved one seems ready, help her to rework relationships with children, grandchildren, and siblings.

- Churches, synagogues, or mosques
- Mental health clinics or counseling centers
- Senior centers or the agency on aging in your area
- Hospitals
- Funeral homes

ADDITIONAL RESOURCES

ORGANIZATIONS AND WEB SITES

AARP

AARP's Legal Services Network

800-424-3410

www.aarp.org/endoflife

AARP Grief and Loss Programs

601 E Street, N.W.

Washington, DC 20049

202-434-2260

Fax 202-434-6474

E-mail: griefandloss@aarp.org

Cremation Association of North America (CANA)

www.cremationassociation.org

FAMSA-Funeral Consumers Alliance

P.O. Box 10

Hinesburg, VT 05461

802-482-3437

www.funerals.org

Federal Trade Commission

Consumer Response Center

Washington, DC 20580

877-FTC-HELP

TDD 202-326-2502

www.ftc.gov

Hospice Association of America

228 Seventh Street, S.E.

Washington, DC 20003

202-546-4759

Fax 202-547-9559

www.hospice-america.org

Hospice Foundation of America

2001 S Street, N.W.

Washington, DC 2000

202-638-5419

800-854-3402

www.hospicefoundation.org

International Cemetery and Funeral Association

1895 Preston White Drive

Reston, VA 20191

800-645-7700

www.icfa.org

Monument Builders of North America

800-827-1000

www.monumentbuilders.com

The National Cemetery Administration

www.cem.va.gov

National Family Caregivers Association

800-896-3650

www.nfcacares.org

National Federation of Interfaith
Volunteer Caregivers

816-931-5442;

www.nfivc.org

The National Funeral Directors Association

13625 Bishop's Drive

Brookfield, WI 53005-6117

414-789-1880

Fax 414-789-6977

www.nfda.org

National Hospice and Palliative Care Organization

1700 Diagonal Road, Suite 625

Alexandria, VA 22314

703-837-1500

Fax 703-837-1233

www.nhpco.org

North American Cemetery Regulators Association

340 Maple Street

Des Moines, IA 50319-9966

515-281-4441

Fax 515-281-3059

The Partnership for Caring

800-989-9455 (24-hour Hotline)

www.partnershipforcaring.org

RWJF Last Acts Campaign

800-844-7616

www.lastacts.org

State Agency on Aging

Administration on Aging

U.S. Department of Health and Human Services

800-677-1116 (locator line)

www.aoa.dhhs.gov

Supportive Care of the Dying

Providence Health System

4805 NE Glisan Street, 2E07

Portland, OR 97213

503-215-5053

Fax 503-215-5054

www.careofdying.org

U.S. Department of Veterans Affairs

800-827-1000

www.va.gov

U.S. Living Will Registry

523 Westfield Ave.

P.O. Box 2789

Westfield, NJ 07091-2789

800-LIV-WILL (800-548-9455)

Fax 908-654-1919

The Well Spouse Foundation

800-838-0879

www.wellspouse.org

BOOKS

Byock, Ira. *Dying Well*. Riverhead Books, 1997.

Kübler-Ross, E. *On Death and Dying*. New York: Macmillan, 1971.

Lynn, Joanne, and Joan Harrold. *Handbook for Mortals: Guidance for People Facing Serious Illness*. New York: Oxford University Press, 1999.

Mitford, Jessica. *The American Way of Death, Revisited*. New York: Vintage, 1998.

Myers, Edward. *When Parents Die*. New York: Penguin Books, 1997.

Nuland, Sherwin. *How We Die*. New York: Vintage, 1993.

Secunda, Victoria. *Losing Your Parents, Finding Your Self*. New York: Hyperion, 2000.

Smith, Douglas C. *Caregiving: Hospice-Proven Techniques for Healing Body and Soul.* New York: Macmillan, 1997.

Tatelbaum, Judy. *The Courage to Grieve.* New York: HarperPerennial, 1980.

Webb, Marilyn. *The Good Death: The New American Search to Reshape the End of Life.* New York: Bantam Doubleday Dell, 1999.

Weenolsen, Patricia. *The Art of Dying.* New York: St. Martin's Griffin, 1997.

York, Sarah. *Remembering Well: Rituals for Celebrating*

Index